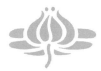

YOGA
AS MEDICINE

the YOGIC PRESCRIPTION for

HEALTH & HEALING

A *Yoga Journal* Book by

Timothy McCall, MD

Photographs by

Michal Venera

• Bantam Books •

YOGA AS MEDICINE
A Bantam Book / August 2007

Published by
Bantam Dell
A Division of Random House, Inc.
New York, New York

Library of Congress Cataloging-in-Publication Data
McCall, Timothy B.
Yoga as medicine : the yogic prescription for health and healing : a yoga journal book / by Timothy McCall.
p. cm.
Includes bibliographical references and index.
ISBN 978-0-553-38406-2 (trade pbk.)
1. Yoga—Therapeutic use. 2. Yoga. I. Title.
[DNLM: 1. Yoga. WB 890 M4776y 2007]
RM727.Y64M43 2007
613.7'046—dc22
2006038917

Printed in the United States of America
Published simultaneously in Canada
www.bantamdell.com
RRH 10 9 8 7 6 5 4 3 2 1

For my mother,

Mary Elizabeth (Betty) McCall,

who didn't get to name me

but who named this book

CONTENTS

Words fail to convey the total value of yoga.
It has to be experienced.

—B. K. S. IYENGAR

HOW TO USE THIS BOOK

THIS BOOK IS DIVIDED INTO THREE PARTS. The four chapters that make up part 1 provide an overview of yoga as medicine, the science behind it, the relationship of stress to health and healing, and a yogic approach to health care. Reading chapter 2, on the science of yoga, is not essential to getting the full benefit of this book. But for those who are skeptical or intellectually curious, chapter 2's reviews of the scientific studies that investigate yoga's healing powers will be of interest. That chapter also provides possible explanations for yoga's benefits that are compatible with Western science, and discusses how science and yoga provide complementary perspectives.

Part 2 contains material that many readers will find useful. Most would benefit from reading chapter 5, "Doing Yoga Safely." Readers wanting more information on this topic, including more details on anatomy, should look at appendix 1, "Avoiding Common Yoga Injuries." Chapter 6 compares different systems of yoga and provides guidelines on finding a good teacher. Chapter 7 details a step-by-step plan for starting and maintaining a yoga practice.

Part 1 of the book also contains a number of Experiential Exercises, in which you can try specific yoga practices and judge the effects for yourself. You'll get much more out of the book if you do these exercises as you read, especially if you're new to yoga. Yoga is more about practice than theory. To understand it, you must do it, and these exercises provide a gentle—yet quite palpable—introduction to the effects of yoga on the body and mind.

Part 3 of the book contains twenty chapters on specific health conditions and concerns, from anxiety to weight loss. Although you may be tempted to go directly to the chapter or chapters that describe conditions you are dealing with, this material will have more meaning to you if you've read all or most of parts 1 and 2. For each of the chapters in part 3, a seasoned yoga teacher describes his or her approach with a specific student who had the condition in question. If you follow yoga, you may recognize many of these teachers as some of yoga's leading lights in the United States. I've chosen a few, however, who are not household names, even in the yoga world. I think you'll find they, too, have very interesting things to say.

Keep in mind that many of the experts could have just as easily been the authority for another condition. For example, just because Shanti Shanti Kaur Khalsa, a teacher in the Kundalini yoga tradition, is the consultant for HIV and AIDS does not imply that her approach is the best for this condition, or that Kundalini yoga might work less well for a different problem. I simply hope to show you over the course of these twenty chapters how some of the top teachers from different traditions work. So even if you don't have chronic fatigue syndrome (CFS), you may be interested in the Viniyoga approach taken by Gary Kraftsow in chapter 14. If you want to know about the traditional Indian medical system of Ayurveda, you might look at Sandra Summerfield Kozak's approach to diabetes in chapter 16.

Keep in mind that the chapters in part 3 are *descriptive,* not *prescriptive.* Judith Hanson Lasater, for example, outlines in the back pain chapter the approach she took with one student who had sciatica and describes why she recommended what she did. This is not necessarily what she would recommend for another student with back pain, and might be quite different from what another teacher might have suggested for the same student. Still, with these caveats in mind, I believe anyone with back pain will find helpful information in the chapter.

You may also benefit from looking at chapters in part 3 that discuss conditions other than your major concern. Depression, for example, can affect your recovery from many conditions, from heart disease to cancer, so many readers will benefit from reading chapter 15. People with fibromyalgia syndrome or CFS may want to read the chapter on insomnia, since poor sleep is often a prominent component of those conditions. People with diabetes, especially the more common adult onset variety (type 2), may want to look at the chapter on weight loss, since overweight plays a big role in that disease.

In addition to the perspectives of the yoga teacher consultants, in each chapter of part 3 I'll provide an overview of the condition in question from my perspective as a Western-trained doctor; discuss how yoga could fit into treatment; talk about special considerations and contraindications; and try to provide a broader holistic approach to the problem. These chapters also include additional ideas from other yoga experts.

I don't want to overwhelm you with Sanskrit, the ancient language of yoga, so I won't be using that many Sanskrit words in this book. Except for a few indispensable words like asana (the poses) and pranayama (the breathing techniques), when I use Sanskrit I'll usually provide the English translation. When describing some yoga poses and other techniques I'll use a combination of English and Sanskrit names, which is what most yoga teachers do. You'll also find a glossary at the end of the book that defines most of the Sanskrit words used in the book, and another on the Sanskrit words used to name the various poses.

Readers looking for more information on the teachers and systems of yoga discussed in the book can turn to appendix 2, "Sources of Further Information." Appendix 3 includes notes and the references for many of the studies cited in the book. The afterword discusses the future of the evolving field of yoga as medicine.

All of the case histories in the book are true. Some students allowed me to use their real names; where indicated, I have changed the students' names, if they requested it or I didn't personally interview the student. In those instances some identifying characteristics were also altered to protect confidentiality. One case, in the chapter on chronic fatigue syndrome, is a composite of several students.

INTRODUCTION: A LEAP OF FAITH

IN THIS BOOK, I'M ASKING YOU TO THINK OF YOGA AS MEDICINE—a concept which is perhaps new and quite foreign to you. Because it is a kind of medicine that can benefit the healthy as well as the sick, I'm going to suggest that you consider starting a regular practice, no matter what your current state of health. You may have seen pictures of yoga contortionists or heard about grueling "power yoga" and "hot yoga" classes that convinced you this isn't something you could possibly do. If so, I hope to show you that virtually anyone can do yoga, including those who start out with little strength, energy, or flexibility, and those who are ill or injured.

I say this not as a lifelong yoga teacher or someone who can readily bend his body into the shape of a square knot—I'm not, not by a long shot. I am a physician, a board-certified specialist in internal medicine, who came to yoga in middle age and found it—and continues to find it—incredibly challenging. But in this challenge, I have seen steady growth in what I can do and how good I feel. My body has changed in ways I wouldn't have believed possible, as has my mental state. The more I put into my yoga practice, the greater the rewards have become.

I signed up for my first yoga class in the same spirit that I'd brought to salsa dancing and tai chi. It was simply something interesting I'd heard about and decided to try. I didn't come in with any kind of faith that yoga would change my life, but it did.

At first my progress was slow. I studied yoga casually for a couple of years, making it to a class every other week or so. Due to my busy schedule, I never seemed to find the time to practice at home, even though my teacher, Patricia Walden, had said many times that fifteen or twenty minutes every day was much more valuable than a longer session once a week.

Like a lot of people who play competitive sports and never pay much attention to stretching, I'd started out incredibly stiff. I had great difficulty with even the most basic poses. With my legs straight, I couldn't touch the floor with my fingertips. I couldn't sit cross-legged without feeling discomfort in my upper back. I had difficulty just straightening my spine, let alone bending it backward. And even though I enjoyed the feeling of peace that class left me with those first two years, my body never became much more flexible. Then I made a decision: I was going to take a leap of faith.

I resolved to get up every morning for one year and practice yoga. I bought a mat, a strap, and a book describing the basic stretching, strengthening, and relaxation poses known as asana (pronounced AH-sah-nah). Even if my schedule was crazy and I could only fit in a few minutes, I'd do it. I started inserting yoga into the cracks in my day. If I was sitting at the computer or had a break between patients, I'd take a minute to stretch my arms over my head or bend forward, place my hands on the desk, and lengthen my spine for a few seconds. If I was on the road, I'd do asanas in my hotel room. I started to pay more attention to my body, noticing the way my shoulders tended to slump as I sat behind the wheel or read a book.

With regular practice, amazing things began to happen. After a few months, my chest started to open up. My friends and family noticed that my chronically slouching posture, from years of studying and computer work, was improving. The knots that I had thought were a permanent fixture in my upper back slowly melted away. I didn't get injured as often as I used to. In the five years before starting yoga, I gave up basketball due to heel spurs and I lost a year of playing tennis due to an inflammation of my elbow. I'd noticed the twinges of pain that heralded a rotator cuff problem in my shoulder. Chronic pain in my Achilles tendon had me worried that I'd suffer the same kind of rupture I'd seen my best friend go through. All of these problems are better now, and I suspect that if I'd been doing yoga all along, I might have avoided many of them completely.

Perhaps even more profound than yoga's physical effect on me were the mental and psychological benefits. Once I developed a regular practice, I noticed a change in outlook. Problems didn't seem to get to me as much. If I dropped a tray of ice cubes and they scattered across the kitchen floor, I didn't blurt out words that would get beeped off network TV. I just laughed, shook my head, and cleaned up. I didn't seem to worry as much. Without even consciously trying, more and more I seemed to be doing what yoga philosophy teaches: to give your best effort without being attached to the result.

Yoga also had an even deeper effect on me. A couple of years after starting yoga, I decided to leave direct patient care and devote myself full-time to research and writing. With the rise of the managed-care approach to medicine, I found it increasingly stressful as well as difficult to do what I thought was right for my patients. As the conveyor belt of care was sped up to cut costs, I wasn't getting the chance to know patients as well as I wanted to, which greatly diminished one of the most satisfying aspects of doctoring. It's not quite true to say that yoga led me to quit my medical practice, but yoga did put me in touch with an inner voice that was telling me, *This isn't working anymore.*

It was ten years ago that I took that leap of faith. Since then I've continued to do yoga poses virtually every day and I've added breathing exercises known as pranayama (prah-nai-YAH-mah), meditation, and other practices to my routine. My body has continued to change. I've gained muscle, lost fat, and become a lot more flexible. When I'm warmed up, I can stand with my legs straight and place my palms flat on the floor. I can do some poses that I used to think would never be possible, though there are still plenty of them—including backbends—that I have great difficulty with. But these markers of physical prowess aren't what really counts.

What's become more important to me is the mental peace that has come, the sense of gratitude, the gradual and sometimes sudden opening of some formerly inflexible area of my body or mind, and the feeling of community I've found with fellow students and teachers. Stepping out of the crazy, fast-paced world to pay close attention to what's happening right then and there puts me in touch with a calm place deep inside me—deep inside all of us. It's like the stillness on the ocean floor that remains undisturbed, no matter how frantically waves crash on the surface.

For the last several years, in addition to deepening my own yoga practice, I've been investigating the use of yoga for people suffering from a variety of medical conditions. My interest was originally sparked by all the stories I heard from people who said yoga had helped them deal with depression or back pain or a difficult transition into menopause.

The process of learning about yoga therapy, however, hasn't been easy. For starters, there is no one place to acquire this knowledge; the yoga world is incredibly Balkanized. There are dozens of competing traditions, many of which don't seem interested in sharing their discoveries with each other or the outside world. Complicating matters further, some of what I've heard from yoga teachers, or read in magazines, quite frankly defies modern understanding of anatomy and physiology, or is grounded in a metaphysics that can be off-putting or virtually incomprehensible. In addition, many yoga teachers with much to offer are shy about touting yoga's therapeutic potential—especially in writing—while others who in my estimation have far less substance boldly claim their brand of yoga can cure any disease.

Not to be deterred, I've read books, attended classes, workshops, and conferences, reviewed the scientific literature, and sought out some of the world's leading yoga teachers and yoga therapists to find out what they're doing and what they find most helpful. You'll hear from many of these teachers in this book. I've also worked with my teacher, Patricia Walden, using yoga to treat people with such maladies as depression, breast cancer, and Parkinson's disease. Although we didn't do rigorous scientific studies, my strong impression based on years of clinical medical experience is that these students benefited enormously.

Patricia teaches a style of yoga known as the Iyengar method, named after the aging master B. K. S. Iyengar, and that's the style we used in the therapeutic work we've done together. In my role as a writer and scientist interested in researching this field, however, I have taken workshops, had private therapy sessions, and learned from teachers in dozens of different styles. One of the most amazing things I have observed is that every system of therapeutic yoga I've looked at seems to help people heal.

Reflecting the multitude of good choices in therapeutic yoga, this book takes a pragmatic approach. It features yoga teachers from many different traditions using a broad range of approaches and tools. Every one of these yoga therapists brings decades of experience to the task.

Not all yoga styles are represented in this book. There are more approaches and teachers out there than it's possible to research or include. Some omissions are deliberate because I do not believe that all systems of yoga, particularly those that are more physically demanding, are appropriate for people with serious disease. (This is not to criticize these styles of yoga for people who are fit and healthy. Many people love them and they have their place.)

Because this book is aimed at a Western audience and because I am a doctor, I use the language and perspective of science as much as possible. I know this is the best way to show physicians and other health care professionals that yoga as medicine could benefit their patients—including many who don't respond well to conventional therapies, who may be among the most frustrating of their patients to treat.

Most conventional doctors have almost no knowledge of the potential medical applications of yoga. But it isn't really their fault. I don't recall hearing a single word about yoga in medical school, in three years of postgraduate training in internal medicine, or in the dozens of seminars and conferences I attended in more than ten years of office-based medical practice. Looking back, it makes me sad to think of all the patients I saw before I discovered yoga who might have benefited from it—many of whom didn't find any relief in what was available.

Although there are more than a hundred scientific studies that have found yoga to be an effective treatment for a variety of medical problems, from heart disease to carpal tun nel syndrome, most of this work is unknown to the average physician. While a few of these studies, mostly those done in the West, have gotten media attention here, the overwhelming majority of the scientific research into yoga takes place in India. Most of this Indian research is difficult or impossible to get access to in this country, which is part of the reason most physicians and most yogis have never heard of it. To learn more, in 2002 I spent more than two months traveling to different yoga therapy clinics and research institutions in India. I'll be sharing some of my discoveries from that trip with you in this book. Since then I have returned twice to continue my research, focusing in particular on the connections between therapeutic yoga and the ancient system of Indian medicine, Ayurveda, which I'll also discuss.

But no review of research, or visits to clinics or studios of master practitioners is sufficient to understand yoga. To really grasp what yoga can do, you need to experience it yourself. That's why I'm urging you to consider taking a leap of faith, like the one I took ten years ago. It was my experience that made me believe in yoga; not any preconceptions. My experience tells me yoga works—in addition, of course, to the scientific evidence and what I've directly observed and heard from others.

My suggestion is to suspend disbelief just long enough to try a few sessions of yoga and let your experience dictate whether to continue. If you find yoga brings you nothing, you won't have lost much. But if you find the experience as eye-opening as I have, you have a whole world to gain.

Yoga is something you learn by doing. I've been practicing for about twelve years, but there are people who have been at it decades longer who greatly surpass me in yoga expertise. Nonetheless, I believe that as a medical doctor as well as a serious student of yoga, I can offer a helpful perspective to people hoping to heal, people doing healing work with others, and anyone who's just curious about yoga's health benefits—unlike Western medicine, yoga can help the healthy as well as the sick to feel better.

If science is the modern world's greatest contribution to knowledge, then yoga is the gem of the ancient world. It is my belief that these two ways of knowing—which seem so different, even at odds with each other—can be reconciled, advancing our understanding more than either discipline alone. Combining the insights of these two great systems can result in an increase in the likelihood of better health, a reduction in bothersome symptoms, and the relief of suffering.

Yoga is not a panacea, but it is powerful medicine indeed for body, mind, and spirit. Above all, yoga is a path. The longer you stay with it and the more heart you put into the journey, the farther it can take you.

PART ONE

YOGA
AS MEDICINE

Yoga is 99 percent practice,

one percent theory.

—PATTABHI JOIS

YOGA AS MEDICINE

Whether you are sick or weak, young, old or even very old,

you can succeed in yoga if you practice diligently.

—SVATMARAMA (HATHA YOGA PRADIPIKA)

 If you are new to yoga, welcome. Yoga can change your life. If you are currently practicing yoga but want to learn more, you probably already know something of yoga's life-changing potential. If you are sick, it can help you feel better. If you are depressed or anxious, tired all the time, addicted to drugs, or bothered by low back pain, yoga can set you on the path to recovery. For those with chronic health problems like arthritis, diabetes, multiple sclerosis, or HIV/AIDS, regular yoga practice can help you live better and, in all likelihood, longer. And for people suffering temporary symptoms—such as tension headaches, hot flashes, or sinus pressure—specific yoga postures, breathing techniques, and other practices can bring relief.

As someone who has been an MD for over twenty years, I can tell you that yoga is quite simply the most powerful system of overall health and well-being I have ever seen. Even if you are currently among what might be called the temporarily healthy, as preventive medicine, yoga is as close to one-stop shopping as you can find. This single comprehensive system can reduce stress, increase flexibility, improve balance, promote strength, heighten cardiovascular conditioning, lower blood pressure, reduce overweight, strengthen bones, prevent injuries, lift mood, improve immune function, increase the oxygen supply to the tissues, heighten sexual functioning and fulfillment, foster psychological equanimity, and promote spiritual well-being . . . and that's only a partial list.

Yoga has a decidedly different view from Western medicine's about what constitutes health—and this may be a big part of why it's so effective. The absence of symptoms is in no way equated with health in yoga. Health to the yogi extends far beyond not having a headache or knee pain—or even being cured of cancer. It is about optimizing the function of every system in your body from the muscles to digestion, circulation, and immunity. It is about emotional well-being, spiritual resilience, and buoyancy, even joy. Yoga teaches that only when these elements are aligned can you maximize your chance for health and healing.

Yoga envisions a web of causation that is much more complex than the limited number of factors most doctors consider. In the case of heart disease, for example, it looks beyond cholesterol and blood pressure to stress and the role of the mind in perpetuating it, your emotional temperament, your connections to other people, and whether you are living your life in accordance with some larger purpose. The idea is that a wide variety of factors can affect your well-being, and the most efficient way to remedy health problems is to work on many areas simultaneously. This is precisely what the practice of yoga does.

In yoga, you do your spiritual work and it affects the body. You stretch and strengthen your muscles and that affects your circulation, digestion, and breathing. You calm and strengthen the nervous system and it affects the mind. You cultivate peace of mind and it affects the nervous system, the immune system, and the cardiovascular system. Yoga says that if you look clearly you will see that everything about you is connected to everything else. From a therapeutic standpoint, this provides the insight that you improve the functioning of any one organ or system by trying to improve all.

Thus a crucial difference between yoga as medicine and conventional medicine is yoga's holistic emphasis on strengthening you throughout your body and mind. If you go to most doctors feeling out of sorts but without specific pain or other symptoms, with the exception of ordering a few tests to rule out the possibility of various diseases, they generally won't have much to offer you. If you're interested in making your nervous system more resilient, boosting immunity, or improving your ability to breathe, they'll have little to suggest.

The opposite is true of yoga. But rather than being in competition with conventional medical care, yoga can complement it. Indeed, in my experience, yoga can help you get the most out of whatever other care you receive, alternative or conventional. As an adjunct to other care, yoga has an advantage over many other modalities that typically get labeled as alternative medicine. It can amplify the benefits and, since yoga can often allow you to use fewer drugs and herbs or use them in smaller doses, the chance of side effects is lessened. In addition, unlike other treatments, which can interfere with each other—the way vitamins can interfere with chemotherapy or some herbs with anesthetics—a properly chosen yoga practice is extremely unlikely to interact in a harmful way with any other treatments.

Yoga appears to be effective in the treatment of a wide variety of health conditions. We'll be reviewing the scientific evidence later but, for now, let's see what people who've tried therapeutic yoga have to say. In 1983–84, the London-based Yoga Biomedical Trust, run by Robin

Monro, PhD, surveyed twenty-seven hundred people, most between the ages of thirty-one and sixty, who used yoga therapeutically. To be included, participants had to have practiced yoga for at least two hours a week for a year or longer. Though the number of people with some of the conditions in question was small, the results (see table 1.1) were impressive: 98 percent of back-pain sufferers found yoga helpful, 90 percent of cancer patients, 82 percent of people with insomnia, and 100 percent of alcoholics. The lowest success rate in the survey was for women with "menstrual problems," two out of three of whom found that yoga helped.

TABLE 1.1 CONDITIONS IMPROVED BY YOGA, SELF-REPORTED

MEDICAL CONDITION	NUMBER OF PEOPLE REPORTING	PERCENTAGE HELPED BY YOGA
Alcoholism	26	100
Anxiety	838	94
Arthritis and Rheumatic Disorders	589	90
Asthma or Bronchitis	226	88
Back Disorders	1,142	98
Cancer	29	90
Diabetes	10	80
Duodenal Ulcers	40	90
Heart Disease	50	94
Hemorrhoids	391	88
High Blood Pressure	150	84
Insomnia	542	82
Menopausal Disorders	247	83
Menstrual Problems	317	68
Migraine	464	80
Neurological and Neuromuscular Diseases	112	96
Obesity	240	74
Premenstrual Syndrome	848	77
Smoking	219	74

Source: The Yoga Biomedical Trust, London

Imagine how much you'd be hearing about a new drug that could accomplish even a fraction of this. Nevertheless, it's my experience that few in the medical community or the general public have any conception of what yoga has to offer. Part of the problem, I'm convinced, is that many people who could benefit from yoga shy away due to misconceptions about what it is and isn't, or who can do it and who shouldn't. So before we get more deeply into the substance of how to use yoga as medicine, I'd like to address those subjects.

Common Misconceptions About Yoga and Yoga Therapy

YOGA ISN'T . . . ONLY FOR THE FLEXIBLE AND FIT

Some people avoid yoga because they think it's only for people who can bend like Gumby. They think it's for the young, strong, and athletic—and if you look at pictures in magazines or sample some vigorous yoga classes you could easily get that impression.

Interestingly enough, if you feel that you couldn't possibly do yoga, then yoga might be especially helpful for you. It's well-known among yoga therapists that people with no experience in yoga often make quicker progress with health problems than students with years of experience. Indeed, it is those who find yoga the most challenging, think they are terrible at it, and can't seem to quiet their minds who have the most to gain.

YOGA ISN'T . . . ONLY FOR THOSE IN GOOD HEALTH

While I was researching yoga therapy in India, I visited centers that treated people with all kinds of physical, mental, and emotional problems: old people, stiff people, people with years of chronic disease, people in pain, people who were too depressed to get out of bed. Yoga has been used successfully on schizophrenics and on children with Down syndrome, cerebral palsy, and autism. Those who are bound to bed or wheelchairs can do yoga modified for their needs and abilities. There are people in their eighties, nineties, and beyond doing yoga, and I'm convinced that if you embrace the practice, you'll increase your odds of making it that far and feeling good when you get there.

Yoga has helped cancer patients and people with heart disease so advanced that emergency surgery was recommended. In almost all instances, yoga therapists encourage their students to continue their coventional medical care. But many yoga students notice after a while they need less of it: medication may be reduced and some drugs become entirely unnecessary, surgery may be delayed and then canceled. In India, I spoke with patients in whom all signs of rheumatoid arthritis or type 2 diabetes disappeared with regular practice. This is not everyone's experience, of course, but it shows what may be possible.

YOGA ISN'T . . . A RELIGION

Yoga is not a religion. Although yoga came out of ancient India it is not a form of Hinduism. In fact, yoga is happily practiced by Christians, Buddhists, Jews, Muslims, atheists, and agnostics alike (see p. 303). There is certainly a spiritual side to yoga, but you don't have to subscribe to any particular beliefs to benefit from it. It's probably more appropriate to view yoga as somewhat akin to Alcoholics Anonymous (AA). Like AA, yoga has a spiritual dimension that you can focus on or totally ignore, depending on what's most useful to you. Like AA, yoga is compatible with any religion, or none, if that's your preference.

Also like AA, yoga allows a "take what you can use and ignore the rest" approach. Meditation, which many people find effective for a variety of problems, originated in yoga and remains an integral part of it. (Although meditation is often thought of as a Buddhist practice, the Buddha himself was a yogi.) But if meditation seems too foreign to you, don't do it. If chanting *Om* strikes you as weird, chant something else, a prayer to Jesus or Allah or for world peace, or don't chant at all. In the thousands of classes I've attended, I've never once seen a teacher object to a student skipping it. I've also found that even those who aren't the least bit interested in spirituality, or whose childhood religious experiences were traumatic, don't have a problem with what goes on in most yoga classes or therapeutic settings. This is one of the beauties of yoga. There are so many practices and so many ways of modifying those practices that virtually anyone's needs can be met.

What Is Yoga?

Yoga is a systematic technology to improve the body, understand the mind, and free the spirit. Yogis tend to be more flexible, stronger, more energetic, thinner, and more youthful than people who don't do yoga. And what's happening on the outside is a reflection of what's happening to every system of the body. With the practice, you are strengthening and calming the nervous system. You are increasing the blood flow to internal organs and bringing more oxygen to your cells. You are clearing the mental clutter that can wreck your life, allowing you to see things more clearly. You are cultivating the spiritual muscles in a way that can make you happier, less anxious, more at peace.

Yoga has a number of tools that can help overcome one of the chief factors undermining the health and well-being of many in the modern world: an out-of-balance stress-response system. Since stress is a factor in a host of medical conditions—from heart attacks to infertility—yoga's role in stress reduction helps explain why it is useful in so many situations. But stress reduction is good for everybody, not just the sick. One yoga class or even a single breathing exercise can leave you feeling calmer and more centered. Chapter 3, "Yoga for Stress Relief," will cover this topic in detail.

TIP Yoga is strong medicine but it is slow medicine. Don't expect overnight cures with yoga (though for many people it does start to yield benefits right away). One major difference between yoga and many other approaches to healing is that yoga builds on itself, becoming more effective over time. This is not true of most drugs or of surgery, which often gradually diminish in effectiveness. In this sense yoga is something like learning to play a musical instrument: the longer you stick with it and the more you practice, the better you get and the more you will get out of it. A corollary to this is that yoga, by and large, is not the proper treatment for acute problems like broken bones, overwhelming infections, or surgical emergencies. These are best cared for in a conventional medical setting, and indeed the treatment of such acute problems is allopathic medicine's strength.

Yoga's health benefits can in part be explained by the fact that the various stretching, breathing, movement, balance, meditative, and strength practices—the elements of what's known as hatha (pronounced HOT-uh, not HATH-ah) yoga—provide many of the benefits of other worthwhile activities like walking, weight lifting, or biofeedback, plus a whole lot more. And unlike such health-club standards as StairMasters, stationary bikes, and treadmills—where the minutes seem to go by painfully slowly—yoga can be fun. Most people who do it regularly discover that yoga gets more interesting over time. I don't know anybody who feels that way about stomach crunches.

There is a continuum of effects from yoga. First, it can relax you. It can also, sometimes in fairly short order, lead to the relief of some symptoms of illness. With sustained practice, particularly of the stretching and strengthening exercises known as asana, and the breathing techniques known as pranayama, the body and breath become stronger. Posture and lung capacity improve, as does bowel function, lymphatic drainage, and the functioning of the immune system. Gradually one feels more balanced, better able to endure the slings and arrows of outrageous fortune.

In fact, yoga is all about balance. Many people have the impression that the physical practice of yoga is about being flexible, but physical flexibility is not the primary goal of asana practice; balance is. Some people who come to yoga, particularly some women, are very flexible; what they need is strength. Other people, including many men, are pretty strong when they first come to yoga, but lack flexibility. Some yoga students are debilitated by fear. Others have trouble staying motivated. Some people can't relax. What the practice of yoga does is challenge you wherever you need it, transforming liabilities into strengths, making you a more balanced person. Asana practice is itself balanced because it involves doing different poses from each of the major categories (see pp. 14–15). Ideally, if your condition allows, your practice will include some vigorous poses which are balanced with relaxation. This is one reason why yoga classes almost always end with Savasana (shah-

VAH-sah-nah), the Deep Relaxation pose. Similarly, you can balance asana with pranayama, meditation, chanting, guided visualization, and other techniques.

Yoga is a series of practices that allow you to steadily gain discipline, strength, and self-control while cultivating relaxation, awareness, and equanimity. While it wasn't originally invented to improve health or to facilitate recovery from serious illness—it was and still is, for those who choose to use it that way, a spiritual path, a way to find happiness and meaning in a chaotic and out-of-control world—there is a growing body of scientific evidence suggesting that yoga has serious therapeutic value. Let's consider a real-world example of someone who is using yoga as medicine to help cope with a medical condition.

Dolores Johnson is a very attractive woman of African and European descent whose parents were first-generation emigrants from a tropical island nation. She looks almost a decade younger than her forty-two years. She's warm, smiles broadly, and has a soft glow in her eyes. There's something in her presence that I've come to associate with people whose lives have been changed by yoga: she seems calm, happy, grateful, and fully alive.

It's very surprising to learn that despite her glow of health, Dolores has been infected with human immunodeficiency virus (HIV) for more than fifteen years. Dolores (not her real name because she can't, as she says, "disclose," at the high-tech corporation where she works, even though discriminating against those infected with HIV is illegal) has been using yoga as part of a comprehensive treatment plan to deal with her infection. When I first met Dolores in 2002, she'd been off all HIV drugs without any decline in her T-cell count—and with her doctor's blessing—for more than a year. She was thriving on a combination of yoga, Chinese herbs, acupuncture, scripture reading, meditation, and prayer.

Besides HIV, some very bad things have happened to Dolores. At fifteen she lost her mother to a painful breast cancer death. Her dad went quickly from a brain tumor two years later. And then, in her late twenties, she learned that her boyfriend Steve (also a pseudonym) had unknowingly infected her with HIV. A letter arrived that informed him that his late wife had been infected by a blood transfusion during her long battle with Hodgkin's disease.

When Dolores and Steve both tested positive for HIV, public ignorance and fear of AIDS was rampant. This was 1990, the year before Magic Johnson went public with his HIV status. They soon married. Because Steve had been infected years before and had gone too long without treatment, his immune system was so damaged that even significant advances in medication couldn't save him. He died in 1999.

A year before Steve died, Dolores took a yoga class when a coworker invited her to come along. She figured it might help her to deal with the stress of nursing her ailing husband at home while continuing to work at a demanding job. At the end of that first class, which was a gentle practice, taught by a teacher trained in the Kripalu style of yoga, Dolores found herself in tears. "I wasn't angry. I wasn't upset," she says. "This felt good." After a while she moved on to more vigorous power yoga classes. She also began to practice at home a few times each week, sometimes with the aid of an instructional yoga video.

Dolores believes the poses have strengthened her muscles, and all the breathing and stretching exercises have helped her immune system. Beyond the physical benefits, though, she says yoga brings her joy. "As I kept taking yoga and learning more about it, I realized how much more power it was giving me to be more confident with myself, with my body and with my connection to the universe, and with my spirituality," she says. "And I really liked that."

Dolores's story is still unfolding, and we will return to it later in the book. But even this much of it gives you insight into the power of yoga to change lives.

The Roots of Yoga as Medicine

India's culture is among the oldest in the world, and yoga is a gift it has handed down to us. According to scholar Georg Feuerstein, yoga may date back to the seventh millennium B.C.E., though no one knows for sure how old it is. Yoga first came to the United States when Swami Vivekananda, a Hindu monk, gave a riveting address about yoga and the unity of purpose of different religions as part of the World's Columbian Exposition in Chicago in 1893.

As science is beginning to validate many of the claims made by yoga practitioners and yoga therapists, you may wonder how such an ancient culture could have arrived at so many truths. The ancient yogis didn't have fancy machines or advanced technology to study the internal organs or the nervous system. Instead, they used the observational powers of the body itself. They manipulated the body in every way they could think of and experimented with various techniques for channeling the breath, and as they did this they explored the effects. They believed that what they learned about themselves helped them better understand the world around them; the more they explored and observed, the more sophisticated their ability to perceive different aspects and subtleties of the body became.

Sitting in caves in the Himalayas, hideouts in the forest, and ashrams in the countryside, guided by the discoveries of the generations that preceded them, aspirants chanted, meditated, and experimented with the body in a dedicated and systematic way for centuries. They learned to stretch the muscles, open the joints, align the bones in various configurations, and observed what happened as a result. They stood on their heads and bent over backward. They mimicked the posture of animals (to this day many yoga poses carry the names of animals). They moved the joints through a much larger range of motion than most people ever use, creating a series of postures designed to systematically work every part of the body and create awareness where there was none.

By experimenting with the breath, the ancients noticed that certain practices could bring a sense of energy and warmth, while others calmed and balanced the nervous system. They figured out ways to raise or lower the temperature of their hands. They developed meditation techniques that allowed them to sit naked outside in freezing winter air and generate so much heat they could dry wet sheets placed over them. With greater awareness, they realized that humans tend to breathe primarily through one nostril at a time, flipping back and forth over the course of the day—a finding recently confirmed by Western science (see p. 62). The yogis learned to control the inhalation, the exhalation, and the pauses between, and through their experiments came to believe that when you control the breath you control the mind. Advanced yogis even achieved feats like stopping their hearts and restarting them or reducing their breathing rate and their need for oxygen to almost nothing. They invented various ways to cleanse the body such as swallowing long pieces of cloth and then slowly extracting them from the intestines. Although most of us would have little interest in trying these practices, in the course of their far-ranging experimentation they discovered things that even the most conventional Westerners would find useful and accessible. Following is a very simple exercise that shows how even a very simple movement can have an effect on the nervous system.

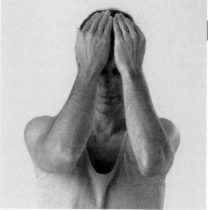

FIGURE 1.1

EXPERIENTIAL EXERCISE: Sit up straight in any comfortable seated position, either on the floor or in a chair. Bring the fleshy part of your palms onto your eyebrows and your fingers onto your scalp (figure 1.1). With the heels of your hands you should be able to feel the thick bony ridge above your eyes. Don't put pressure on the eyeballs themselves. Close your eyes. Without actually moving your hands much, gently tug the skin on your forehead up so the eyebrows move slightly toward the hairline. Stay for fifteen to thirty seconds, tuning in to how you feel. Do you feel relaxed? Are you more alert? Do you notice any difference at all? Now with your hands in the same position, move your eyebrows slightly down toward your cheeks. Stay there for fifteen to thirty seconds, observing any differences. Did your breath slow down and get a little deeper? Was the relaxation more profound than when you were tugging the eyebrows up? Repeat these two exercises as many times as you wish.

Although the effect is subtle, what most people discover when they tug their eyebrows in an upward direction is that the experience is neutral or slightly stimulating. In contrast, almost everyone finds the second part of the exercise when the eyebrows move downward to be very relaxing. The breath slows and the nervous system starts to relax almost immediately. It's pretty much automatic.

Now try another exercise that utilizes the relaxing effects of moving the eyebrow tissue down toward the cheeks. This is a simple restorative pose that can be used for such disorders as anxiety, headaches, and insomnia. You may notice that it's a bit like what many children did in kindergarten, back when naps were part of the program.

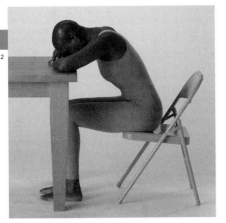

FIGURE 1.2

EXPERIENTIAL EXERCISE: Sit in a chair facing a table. Place your forearms on the table, and cross your arms. Bend forward and rest your forehead on your hands or wrists so the inner edge of the forearm closest to you is just above your eyebrows (figure 1.2). Using your forearm, gently move the flesh between your eyebrows in the direction of your nose. Rest for one to five minutes in the pose. Notice if your breath deepens and slows. Try to let go of effort and pay attention, and not fall asleep. If you fall asleep it's a sign that you need more sleep than you're getting.

The direction of the "energy" of the eyebrow skin and its effects on the nervous system is just one of literally thousands of discoveries that yoga masters through the ages have made that many modern Western doctors still don't know about. The yogis didn't so much invent these effects as uncover them and then come up with practices that exploited this built-in circuitry. Thus yoga therapy takes advantage of innate body systems that can help you heal.

It is yoga's ability to bring awareness to different parts of the body and use that awareness to influence autonomic functions—such as heart rate, brain waves, and blood pressure—that makes yoga such powerful medicine. You can use it to reduce your levels of stress hormones, like adrenaline and cortisol, which could have beneficial effects on conditions ranging from diabetes to insomnia to osteoporosis. You could lower your blood pressure and with it the risk of heart disease and stroke. You can learn to slow the mind down, lessening anxiety and depression. You can relax the muscles in the back and neck, potentially improving such conditions as headaches, carpal tunnel syndrome, and arthritis.

Although many Westerners (and these days, many Indians) come to yoga to reduce stress or improve their health, these were not the goals of the ancient yogis. They viewed yoga as a path to spiritual enlightenment. To them, better health was simply a side effect of treating your body as a sacred gift from God. Living a moral life, engaging in stretching and strengthening exercises, pranayama, and meditation were all part of the path to higher consciousness. Disease was seen as an obstacle to spiritual enlightenment and thus strengthening the body and ridding it of illness was part of that path.

The Yoga Therapy Toolbox

When people in the West refer to yoga they typically mean only the practice of the various physical postures. This misunderstanding is natural, since the asanas make for the most interesting photographs in books, magazines, and newspapers. But as Patanjali, the great codifier of yoga, defined it more than fifteen hundred years ago, yoga has eight constituent parts. The eight limbs of yoga, as found in Patanjali's *Yoga Sutras*, are:

1. The Yamas: Ethical guidelines (see table below).

2. The Niyamas: Spiritual observances (see table below).

TABLE 1.2 ANALOGOUS TO THE 10 COMMANDMENTS, THE FIVE YAMAS AND THE FIVE NIYAMAS ARE THE "DON'TS AND DO'S" OF YOGA.

YAMA	
Ahimsa	Non-harming
Asteya	Non-stealing
Satya	Truthfulness
Brahmacharya	Sexual restraint
Aparigraha	Non-hoarding (i.e., don't be greedy)

NIYAMA	
Sauca	Cleanliness, purity
Santosha	Contentment
Tapas	Discipline
Svadhyaya	Self-study
Ishvara Pranidhana	Devotion to God

3. Asana: Physical postures. Asana constitute a systematic way to take the body through its entire range of motion. As they gradually increase the freedom of movement, the asanas build flexibility, strength, and balance in every area of the body. The postures themselves can be divided into several categories with differing effects. Included are standing poses, forward bends, backbends, side stretches, twists, inversions, meditative poses, and relaxation poses (figure 1.3).

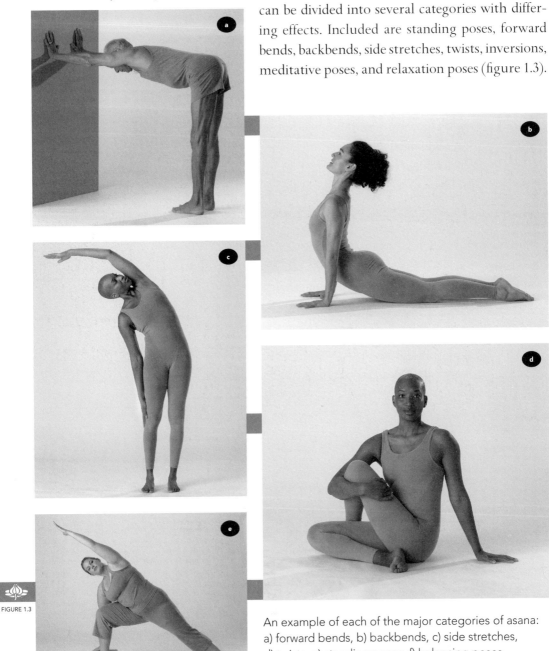

FIGURE 1.3

An example of each of the major categories of asana:
a) forward bends, b) backbends, c) side stretches,
d) twists, e) standing poses, f) balancing poses,
g) inversions, h) relaxation poses, i) meditative poses.

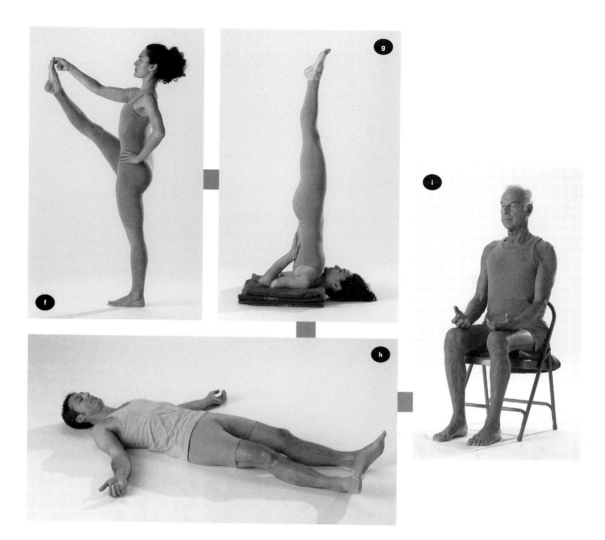

Many poses combine these different elements. Parsvottanasana (figure 1.4), for example, is a standing pose that involves forward bending at the hips, twisting of the pelvis, and inverting the head relative to the trunk, challenging your balance.

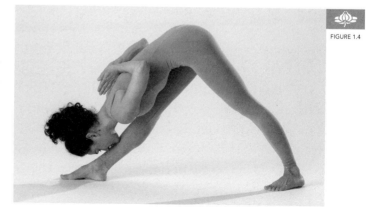

FIGURE 1.4

4. Pranayama: Breathing exercises. These include a wide variety of practices that can either energize or relax you. Pranayama practices can quiet the mind, calm the nervous system, and set the stage for meditation. Here's an exercise called Bhramari (BRA-mar-ee) that I first learned at the Vivekananda ashram in Bangalore, India. The literal meaning of the word *Bhramari,* according to the Tantric yoga teacher Rod Stryker, is "the sound of the bees." According to the *Hatha Yoga Pradipika,* a classic Tantric text and the earliest known work on hatha yoga, as a result of this practice "the mind becomes absorbed in bliss." Here is how Rod recommends doing Bhramari.

EXPERIENTIAL EXERCISE: BHRAMARI. Sit on the floor in a cross-legged position, with your spine straight. If you prefer you can sit up straight in a chair. Close your eyes and take a few slow, deep breaths. Then, after a full inhalation, begin making a gentle buzzing sound as you slowly exhale. The sound should come from as low in the throat as possible and should be soothing. As you're exhaling, feel the vibration of the sound rising out of the back of your throat, through the roof of the mouth, and up to the brain itself. Gradually allow your attention to become completely absorbed in the sound of the vibration. As thoughts come up, relax more deeply into the sound. When you run out of air, inhale slowly and deeply. Repeat the cycle. If you feel short of breath at any time, return to regular breathing until you are breathing normally again. You can then resume the practice. If you're comfortable doing so, you can gradually increase the length of exhalation. Continue the practice for one to five minutes.

5. Pratyahara: While often translated as "withdrawal of the senses," pratyahara is perhaps more accurately thought of as turning the senses inward. It's the ability to turn off the external messages from your eyes, ears, and other sense organs, and tune in to your internal environment. Instead of listening to the sounds in the room you're in, for example, you focus on the internal sound of your breath as you just focused on the humming sound of Bhramari. Try this exercise of Ujjayi (oo-JAI-ee) breath. It can be used as a stand-alone pranayama, or practiced throughout a series of asana.

EXPERIENTIAL EXERCISE: UJJAYI BREATH. Sit in any comfortable position or lie on your back, supporting your head on a folded blanket or pillow. Inhale and exhale through your mouth while imitating the deep, sibilant breath sound that the character Darth Vader made in the movie *Star Wars.* If you are unsure of how to do this (or never saw the movie), imagine you are trying to fog your glasses before cleaning them. Keeping your mouth open, take several slow, deep breaths, making the sound on both inhalations and exhalations. Now close your mouth and continue to make the whooshing sound as you breathe through your nose. Feel the air as it passes the back of your throat. It's the narrowing of your vocal cords that allows you to precisely control the amount of air moving in and out, the way a nozzle on a hose regulates the flow of water. Now close your eyes and focus your attention on the sound of the breath in your throat. Allow this attention to take you away from any sounds around you. Imagine that the breath is as loud as if you were in an echo chamber. When you first learn Ujjayi, you will breathe with an audible noise. But as you progress with the practice, the sound may become so subtle that someone sitting next to you would not hear it. Even with this quieter and more subtle version, you can still use the focus on the sound to keep your sense of hearing directed internally. Continue the practice for a minute or two.

6. Dharana: Concentration, the ability to maintain your focus. Most of what we call concentration in the West is a pale imitation of what happens in yoga. You may have noticed if you did the last exercise that you kept forgetting about the sound of your breath and your thoughts drifted elsewhere. Even in a minute or two you might have seen how much room for improvement you have.

7. Dhyana: Meditation; relaxed concentration where the stream of thoughts in the mind slows. Technically speaking, meditation can't be taught. What is typically called meditation are concentration exercises, but if you practice concentration, meditation may occur spontaneously. That said, drawing the attention inward and focusing has value and measurable benefits on health even if from a technical standpoint you don't achieve true meditation.

8. Samadhi: Blissful absorption. Yoga experts differ in their definition of samadhi (sah-MAH-dee). Some feel it is something that can be tasted, albeit fleetingly, in asana and pranayama and even in the course of everyday life, while others consider it to be the pinnacle of yoga, experienced only by masters. It is sometimes said that if you can follow twelve breaths from beginning to end without interrupting thoughts you will reach samadhi. As you've probably already experienced, following even one breath with absolute attention and no interrupting thoughts is not easy.

In addition to these eight limbs there are many other yogic tools that can be used in yoga as medicine. These will be discussed throughout the book.

Chanting of Mantra	Diet
Yogic Seals and Gestures (Mudra)	Herbs
Energetic Locks (Bandha)	Community (Sangha)
Direction of Gaze (Drishti)	Props, like blankets, mats, and blocks
Geometric Designs (Yantra)	Hands-On Adjustments and Assists
Cleansing Exercises (Kriya)	Ritual
Selfless Service (Karma Yoga)	Yoga Philosophy (Jnana Yoga)
Devotional Practices (Bhakti Yoga)	Intention (Sankalpa)
Imagery	Faith

All together, there are hundreds of different yoga tools. Indeed, there are hundreds of different asanas alone. The various tools have different effects and can be combined in a limitless number of ways. Different styles of yoga and different teachers vary in which tools they use, how they teach them, and how they combine the different tools.

Yoga as Medicine vs. Taking a Yoga Class

Yoga therapy is not the same thing as taking a yoga class. Indeed, if you have a serious medical problem and wander into a randomly chosen class, you could easily wind up worse off than when you started. Distinctions among styles of yoga and levels of expertise among yoga teachers are lost on many people, including a lot of physicians, which can be a problem. For example, a doctor who had read Marian Garfinkel's widely reported study on yoga's effects on carpal tunnel syndrome (CTS) in the *Journal of the American Medical Association,* and suggested that a patient try a yoga class, might do more harm than good. In many yoga classes, students do several repetitions of the sequence of poses known as a Sun Salutation. At several points during a Sun Salutation, you put much of your body weight directly onto the hands with your wrists cocked back—not a good idea if you've got CTS.

In her study, Garfinkel, a highly experienced teacher with many years of training, carefully chose the yoga postures subjects used and depending on how they responded, modified the protocol for each individual. In choosing the regimen, she avoided the many poses that could actually make CTS worse or modified them to make them safer (figures 1.5a & b).

In some ways, therapeutic yoga can be more like an appointment with a physical therapist or rehabilitation specialist than a yoga class, and as such is best taught by someone with a lot of experience. The average yoga teacher in a health club, where most Americans

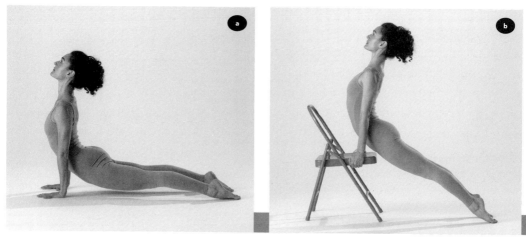

FIGURE 1.5

The yoga pose Upward-Facing Dog, often taught as part of Sun Salutations, as it is usually performed. The weight on cocked wrists can exacerbate symptoms of carpal tunnel syndrome (figure 1.5a). The same pose adapted for Marian Garfinkel's study on CTS. Notice the neutral position of the wrist (figure 1.5b).

take yoga classes, isn't likely to know enough to teach therapeutic yoga well, especially not in a group setting. Even some teachers in dedicated yoga studios won't know enough about which poses present safety concerns. (For more on contraindications—medical reasons to avoid particular practices—see chapter 4 and appendix 1, "Avoiding Common Yoga Injuries," as well as the chapters on specific conditions.)

For people with serious conditions, yoga therapy is generally taught one-on-one or in small groups. While general yoga classes may be great preventive medicine for people who are fit, many are too demanding for someone with a serious medical condition. If you have any doubts, be sure to speak with the teacher about what techniques she employs and whether she has experience in working with people who have had similar problems. If you have a medical condition and do take a general class, always try to err on the side of safety. If you're not sure whether a pose is good for you, don't do it. And certainly, if you notice pain, dizziness, shortness of breath, or other worrisome symptoms you should come out of the posture and tell the teacher. Good teachers will respect your decision to stop and will sometimes have suggestions on modifying the pose to make it safer for you.

Therapeutic yoga tends to be gentle and nurturing, though it also can be challenging. It places a heavy focus on bodily awareness, and in some systems on postural alignment, with movement tied to relaxed, rhythmic breathing. Much more than in physical therapy, students of therapeutic yoga are taught to tune in to subtle sensations of their muscles and joints, as well as the inner experience of the mind. Another difference is the heavy emphasis on relaxation. In fact, when patients are gravely ill, undergoing chemotherapy, or in the postoperative period, the entire practice may consist of breathing and relaxation until the patient gains enough strength to take on more.

The approach tends to be hands-on, tailored to the individual based on needs, abilities, and responses, as well as the teacher's or therapist's observations and any contraindications. Props such as blankets, bolsters, and straps may be employed to make postures more comfortable and safer, or postures themselves may be modified. Once students have begun to work with a yoga therapist, they are encouraged to develop a home practice, which appears to be critical to the effectiveness of the intervention.

Yoga as a Technology for Life Transformation

Although medical knowledge is constantly being refined, the basics of what we know about getting and staying healthy haven't changed much in recent years. Just about everybody knows you shouldn't smoke, and that you should eat lots of fruits, vegetables, and whole grains, get some kind of regular exercise, and keep your stress levels from spiraling out of control. The difficult part isn't knowing what to do, it's actually doing it.

In my medical practice, I saw that even patients who really wanted to change and made valiant efforts had a tough time sticking with the program. The more I've studied yoga, the more I've become convinced that it offers something doctors and public health authorities are missing: a way for people to implement the changes they want to make.

Yogis realized thousands of years ago—and what scientists are just now catching on to—that changing dysfunctional habits is largely a matter of the mind. The mind is a subject that yogis have studied systematically and that until recently medical researchers pretty much ignored. Yoga can make the critical difference in your health and well-being by giving you greater control of your mind, as well as greater understanding of the tricks it can play. This, perhaps more than anything, is what leads to life transformation.

Critical to understanding the mind's contribution to perpetuating bad habits is what the ancient yogis called samskaras. Samskaras (sahm-SCAR-ahs) are habits of action and thought that get deeper all the time, like grooves in a muddy road. From a yogic perspective, every time you do or think something, you increase the likelihood that you will do or think it again. That's true of both desirable and undesirable thoughts and actions.

When I was in medical school in the 1980s, we were taught that the brain wasn't capable of much change in adulthood. The number of neurons was fixed early in life and declined from there on. Connections between different brain cells were formed during certain critical periods early in life and after that the architecture couldn't be modified.

With advances in understanding and technology, scientists now talk about "neuroplasticity." The brain, they have realized, is plastic, meaning it is capable of change. When you perform a new action, brain cells called neurons form new connections, and the more frequently you do it, the stronger these neural links become. This, in essence, is the neurobiological explanation of samskaras.

In the *Yoga Sutras,* Patanjali gives a formula for success in yoga: practice regularly without interruption over a long period of time. This sounds like the perfect formula to create deep new behavioral grooves taking advantage of neuroplasticity. The yogic model is that by creating new samskaras, and systematically strengthening them through repetition, you create habits so strong they can compete and replace older, dysfunctional ones. As Swami Vivekananda put it, "The only remedy for bad habits is counter habits."

> **TIP** Even if you are too sick to do your yoga practice, yogis believe that there is value in simply imagining it in a step-by-step fashion. The more details you bring into the visualization the more effective it's likely to be. The benefit of practicing in your mind's eye is that any groove you've created through regular practice isn't weakened by your absence from the mat; instead, it is deepened.

The Yoga of Action: Tapas, Svadhyaya, and Ishvara Pranidhana

Patanjali outlined a system of self-transformation that he called kriya yoga, the yoga of action. Kriya yoga comprises three elements: tapas, svadhyaya, and Ishvara pranidhana, which you'll notice are also the final three niyamas.

Tapas is the Sanskrit word for heat and shares a root with the English word *taper,* a type of candle. To the ancient yogis, the human body without yoga is like an unbaked clay pot, and regular yoga practice is the kiln that gives the body the strength and resilience to withstand the wear and tear it is subjected to. The key, Patanjali said, is regularity of practice. Tapas, the fire, or dedication that fuels practice, is what keeps you going even if you don't always feel like it.

If mustering the willpower to practice regularly seems like too much for you, don't despair. One of the most amazing things about yoga is that it is both a discipline and a tool that promotes discipline. There's something about doing yoga every day that makes you want to do it every day, and this tapas, which tends to grow over time, can be extended to other aspects of your life.

Certain yoga asanas are known to build tapas. If you aren't feeling motivated, it's often a good idea to begin your practice with some of these postures. Try the following exercise that I learned from my teacher, Patricia Walden.

FIGURE 1.6

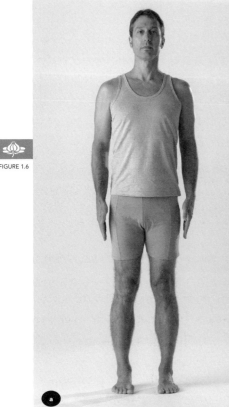

EXPERIENTIAL EXERCISE: Stand with your feet hips' width apart or sit up in a chair (figure 1.6a). Take a moment to notice the way you feel. Tune in to your body and your general level of energy. Now slowly inhale and lift both arms out in front of you, and then over your

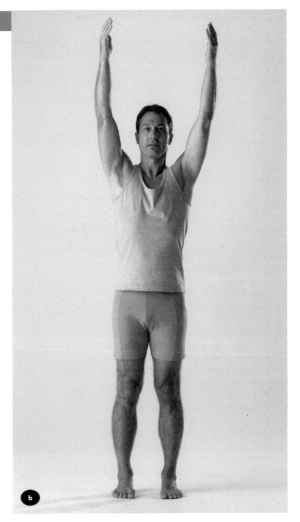

head (figure 1.6b). As you exhale, bring your arms back down. Repeat the arm movements, moving with your breath, five more times. Afterward, stand where you are or continue sitting, and close your eyes. Notice any warmth in your chest. Observe how your arms feel. Are they heavy? Do you feel life in your shoulders? Is there a tiny bit more awareness now when you tune in to your body? How about your energy level? Many people find that they're energized even though they've just exerted themselves. If you experienced this, you have tasted tapas.

Another practice that's known to build tapas is one of the most well-known postures of hatha yoga, Downward-Facing Dog (figure 1.7). If your enthusiasm is flagging, sometimes staying a minute or two in this pose (assuming you've built up the strength to do so) can give you enough tapas to want to continue your practice.

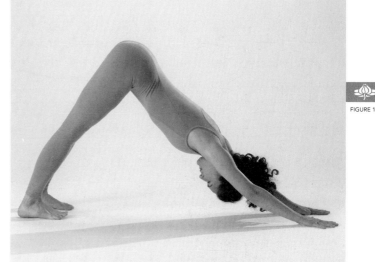

FIGURE 1.7

The ancient yogis realized that while tapas is a phenomenon of the body, it is also about the mind. Imagine you had already held Dog pose about as long as you felt you could and wanted to come back down. What if someone said that they'd pay you a million dollars to hold the pose for thirty seconds longer? It's amazing how the strength can somehow be found when the mind wants something. Once you grasp that you have the ability to redirect your mind, you discover that even though your mind can make all kinds of excuses for not doing something, you can overrule those objections and decide to do it anyway. This is tapas.

Svadhyaya, or self-study, the second element of kriya yoga, is the growing ability to sense what's happening in your body and mind when you do your yoga practice; this, too, can be extended off the mat. You begin to be able to feel when the hamstring muscles in the back of your thighs are being stretched in a forward bend, or if your breathing is getting a little strained in Dog pose. As you continue your practice, your ability to monitor the state of your body, breath, and emotions becomes progressively more refined. After a while, you may find yourself realizing that you always feel groggy or congested after eating certain foods, even if you like their taste, or that certain TV programs consistently leave you feeling more restless and unhappy. Once you really feel the effects of the choices you make in life, you may end up wanting to make different choices.

Ishvara pranidhana is the third element of kriya yoga. Its literal meaning is "devotion to God," which can be interpreted as "faith in a higher power." I like to think of it as "giving up the illusion of being in control of what happens." Yoga says give your best effort but realize that you can't control the result. That's in God's hands, as the *Bhagavad Gita* teaches.

Thus a yogic approach to weight loss would not be "I'm going to lose fifty pounds in the next two months," but rather something like "I intend to walk every day for half an hour and eat slightly smaller portions, especially at dinner." The first approach is results oriented, geared to an outcome that you can influence but ultimately can't control, and can therefore become a formula for frustration and even fatalism. The second approach is the yogic tool of intention, or sankalpa. Setting an intention is formulating a plan of action. It's what you tell yourself you're going to do. "Take care of the present," the twentieth-century yoga master Ramana Maharshi said. "The future will take care of itself." For more on this topic, please see chapter 7.

Taking It Home

To deepen samskaras, the key is repetition. In the case of yoga, this means practice, ideally every day. This is what will most efficiently forge new neural pathways and strengthen grooves you've already begun to dig. Yogis find that setting an intention to practice daily for a specific amount of time can help it happen. Be realistic, though, and shoot for an amount that you are likely to be able to do, perhaps fifteen or twenty minutes a day to begin. While yoga classes can be valuable, I advocate a personal practice, usually done at home, as the best way to deepen the grooves because few people have more than a few hours each week they can dedicate to yoga. If it takes, say, half an hour to get to a class, half an hour to get home, and extra time to change your clothes, pack your mat, and whatever else you need to do, a single ninety-minute class could easily consume three hours. In that same amount of time you could do a twenty-minute practice six days a week and an hour-long session once a week. If you can afford the time, weekly classes combined with a daily home practice is ideal.

At first, a daily practice of even twenty minutes a day may seem like a lot. If so, why not try taking just a step in the direction of yoga? Could you try some of the exercises in this book? Could you commit yourself to a few minutes of yoga practice a day, even only to taking a single conscious breath, until the groove and your sensitivity to the benefits of yoga deepen? You may feel so much better that you'll simply find yourself making the time you need, even wanting to increase it. That's a sure sign that some kind of transformation is under way.

Keep in mind that despite your best attempts, you may be unable to live up to your intention. If so, that's okay. The first step to life transformation is to see what is—to acknowledge, at least to yourself, where you are right now. You may not be able to create change immediately, but all change begins with seeing clearly. If your first attempt doesn't work out, you might want to scale back your intention a bit or simply try again.

If you're still not sure, consider what Dolores has to say. Keep in mind that yoga was completely foreign to her when she took her first class. Her advice: "Step out on faith. Try it. You might think it's a risk, but there's gain." She adds, "Yoga feels good. Yoga makes you feel good. If I could tell somebody one thing, that's it."

As a doctor who has spent the last decade investigating the field, I'd add that when done with awareness and proper instruction, yoga is extremely safe. It's fun. It's surprisingly effective, and the more you do it, the more effective it becomes. Yoga can make your life better in so many ways, including some you might not predict.

But you don't have to believe me. Try it for yourself and see what you think. That's the yogic way.

THE SCIENCE OF YOGA

There is not one muscle in the body over which man cannot establish a perfect control.

The heart can be made to stop or go on at his bidding, and each part

of the organism can be similarly controlled.

—SWAMI VIVEKANANDA

Swami Rama, a yoga guru raised in the Himalayas, sat in the lotus position on an armchair just wide enough to accommodate his knees, wires running from his chest to an electrocardiogram (EKG) machine. With him in the biofeedback laboratory at the Menninger Clinic in Topeka, Kansas, was Dr. Elmer Green, the lab's director. The year was 1970. In the control room, Green's wife, Alyce, and a group of researchers and lab technicians monitored the EKG output. Near the end of three days of testing, it was time for the yogi to "stop his heart."

Rama had already displayed body control far beyond anything the scientists had ever seen. His first day in the clinic, he'd demonstrated a remarkable ability to change the temperature of his hands. By selectively widening and narrowing the two major arteries in the wrist—a normally involuntary process he could control using his mind alone—the guru was able to create a temperature difference of about ten degrees Fahrenheit between areas of his palms just inches apart. According to Dr. Green, "The left side of his palm, after this performance, which was totally motionless, looked as if it had been slapped with a ruler a few times—it was rosy red. The right side of this hand had turned ashen gray."

Later, the swami demonstrated his ability to change his electroencephalograph (EEG) readings to any of the four major brain-wave types then recognized in Western science: alpha, beta, theta, and delta. (Recently scientists have described a fifth type, gamma waves, present in some long-term meditators.) After keeping himself in a pattern of delta waves (usually associated with deep sleep and no awareness), Rama was able to accurately recall things that the technicians had whispered to one another when they thought he couldn't hear them. They themselves had forgotten some of what they'd said until he reminded them. He had told the Greens beforehand that they would think he was asleep but that he'd be fully conscious the whole time.

Still, both Alyce and Elmer Green were nervous about the yogi's intention to stop his heart; that was another thing completely. Swami Rama had insisted, however, so they were moving forward. Rama had told them he could do this comfortably for three or four minutes and asked how long they would need to get adequate test results. Elmer told him ten seconds would be "quite impressive," and Swami Rama agreed to this limitation.

After warming up by slowing down and speeding up his heart rate, the yogi told Elmer, who was in the room with him, "I am going to give a shock. Do not be alarmed." Elmer took this to mean that he was going to give himself some kind of neural shock but soon realized he had meant that he was going to shock the lab personnel. He was right. After eight seconds of hurried consultation among the staff, who were worried about what they were seeing on the EKG, Alyce said, "That's all," over the intercom from the control room. Shortly thereafter, the swami released the contraction of his abdominal muscles he had been holding and his heart returned to normal beating. From the glint in Rama's eye, Elmer could tell that the swami thought the test had been a success.

When the scientists looked at the EKG afterward, however, it turned out that the swami's heart rate hadn't gone to zero, the ominous flatline they'd expected (the guru later told them he could have done that, too, by putting his body into a kind of hibernation). Instead, from one beat to the next, his heart rate had jumped from seventy beats per minute to about three hundred. Later, the guru told Elmer Green that when he "stopped" his heart this way he could feel "fluttering" in there.

When cardiologist Marvin Dunn of Kansas University Medical Center examined the EKG, he saw that Rama had gone into an abnormal rhythm known as atrial flutter at pretty much the maximum rate the heart is capable of. Dr. Dunn explained to Green that when the heart beats so quickly, it doesn't have enough time between contractions to fill with blood, so almost nothing is pumped out. As a result, the pulse disappears and the person usually passes out. He asked, "What happened to this man?" "Nothing," Green answered. "We took his wires off and he went upstairs and gave his lecture."

Swami Rama had induced the changes in his heart rhythm by a series of actions that included some combination of breathing techniques, muscular contractions, and mental focusing, although he didn't reveal precisely how he did it to the scientists, or even his most senior students. He agreed to perform such feats only because he thought it might lead scientists and skeptical Westerners to take yoga more seriously. Swami Rama often reminded students that attaining such yogic powers was not the aim of yoga. In his words, the real goals of yoga were to attain serenity and total freedom from suffering. Unfortunately, as persuasive as the swami's demonstration may have been, most scientists and doctors don't seem to have noticed his efforts.

SOME OF THE HEALTH CONDITIONS SHOWN BY
SCIENTIFIC STUDIES TO BENEFIT FROM THE PRACTICE OF YOGA

Alcoholism and Other
  Drug Abuse
Anxiety
Asthma
Attention Deficit Hyperactivity
  Disorder
Cancer
Carpal Tunnel Syndrome
Chronic Obstructive Pulmonary Disease
  (e.g., Emphysema)
Congestive Heart Failure
Depression
Diabetes
Drug Withdrawal
Eating Disorders
Epilepsy
Fibromyalgia
Heart Disease
High Blood Pressure
HIV/AIDS
Infertility
Insomnia
Irritable Bowel Syndrome
Menopausal and Perimenopausal
  Symptoms

Mental Retardation
Migraine and Tension Headaches
Multiple Sclerosis
Neuroses (e.g., Phobias)
Obsessive-Compulsive Disorder
Osteoarthritis
  (Degenerative Arthritis)
Osteoporosis
Pain (Chronic)
Pancreatitis (Chronic)
Pleural Effusion (Fluid Collection in
  the Lining of the Lung)
Post–Heart Attack Rehabilitation
Postoperative Recovery
Post-Polio Syndrome
Pregnancy (Both Normal
  and Complicated)
Rheumatoid Arthritis
Rhinitis (Inflammation of the Nose)
Schizophrenia
Scoliosis (Curvature of the Spine)
Sinusitis
Tuberculosis
Urinary Stress Incontinence

Science Studies Yoga

Yogis are convinced of the healing benefits of yoga, based largely on direct experience and their observations of others. While this may not meet the criteria of scientific proof, their assessments should be taken seriously because the practice of yoga directly cultivates the ability to perceive internal states. Very experienced teachers, who have gone deeply into their own practices, also develop an uncanny ability to observe others.

Moreover, as the table on p. 28 suggests, there is an ever-growing body of scientific evidence that yoga can be useful for a wide variety of medical conditions, helping people to feel better, to heal after major illness or surgery, and to live better with chronic disease. We'll discuss some of these studies in more detail in the chapters on specific conditions later in the book.

Unfortunately, most doctors don't know about this research. I certainly didn't before I started poring through the scientific evidence in both Western and hard-to-find Indian scientific journals. While the methodology of older studies, particularly those done in India, is not up to current standards, and more, and more rigorous, research is needed, the situation is improving with more and better research being published in both India and the West. We can expect more evidence in the years to come from studies currently under way evaluating yoga's effects on everything from breast cancer to back pain.

Talking About Science and Yoga

In their efforts to explain yoga's benefits, yoga teachers and practitioners tend to speak of chakras (energy centers), prana (vital force), and nadis (channels through which prana flows). While these concepts may be useful in understanding yoga, they are completely unpersuasive to most Western scientists. Indeed, most Western scientists find such explanations off-putting.

Worse, some yoga teachers make outrageous claims for the system they promote or dress up their theories about how it works in pseudoscientific language. One well-known teacher told me she could "cure" allergies within two weeks, and asthma in four. Another famous guru claims his system can cure all diseases. My response is to quote the astronomer Carl Sagan: "Extraordinary claims require extraordinary evidence." In contrast, many of the top yoga therapists I've observed quite intentionally understate what yoga can do. They don't want to be seen as selling snake oil.

My advice is to not get too caught up in the words or worry about the occasional far-fetched claim. If notions like chakras and prana turn you off, just think of them as metaphors. We use this kind of metaphorical thinking in the West all the time. There may not literally be an id, ego, and superego in the brain, but these psychoanalytic concepts can still be an interesting way to think about how the mind works. Good metaphors can help us understand, as yogis put it, "what is."

The fact is, all kinds of nutty things are said about yoga. Some critics will try to use the most extreme pronouncements of ancient yogic texts or of modern teachers to discredit the entire field. If you fall prey to this kind of skewed logic, you risk missing something that could really make your life better.

How Yoga Works

Many of yoga's benefits can be explained in ways that conform with Western ways of knowing. Here are forty ways that yoga facilitates better health, both as prevention and as treatment, that are supported by evidence. While it would have been possible to choose others, the mechanisms of action selected provide a broad overview of how yogic tools including asana (poses), pranayama (breathing techniques), and meditation can improve health.

40 WAYS YOGA HEALS

1. Increases Flexibility
2. Strengthens Muscles
3. Improves Balance
4. Improves Immune Function
5. Improves Posture
6. Improves Lung Function
7. Leads to Slower and Deeper Breathing
8. Discourages Mouth Breathing
9. Increases Oxygenation of Tissues
10. Improves Joint Health
11. Nourishes Intervertebral Disks
12. Improves Return of Venous Blood
13. Increases Circulation of Lymph
14. Improves Function of the Feet
15. Improves Proprioception
16. Increases Control of Bodily Functions
17. Strengthens Bones
18. Conditions the Cardiovascular System
19. Promotes Weight Loss
20. Relaxes the Nervous System
21. Improves the Function of the Nervous System
22. Improves Brain Function
23. Activates the Left Prefrontal Cortex
24. Changes Neurotransmitter Levels
25. Lowers Levels of the Stress Hormone Cortisol
26. Lowers Blood Sugar
27. Lowers Blood Pressure
28. Improves Levels of Cholesterol and Triglycerides
29. Thins the Blood
30. Improves Bowel Function
31. Releases Unconscious Muscular Gripping
32. Uses Imagery to Effect Change in the Body
33. Relieves Pain
34. Lowers Need for Medication
35. Fosters Healing Relationships
36. Improves Psychological Health
37. Leads to Healthier Habits
38. Fosters Spiritual Growth
39. Elicits the Placebo Effect
40. Encourages Involvement in Your Own Healing

1. Increases Flexibility. Anyone who has ever taken a hatha yoga class knows that yogic postures ask you to stretch in ways you never would have thought of; anyone who has hung in with asana practice has also observed that tight areas open up over time and poses that were once impossible become possible. While it seems obvious, scientific studies have documented the increased flexibility of muscles and the increased range of movement in different joints that come with yoga practice. The question remains: How might this benefit health? Consider just a couple examples from a potentially very long list: A lack of flexibility in the hips can put strain on the knee joint, due to improper alignment of the thigh and shin bones. Back pain can be caused by tightness in the hamstrings—muscles in the back of the thighs—that leads to a flattening of the lumbar spine.

2. Strengthens Muscles. Muscle weakness contributes to numerous problems, including arthritis, back pain, and falls in the elderly. Many of the physical limitations that people associate with aging, including weakness and progressive disability, are due to a loss of muscle, a condition recently dubbed sarcopenia. Studies have shown that even people in their eighties and beyond can make rapid gains in function when they adopt a regimen to build muscle. Asana practice not only strengthens muscles but does so in a functional way, attending to every area of the body, balancing strength with flexibility. In contrast, some weight lifters have routines that aren't well balanced and result in uneven strengthening and a loss of flexibility. Similarly, many people do stomach crunches to protect the back but strong abdominal muscles tend to tug the pubic bone up, flattening the lower back, which actually makes some back problems worse. In addition to strengthening muscles, yoga appears to build endurance and delay the onset of fatigue.

3. Improves Balance. While strength can help an old person avoid a fall, you're also a lot less likely to trip on the way to the bathroom in the middle of the night if you've improved your balance by regularly practicing asana like the Tree pose (figure 2.1). Better balance may not seem like a big deal until you consider that falls are a leading cause of hip fractures, the loss of independence, and admission to a nursing home. Yoga also helps you use your body in an overall more balanced way, left to right and front to back, which can help minimize the muscle imbalance that so often leads to bothersome symptoms and injuries.

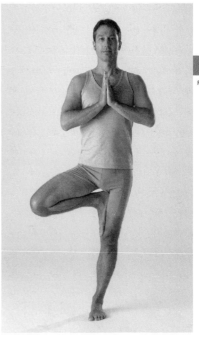

FIGURE 2.1

4. Improves Immune Function. Many yoga practices are likely to improve immune function but, to date, meditation has the strongest scientific support. Meditation appears to increase immunity in instances where that's helpful, as well as lower it in the case of autoimmune diseases, marked by inappropriately aggressive immune function. Jon Kabat-Zinn, PhD, former director of the University of Massachusetts Stress Reduction Clinic, conducted a study of people with moderate to severe cases of the autoimmune skin disease psoriasis. Those who listened to a guided meditation tape while they received the standard treatment of ultraviolet light therapy were almost four times as likely to have complete clearing of their skin. Says Kabat-Zinn, "The power of that study is that it shows that the mind can influence a healing process all the way down to the level of what has to be gene expression and cell replication." More recent research by Kabat-Zinn and Dr. Richard Davidson at the University of Wisconsin examined a group of high-tech workers who learned simple meditation techniques and yoga postures. The group developed a higher level of influenza antibodies in their blood after getting a flu shot than a control group, an indication of better ability to fight the infection.

5. Improves Posture. Many back, neck, and other muscle and joint problems can be caused or made much worse by poor posture, something that yoga can very effectively improve. Think of your head as a bowling ball, big and round and heavy. When that ball is balanced directly over an erect spine it takes much less work for the neck and back muscles to support it than when it's held several inches forward, a common postural habit (figure 2.2). The head-forward position can lead to back pain, and contribute to such problems as headaches, arthritis, carpal tunnel syndrome, and even fatigue. Hold up that bowling ball for eight or twelve hours a day and you may have less energy to do whatever else you need to do. More surprisingly—to people who aren't yogis—there's even scientific evidence that poor posture contributes to premature death. As part of a larger study looking at osteoporosis, Dr. Deborah Kado at UCLA followed over thirteen hundred older patients who had excessive kyphosis, a C-shaped slump of the upper back, for more than four years. She discovered that the slumpers were 44 percent more likely to die during the period of the study. Even more surprising, perhaps, was that those with poor posture were 2.4 times more likely to die of atherosclerosis-related conditions like heart attacks, which would put poor posture up there as a risk factor with smoking and elevated cholesterol. The precise mechanism of how bad posture could increase the death rate from heart disease isn't known, but yogis believe that slouching compresses the heart and potentially compromises its blood supply. The lungs also have less room to expand if your chest is hunched over, which means you can't bring as much oxygen into your body, the fuel the heart depends on (see next page). This notion is backed by an experiment done in Italy which

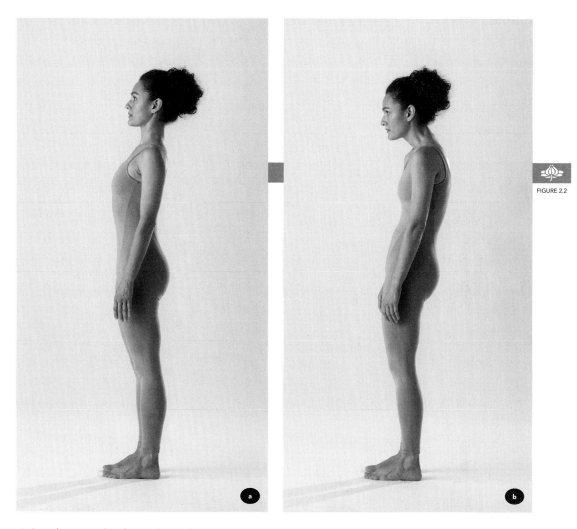

FIGURE 2.2

a) Good posture b) The C-shaped spine, a common postural habit. The farther forward the head is held relative to the spine, the greater the strain on the neck and upper back.

found that people with excessive kyphosis were 2.5 times more likely to have shortness of breath, with the degree of compromise being proportional to the severity of curvature of the upper back. Both studies were published in 2004 in the *Journal of the American Geriatrics Society.* New research suggests that excessive kyphosis is not only a result of spinal fractures, but may cause them as well. A pilot study, published in the *American Journal of Public Health,* suggests that a twelve-week program of yoga poses, modified to meet the patients' needs, improves posture, postural awareness, height, head position, functional skills, and well-being in women age sixty and older with excessive kyphosis.

EXPERIENTIAL EXERCISE: This exercise requires a six- to ten-foot yoga strap, depending on your size (in a pinch, two men's ties, knotted together, can substitute). Place the strap over your upper back and hold one end in each hand (figure 2.3a). Drape each end of the strap over the its respective shoulder (do not cross the strap in front of your body), then cross the straps in back, holding one end in each hand (see figure 2.3b). The strap

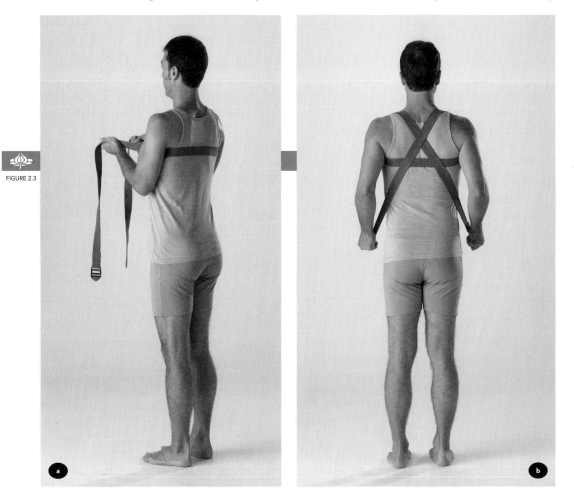

FIGURE 2.3

should be moderately tight and not kinked or twisted. Once the strap is in the correct position, lightly tug on each end in a downward direction. If the strap is positioned correctly, you will feel traction on the trapezius muscles in your upper back near your neck. You may also be able to sense how your shoulder blades are being pulled in toward the ribs. Walk around the room while continuing to gently pull the ends of the strap. Do you notice how different it feels to walk when you are aligned this way? Do you feel lighter on your feet? If so, you've just had a sneak preview of what improved posture could bring you.

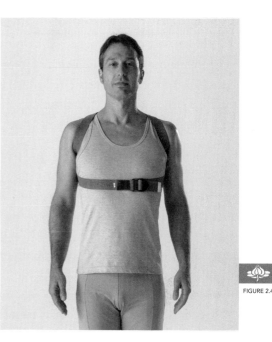

TIP For people who tend to slouch, a rope jacket is something you can wear when you are sitting at a desk. All you do is put it on as shown at left, then simply buckle the strap in front (figure 2.4).

FIGURE 2.4

6. Improves Lung Function. Yoga does this through both posture and breathing. A slumping posture pushes the bottom ribs into the abdomen, restricting rib movement and further limiting the amount of air taken in. If you don't bring a good amount of air to the base of the lungs, you compromise the ability to replenish this blood-rich area with oxygen and remove gaseous waste products. The better posture that yoga encourages will open the region of the lower ribs, and learning to use the abdominal muscles to exhale more fully (see chapter 8) will allow you to take in more air on the subsequent breath. Yoga practice has been shown to improve vital capacity (the total amount of air you can blow out), how much you can blow out in one second, and breath-holding time, as well as the peak flow rate, which helps explain why yoga appears to be useful in asthma.

7. Leads to Slower and Deeper Breathing. Yogis, compared to other people, tend to take fewer breaths of greater volume. Slower breathing is calming to the nervous system. Yogic breaths are also much more efficient. This effect was shown in a study, published in 1998 in the prestigious British medical journal *The Lancet,* done on people with breathing problems due to congestive heart failure (CHF). In advanced CHF, fluid can accumulate in the lungs, interfering with normal oxygenation, creating a feeling of suffocation. The natural response is to get agitated and breathe very quickly to try to get in as much air as possible, but it turns out that this is counterproductive. Many rapid, shallow breaths actually deliver less air to the alveoli, the tiny air sacs in the lungs where oxygen exchange happens, than a few slower, deeper breaths. After one month of practicing a yogic technique known as complete breathing, patients in the study dropped from an average of 13.4 breaths per minute to 7.6, while their exercise capacity increased significantly, as did the oxygen saturation of their blood. Indeed, patients who started out feeling so short of breath that they were breathing more than twenty times per minute wound up with higher levels of oxygen in their blood by taking only six yogic breaths per minute.

8. Discourages Mouth Breathing. Yoga promotes breathing through the nose on both inhalation and exhalation. The nasal passages filter, warm, and humidify the air, removing some of the pollen and pollutants you've inhaled before they get to your lungs. Warm, moist air is less likely to set off an asthma attack. Mouth breathing dries out your mouth, and is felt by dentists to contribute to a misaligned bite, bad breath, and other problems. There is also some evidence that mouth breathing at night contributes to snoring and possibly sleep apnea, a common and potentially deadly condition in which people repeatedly stop breathing while asleep. Because the nasal passages are narrower than the mouth, there is more resistance to air flow in them, which tends to slow the breath, calming the nervous system and the mind. (For more on mouth breathing, see chapter 10.)

9. Increases Oxygenation of Tissues. More oxygen to the lungs may translate into more oxygen to the brain and other tissues, including those areas that are in the process of healing. Yogic relaxation has been shown to increase blood flow to the periphery of the body, such as the hands and feet. Yoga has also been shown to increase levels of hemoglobin and red blood cells, the carriers of oxygen to the tissues. People who breathe quickly and shallowly eliminate more carbon dioxide from their lungs than is desirable, causing the pH of the blood to rise (that is, it becomes more alkaline). In response, hemoglobin holds on to oxygen more tightly, meaning less gets to the tissues in need. While it has not yet been documented scientifically, twisting poses are thought to wring out venous blood from internal organs, allowing more oxygenated blood to flow in once the twist is released (a phenomenon some yogis call "wring and soak"). There is also evidence that when muscles are chronically tight, blood flow through them may be restricted. Some areas may build up metabolic waste products, potentially contributing to soreness. Less oxygen and nutrients being delivered to the tissue inhibits normal functioning, and we might therefore expect the muscle to be less strong, less efficient, and more prone to injury than it might otherwise be.

10. Improves Joint Health. The cartilage in joints such as the knee acts as a shock absorber and allows the bones to glide smoothly over one another. Functioning something like a sponge, this cartilage is nourished by synovial fluid, which is squeezed out with movement, allowing a fresh supply to be soaked up. If range of movement is limited, areas of the cartilage degenerate due to a lack of sustenance, and become unable to cushion the bones as they move. Along with increasing range of movement, asana practice can also help improve the alignment of bones, potentially reducing the wear and tear. By increasing the range of motion in a joint, and taking you out of familiar movement patterns—and the literal grooves in the joint surface that can result—there tends to be less wear and tear in any one area.

11. Nourishes Intervertebral Disks. Like joint cartilage, the cartilage that makes up the spinal disks lacks an independent blood supply and requires movement to deliver nutrients from nearby blood vessels. A well-balanced asana practice that includes backbends, forward bends, and twists, as well as a gentle elongation of the spine, helps prevent the drying out and degeneration of these disks, helping them do their job as shock absorbers between the vertebrae. Cushioning the vertebrae protects the nerves exiting the spinal column from compression and impingement.

12. Improves Return of Venous Blood. Since veins, unlike arteries, can't push blood along, they depend on the movement of adjacent areas of the body, such as happens in asana practice, to move blood back from the periphery to the center. Upside-down poses encourage venous blood from the legs and pelvis to flow back to the heart. Improved return of venous blood could help with such problems as swollen ankles. With better return of blood to the heart, the heart doesn't have to work as hard.

13. Increases Circulation of Lymph. In addition to arteries and veins, there is a third system of vessels that circulates fluids throughout the body. That system carries lymph, a fluid rich in lymphocytes and other immune-system cells. The lymphatic system fights infection, kills rogue cancer cells, and disposes of some toxic waste products of cellular functioning. Like veins, lymphatic vessels lack the muscles in their walls that arteries use to propel blood. When you contract and stretch muscles, move organs around, and come in and out of yoga postures, lymph flow improves and with it lymphatic system function.

14. Improves Function of the Feet. The Chinese have a saying, "Aging begins in the feet," and yoga teaches that the feet are the foundation of good posture. When they aren't working properly, it can lead to problems in the ankles, knees, hips, lower back, and beyond, as the uneven forces are transferred upstream. Experienced practitioners of alignment-based yoga styles (see chapter 6) gradually develop greater distance between their toes and between their metatarsals (the long bones of the feet), widening and stabilizing their base. Many common foot problems, like fallen arches, can be improved and sometimes even corrected by regular practice of yoga standing poses.

15. Improves Proprioception. Proprioception is the ability to feel where your body is in space, even with your eyes closed. Most people with bad posture or dysfunctional movement patterns aren't aware of what they are doing wrong, and their lack of awareness prevents them from making changes. The regular practice of asana, however, steadily builds the ability to perceive what your body is doing. Body awareness is part of the larger concept of awareness that is central to all yoga practice. With awareness comes the possibility of making different choices. As you become more sensitive to internal processes, you become more likely to notice subtle symptoms of serious disease at a stage when it may be more susceptible to treatment. Years ago, yoga teacher Judith Hanson Lasater told her husband, "I have pneumonia in my right lung." He looked at her skeptically and said it was just a bad cold. "I'm a professional breather," she said, "and I cannot inflate my right lung." An X-ray proved she was right. Similarly, if you notice tightness in your neck and address it early with simple yoga stretches, you might never get that full-blown migraine. Awareness can also temper your stress response. As soon as you sense it kicking in, you might use a breathing technique to slow it down. Yogic awareness also allows you to tap into emotions earlier, to recognize, as Buddhists put it, "the spark before the flame." This gives you more chance not to react impulsively out of anger or fear, to analyze feelings before a cascade of biochemical events sweeps you away and you do something you might regret later on.

16. Increases Control of Bodily Functions. With greater awareness comes more control over the body. While few people could aspire to the extraordinary control exerted by Swami Rama, many people could use simple yoga techniques to lower their blood pressure a few points, bring more blood flow to their pelvis if they're battling infertility, or induce relaxation if they're having trouble falling asleep.

17. Strengthens Bones. Many yoga poses involve weight bearing, which strengthens bones and helps ward off osteoporosis. Such standing poses as Warrior II (figure 2.5) require weight

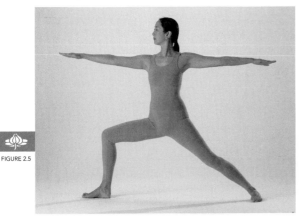

bearing in the legs. Unlike most other forms of exercise, such poses as Downward-Facing Dog and arm balances place weight on the wrists, a frequent location of osteoporotic fractures. An unpublished study done at California State University, Los Angeles, found that six months of yoga practice, focusing on standing poses, significantly increased bone density in the vertebrae in eighteen women between the ages of eighteen and sixty-five, compared to controls who maintained their usual physical activity. In addition, yoga's documented ability to lower levels of the stress hormone cortisol (see point 25) may help keep calcium in the bones because excess cortisol both decreases bone formation and increases its breakdown.

18. Conditions the Cardiovascular System. From lowering the risk of heart attacks to relieving depression, aerobic exercise is a powerful force for prevention and healing. Not all asana practice is aerobic, but when done vigorously it certainly can be. Even yogic exercises that don't bring your heart rate into the aerobic range can improve your cardiovascular conditioning. Studies have found that yoga practice lowers the resting heart rate and increases the maximum uptake of oxygen as well as endurance during exercise, all indications of improved aerobic conditioning. One study of forty young men in the Indian army found that a group practicing yoga one hour per day had similar gains in aerobic capacity to another group doing conventional exercise, but the yoga group alone showed significant reductions in perceived exertion on maximal exercise. In people with heart disease, a comprehensive lifestyle program that included yoga resulted in an improvement in the heart's pumping ability. One study found that subjects who practiced just pranayama could work harder with reduced oxygen consumption.

19. Promotes Weight Loss. Several studies have found that people who begin regular yoga programs lose weight. In addition to weight loss, one study found significant reductions in fat folds—at the back of the arms, beneath the shoulder blades, and in several other locations—as well as in body circumference. Beyond the calories burned by practicing yoga, there can also be a spiritual and emotional dimension to overweight that yoga addresses; this may be part of the reason that many people find that yoga works for them when prior attempts at weight loss have failed. A final way that yoga may aid in reducing overweight is the consciousness it can bring to eating (see chapter 27).

20. Relaxes the Nervous System. When people talk about stress reduction, they often mean changing the balance between the two branches of the autonomic nervous system (ANS), switching it from a hypervigilant state, mediated by the sympathetic nervous system (SNS), to relaxation, mediated by the parasympathetic nervous system (PNS). The ANS regulates the function of internal organs such as the heart, lungs, and intestines; it is sometimes dominated by the SNS and sometimes by the PNS, depending on the circumstances. The SNS, the "fight or flight" response, becomes more dominant in emergencies. When there is no perceived emergency, the PNS dominates. The PNS is calming and restorative; it lowers the breathing and heart rates, decreases blood pressure, and increases blood flow to internal organs such as the intestines and reproductive organs, allowing you to "rest and digest." These effects, which are the opposite of fight-or-flight, constitute what

Dr. Herbert Benson has dubbed "the relaxation response." The system he popularized to elicit it, which involves closing the eyes, following the breath, and repeating a word or phrase, is directly modeled on Transcendental Meditation (TM), a type of yogic mantra meditation, though other yogic tools including asana and pranayama can similarly shift the balance of the ANS. Conventional medicine is increasingly recognizing the role of stress in a wide variety of medical problems—not just the obvious ones like migraines and insomnia—as we'll discuss in chapter 3.

21. Improves the Function of the Nervous System. To say that yoga simply relaxes the nervous system is an oversimplification. Many yogic practices, like backbends and strong pranayama techniques, actively stimulate the SNS, so yoga's benefits can't be reduced to just relaxation. What you want is an ANS that's finely tuned to respond to whatever stresses life brings, shifting the relative activation of the PNS and SNS as needed. My guess is that yoga, by a combination of stimulating and relaxing practices, tones the nervous system to give it this flexibility. Researchers analyze the function of the ANS by looking at such factors as how well the body senses and adjusts to changes in body position (baroreceptor sensitivity) and whether the heart maintains a healthy though subtle variation in its rhythm (heart rate variability). Yoga appears to improve both of these measures.

Yogic Tool: **CHANTING.** A study by Italian researcher Luciano Bernardi and colleagues, published in the *British Medical Journal,* found that chanting could have profound effects on the nervous system. They compared the effects of chanting either a yogic mantra or the Ave Maria, typically said once for each bead of a rosary. (The rosary was introduced to Europeans by returning crusaders who learned about it from Arabs who had been introduced to it by Indian and Tibetan yogis. In yoga they are called mala beads, and reciting mantra while you finger them is known as japa.) The researchers found that it takes about ten seconds to recite either, including an inhalation in between, resulting in a breathing rate of six times per minute. This rate turns out to have calming, powerful effects on the body. There were also improvements in two measures of the health of the nervous system: baroreflex sensitivity and heartrate variability. Abnormal findings on these two measures are strongly correlated with a poor prognosis for people with heart disease. Chanting tends to increase the length of the exhalation relative to the inhalation, calming the nervous system. Other studies suggest the vibrations generated in the head from humming sounds, as when you chant Om, help keep the sinuses open.

22. Improves Brain Function. Yoga has been shown to improve coordination, reaction time, memory, and other measures of effective brain function. When you study yoga, you are learning completely new ways to move the body, and coordinating different actions simultaneously. Beyond all the variety in asana, there are breathing techniques, visualizations, mantras, and different kinds of meditation. Each of these activities causes the brain to build new synapses, the connections between neurons. Scientists now believe that continuing to learn new things into older age is one key to increasing neuroplasticity and maintaining brain function. Yoga also teaches you to focus your attention.

23. Activates the Left Prefrontal Cortex. Using a sophisticated type of brain scan called a functional MRI, Richard Davidson found that the left prefrontal cortex shows heightened activity in people who meditate, a finding that has been correlated with greater levels of happiness, better immune function, more flexibility in outlook, and a temperament that is harder to anger or fluster. The most dramatic left-sided activation Dr. Davidson has seen was found in a Westerner trained as a Tibetan monk. The calm demeanor and softness in the eyes you see in some spiritual masters seems to have physiological correlates in the brain.

24. Changes Neurotransmitter Levels. A study at Benares Hindu University found that three- and six-month practices of yoga lessened depression. The practice consisted of relaxation poses, inversions, and other asana, pranayama, and meditation. The yoga group and a comparison group treated with an antidepressant showed similar improvements in neurotransmitter levels, both experiencing a significant rise in serotonin levels and a decrease in levels of cortisol and monoamine oxidase. Such changes may help to improve mood.

25. Lowers Levels of the Stress Hormone Cortisol. The adrenal glands secrete the stress hormone cortisol in response to an acute crisis. When people are regularly stressed, their cortisol levels may be chronically elevated. As chapter 3 will detail, persistently elevated levels of cortisol can have adverse effects on the immune system, on body weight, and on memory.

26. Lowers Blood Sugar. Yoga has been found to lower fasting blood sugar in people with diabetes, as well as levels of hemoglobin A1c, a measure of longer-term control of blood sugar. The effect may in part be due to lowering cortisol and adrenaline levels. Higher blood sugar levels increase the risk of such common diabetic complications as heart attacks, kidney failure, and blindness. Yoga may also help lower high blood sugar levels via weight loss and appears to improve sensitivity to the effects of insulin.

27. Lowers Blood Pressure. High blood pressure contributes to many medical problems including heart attacks, kidney failure, and strokes. Activation of the stress response elevates blood pressure via such mechanisms as constricting arteries, conserving salt and fluids, and increasing the contractile force of the heart muscle. The exercise and the weight loss that commonly accompanies regular yoga practice also tend to independently reduce blood pressure. Yogic relaxation, in particular, appears to be effective, as described in chapter 20.

28. Improves Levels of Cholesterol and Triglycerides. Numerous studies have documented yoga's ability to lower the levels of blood fats, including LDL (the so-called bad cholesterol) and triglycerides, which are associated with many health problems including heart attacks and pancreatitis. A number of different mechanisms may be at work. Yoga's well-known ability to act as an antidote to stress, for one, may help reverse stress's tendency to boost cholesterol levels and worsen the ratio of total to HDL cholesterol (the good cholesterol). The weight loss and conditioning that mark regular yoga practice tend to drop triglyceride levels and boost HDL, high levels of which protect against heart attacks by acting as a fat scavenger within the bloodstream.

29. Thins the Blood. The final precipitant of most heart attacks and strokes, two of the three top killers in the modern industrial world, is blood clotting. Clots, formed when thousands of microscopic blood platelets stick together, tend to lodge in arteries already narrowed by fatty plaques of atherosclerosis. Heightened blood clotting increases the odds of survival if you're mauled by an animal or shot by an arrow, but in the modern world, most of the arrows are psychological, so thicker blood isn't helpful at all. Yoga reduces the tendency of platelets to aggregate into clots, as well as cuts the level of fibrinogen and encourages the breakdown of fibrin, two clot-promoting proteins.

30. Improves Bowel Function. Stress is a big contributor to intestinal problems, from ulcers to irritable bowel syndrome. Perhaps the most universal indication that stress can affect the guts are the "butterflies" just about everyone has felt at one nerve-racking time or another. Stress can lead to constipation or diarrhea. Head-forward posture contributes to constipation by compressing the large intestine and interfering with normal movement of stool. Aside from acting as an antistressor and improving posture, asana practice can be beneficial in helping move food and waste products through the bowels.

31. Releases Unconscious Muscular Gripping. Have you ever noticed yourself, for no apparent reason, clenching your teeth, or holding a pencil, a telephone, or a steering wheel with a death grip? Unnecessary, unconscious gripping can lead to chronic tension in the wrists, arms, shoulders, neck, and face, and to muscle fatigue and soreness, which in turn can worsen your stress level and mood. Yoga can teach you, in the words of senior Iyengar teacher Mary Dunn, to "take the tension out of attention," to balance effort and relaxation. Through the awareness you build up in yoga practice, you begin to notice which muscles you contract unnecessarily. It might be your tongue, or the muscles of your face and neck. If you simply tune in, you may be able to release some unnecessary holding right away. With muscles like the quadriceps (the large muscles at the front of the thighs), the trapezius (the kite-shaped muscles that extend from the neck to each shoulder and to the middle of the back), and those in the buttocks, however, it may take years of asana practice to learn how to let them relax.

32. Uses Imagery to Effect Change in the Body. Visualization and imagery play an important role in yoga practice and can help facilitate bodily and mental changes. Imagine biting into a lemon and your lips pucker and salivary juices flow. Think about contracting your biceps without actually doing it and sophisticated electrical monitoring of muscle cells will show a partial contraction. Crazy as visualization may seem, science is confirming what yogis have known for thousands of years. Dr. Vinoth Ranganathan of the Cleveland Clinic conducted an experiment in which volunteers were trained to imagine contracting specific muscles in their arms for fifteen minutes, five days a week. At the end of twelve weeks of this regimen, tests showed that the people who imagined the exercises had developed statistically significant increases in strength in those muscles compared to the control group.

33. Relieves Pain. Various studies have found that asana, meditation, or a combination of the two reduces pain in people with arthritis, back pain, fibromyalgia, carpal tunnel syndrome, and other conditions. New brain-imaging techniques have found that seasoned meditators can decrease the signals between the thalamus, a part of the brain that transmits pain messages, and the higher brain centers of the cerebral cortex. Jon Kabat-Zinn finds that mindfulness meditation can improve the ability to tolerate pain by teaching you to separate the pain itself from your thoughts and emotions about it (which otherwise can fuel the fire). Not just an end in itself, pain relief may facilitate healing by lifting mood, encouraging activity, and reducing the need for medication.

34. Lowers Need for Medication. Studies have shown that yoga allows some people with asthma, heart disease, high blood pressure, type 2 diabetes, and obsessive-compulsive disorder to lower their dosage of medications and sometimes to get off of them entirely. Since all drugs have side effects, ranging from impotence due to blood pressure medications to dangerously low blood sugars from diabetes drugs, it's generally a good idea to take as few medications as possible or, if they prove necessary, to use the smallest effective dose. Using fewer drugs also lessens the chance of potentially dangerous drug-drug interactions and—of course—saves money.

35. Fosters Healing Relationships. Just as a good doctor-patient relationship can be healing, a good partnership with a yoga teacher can confer therapeutic benefit. Often teachers adjust students or touch them in ways to facilitate relaxation or moving more deeply into a posture. This is what doctors used to call "laying on of the hands," which unfortunately with the boom in high technology has mostly been replaced with what I call "laying on of the drugs." Part of the benefit of a good relationship with a teacher is related to the distinctly unscientific concepts of love and caring, which while hard to measure, undoubtedly facilitate healing. In a similar way, the sangha, or community of yoga teachers and students that forms around studios and other places people practice, provides the kind of social support which scientific evidence suggests benefits health.

36. Improves Psychological Health. Yoga has been shown in a variety of studies to improve a number of measures of psychological health, including mood, self-esteem, and sense of equanimity. Yoga also lowers levels of anger, and, perhaps as a result of this as well as some of the other changes listed, fosters better relationships with others. In addition to its value in improving the quality of life, there is evidence that psychological well-being has a huge impact on physical health. Studies suggest, for example, that chronic anger and hostility are as strongly linked to heart attacks as such well-known risk factors as smoking, diabetes, and elevated cholesterol.

37. Leads to Healthier Habits. The psychological health and sensitivity to the body that regular yoga practice facilitates encourages people to make healthier choices, a finding documented for students of TM, which also appears to be common among committed yoga practitioners. People who take up yoga may start to walk regularly, eat better, or quit smoking after years of failed attempts. As their practice deepens, their habits tend to become even healthier. After one year of yoga, a student might decide to cut down on red meat. After five years, he might cut it out entirely.

38. Fosters Spiritual Growth. The regular practice of yoga, particularly when it is done with the intention of self-examination and betterment, often puts practitioners in touch with a different side of themselves. Among the spiritual aspects that yoga fosters are feelings of gratitude, empathy, forgiveness, and the sense that you're part of something bigger than yourself. While better health is not the goal of spirituality, numerous scientific studies have documented that it has this effect. A final area where the spiritual side of yoga can help is with suffering. From a yogic perspective, suffering, or duhkha, is different from pain. Pain can't always be avoided, but how much you suffer as a result depends on your state of mind. Thoughts and emotional reactions to painful experience, yoga teaches, can fuel the fire of discontent and undermine healing. Learning to quiet the restless mind and tune in to its tricks and habits is the path to transcending suffering.

39. Elicits the Placebo Effect. Just believing you will get better can make you better, as countless case histories and scientific studies have demonstrated. Unfortunately, many conventional scientists act as if something that works by eliciting the placebo effect some-how doesn't count. But people who are suffering tend to be pragmatic. They just want to be helped. If chanting a mantra facilitates healing, even if it is "just" through the placebo effect, why not do it?

40. Encourages Involvement in Your Own Healing. In much of conventional medicine, patients are passive recipients of care. In yoga, the essential element is not what is done to you but what you do for yourself. Yoga gives people something tangible they can do and most people start to feel better the very first time they try it. They also observe that the more they commit to the practice, the greater the benefits tend to be. This not only in-volves them in their own care, it gives them the message that there is hope, and hope itself can be healing—and self-perpetuating. If you believe that yoga really can help you, you are much more likely to practice every day. And if you do that, it is much more likely to work (and not just because of the placebo effect).

As you read through these forty ways yoga benefits health, you probably noticed a lot of overlap. While for the purposes of understanding you can separate the mechanisms un-derlying the physiology and psychology of health, in reality they are densely interwoven. Change your posture and you change the way you breathe. Change your breathing and you change your nervous system. This, of course, is one of the great lessons of yoga: every-thing is connected—not just your hip bone to your knee bone but you to your community and the world. Interconnections are vital to understanding how yoga works, because yoga is a holistic system that taps into dozens of mechanisms that may have addi-tive and even multiplicative effects. This kind of synergy may be the most important way of all that yoga heals.

Better still, most of the direct effects of yoga—strength, flexibility, balance, the ability to calm the nervous system—grow in magnitude with continued practice, as do the heal-ing benefits. Working like compound interest, gains accrue over years and even decades. Most yoga experiments done in the West, however, due to financial and logistic concerns, are conducted for a very short time, often eight to twelve weeks. It's impressive that so short a time has been sufficient to document benefit in many cases, but any experienced yogi will tell you twelve weeks is a drop in the bucket. Thus it's likely that most yoga stud-ies to date have systematically underestimated yoga's healing power. Yoga is strong medi-cine but slow medicine. A drug may be faster out of the blocks but yoga is often the tortoise that wins the race to better health.

Integrating the Best of Yoga and Western Science

Modern medicine and yoga have completely different methods of deciding on the best treatment for a particular patient. In medicine, particularly in recent years, doctors have looked to the results of large controlled studies. They judge which of the treatment options tested helped a greater (and statistically significant) percentage of patients. From there, they extrapolate the result back to you. While far from perfect, this approach has helped millions of people and advanced understanding in countless ways.

Most yoga experts, on the other hand, believe that yoga therapy must be personalized to be maximally effective. There can be no standard treatment for all people with back pain because back pain has many causes, and each happens in the unique context of the body, mind, life history, and present circumstances of the person suffering the problem. A yoga therapist weighs all of these factors in developing a treatment plan. From a yogic perspective, it doesn't matter if a certain pose helps nine out of ten people with back pain. A good teacher will watch you do the pose and should be able to tell whether it's likely to help you or whether you need something different.

The best yoga therapy I've observed appears to be an art as much as a science. Skilled teachers might plan a basic regimen for a given person with a particular set of problems, and that regimen might be similar to one for someone with a comparable set of problems. But based on the student's progress and on the teacher's observations, the regimen will often be modified during the course of treatment. In medical classes at the Iyengar Institute in Pune, India, B. K. S. Iyengar, legendary for his therapeutic prowess, would sometimes put a student in a pose, take one look, and immediately take the person out of it. Whatever his theory for choosing the posture—and Iyengar is a master at designing poses and sequences of poses to elicit specific effects—as soon as he saw the result, he knew it wasn't right. Perhaps the student's complexion paled, her eyes glazed over, or her breathing seemed more constricted. Standardized protocols, used in most scientific investigations, do not allow for this kind of observation or improvisation.

Most of the experienced therapists I observed insist there can be no standardized anything. Geeta Iyengar, the guru's daughter and now the principal teacher at the Institute, told me that sometimes what worked with a student yesterday won't work today. If the student just strained her back or had a particularly stressful day at work, the entire program for her underlying condition may need to be changed. If yogis are correct that personalized yoga protocols are much more effective than the one-size-fits-all approaches favored in medical research, once again, most published studies on yoga will have underestimated yoga's effectiveness.

Of course, yogis would argue that much of what yoga does can never be measured by science. Healing, transcending the suffering (duhkha) that marks human existence, takes place primarily on a spiritual plane. Unfortunately, there's no "spirituogram" that can quantify this aspect of yoga, so science doesn't look there. As with any holistic endeavor, measuring the constituent parts is not the same thing as understanding the sum of those parts. Reductionist science may tell us that yoga decreases systolic blood pressure and cortisol secretion, increases lung capacity and serotonin levels, and improves the functioning of the autonomic nervous system, but that doesn't begin to capture the whole of yoga.

Modern science is a wonderful tool that continues to discover life-saving treatments, but in many ways it doesn't know how to make you happy, find meaning in your life, or feel connected to others—precisely the things many people feel are the most important. Beyond improving the quality of your life, these factors can have a profound effect on whether you get sick and how likely you are to recover. Science has also largely failed at the task of giving people the mental strength to make the kind of changes, like exercising and eating better, that would make them healthier. This is the tapas, described in chapter 1, that the regular practice of yoga builds.

While yoga can make the tools of modern medicine more effective, it's also true that science can help yoga. While research has already documented the efficacy of yoga for a number of conditions, much more needs to be done. Preliminary results should be confirmed. Larger, longer studies would be desirable. Research could help sort out which yogic tools appear to work and better explain, especially with cutting-edge technology like functional MRI scanning, how yoga does what it does. Medical knowledge can also aid yoga teachers in figuring out which practices are likely to be safe and which may be ineffective or too risky for some students. "Yoga does not quarrel with science," said physician and yoga master Swami Sivananda. "It supplements science."

Ultimately, science and yoga should not be seen as competing. What yoga does well complements modern medicine's strengths, providing more options for people in need of healing. While it's true that yoga and medicine provide very different perspectives on health and disease, viewing the world through both paradigms can help you see reality more clearly and make more skillful choices. Nothing could be more yogic than that.

C H A P T E R   3

YOGA FOR STRESS RELIEF

The mind makes a man its slave;

again the same mind liberates him.

—SWAMI SIVANANDA

 Stress is not all bad. Being nervous, worried, and on edge has survival value. As you've probably heard many times before, you wouldn't even be here to read this if your ancestors hadn't had a well-honed stress response system to survive marauding invaders and hungry predators. Even getting out of bed in the morning demands a surge in blood pressure that wouldn't occur without your built-in stress response system, which relies on activation of the sympathetic nervous system (SNS) and the release of stress hormones, including adrenaline and cortisol.

When you perceive a threat—anything from a confrontation with an angry motorist to an unexpected tax bill from the IRS—your SNS is activated almost immediately. Your blood pressure goes up and your heart beats harder, bringing extra blood to the large muscles of the legs and arms to allow you to defend yourself or flee from trouble (hence the term fight-or-flight). Blood clots more easily in case you are injured. White blood cells stick to the walls of capillaries, ready to be mobilized if any wounds incurred get infected. Energy sources, including sugar and fats, are mobilized to give you plenty of fuel. If you've ever had a near miss—like almost getting hit by a bus—you know that the stress response kicks in almost immediately, then takes a while to wear off.

If your stress response system is functioning well, once the threat has passed, your body shifts into a restorative mode in which the parasympathetic nervous system (PNS) dominates over the SNS. Your blood pressure and heart rate return to normal. Stress hormone levels drop, as do blood sugar levels and measures of blood clotting. In the modern world, most of the "threats" we face are no longer physical. Typical contemporary stressors—worries about relationships, problems at the job, and abstract concerns about money, security, happiness, and fulfillment—tend not to be resolved quickly, so the stress response system either stays activated or is repeatedly reactivated. When that's the case, your built-in protection system can turn on you and cause disease.

The Link Between Stress and Disease

When someone mentions a stress-related health problem, you might think of an ulcer, trouble falling asleep, or tension headaches. Stress can indeed contribute to these problems, but scientific evidence is showing that stress fuels some of the biggest health problems of our time, including type 2 diabetes, depression, osteoporosis, heart attacks, and strokes, as well as autoimmune diseases like multiple sclerosis (MS) and rheumatoid arthritis. While there isn't a lot of evidence that stress causes cancer, it appears to increase the odds of dying from the disease. All told, it could be argued that stress is the number one killer in the Western world today.

There has been much reported in recent years about an epidemic of obesity, most tragically among children, who may end up overweight for life. New evidence suggests that the biggest predictor of overweight in children is their stress levels. A study published in the journal *Health Psychology* found that stressed-out children eat more than twice as much at meals than less-tense classmates, snack more, and make far more unhealthy food choices. They also showed one of the hallmarks of unhealthy eating: skipping breakfast, which sets the stage for overeating later in the day. Overeating may be in part due to the effects of cortisol. Yoga has repeatedly been found to lower levels of this stress hormone.

CORTISOL: A KEY PLAYER IN STRESS-RELATED DISEASE

The elevation in cortisol levels that results from stress undermines health in numerous ways. High cortisol levels have been linked to increased fasting blood sugar, high systolic and diastolic blood pressure, high triglyceride levels, as well as insulin resistance. Each of these is an independent heart attack risk factor, and together they act synergistically to multiply the danger. Cortisol appears to be intimately involved with stress-related eating; high levels are linked with what scientists studying rats call "food-seeking behavior," and binge eating in humans. If you do overeat, cortisol ensures that the extra calories are converted into fat deposited in the most dangerous place of all from a health standpoint, the abdomen. Excess intra-abdominal fat greatly increases the risk of type 2 diabetes and heart disease, two of society's biggest killers. But this is only a partial catalog of cortisol's effects.

Elevated cortisol also lowers bone density, has been linked to depression, and appears to affect immune function. When you respond to an acute crisis with a surge in cortisol you get a temporary boost in immune function. But when cortisol levels remain chronically high, they have a deleterious effect on the body's built-in defenses. This is no surprise: cortisone and other drugs related to cortisol are used medically to suppress the immune system. Scientists have linked chronic stress with how likely you are to develop a cold if exposed to a virus, and how severe the symptoms will be. High levels of stress are known to reactivate herpes infections and to make your immune system less likely to respond to a vaccine. Cortisol appears to be the major player in this immune suppression.

Cortisol has even been linked to memory loss. One reason that stressful events are so strongly imprinted in the mind is high cortisol levels. Chronically high cortisol levels, however, can undermine memory and lead to permanent changes in the brain. Some studies link the tendency toward stress to the subsequent development of Alzheimer's disease (although there is no proof of a causal connection). Chronic stress, however, probably does accelerate the decline in mental function in someone who has the disease and may contribute to other forms of dementia.

The list below summarizes the ways stress can undermine health. (Notice that many of these effects are the opposite of the results of yoga, as described in chapter 2.)

HEALTH EFFECTS OF STRESS

Impaired Function of the Immune System	Increased Cholesterol
Increased Inflammation	Increased Triglycerides
Decreased Bone Density	Increased Blood Clotting
Problems with Memory	Impaired Wound Healing
Increased Appetite	Poorer Sleep
Weight Gain	Increased Sensations of Pain
Fat Deposited in Abdomen	More Fatigue
Increased Resistance to Insulin	Worsening of Mood
Increased Blood Sugar	Adoption of Less Healthy Habits

Yoga's Take on Stress

Whatever the external causes, stress is often fueled by your thoughts. The mind can even produce stress worrying about problems that almost certainly won't occur. Some of Mark Twain's biggest disappointments, he quipped, never happened.

The good news is that healing and just plain feeling good about your life can also be facilitated by your thoughts. As much as anything, yoga is a technology that teaches you how to stop your mind from working against you. Yoga turns the mind into your ally. In the words of Patanjali, "Yoga slows down the fluctuations of the mind." By turning down the volume on what I call tape loops—mental samskaras—you can get in touch with a more blissful place inside. At first you may only notice it toward the end of a yoga session, but if you maintain the practice, you become more and more aware of a calm place at your core throughout the course of the day. Over time yoga helps you realize that much of what you routinely get upset about is not that important. That may be the best stress reduction method of all.

One yogic tool that intentionally uses thoughts to change the body and mind is guided imagery. While you relax in either a seated position or lying down, a teacher (in person or on tape) guides you to different places in your imagination. The images can be visual, auditory, tactile, or metaphorical. Try the following exercise, led by Rod Stryker, and see if it affects the way you feel. Don't move through it too quickly. When Rod teaches it to a class, the pace is leisurely. He pauses frequently between instructions, taking six to eight minutes from beginning to end.

EXPERIENTIAL EXERCISE: GUIDED RELAXATION. As with all relaxation exercises, first turn off any music, television, phones, or anything else likely to distract you. Sit in a comfortable, upright position or lie down. When you are settled, imagine that a wave of relaxation is spreading through your entire body. Let go of any holding in your jaw. Let your lips part and your upper and lower teeth separate slightly. Without changing your facial expression, imagine the feeling of a smile. Grow that radiant, open innocence, the joyousness behind a smile. After a moment, bring the feeling of a smile to your heart and linger there in your imagination. Then feel a smile in both lungs and in the space between your shoulder blades. From there bring the feeling of a smile to your abdominal organs and digestive system, your lower back, your pelvis and reproductive organs, and both legs. Finally feel your whole body as one large, open, radiant smile. Feel yourself as the embodiment of a smile, your whole being renewed, reverberating with the presence of a smile. Every cell is smiling.

Did you notice any changes from doing this exercise? Do you feel more relaxed? Has your breathing slowed down or gotten deeper? Is your mood lighter? It's possible that you didn't feel much. People differ in which images work best for them. If you are a more visual person, you might respond better to images of a beautiful scene in nature. Images can also combine sense modalities. An imagined beach scene, for example, might conjure up the sound of the waves, the smell of salt water, and the sensations of warm sun and ocean breeze. If you are interested, you might experiment with various imagery exercises aimed at different senses to see which ones appeal to you most.

Yoga practices like this can be profoundly relaxing, even joyful. The power of yoga, however, goes beyond how you feel while you do it and immediately thereafter. Yoga also holds the possibility of being transformative.

SAMADHI ON THE BEACH

Most people have experienced a feeling of deep calm at the ocean, or in another natural setting. They get so absorbed in the beauty and the power that surrounds them that they lose all self-consciousness. For just a moment, the constant chatter of the mind slows down. Sometimes in a moment like this people find clarity. Maybe they realize that they aren't happy in their job or in their personal life and need to make a change. It's not that they make a decision, exactly. It's more like they recognize a message coming from inside that they couldn't hear in the din of their everyday lives.

The psychologist Mihaly Csikszentmihalyi has written extensively about a phenomenon he calls flow. Flow is the effortless sense of being in the moment. From a yogic perspective, it's also a place where healing can occur. It might happen while doing your work, sitting on the beach, listening to a symphony, or if you are very lucky, even in the middle of a traffic jam. If you've ever had an experience like this—even if you've never done yoga—you've already had a glimpse of what the practice of yoga could bring you.

The experience of complete absorption is what the ancient yogis called samadhi, a Sanskrit word meaning "still mind" and the eighth limb of Patanjali's eight-limbed path. Samadhi, Rod Stryker says, happens when you are completely engaged in what you are doing; there are no thoughts of anything else, and time disappears. Samadhi is a blissful state, beneath words, that yoga teaches is your birthright. It's built right into your circuitry, though you may need to learn how to access it.

Yoga is a method, or a collection of methods, to get to samadhi. Yogis believe that when you quiet the mind, you come to realizations about what's true and what's not true, what's important and what isn't. As blissful as samadhi can be, its greatest benefit is not the experience itself: it's what the experience teaches you about how to live your life. The kind of samadhi in everyday life described above is, from a yogic perspective, only the beginning. Patanjali described several levels of samadhi. Deeper states of samadhi, and the insights that accompany them, yogis believe, come only through the regular practice of meditation. Still, even a moment of samadhi on the beach can change you, and may whet your appetite for more.

CALMING THE MONKEY MIND

In contrast to the inner quiet of complete absorption in the moment is the more usual state in which the mind's tape loops just won't stop. In most people the mind constantly roams from topic to topic, provides a running commentary on how things are going, interspersed with a seemingly random stream of thoughts: worries, to-do lists, snatches of song lyrics, sexual fantasies, images from the media, and assorted memories. This is what yogis call the monkey mind. It's kind of like a hyperactive kid, flitting from thought to thought, never concentrating on any one thing for very long. Much of what fills the monkey mind are mental samskaras: repetitive, automatic thoughts about what you fear, desire, or hate. The monkey mind rarely attends to the present moment. It would much rather obsess about past resentments, relive old glories, worry about the future, or fantasize about how life could be different.

When you spend all of your time listening to your internal tape loops, you can't fully attend to the present. You don't hear what your spouse just said. You don't fully taste your food. You quite literally don't smell the roses. Since many people have never experienced anything else, they think a constant inner dialogue is normal. Others may not be consciously aware of how often they are lost in their internal world of thought. To further explore this idea, please try this simple meditation exercise.

EXPERIENTIAL EXERCISE: MEDITATION ON THE BREATH. Sit up straight, either on the floor or in a chair. If sitting is not possible, lie on your back. Gently close your eyes and begin to follow the breath, but don't make any effort to change it. Try not to drift into sleep. Bring your attention to the sound of the breath flowing in and out. Notice the air as it brushes the inside of your nose. Pay attention to the entire inhalation right up until it ends and the exhalation starts. Tune in to the exact moment of transition. Focus on the fine details of how the breath feels in your nostrils and listen to the sound it makes. Notice if the in breath and out breath are equally smooth and of similar length. If you notice that your attention has wavered, simply return your focus to the breath once again. Stay with the practice for two to five minutes.

After you've finished, think about how the exercise went. Were you able to keep your focus on the breath? Did your thoughts tend to wander? Were you thinking about a pain in your back or an itch on your nose? Did your mind jump to what you need to do later today or tomorrow? Were you judging yourself?

If your mind was all over the place in this exercise, don't worry. You are in very good company. Almost everybody's mind is like that almost all the time. It's only when you sit in one place, close your eyes, and try to focus that you begin to see it clearly. Very few people can maintain one-pointed concentration for the duration of even a single breath. Part of the usefulness of this meditation exercise is that when you try to be quiet, you can clearly see how busy your mind is.

Modern humans spend almost all of their waking life in the land of words and concepts. These are important, of course, but through yoga you learn that you shouldn't spend all of your time there. Yoga teaches that the real you lies beyond that endless verbal stream. It's not that you want to abandon rational thought. You just want to be able to turn it off for brief periods, so that you can tune in to direct experience and the unselfconscious self that lies beneath the surface. What the ancient yogis invented were a series of techniques to lessen the distraction of the nonstop verbal parade so that the mind can become clearer and more perceptive.

From a health standpoint, besides distracting you and sometimes making you miserable, the monkey mind tends to keep the SNS activated, which is just the opposite of what most people in the modern world need. The feelings of calm, connection, and meaning we experience when we fully occupy the present tend to shift the balance toward the PNS, potentially undoing some of the damage.

STRESS AND THE BREATH

Breath is perhaps the most important tool in yoga practice. The ancient yogis discovered that the breath, which is normally automatic, has profound effects on the nervous system if consciously controlled, with the potential either to increase activation or to promote relaxation, depending on the practice. Through yoga practice, you come to realize how your breath affects how you feel and how you can use it to alter your state of being. Much of the focus in yoga is on slowing and deepening the breath, but it's also about making the inhalation and exhalation as smooth as possible with no major bumps or hiccups. Controlling the fluctuations of the breath, yogic lore teaches, helps calm the fluctuations of the mind (see box on p. 55).

Feeling stressed can have a number of effects on the breath, most of them not good. From a yogic perspective, breathing in dysfunctional ways can be both a consequence *and* a cause of stress; you may breathe erratically when you feel stress, *and* choppy, inefficient breathing causes tension and unease. Just slowing the breath down and making it more regular begins to lessen feelings of stress within seconds. This wisdom is reflected in the common injunction to someone on the verge of losing self-control: "Take a deep breath."

SLOW, DEEP BREATH

↓

RELAXED NERVOUS SYSTEM

↓

CALM MIND

↓

A SENSE OF CONNECTION   COMPASSION   INTUITION   CREATIVITY   HEALING

In yoga, the breath is used to relax the nervous system, which in turn calms the mind. When the mind is still, yoga teaches, you have access to deeper wisdom from within, and both creativity and healing are facilitated.

DIAPHRAGMATIC BREATHING

Crucial to understanding yogic breathing is appreciating the role of the diaphragm, the most important of the muscles that help move air in and out of the lungs. The top part of this large, thin muscle is shaped something like the dome of an umbrella, and separates the chest from the abdomen. The heart and lungs sit right on top of it and the liver, stomach, and other abdominal organs just below it. Its top part connects to the inside of the lower ribs in both the front and back. On the diaphragm's underside, a thick tendon connects it to the lower spine. When the diaphragm contracts to initiate the in breath, its dome moves downward. If your abdomen is relaxed, the pressure will make the belly gently expand outward and the lower regions of the lungs expand downward. If you tune in, you may notice a subtle sensation of pressure between the navel and the breastbone when you inhale, which resolves as you breathe out. You may also notice a subtle flaring of the lower ribs on inhalation, also facilitated by diaphragmatic movement, that allows you to take in more air.

In a normal, healthy breath, the abdomen tends to puff out as you inhale. As the diaphragm moves down to allow more room for the lungs to fill, the abdominal organs get gently compressed and the belly tends to move out. Then when you exhale, the diaphragm relaxes and moves back up and the belly tends to move in a bit. One type of inefficient breathing that can be a marker of stress is what yogis call reverse, or paradoxical, breathing.

Instead of using the diaphragm to take in air in the most efficient manner, paradoxical breathers work against themselves, contracting this large muscle when they should be relaxing it and vice versa. Reverse breathers pull in the abdomen when they breathe in and let it out when they exhale. The breath tends to be short and staccato, with a quick lift of the rib cage on inhalation. If you try it, you may notice that this type of breathing is similar to the sudden breath you take when you are startled. The effect on the nervous system of habitually breathing this way is a bit like getting startled thousands of times a day.

EXPERIENTIAL EXERCISE: BREATHING ASSESSMENT. You can assess whether you are a normal or a reverse breather either sitting in a chair or lying on your back. If you lie down, you may want to bend your knees and put a pillow beneath your head for comfort. Place one hand on your abdomen and the other over your lower ribs. As you gently inhale and exhale, notice which way your hands are moving. Don't try to change anything right now, just notice. In normal breathing, the abdomen puffs out gently with the inhalation and moves back in as you exhale, while the rib cage doesn't move as much. In reverse breathing, the belly moves in on the inhalation and out on the exhalation, and there is more movement occurring in the upper rib cage.

If it turns out you are a reverse breather, don't worry. This is something you can change over time. Better still, if you're a reverse breather who suffers from anxiety, insomnia, high levels of stress, or any other condition made worse by stress, you may have just discovered something you can change that could significantly lower your stress levels. Bringing more awareness to the breath and learning some simple yogic breathing techniques, such as the one that follows, could start to help you almost immediately.

EXPERIENTIAL EXERCISE: BELLY BREATHING. If you're able, lie on your back for this exercise. First observe a few natural breaths. Then inhale, and on the next exhalation gently contract your abdominal muscles, bringing your navel in the direction of your spine. With little or no muscular effort, let your abdomen gently lift as you inhale. Breathe this way for a minute or so, then pause to observe any changes in your mind or body. Most people find themselves feeling much more relaxed. You can try this exercise in a sitting position, too. If the seated belly breath works for you, you can use it anytime you wish—at your desk at work, at a stoplight when stuck in traffic, or in an airplane flying through turbulent weather.

SENSORY OVERLOAD AND STRESS

Yoga teaches that just as what you eat has a tremendous effect on the health of your body, what you take in through your sense organs feeds your mind. Until the twentieth century, people generally had to slow down when it got dark in the early evening and remain that way until early the next morning. With the invention of electric light all that changed. Now computers, TVs, beepers, PDAs, cell phones, neon lights, and car alarms, to name a few, bring an avalanche of sights and sounds that may be much more jarring to the nervous system than most people assume. Studies suggest that noisy workplaces—even when workers believe they aren't bothered by the sounds—can activate the body's stress response system. Thus sensory overload is likely to be exacerbating already sky-high stress levels in the modern world. No wonder it's so hard for most people to concentrate.

Pratyahara, the fifth limb of yoga's eight-limbed path, is the turning inward of the senses. By selectively increasing your attention to internal phenomena like the breath, you can learn to tune out external phenomena. You still hear outside sounds, but like the din of voices in a crowded cafeteria, they become sensations you can allow to fade into the background. Rod Stryker says, "One of the reasons that we experience so much fatigue is that the senses are just overwhelmed with too many stimuli. The more we can turn our awareness inward, turn the senses internally, the more they are replenished and rejuvenated. That internalization of attention is also the bridge to the healing power of yoga."

Try this exercise that can facilitate pratyahara.

EXPERIENTIAL EXERCISE: PALMING EXERCISE. Sit in any comfortable seated position, with your spine in an upright position. Begin by rubbing your palms together to gen-

erate heat for fifteen to twenty seconds. Then place your palms over your closed eyes. Do not put any pressure on the eyeballs themselves, which are sensitive structures. Instead, press on your brow and on the cheeks outside the bony rims of your eye sockets. Continue to keep your chest upright but allow your head to gently tip forward (figure 3.1). Start to tune in to the breath. Notice the color and texture of any visual patterns beneath your hands. Allow those visual images to fade to black as the muscles of your face let go. Stay for one to five minutes. When you stop, notice whether you feel any more relaxed and are able to see with less tension in your eyes.

It is also possible to learn to bring relaxation to your eyes using awareness and imagery. If you notice yourself staring during your yoga

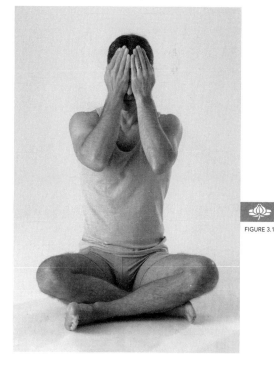

FIGURE 3.1

practice or at any other time, simply try to soften your focus. Tune in to any tension in the muscles surrounding the eyes and try to let it go. The following imagery exercise is based on something I learned from B. K. S. Iyengar's son Prashant.

EXPERIENTIAL EXERCISE: EYES ON THE SIDES OF YOUR HEAD. Stand in Mountain pose (Tadasana). Balance effort with relaxation as you press your feet into the floor and lift your chest (figure 3.2). Keep your breath smooth and release any gripping in your shoulders and neck. Look straight ahead. After a few seconds, imagine that you have eyes on your temples that can see out to the sides. As you breathe, try to perceive what those eyes would be seeing. Don't pull the images toward you, just let them passively seep in. If you feel a wave of relaxation come over you with this exercise, it's likely you're holding tension in your eyes and facial muscles all day long.

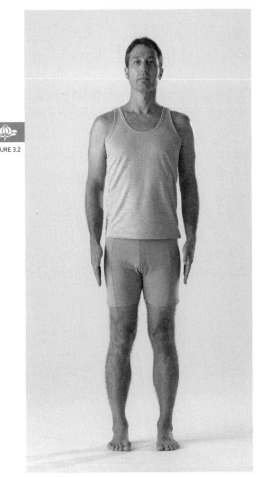

FIGURE 3.2

Yoga Practices for Stress

ASANA

The regular practice of yogic postures can be a fabulous way to lower stress when you feel overwhelmed, and as preventive medicine. Besides changing the balance of the nervous system, asana reduces muscle tension. From a yogic perspective, stress can cause muscle spasms and the reverse is also true: tight muscles can raise your stress levels. Thus a varied asana program is an effective way to gradually lessen this chronic source of stress, even if some of the postures don't necessarily feel relaxing while you are doing them.

The practices that follow, on the other hand, can bring a sense of profound relaxation, sometimes almost immediately. If your nervous system is too aroused from stress or over-stimulation, however, you may not be able to settle into relaxation right away. In that case, yogic postures can be a wonderful prelude, allowing you to burn off steam, setting the stage for deep relaxation.

SAVASANA: YOGIC DEEP RELAXATION

Savasana, Sanskrit for Corpse pose, is sometimes called Deep Relaxation (figure 3.3). It's typically the last posture of a yoga class. While it looks easy, yogis insist Savasana is the most difficult pose to do well—and the most impor-tant. Savasana is nothing like taking a nap or lying around on the couch. Those activities tend to bring dullness to the mind,

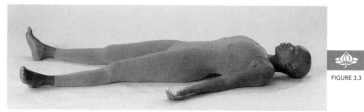

FIGURE 3.3

what yogis refer to as a tamasic state. In Savasana, you are not spacing out, you are tuning in with evermore subtlety to what is going on. This is a sattvic, or clear, state of mind. As Swami Vivekananda put it, "A fool enters into sleep and comes out as a fool while a fool enters into samadhi and comes out as a wise man. One is unconsciousness and the other is super-consciousness."

CAUTION The position of the head is crucial in Savasana and other relaxing poses. If your chin is ele-vated relative to the forehead (see figure 3.4a), the position tends to be stimulating. If your chin is even with the forehead or slightly lower, it's easier to relax.

a) The position of the chin is higher than the forehead, undermining some of the relaxing effects of Savasana.
b) In order to correct the problem, it may be necessary to elevate the head with a pillow or folded blanket.

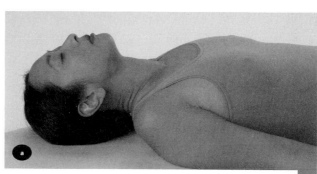

FIGURE 3.4

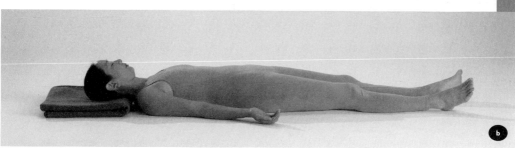

EXPERIENTIAL EXERCISE: RELAXATION (Savasana). Lie flat on your back. Allow your arms and legs to gently splay out from your body symmetrically. Let your palms face the ceiling and your feet roll out to the sides. If you have any back discomfort, bend your knees and place a blanket or pillow under them. (If you are pregnant and beyond the first trimester, please see p. 101 for advice on how to modify the pose.) After thirty seconds or so, make any final adjustments you need to be comfortable; after that try to stay absolutely motionless, as any movement can interfere with deep relaxation. Allow your eyes to gently close. Imagine that your body is getting heavier, sinking more deeply into the floor. Feel the heaviness of your hip bones, the backs of your heels, and your shoulders. Imagine that the surface below you is made of soft rubber and that at all points of contact your body is actually sinking an inch or two into the floor. Try to relax your jaw completely so there is a slight space between your upper and lower teeth. Your tongue, where most people unknowingly hold a lot of tension, should completely relax, to its root. When the tongue is tense it bunches up. Allow your tongue to feel as flat as a dog's, so that there is a feeling of space between the bottom and top of your mouth. Because old habits die hard, it's useful to return your awareness to your tongue again and again during the course of relaxation to see whether you've gone back to tensing up. See, too, if letting go in your tongue helps you relax your throat, and whether that in turn helps you find any release in the chest. Stay in the pose for five to fifteen minutes (the longer, the more beneficial). As you relax into the posture try to simply notice your breath. Don't try to control it, just follow it in your mind. If you can learn to let go, you may discover that your breath becomes a little shallower as you ease into relaxation. It will still be regular but not as deep as when you first began. Ideally, you should not fall asleep in Relaxation pose. The goal is a state of relaxed

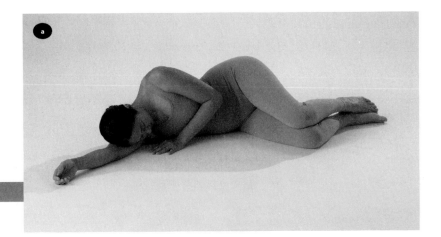

FIGURE 3.5

awareness. If you do fall asleep, it's a sign you are sleep deprived. Sleeping in Relaxation pose isn't yoga but the sleep may be useful.

If the room is at all cool, be sure to dress warmly or cover yourself with a blanket. When you relax deeply, your body temperature tends to drop slightly. Feeling cold, however, can activate the SNS, which constricts the arteries in the feet and hands to retain body heat, but also counteracts the mental relaxation you're looking for.

How you come out of Relaxation pose is crucial. Despite being instructed to the contrary, many students abruptly sit up as soon as the teacher says come out of the pose. Doing so can negate some of the benefits. If you've just spent fifteen minutes coaxing your nervous system into a state of relaxation, coming out abruptly can give you a jolt of adrenaline, leaving you considerably less relaxed. The proper technique involves bending the knees toward your chest, then rolling onto your right side (figure 3.5a). If possible, keep your eyes closed at this stage, as it tends to keep your senses directed inward. Stay on your side for a minute or so, and when ready, use your arms—not the muscles of your back—to slowly push yourself to a sitting position, bringing your head up last (figure 3.5b).

If Savasana is hard for you, be patient. Even relaxation expert Judith Hanson Lasater admits, "I couldn't do Savasana at first." She finally figured out that Savasana is not something you do. "It's a *noticing* practice," an exercise in mindfulness. You notice your hand is tense, your jaw, your belly, "and then, as you become aware of it, of course, it dissipates."

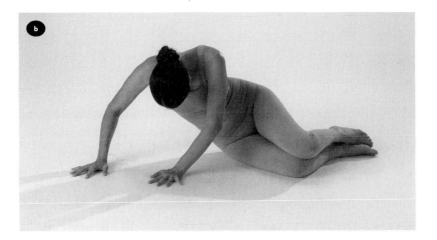

LEFT/RIGHT BREATHING

Using their heightened awareness, ancient yogis detected what scientists now refer to as the nasal cycle. Humans (and other animals) cycle alternately from breathing through one nostril to breathing through the other, for periods ranging from a few minutes to a few hours. This pattern continues even during sleep. In one area of investigation, yogis compared the effects of left-nostril breathing, right-nostril breathing, and breathing through both simultaneously. One reason for turning to the right as you come out of Savasana is that lying on your right side promotes breathing through the left nostril, which encourages relaxation.

According to ancient yogic teachings, the left nostril is connected to ida, a hypothesized energy pathway, or nadi, which travels alongside the spine, and is cooling, restorative, and feminine in nature. It more or less corresponds to yin in traditional Chinese medicine. The right nostril is governed by pingala, a complementary nadi, which is warming, energizing, and masculine, roughly equivalent to yang. More and more scientific research is supporting the notion that breathing through different nostrils has very different effects on the body.

RIGHT-NOSTRIL BREATHING	LEFT-NOSTRIL BREATHING
Stimulates Sympathetic Nervous System (Fight or Flight)	Stimulates Parasympathetic Nervous System (Relaxation Response)
Stimulates Left Hemisphere of Brain	Stimulates Right Hemisphere of Brain
Increases Verbal Performance	Increases Spatial Performance
Increases Blood Sugar Levels	Lowers Blood Sugar Levels
Increases Rate of Blinking	Reduces Rate of Blinking
Decreases Intraocular (Eye) Pressure	Increases Intraocular Pressure
Increases Heart Rate	Decreases Heart Rate
Inflates Right Lung Preferentially	Inflates Left Lung Preferentially

A yogic practice that is believed to balance the sympathetic and parasympathetic branches of the autonomic nervous system is Nadi Shodhana, alternate nostril breathing—out and then in through one nostril, then out and in through the other, repeating this pattern for the duration of the practice (see p. 287). Masters believe that during meditation the breath should flow evenly through the two nostrils, and Nadi Shodhana, because of its balancing effects, is considered the perfect prelude to meditation.

RESTORATIVE YOGA: SUPPORTED SAVASANA

A number of restorative yoga postures invented by B. K. S. Iyengar are among the most powerful and effective ways to relax. You position your body in a yoga pose but various props, such as bolsters, blankets, blocks, and straps, do most of the work for you. Your job is to simply settle into the pose, draw your senses inward, and, as always in yoga, keep your focus clear but soft.

Judith Hanson Lasater became a specialist in restorative yoga after suffering a personal tragedy that left her unable to do her normal yoga practice. She had learned supported poses working with Iyengar and used to teach them. "Then my twin brother got very sick, and eventually died. During that whole year period I was so distraught, all I did was restorative."

Even the pose Savasana can be done in a more supported fashion by lying back over a bolster (figure 3.6). By letting the prop hold you in the posture, the rib cage expands naturally. You tend to breathe more deeply, slowly, and regularly. Yogis find the pose to be energizing, due to the effects of the slight backbend, but also restful, since you're lying down and it requires so little effort to stay in the pose.

Some people who are too sick to do regular asana can do restorative postures. If you are bedridden, rather than just lie there, why not prop yourself into a supported Savasana or other pose once or twice a day? I highly recommend that anyone with chronic disease incorporate it into their treatment plan, no matter what other measures or other style of yoga they are practicing.

Supported Savasana

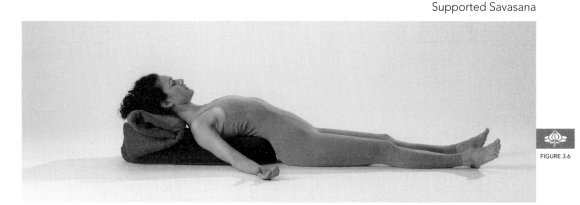

FIGURE 3.6

Although you can improvise with pillows and blankets at home, I think anyone with a serious medical condition should consider buying a few high-quality props for restorative yoga. One I particularly recommend is a cylindrical bolster like the one shown in Supported Savasana. I prefer ones that have a firm stuffing such as cotton batting as opposed to those filled with foam. The number of uses you will find for this prop is amazing.

RESTORATIVE YOGA: LEGS-UP-THE-WALL POSE (VIPARITA KARANI)

One of my favorite restorative poses is Viparita Karani, also sometimes called "Legs-Up-the-Wall," which elicits the relaxation response, a form of resting while you are awake, that is a different physiological state from sleep. If you feel tired in the afternoon, try this pose. Viparita Karani and other restorative poses generally won't leave you feeling groggy and won't interfere with falling asleep at night (unless you fall asleep in the pose) which naps unfortunately can do. Legs-Up-the-Wall can be done with the hips on the floor, but for an even greater effect, try the Iyengar practice of elevating the pelvis on a bolster or a stack of folded blankets.

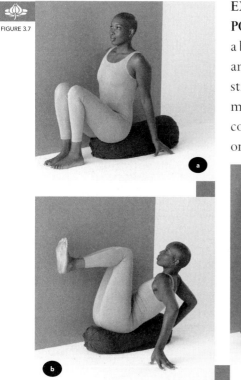

FIGURE 3.7

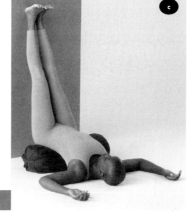

How to Get into Supported Viparita Karani

EXPERIENTIAL EXERCISE: LEGS-UP-THE-WALL POSE (Viparita Karani). Set up for the pose by placing a bolster or a stack of folded blankets parallel to the wall and approximately six inches away from it (if your hamstring muscles at the backs of your thighs are tight, you may need to move the prop farther from the wall). To come into the pose, sidle up to a wall and sit on and to one side of the bolster or blankets (figure 3.7a). Place your hands on either side of the bolster and swing your legs up the wall (figure 3.7b). If you are on a bolster, your tailbone should rest just over the front edge of the bolster so that your sacrum, the triangular bone at the base of your spine, angles down toward the floor. This maintains the normal inward curve in your lower spine and makes the pose more relaxing. Place your arms in "cactus" position as show in figure 3.7c, or palms up alongside you, as in Savasana. Rest in this pose for five to fifteen minutes. If you start to lose circulation to your feet, come down earlier or simply cross your legs, keeping your hips where they are. To come down from the bolster, bend your knees and use your feet to push off the wall to bring your buttocks to the floor in front of the bolster. From there, use your arms to help you sit up.

A SEQUENCE OF RESTORATIVE POSES
WITH CUMULATIVE EFFECTS

As powerful as individual poses are, the cumulative effects of doing a well-designed sequence of these postures can be even more profound. This restorative sequence was designed by Patricia Walden. In Supported Downward-Facing Dog pose (Adho Mukha Svanasana) and in Half-Standing Forward Bend (Ardha Uttanasana), the head is supported to increase the calming effect. In Supported Bridge pose (Setu Bandha) and Legs-Up-the-Wall pose (Viparita Karani), Patricia recommends belting the thighs with a yoga strap for added relaxation (not shown). Similarly, the strap looped around the legs, and the yoga blocks or folded blankets placed under the thighs in Supine Cobbler's pose (Supta Baddha Konasana) allow the hips to release tension.

a) Supported Dog pose (Adho Mukha Svanasana)

b) Supported Half-Standing Forward Bend (Ardha Uttanasana)

c) Supine Cobbler's pose (Supta Baddha Konasana)

d) Supine Cross-Legged pose (Supta Svastikasana)

e) Supported Bridge pose (Setu Bandha)

f) Legs-Up-the-Wall pose (Viparita Karani)

g) Relaxation pose (Savasana)

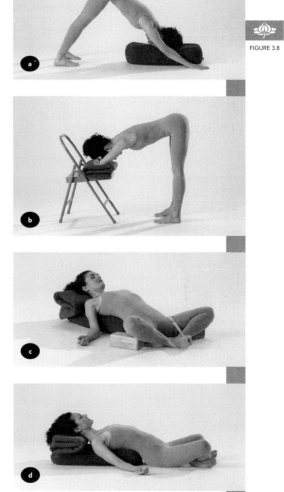

FIGURE 3.8

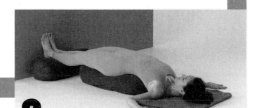

FIGURE 3.9

If time allows, Patricia suggests adding two variations to Legs-Up-the-Wall pose for even deeper relaxation. After lying with your legs up the wall for five minutes, unbuckle your belt, and leaving your hips on the bolster, cross your legs against the wall (figure 3.9a) as if you were in a seated position. After a minute or two, switch the cross of your legs and stay there an equal amount of time. Then uncross your legs, and push your feet into the wall to shimmy your buttocks just over the edge of the bolster and onto the floor. From that position, cross your legs and rest them on the bolster (figure 3.9b), stay a while, then cross your legs the other way. This sequence is known as Viparita Karani with cycle.

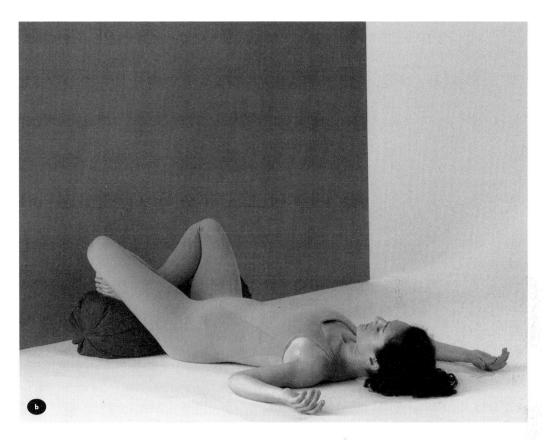

(b)

If you do this or another restorative sequence, try to maintain any calmness you achieved in one pose during the transition to the next. At first you may only want to stay a minute or two in each pose, gradually building up to as much as fifteen minutes in subsequent sessions. Some people buy timers so that they know when to move to the next pose. If you do this be sure to get one with an alarm that won't be jarring (which could potentially undo some of the restorative benefits).

YOGA NIDRA

Yoga Nidra, Sanskrit for yogic sleep, is an intricate form of guided relaxation, taking you on a journey through dozens of different visualizations, normally while you lie in Savasana. A teacher or a recorded voice guides you through the practice, which can run anywhere from a few minutes to more than three-quarters of an hour. Because you attend to the voice and bring attention to the different areas of the body and different images as you're directed, your mind stays occupied. This is a particular advantage for people who tend to brood or get anxious if they try to relax without guidance. Since Yoga Nidra requires very little effort, it is a practice that is suitable for almost anyone, including those who are seriously ill and who may not have the energy for asana or even seated meditation.

Yoga Nidra, Rod Stryker says, gives the benefits of the deepest sleep without the dullness of being unconscious. A lot of what most people think of as relaxation, he says, is only partial. Yoga Nidra involves not just relaxing the body and mind, but also the nervous system and the subconscious mind in a systematic fashion. "Different tools were developed over the millennia for achieving this state," according to Rod, "and what we have today is a compilation of the different types of techniques that have been used." Rod is currently involved in two research projects in which scientists are evaluating the healing potential of the practice. The best way to do Yoga Nidra is in a class setting or at home along with one of the several CDs available (see appendix 2).

MEDITATION

In many forms of meditation, you attempt to fix your concentration on one thing, what the yogis call one-pointed attention. The thing you concentrate on could be your breath, a sound or a phrase (mantra), a candle, a geometric design (yantra), an image of a deity or guru, or of a light emanating from the center of your body. Simply choose something that has a resonance for you and try to stick with it throughout a sitting. Flitting back and forth between different focal points is less likely to result in a meditative state.

A big obstacle to meditation is that many people feel intimidated by the concept of meditation or what they consider their failed attempts to do it. Their minds are so busy that they conclude they are wasting their time. In fact, tuning in to the fluctuations of the mind is the first step toward actually meditating, and can be a form of meditation itself, as in mindfulness practice. Remember that from a yogic perspective, to effect change you first need to see clearly what is. And for most people, what is, is that they can't fix their attention on any one thing for more than a few seconds. Thoughts butt in like intrusive neighbors. But that's how everyone feels at first, and even experienced meditators find their minds wandering again and again.

Part of learning to meditate is to notice all the judging in your mind. *I'm no good at this. This isn't working. I can't meditate.* Those are all just fluctuations of the mind, the chatter that keeps you away from direct experience. If it's cropping up in your meditation practice, it's undoubtedly happening in the rest of your life, and recognizing that is one of the fruits of the practice. Meditation is like playing a musical instrument. If you spend your whole time on the violin thinking about how lousy you are, your experience will be torturous. Your internal monologue will distract you from what's actually going on and you will miss the opportunity to really hear what you are doing. But play your scales over and over in spite of your doubts and you may discover an ease coming to your practice that had formerly eluded you.

Studies suggest that many of the physiologic benefits of meditation—lowering blood pressure, heart rate, stress hormone levels, and the like—accrue even to those who don't think they are doing it well. In his research, Jon Kabat-Zinn has found that a program which includes mindfulness meditation along with some asanas seems to help people independent of their medical or psychiatric diagnosis. "We work with people with a wide range of different kinds of conditions, all mixed up in the same room," he says. "Whether it's headaches, or high blood pressure, or irritable bowel syndrome, or trying to get back in shape after coronary bypass surgery, or cancers, many different kinds of cancers, the mind-body response is—in terms of symptom reduction, in terms of attitudinal change—the same."

Here's an ancient meditation technique based on the sound of the breath. To yogis the breath itself can be a mantra. They hear in the in breath the sound *so* and in the out breath *ham,* pronounced hum. In Sanskrit, the words *so ham* mean "I am that," reminding them of their connection via the breath to the entire universe.

EXPERIENTIAL EXERCISE: SO HAM MEDITATION. Sit in a comfortable upright position or, if necessary, lie down. Close your eyes and start to tune in to the sound of your breath. Imagine that the in breath makes the sound *so* and that the out breath makes the sound *hum*. As the breath comes into your nose, hear in your mind *soooooo* for the entire duration of the inhalation, and *hummmmmm* for the entire exhalation. If your attention wavers, don't judge yourself but simply return your focus to the sound of the breath. To deepen the practice, you could also try to maintain your internal focus at the third eye, located in the middle of the brain behind the spot on the forehead where many Indian women place a decorative bindi. Stay for five minutes or longer (any amount is good but many yogis believe that the deeper benefits of the practice come with daily sessions of at least twenty minutes).

Meditation may seem like work at first and not as relaxing as many of the other practices mentioned in this chapter. But if you stick with it and practice—even if you have doubts and even when you don't feel like it—over the long run, meditation can be the most powerful stress-reduction technique of all. Shanti Shanti Kaur Khalsa points out that there is a "difference between the sensations you have during something and the outcome. You can not enjoy meditation but be transformed by it." Or, as most people who hang in eventually discover, you can be transformed by meditation *and* enjoy it immensely. And if you believe the ancient sages, meditation is the key to transformation.

Making Time to Relax

Some readers, particularly those from the United States—the most overworked nation in the world—may say, "That's all well and good but where am I supposed to find the time to relax?" The only way it will happen is if you make it a priority. In the last thirty years, US productivity has doubled. Part of that has come from the almost two hundred additional hours the average person now works annually. Unless individuals and society are willing to examine some of the assumptions that foster this inherently stress-provoking way of life, they are unlikely to solve their problems with stress and stress-related disease. It requires tapas—yogic discipline—to schedule and make time for relaxation, especially if your samskara, your habit, is to always do more and go faster.

Periodically getting away from it all is another vitally important way to cut stress that's too often neglected. Many Westerners, including more Europeans of late, rarely if ever take vacations. If they do, they bring along work, cell phones, and laptops that ensure they can't really let go. Although it's not one of the commonly cited risk factors for heart attack, failing to take vacations may be more dangerous than smoking or high cholesterol. In the famous Framingham Heart Study, women who skipped vacations for six years in a row were eight to sixteen times more likely to develop heart disease. Add yoga to your vacations, of course, and you'd only increase the benefit.

Making time for relaxation could be as simple as fitting it into the cracks in your day or substituting one habit for another. Could you lie for five to fifteen minutes in Savasana once a day rather than watching TV, reading the paper, or talking on the phone? Could you close the door to your office and put your legs up the wall when you feel sleepy in the afternoon instead of taking a coffee break? Nischala Joy Devi says a few minutes of deep relaxation a day can remind you that even when you're busy on the outside, there's a quiet place within. Do the practice as if your life depends on it, she tells her students, "because it does."

BRINGING A YOGIC PERSPECTIVE TO YOUR HEALTH CARE

The part can never be well unless the whole is well.

—PLATO

Yoga usually gets lumped into the world of "complementary and alternative medicine," but the boundary between alternative medicine and conventional medicine is an artificial one; there are practices which could fall on either side of the line. Historical flukes and the politicization of science and medicine have trumped merit in determining which kinds of health care were accepted into the mainstream and which were relegated to alternative status. So using thyroid hormone pills, an exact chemical replica of naturally occurring human hormone, is conventional medicine, but supplementing with melatonin, another human hormone, is alternative. If a chiropractor adjusts your back, that's alternative, but if an osteopath does it, it's conventional. At one point, homeopathy was considered part of conventional medicine, but the medical establishment has had a change of heart about that one.

A much more valuable distinction is between holism and reductionism. The reductionist approach tries to reduce the complexity of illness to one factor, and then tries to attack it with a "magic bullet"—drugs or surgery. It could also be an herbal remedy, because magic-bullet thinking is prevalent in both alternative and conventional medicine. A common example of reductionism is the conventional approach to heart disease, which at its worst reduces this enormously complex field to little more than "take this drug to lower your cholesterol." When the magic bullets are strong enough, you're not required to consider the ways that your diet, your exercise habits, your stress levels, and other factors may be contributing to your health problems.

In contrast, holism involves looking at all sides of a problem, and trying to intervene at as many points as possible and as gently as possible. Viewed holistically, almost all problems are multifactorial. A truly holistic approach looks at all the different systems of the body and tries to optimize them, using whatever combination of measures is most likely to be effective and safe. Some MDs, of course, take a more holistic approach than others.

Also, be aware that many therapies categorized as alternative are reductionist, not holistic measures. The alternative remedy for heart disease, chelation therapy, in which a synthetic chemical is infused into a vein, may or may not be effective, but there's nothing holistic about it. Similarly, when vitamins are taken in megadoses, they are really functioning as drugs. Taking something from nature, isolating one component, and concentrating it is reductionism. Some herbal extracts, in which one component of the herb has been isolated, aren't exactly herbs anymore. They're more like drugs, even if they're derived from natural sources. A whole herb (and some less concentrated extracts), on the other hand, tends to contain hundreds of different chemicals which work together synergistically, making it a more holistic remedy.

I'm not saying you should never use reductionist therapies. They are valuable tools in the right circumstances, and can be used, selectively, as part of an overall holistic approach. Just understand that they tend to have a higher risk of side effects than more holistic measures (not that the latter are risk-free by any means). Similarly, if you are favorably disposed toward alternative medicine, don't let that allow you to ignore the risks of reductionist tools that happen to have been labeled alternative.

The following table contrasts the generally reductionist strategies found in conventional medicine with yoga's holistic approach.

TABLE 4.1

SOME DIFFERENCES BETWEEN THERAPEUTIC YOGA AND CONVENTIONAL MEDICINE

CONVENTIONAL MEDICAL APPROACH	YOGA AS MEDICINE APPROACH
Reductionist	Holistic
Faster in onset	Slower in onset
Effects tend to wane over time	Effects tend to increase over time
Best at dealing with acute problems (accidents, emergencies)	Less good at dealing with acute problems

Less good at dealing with chronic problems (diabetes, arthritis)	Very good at dealing with chronic problems
Less good at dealing with psychosomatic illness (stress, irritable bowel syndrome, headaches, etc.)	Excellent at dealing with psychosomatic illness
Good at dealing with pain (at least in theory) but poor with suffering	Can help with pain and excellent at dealing with suffering
Therapies usually rely on one major mechanism of action	Therapies rely on many simultaneous mechanisms of action
Treatments standardized	Treatments tailored to the individual
Often ignores possible healing synergies	Relies on additive and multiplying effects of multiple interventions
Side effects usually negative	Side effects often positive
Doctor controlled	Patient controlled
Patient is mostly the passive recipient of therapy. Patient can be unconscious.	Patient actively does the treatment (with some guidance). Consciousness required
Usually little learning involved	Involves learning
High-tech	Low-tech
Many treatments must be given in hospital or clinic	Treatments can be done at home
Disdains anecdotal evidence	Relies on direct experience of patient
Relies on diagnostic tests over direct exam of the patient	Relies on direct observation of the patient
Expensive and may require continued expenditure over time	Inexpensive; once you learn yoga and buy props, it's free unless you decide to study more
Minor emphasis on prevention	Major emphasis on prevention
The absence of symptoms or signs of disease, and normal lab tests are equated with health	Health is defined as a high level of physical, emotional, and spiritual well-being

TIP One reason yoga is such a powerful force to improve health is that *you* do it. Others may help you get there but you need to do the work, or nothing happens. Good holistic healers, whether alternative or conventional, actively involve patients in their own care. In addition to any treatments they administer, they're likely to suggest measures like yoga, walking, meditation, dietary changes, or writing your feelings in a journal. These measures can empower you in ways that passively receiving drugs and surgery do not. I am absolutely convinced that taking an active part in your own care not only improves how you feel, it improves your chances of recovering.

HOLISM IN ACTION: DOLORES

In chapter 1, I told the story of Dolores, who used yoga, traditional Chinese medicine (TCM) including herbs and acupuncture, and her Christian faith to help her cope with an HIV infection. Different parts of her regimen strengthened her physical body, reduced her level of stress, met her emotional and spiritual needs, and helped mitigate the attack on her immune system by the virus.

When we first met, Dolores had been off all conventional medications for more than a year and was feeling well. Meanwhile her doctors were monitoring her T-cell count—a measure of immune function—as well as the amount of HIV in her blood. Eventually, they found that her T-cell level began dropping from normal to just slightly below that—though not yet dangerously low—and that her HIV level simultaneously began to creep up. At her doctor's suggestion, she went back on medication, taking some of the newer drugs that have been developed in recent years.

Dolores had initially stopped the medication because she developed a common side effect of the powerful drugs used to fight HIV, a fat distribution problem. She began to notice that she was losing a little fat on her face, knees, and elbows. She was sure it was because of her medication. Her doctors assured her she looked fine. "No I don't," she told them. "I can tell the difference in my body." She went off her meds with her MDs' approval for a total of a year and a half and there was no more progression of her fat maldistribution problem. Now she takes three different drugs. So far she is tolerating them well; the new drugs appear to have fewer side effects than the old ones. Her T-cell count has bounced back up and the amount of HIV in her blood is again below detectable levels.

In addition to going back on medication, however, Dolores has continued to explore other avenues to health and healing. Yoga has had a major impact on how she eats. While most Westerners probably don't consider diet a part of yoga, yogis view it as essential. Their intensive self-study allows them to feel the impact of the food they eat on their state of mind as well as the quality of their practice. "When you start to open up all those channels inside," Dolores says, you start to realize the connection between what you eat and how you feel. Growing up, Dolores never thought about healthy eating. Now, she says, "I'm not a vegetarian or a total health nut but I do watch what I eat." Whenever she can, she chooses organic.

In addition to taking care of herself, Dolores strives to care for others. Service, what yogis call *karma yoga,* is a big part of Dolores's spiritual path. Working with her church, she has been instrumental in setting up a literacy project for adults in the community. She says, "You've got to be able to share and give back." Recently, Dolores has started to attend night school, as part of her desire to leave her job in the corporate world so that she can become a teacher. This change reflects the process that yogis call finding your *dharma,* your life purpose or work (in the broadest sense). Many people discover that when they begin to quiet their minds, they have more access to their intuition, their inner wisdom. "It opened up my creativity more, it opened up awareness, leading me to do what I'm supposed to be doing here. I want to teach, and share, and continue to help where I can."

Yogic Tool: **BHAKTI YOGA.** Bhakti, or devotion, is considered one of the major paths in yoga. Repeated studies have found that people who are religious are healthier. The combination of meditation and prayer, Dolores says, has been a key to her healing. Even though her prayer is based on her Christian faith, this kind of devotional practice is entirely consistent with Bhakti yoga. Her religious faith has also become a major source of community in her life, what yogis call sangha. "I've found a church that I absolutely love," Dolores recounts, "and I've been a member for almost two years. It's a small, old church with a great pastor. I feel like I found my home, spiritually."

A YOGIC APPROACH TO HEALTH CARE

If you think about it, Dolores's approach to her health is profoundly yogic. Like the Tantric masters of old, she has embraced any tool which might help her. Unlike people who are turned off by the excesses of modern medicine and shun it entirely, she knows that it has made major breakthroughs in understanding how the body works—and, specific to her case, how the AIDS virus can be controlled. Even during the year and a half that Dolores wasn't taking any drugs for her HIV, she was still being monitored by her physicians, and when it seemed appropriate, she agreed to go back on drug therapy. But Dolores has not limited herself to conventional medicine. She found help in acupuncture, Chinese herbs, psychotherapy, and a number of yogic tools including asana, meditation, service, and prayer. She simultaneously took steps to improve her body, her mind, her emotions, and her spirit. She also used her ability to tune in to her body to detect a serious medication side effect before much damage was done. Both that ability and the confidence to assert herself when her doctor initially dismissed her complaint are an outgrowth of her yoga practice.

Dolores has taken a holistic approach to her health, which teaches that you treat a problem by dealing with every factor that might be affecting it. Some conventional doctors may doubt that you could relieve low-back pain by working on your emotional well-being, but once you see clearly—in a way that the practice of yoga facilitates—it becomes obvious. Thus the path of yogic healing involves invoking as many discrete mechanisms as you can to try to effect change in the whole.

BRINGING YOGIC AWARENESS TO HEALTH CARE DECISIONS

Using their finely developed internal awareness, ancient yogis discovered a number of extraordinary things. An advanced practitioner like Swami Rama (see chapter 2) spent decades honing his ability to perceive internal states, much the same way a concert violinist perfects his or her ability to hear and produce fine nuances of sound. Before he could begin to control something like his heartbeat or brain waves, he needed to be able to accurately perceive what was going on inside. If Swami Rama found that a practice or a food had a certain effect, that's more than just idle speculation; it's as if Yo-Yo Ma perceives that his cello is out of tune. The insights of yoga come from masters of such rarified perceptive abilities.

Yoga teaches that the more you cultivate your awareness of your body in your yoga practice, the more you come to trust your perceptions. You'll begin to tune in to feedback from your body on any number of matters related to your health and well-being. You may notice, for example, that trying to unwind by watching television leaves you more restless and depressed, but a walk in your neighborhood leaves you feeling both relaxed and energized. With this information, you might make a different choice in the future. You can also use your heightened awareness to decide which foods to eat and which to avoid, which yoga postures and other practices agree with you, which drugs and herbs to take, which forms of bodywork you use, even which friends you spend time with.

Say, for example, that you think nightshade vegetables like eggplants and tomatoes might be exacerbating your arthritis symptoms, or that dairy products are leading to a buildup of mucus, two ideas generally dismissed by conventional medicine. Rather than say "there's no evidence for that," the yogic approach would be to conduct a little experiment and come to your own conclusion. Cut out the food for a couple of weeks and notice the effect. Then reintroduce it and see how you feel. If your experience tells you that you felt better without the food, that's an important piece of information. If you repeat the experiment and get the same results, the case against the food in question gets even stronger.

You can assert more control over your health care by using your yogic awareness to help monitor the course of your medical conditions. I suggest keeping a diary of your symptoms and the factors that might affect them. In a host of conditions from migraines to asthma, what you eat, how much exercise you get, how much stress you are under, and how well you sleep can affect your symptoms. Writing brief notes in your journal helps facilitate self-study, svadhyaya. See if you can make correlations between your symptoms and whatever else is happening in your life. If there are parameters you can measure, like your blood pressure, your blood sugar if you have diabetes, or your peak flow rates in asthma, I recommend checking them regularly and writing them down, too, to give you more information for analysis. Be sure to look back periodically at what you've written. You may be able to detect trends that affect future decisions.

AHIMSA IN HEALTH CARE

Ahimsa, the principle of nonharming, forms the foundation of yoga and is also fundamental to a yogic approach to health care. You might think that you would always want the most powerful treatment for any condition you have, but often that's not a good idea. A better treatment balances likely benefits with the risk of side effects. Less powerful treatments are often the best place to start if they have a track record of safety. OxyContin may be a powerful pain reliever but it's generally not the right drug for a headache. You don't want to ring a doorbell with a sledgehammer.

One major advantage of traditional medical systems like Ayurveda (see p. 82), Tibetan, Japanese, and Chinese medicine is that in the hands of skilled practitioners they are both effective and generally extremely safe (though simply taking isolated remedies from these systems without expert guidance can be risky). Another selling point for traditional systems like Ayurveda and traditional Chinese medicine is that they can detect and treat imbalances in the preclinical phase, that is, before a specific disease can be diagnosed by Western doctors. These systems can also help people whose symptoms don't match any known medical disorder. Finally, treating imbalances may improve other symptoms beyond those for which you are seeking care.

Newer healing approaches that appear to be extremely safe include homeopathy and energetic work such as Reiki and therapeutic touch. Though still hotly debated, these methods do have some support for their effectiveness in research, as well as many anecdotal reports. As long as they are safe, it can even make sense to use therapies with absolutely no scientific evidence of efficacy. Many doctors make the logical error of rejecting tools for which scientific proof is lacking even though they might work and appear to be safe. This is especially unfortunate considering that many safe alternative therapies that many people find effective simply have never been studied.

I believe that one of modern medicine's biggest blind spots is bodywork, including various styles of massage therapy, shiatsu (Japanese acupressure), myofascial release, Rolfing, Trager work, Thai yoga massage, reflexology, and craniosacral therapy. Ayurveda, too, has its own very rich tradition of massage and other bodywork techniques, but most Western physicians know nothing about it. While not bodywork per se, the Alexander Technique and the Feldenkrais method are two additional approaches that appear to have powerful healing potential. Although there isn't a lot of scientific support for most forms of bodywork, I have found several varieties extremely helpful in my own case and hear similar reports regularly. Some doctors reject various forms of bodywork such as reflexology because the explanations proponents give don't sound logical—a mistake I used to make myself. What I didn't understand is that people may be completely off-base in their explanations of how something works and yet be absolutely correct in their perception that it does. Since there are hundreds of different bodywork techniques and very little research under way, if you wait for scientific evidence before trying it, you probably won't be using this array of powerful therapeutic modalities in this lifetime.

My experience is that there are synergistic benefits to supplementing yoga with different types of bodywork. The proprioceptive abilities—your ability to feel what's happening in your body—that you gain from steady yoga practice can help you go deeper into the experience of what the practitioners are doing with their hands. The ability to feel what's happening in your body with greater-than-normal sensitivity can also let you determine whether the bodywork is having a beneficial effect. This, again, is not something that has been validated by science, but experienced yogis can feel it—and the experience is very persuasive. Once you've developed your "felt sense," you become sensitive to variations in the quality of different bodyworkers and can better appreciate how extraordinarily gifted the best ones are. The ones with really good hands get a reputation; if you ask around, you can usually find out who they are. It's an especially good idea to solicit the opinions of yogis or other people who have developed their own perceptive abilities.

YOGA AND ENVIRONMENTAL HEALTH

One of the niyamas, the second limb of yoga as outlined by Patanjali, is purity, or cleanliness. In the modern world, one of the biggest challenges to purity as it affects health has to do with environmental pollution. Since pollutants make it into the food you eat, the water you drink, and the air you breathe—and can't be avoided entirely no matter what you do or where you live—this is an issue that touches everyone. Still, awareness of the potential risks and a plan to limit exposures when possible may lessen the damage.

Evidence is accumulating that pesticides, herbicides, fungicides, and other biotoxins found in commercially raised food can endanger health. People are exposed to these chemicals not only by eating contaminated food, but by working in gardens, walking on lawns, and even breathing the air. A yogic perspective would suggest that the potential damage to human health from these contaminants has probably been grossly underestimated. Reductionist science generally only studies the effects of one thing at a time. But when assessing the effects of a single pesticide or toxin—if they are studied at all—scientists ignore the potentially crucial factor of additive and even multiplicative effects of multiple exposures to hundreds of different chemicals. When you understand the density of the interconnections among different forms of life in ecosystems, and the overlap between the biological systems of our bodies and those of the targeted pests, the idea that something strong enough to destroy pests will, somehow, have no effect on us seems far-fetched.

> **TIP** A vegetarian diet, particularly if you eat organic as much as possible, limits toxic exposure. Many pesticides, herbicides, and other toxins are concentrated as you move up the food chain: when eating meat and dairy products—high on the food chain—choose food from organically raised animals. Among fish, be aware that tuna and swordfish, big fish that eat little fish, are much likelier to have dangerously elevated levels of mercury. Little fish like sardines are safer. Vegetables, legumes, fruits, and grains are even lower on the food chain. To avoid pesticide residues in your food, it's especially important to buy organic versions of those foods most likely to be contaminated. For produce, be guided by the Environmental Working Group, which in 2003 created rankings based on US government tests. The produce with the highest levels of pesticides were peaches, strawberries, apples, spinach, nectarines, celery, pears, cherries, potatoes, and sweet bell peppers. Washing and peeling fruits and vegetables will remove some but not all toxins. Crops grown locally and eaten in season are less likely to be sprayed postharvest and thus, even if not organic, may have lower pesticide levels. Organic fruits, vegetables, and grains may also have higher vitamin and mineral levels than conventionally grown crops.

Yoga suggests that you look beyond the effect your diet has on your health and state of mind and consider its broader karmic implications. Karma sometimes gets expressed as "What goes around comes around." The Bible similarly advises that you reap what you sow. Independent of the health effects pesticides have on you, there is little doubt that these chemicals poison farm workers, pollute groundwater, and may harm other beings in complex ways that are next to impossible to fully assess. Yogic principles would thus suggest that buying organic will help make the world a better place for you and others to enjoy. Similarly, if you eat meat or dairy products, favor those from animals raised humanely.

Air pollution is another factor in health. Outdoor pollutants such as smog, ozone, and diesel exhaust have been linked to a host of health problems, but often a bigger danger is the toxic air inside your own home. The Environmental Protection Agency estimates that the levels of various pollutants indoors typically run two to five times levels outdoors—and sometimes more than a hundred times higher. This is especially disturbing since many people, especially if they are ill, spend most of their time indoors. Besides upping the risk for conditions like asthma, cancer, and heart disease, indoor air pollution can cause a range of unpleasant symptoms, including headaches, burning eyes, nausea, and fatigue. Ironically, the "tighter" newer buildings, designed to improve energy efficiency, pose the biggest problem. Reduce your risk by minimizing the use of solvents, aerosol sprays, and other chemicals in your home, and by not smoking or allowing others to smoke inside. Air filters and houseplants can remove some toxins from the air.

Yogic Tool: **NETI KRIYA.** Rinsing the nasal passages with a saline solution, an ancient yogic kriya, or cleansing technique, can be useful in lessening the impact of air pollution. (The word *kriya,* which means an action or work, has several others uses in the yoga world.) I remember that when I first saw pictures of Neti Kriya, I thought it looked weird. Now I do it every day and find it pleasant. David Rabago, MD, and colleagues from the University of Wisconsin have done several studies on Neti Kriya. They have found that many patients have initial trepidation, but if properly instructed find Neti Kriya improves the quality of their life and reduces sinus symptoms. I have nasal allergies, so it's a particularly good idea for me, but it's also potentially helpful if you've got asthma or sinus headaches. Performed using a small ceramic pot with a narrow spout (see figure 4.1), Neti Kriya may help remove some toxins before they are absorbed into your system. Rinsing your nasal passages with saline can remove pollutants, cold viruses, allergy-inducing substances like pollen, and other material that winds up in your nose. If you come down with a cold, pollen counts are high, or you live or work in a heavily polluted area, it may be wise to use your neti pot more than the customary once a day.

Here's how to perform Neti Kriya. First, prepare the saltwater solution. With either too much or too little salt in the water, the solution can be irritating to the nasal passages. Shoot for a salinity similar to that of tears. Typically that requires a quarter teaspoon of noniodized salt for every eight ounces of warm (not hot) water. Slightly higher concentrations of salt—which may be more effective at removing debris—are well tolerated if the fluid is buffered with a pinch of baking soda. With your head tipped to one side, pour the liquid from the neti pot into your upper nostril. After flowing through that nostril, the liquid exits via the lower nostril. You can do this one or more times on each side. Breathe through your mouth during the entire procedure. Afterward, gently blow your nose—or if you know Kapalabhati breathing (see chapter 16), do a few of those—to clear the excess fluid from your nasal passages. Do you notice you can breathe more freely afterward?

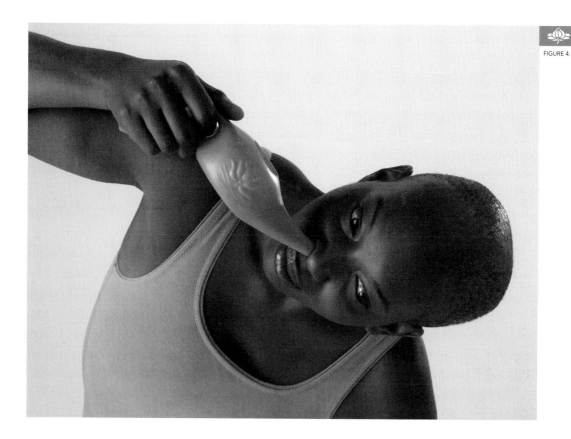

FIGURE 4.1

If you're used to meditating or doing pranayama, you might try Neti Kriya before your next session to see if it adds any subtlety to your practice.

Because repeated rinsing of the nasal passages with salt water can dry them out, Ayurvedic physician Dr. John Douillard recommends using a cotton swab to apply a small amount of warmed sesame oil, ideally organic cold-pressed, to the entrance of each nostril on a regular basis. After application, take a few quick, deep inhalations until you can taste the oil at the back of your throat. This is particularly helpful in fall and winter, when the air is dry.

CAUTION Neti Kriya may not work in people with nasal polyps or other obstructions (water can get stuck), and it could even be dangerous for those with congestive heart failure, kidney failure, or other conditions in which fluid retention is a problem, because the sodium in the saline solution could be absorbed by the body and lead to such fluid retention. For most people with high blood pressure, the small amount of salt that ends up getting absorbed into the body is probably not enough to raise the pressure much.

In ancient India, yoga wasn't even viewed as a therapeutic modality by itself. That was the province of yoga's sister science, Ayurveda. From an Ayurvedic perspective, people have different constitutions that influence the choice of treatments, including dietary approaches, herbs, various purification techniques, and such yogic practices as asana, pranayama, and meditation. Ayurvedic scholar David Frawley points out that in America, partly due to a historical fluke, yoga arrived many decades before Ayurveda did, and thus has developed its own therapeutic tradition influenced by but separated from an Ayurvedic point of view. He argues that if you are to understand what the ancient yogis thought, some knowledge of Ayurveda is essential. And as a powerful form of complementary medicine, Ayurveda also offers tools that can complement yoga therapy.

From the perspective of Ayurveda, each person has a particular constitution or prakriti, a balance of three doshas, that needs to be considered when planning a treatment (see table 4.2). The literal translation of dosha is "that which becomes unbalanced." People who are creative, in constant motion, and perhaps a bit impulsive are from an Ayurvedic perspective showing signs of vata, or air. The slang "space cadet" invokes a similar metaphor, implying a scattered focus of attention. Pittas are fiery types, prone to passion and anger and the drive to succeed. The final dosha is kapha, signifying earth and water. Kaphas tend to be strong, slow to move, and sometimes a bit lazy, though once they get going, can be very hard workers. Ayurveda sees each person as being a blend of all three doshas, though often one dosha dominates. It's also common to have two nearly equal constitutional tendencies, for example to be vata-pitta, and a few people are tridoshic with a balance of all three. Different diseases are thought to reflect certain doshas. Degenerative arthritis, for example, is considered related to vata and adult diabetes to kapha. The doshas, Ayurveda teaches, are also influenced by the climate, the season of the year, and your age.

TABLE 4.2 THE THREE AYURVEDIC CONSTITUTIONS OR DOSHAS

CONSTITUTION	CHARACTERISTICS	TYPICAL MEDICAL PROBLEMS
Vata	Move quickly, flexible, creative, distractible	Insomnia, anxiety, dry skin, constipation, osteoarthritis
Pitta	Intense, driven, passionate, intelligent, workaholic	Anger, heartburn, acne, inflammation, heart disease
Kapha	Move slowly, stable, strong, lazy, tremendous stamina	Overweight, type 2 diabetes, depression, sinus infections

Sandra Summerfield Kozak has found that your Ayurvedic constitution can help you determine which yogic practices are likely to be most helpful to you, and which ones more problematic. It is an interesting paradox that what people are drawn to—in terms of diet, lifestyle, and even the type of yoga they gravitate toward—may not be what they most need. The yogic approach for someone of vata dosha is to ground them. Using asana such as standing poses, they would be taught to sink their feet into the ground, to always balance lifting the body with downward movement. Squatting and seated poses such as forward bends and twists are also said to be beneficial for calming vata. Practices like meditation, pranayama, and very active asana practices, in which you flow quickly from pose to pose, however, can exacerbate vata tendencies, and are riskier to people who aren't yet grounded. Fiery pittas benefit from a calming and restorative yoga practice, though they may be more attracted to very vigorous and challenging types of yoga. If such a practice is not balanced with a heavy dose of relaxation, the person's fire may burn hotter: anger might flare, or their heartburn could get worse. Sandra asks both pittas and vatas to work at 75 percent of their capacity. If they are physically capable, kaphas benefit from just the kind of vigorous practices that many pittas and vatas gravitate toward. Left to their own devices, however, kaphas tend to choose a gentler practice that, while pleasant, may not challenge them in some ways they need.

Yogic dietary advice tends to be heavily influenced by Ayurveda, in which diet is a centerpiece of the therapeutic strategy. From an Ayurvedic perspective, the right foods for each constitutional type can be grouped by taste. Pittas, according to Swami Shivananda, a Dutch physicist turned yogi and Ayurvedic practitioner, should choose mostly foods with bitter, astringent, and sweet tastes. Vatas should favor foods that are sweet, salty, and sour. Ideally, kaphas should eat foods that are spicy, bitter, or astringent. Bitter foods include broccoli rabe and most leafy greens. Sour or acidic tastes include lemons, limes, yogurt, and kefir. Examples of astringent foods are asparagus, artichokes, sprouts, potatoes, and pomegranate. In Ayurveda, sweet refers to naturally sweet foods such as fruit, not refined sugars, which are frowned upon in excess. As with yoga practices, what people are drawn to may not be what's best for them. Pittas often like spicy foods, which increase their fire. Ayurveda recommends that vatas eat warm foods that are smooth in texture to calm their restless minds, but they often prefer corn chips, salads, and granola. Kaphas often love sweet and rich desserts, but these can exacerbate their tendency toward weight gain. The swami points out that you don't need to avoid less-favored foods entirely, but simply recognize that an excess could put you out of balance.

Keep in mind that although Ayurveda divides people by constitutional tendencies, it recognizes that everyone has characteristics of all three, and figuring out what's best for you is a matter of trial and error combined with careful observation. As you gain enough sensitivity to judge the effects different foods have on you, you will come to your own conclusions about which foods are best. You may also notice that over time or at different times of the year, your optimal diet may change.

THE YOGIC APPROACH TO DIET

Although people sometimes don't realize it, proper diet is an integral part of yoga. Food is your sustenance, the source of the thousands of ingredients your body needs to keep you alive and healthy, but it can also be the source of substances that may be harming you. Diet can play a huge role both in causing and perpetuating disease, as well as in helping to remedy the situation if you are already sick. Using your diet as a tool for health and healing is so consistent with the philosophy of yoga as medicine—and is stressed so much in this chapter—precisely because it's safe and effective and is something you can do for yourself.

Some of the yogic thinking on diet is based on philosophical ideas about nonviolence and compassion and, as a result, most yogis—though not all—are vegetarians. Whatever the motivation, the health advantages of a vegetarian diet include a lower risk of heart disease, type 2 diabetes, obesity, and colon cancer. Vegetarians generally have lower blood pressure and cholesterol readings as well. From a yogic perspective, food is meant to contribute to balance and a sattvic, or clear, state of mind.

From a yogic and Ayurvedic perspective, fresh food is best, because food loses prana, or life energy, when it is canned or processed (even when it is just refrigerated and reheated). The idea that fresh food is best finds support in Western science, too. Not only is the vitamin content higher, but the food tastes better. When my mother was a girl in Vermont, they'd put the water to boil on the stove before they went out to the field to pick the corn, so they could drop the corn into the water the second they got back. They could actually taste the difference in freshness if the picked corn sat while the water boiled.

Most processed food has large amounts of salt, sugar, and unhealthy fats added to it, while much of the fiber and many of the vitamins and healthy phytochemicals (plant chemicals) have been lost in manufacturing and storage. Though some of these may have been added, as you'll see on the label, what you get is not the same as eating fresh vegetables, whole grains, fruits, seeds, and nuts. These foods are brimming with natural vitamins and phytochemicals, including many that don't get added to the processed form, and many we've yet to recognize, all of which may act together synergistically.

In the modern world, it may be difficult to avoid eating canned, processed, or reheated food, but the principle holds: eat fresh food whenever possible, the fresher the better. Produce grown near where you live can be delivered faster, and is therefore preferable. Best of all (if you can't grow your own) is to buy at a farmers' market and actually meet the people who planted and nurtured the crops, or raised the animals. But also keep in mind that vegetables and fruits frozen immediately after harvest have higher vitamin content than fresh food that sits around for days.

While your focus should be on eating a diet that is high in vitamins and other natural antioxidants, there is strong evidence for the safety and effectiveness of taking a multivitamin every day (though men and postmenopausal women should avoid multivitamins that contain iron unless their iron levels are low). Some people (especially postmenopausal women) also need to take supplemental calcium to keep their bones strong, and growing evidence suggests that many people could benefit from supplemental vitamin D as well. I personally choose to take small daily doses of a few antioxidants and omega-3 fatty acids, but I've based my choices on educated guesses rather than hard science. In the real world, you often have to make decisions before much evidence is available. All you can do is learn as much as you can and make your best guess, trying to always err on the side of safety. Supplements that contain several of the related forms of a vitamin—a pill containing "mixed carotenoids," for example, instead of plain vitamin A or beta carotene—are a little more like whole food and might turn out to be more effective and less toxic.

You may have heard the saying "You are what you eat." From a yogic perspective, however, you are not just *what* you eat but *how* you eat. Yoga encourages you to be aware of every bite you put in your mouth, noticing its taste, texture, and temperature. Yogis suggest you think about where your food came from and feel gratitude toward those who grew it and prepared it (including yourself if you were the chef). To facilitate awareness and better digestion, yoga says, eat slowly in a nondistracted fashion. It is best not to read or watch television while you chew, but instead to attend to the meal in front of you. Fill your belly only to three-quarters, sit down for your meal, and don't eat on the run. The more you can make eating a form of meditation, the healthier it is likely to be. This is not always possible, but the more you can do it, the better. Such awareness tends to prevent overeating and can make a big difference in your weight (see chapter 27).

 TIP Using only asana, the most common form of yoga practiced in the West, and not other yogic tools is a bit like using only drug therapy without diet, exercise, and stress reduction to try to bring your blood pressure or cholesterol down. That said, for many Westerners, asana is a good place to start, and yoga poses all by themselves can be powerful healing tools. For those who are ready for more, however, I encourage starting basic pranayama like Bhramari and gentle Ujjayi (see pp. 16–17) and meditation immediately. Ultimately, a fully synergistic, multipronged yogic approach involving asana, pranayama, meditation, diet, philosophy, service, and other tools, is likely to take you much farther on the journey to health and healing.

What I've been talking about in this chapter might be called a Tantric approach to health care. Contrary to popular belief, Tantra is not primarily about sex. Tantric masters sought the same freedom as other yogis, but they were relentlessly pragmatic and willing to employ any tool that might help them achieve their goals, even those shunned by classical yogis. Yoga as medicine is similarly pragmatic, integrative, and willing to embrace any healing modality that is safe and might help, regardless of whether it is labeled conventional or alternative, reductionist, natural, or even unscientific and metaphysical.

Dolores adopted such an inclusive yogic approach, and it has not only bolstered her health but transformed her entire life. "It all started with yoga," she says. You could even argue that it was her journey into yoga that brought so much love into her life. Yoga teaches that you tend to attract the energy you put out, whether that's anger, negativity, and violence, or generosity, compassion, and love. That's karma again. Dolores has clearly chosen the path of love: love of God, love of her community, and love of herself, and now nearly everywhere she looks, she finds love coming back to her.

PART TWO

THE PRACTICE OF YOGA

In the beginning you have to
make room for yoga in your daily life,
and give it the place it deserves.
But after some time, yoga itself
will pull you up by the hair
and make you do it.

—VANDA SCARAVELLI

DOING YOGA SAFELY

Do not contract your brain when you stretch your body.

—B. K. S. IYENGAR

Just weeks before my first trip to India to investigate therapeutic yoga in its birthplace, I developed an unusual tingling in my right hand. After a few minutes during which I thought of scary things like a brain tumor and multiple sclerosis, I decided it was probably something a lot more common and a whole lot less serious: carpal tunnel syndrome. It turned out to be a related condition called thoracic outlet syndrome, in which nerves and blood vessels that run to the arm get compressed in the chest or the neck.

I figured that the thoracic outlet syndrome (TOS) must have been related to the asymmetry in my chest that yoga had made me aware of. Looking back, I find it fascinating that in all my years of medical training and practice, no physician had ever noticed this structural imbalance, which is completely obvious to any good yoga teacher. Over the next month, I modified my practice, avoiding poses that seemed to make it worse. By the time I left for India the symptoms had lessened, though the numbness bothered me several times during the long plane flights to Bangalore.

I quickly came to appreciate that, in a funny way, the symptoms were a gift. I had planned to visit various yoga therapy centers to observe their work. Now instead of just watching, whenever possible I would submit myself for evaluation and treatment by the various experts I'd arranged to observe. This would allow me to try their suggestions and see what worked for me. While this wasn't a controlled scientific experiment, my experience had taught me that such direct hands-on exposure can teach you things you might not otherwise understand.

One of my first surprises came in Chennai (Madras), where I spent a couple of weeks at the Krishnamacharya Yoga Mandiram (KYM), a yoga therapy center run by T. K. V. Desikachar, the son of the legendary Krishnamacharya. The teachers there told me that I should immediately stop doing Headstand, Shoulderstand, and Plow pose—poses emphasized in Iyengar yoga, which is my primary practice. In fact, I had been steadily increasing the amount of time I stayed in Headstand, and in recent months had gotten up to ten minutes a day. The teacher at the KYM said Headstand and the other asana they wanted me to stop could be causing or contributing to my problems by compressing my neck and spine, something I had not figured out on my own. To address the problem, they recommended a series of gentle backbends and other poses designed to open up my chest. A few days later, sitting in a seminar on yoga therapy, it occurred to me that for the first time in a month my arm hadn't gone numb once all day.

Looking back, I realized I never had really enjoyed Headstand, Shoulderstand, and Plow pose (see figure 5.1). Plow pose in particular made me feel claustrophobic, not a sensation I'd experienced much before. Unpleasant as I found them, I just tried to tough it out and do the poses with the rest of the class, because of the purported benefits. The claustrophobia I now believe was a clear indication that something wasn't right. Interestingly, Headstand is rarely taught by Desikachar and his followers due to safety concerns. But for many people, if it can be performed safely, Headstand can indeed be highly beneficial, which is why Krishnamacharya himself called it the king of the asanas.

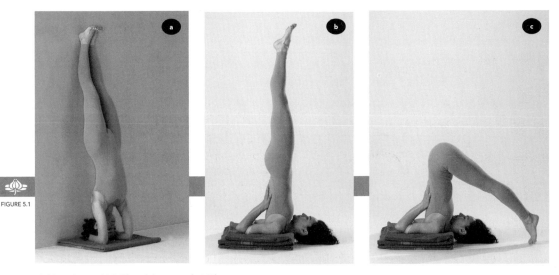

FIGURE 5.1

a) Headstand b) Shoulderstand c) Plow pose

First Do No Harm

Ahimsa, the first of Patanjali's yamas and the foundation of yoga, corresponds to the chief guiding principle of medicine as articulated by Hippocrates: *First do no harm.* In practical terms, this means that when you do yoga, always err on the side of safety. Go slowly, respect your body's limits, and listen to its innate wisdom. The more you do yoga, the more you'll have access to that intuitive sense of what's good for you and what isn't. My body, of course, had been speaking to me but I'd chosen to ignore what it was saying. It had to raise its voice, with the TOS, to get my attention.

As with any physical exercise, the practice of yoga postures is not risk free. You could strain a muscle, inflame a joint, or fall over and hurt yourself. But done carefully, yoga is one of the safest forms of physical activity you can pursue. If you follow basic precautions, get good instruction, and do your practice with awareness, the risks are small, especially compared with the potential benefits. Of course, those could be big "ifs" if you are the kind of person who gets competitive in a yoga class.

Some yogic practices are not appropriate for everybody. This is especially true for people who come to yoga because of health conditions. Various medical problems make the likelihood of injury from certain yogic practices too great. Doctors speak of such practices as being contraindicated. If you have any doubt about the appropriateness of any posture, breathing technique, or other practice, be sure to speak with both your doctor and a knowledgeable yoga teacher—and always err on the side of caution. We'll review contraindications in more detail in the chapters on the different conditions in part 3. Much of this, though, is common sense. If something hurts, don't do it. If a pose becomes uncomfortable, come out of it.

If you have health conditions or take medication that could affect your safety in a given pose, let your yoga teacher know. Approach the teacher before class, or if time or privacy is a concern, ask if you could either write or call. If you don't feel comfortable giving your

 TIP It is not uncommon when people begin to practice yoga regularly that their need for medication decreases. You need to be especially careful if you are taking drugs for high blood pressure or diabetes, because a dose that had been effective could lead to a dangerously low level of blood pressure or blood sugar. The change generally happens gradually over weeks or months, but could happen sooner if you ramp up your practice quickly. It's not advisable to stop any drug or change the dosage without speaking with your physician. But if you are alert to changes in your blood pressure or blood sugar levels, and let your doctor know about them, you can help avoid potential problems.

teacher the specifics you could say "I'm prone to dizziness from my medication so I need to come out of poses slowly," without having to reveal what the medicine is or what you're being treated for.

A big part of keeping yourself safe with yoga is tuning in to how you feel both during and after practicing. Your body might be sore, for example, the day after a strong practice. A little achiness in muscles is fine but it should quickly resolve. However, joints should never hurt more than usual either during or after practice. If they do, it's a sign that you are doing something wrong, for example with poor alignment of your bones, or doing more than you are currently ready for. Some students may feel fine physically after a practice, but may feel spaced out, or agitated and unable to sleep. This again is a sign of having overdone things and should prompt close scrutiny of your practice.

Trying Too Hard

During my stay in Pune, while studying at the Iyengar Institute, I took a class with Prashant Iyengar, son of the famous master. Prashant told us that if we looked around at the hundreds of pictures of his father that lined the studio, we would see "many poses, but one face," meaning that no matter which pose he did, his facial expression never varied. Guruji, as Prashant refers to him, always showed a kind of inner relaxation even as he performed the most difficult asana. But as Prashant scanned the room of students attempting the relatively simple posture he was teaching that day, he saw "one pose, many faces," as students grimaced and bugged their eyes out, or otherwise strained to get it right.

> **TIP** In the *Yoga Sutras*, Patanjali stresses the need in a yoga pose to balance effort (sthira) with ease (sukha), stability with relaxation. The breath is often the most reliable signal of how you are doing in this regard. At all times in your practice you ought to be able to take slow, deep, regular breaths. If you are doing more than you should, it will almost always be reflected in quick and sometimes erratic breathing. If you follow your breath closely, not only can it calm your mind, it can also keep you out of trouble.

Students often push to achieve the outward form of an asana—trying to emulate their teachers or a photo from a magazine—even when their body and breath are telling them they aren't ready yet. That is not a balanced action, not tuning in. It's imposing something from the outside. Viniyoga teacher and bodyworker Leslie Kaminoff says that achieving the so-called classical form of a posture is simply not realistic for many people. Due to anatomical variations, yoga poses readily done by some people are simply impossible for others. He says, "Some people unnecessarily torture themselves over their inability to perform certain asanas without realizing that it's something inherent in their body proportions or shape." If you have thick arms or legs, or if your limbs are short in proportion to your trunk, for example, you may never be able to clasp your hands behind your back in certain twists, or thread one leg behind the other in Eagle pose. Trying to make the impossible happen is a setup for frustration and injury. If you find yourself discouraged, that, too, offers a chance to build awareness through self-study. Why, you might ask, are you so worried about how far you go into a pose? Is it about how you look? Do you feel competitive with others? Such concerns have nothing to do with real yoga and they can undermine its healing power. Far more important than outward form, Leslie believes, is whether, as a result of your yoga, you are able to breathe more effectively or move around in a more pain-free way.

Striving to do what your body is not ready for or not anatomically equipped to perform sets you up for injury. Yoga teacher Roger Cole says that if you don't force things, you're going to prevent 99 percent of yoga injuries. For safety's sake, slow and steady should be the rule. Build up what you do over time and be patient. Even if you—or someone else—thinks you should be progressing more quickly than you are, you can only move forward when your body and breath indicate that the time is right.

Playing the Edge

Generally, in any yoga pose you are holding for more than a few seconds, you want to move into the pose until you encounter the first resistance to further motion. At that point you should stop and breathe slowly, deeply, and smoothly. After a short while, something may release, signaling that it is okay to move more deeply into the pose. This process can be repeated several times. Yogis refer to this as working or playing "the edge." The resistance to movement often comes from muscles that reflexively tighten to prevent injuries. The more quickly and forcefully you move, the more likely the muscle will contract and frustrate your efforts. It's one of your body's natural protective mechanisms. If you try to force your way through that resistance, you may tear muscle fibers. If you breathe and soften, you may find unexpected opening.

Good Pain vs. Bad Pain

In yoga, the "no pain, no gain" philosophy just doesn't cut it. If you are hurting it is a sign that you are doing something wrong, or simply doing too much. However, some yoga practices that are safe are nonetheless very intense. When the hamstrings in the back of your thigh stretch in a standing forward bend, for example, it can cause a sensation that may tempt you to come right out of the pose. Often if you back off just a little and deepen your breath, you can work to deepen the stretch and it will be safe to continue doing the pose. If, however, you noted a sharp pain in the back of the knee while doing the forward bend, that might indicate compression of the joint's internal structures, or strain on its supporting ligaments, and your best bet would be to come out right away. "Working through" any sharp or sudden pain, or any discomfort coming from a joint, is a bad idea. Leslie Kaminoff says, "If you're getting pain from within a joint structure, that's not good pain. There's nothing in there you want to be stretching or changing. Stop. Check your alignment, and try to do it in such a way that you don't get that joint pain." If that's not possible, it's an indication you shouldn't be doing the pose at all.

In general, any discomfort in yoga stretches should be mild to moderate and should be primarily located in the belly of the muscle, instead of near where the tendons attach to the bones. Since you may not know which muscles are where, much less where their tendons attach, it's best to speak with a teacher about any symptoms you're unsure of—and in the meantime to err on the side of caution. As you deepen your awareness with ongoing practice, you will increasingly be able to judge what's safe on your own.

Contrary to popular belief, people who are flexible are at the greatest risk of injury in yoga. They sometimes injure themselves by moving their joints much farther than is safe. In a backbend, for example, someone with a mobile lumbar spine may arch their lower back to an unhealthy degree while not bringing enough movement to the mid or upper back. Many flexible students also have poor body awareness; they can move, but can't assess what they are doing with any accuracy. This can contribute to dangerous misalignment of joints. Yet another risk factor is that the muscles of flexible students tend to be weak. Weak muscles don't protect joints as well and may be more susceptible to tearing. Rather than trying to go as deeply as possible into every pose, people who are highly flexible need to back off of advanced asana and instead focus on practices that build strength.

Staying Safe in a Yoga Class

Watch out for peer pressure. Nobody wants to feel like he or she can't do what everybody else is doing. While natural, such feelings have no place in yoga practice. Yoga is about tuning in to your inner landscape, not showing off or worrying what others will think. The desire to persevere with a pose that your body is indicating is not right (or not yet right) for you ought to elicit some serious self-study, svadhyaya. If you sense you are better off not doing something, share your concerns with the teacher. You can always do another pose until the rest of the group finishes. Good teachers will suggest an alternative. If the teacher doesn't want you to do a particular pose or breathing practice, that's a request that you should honor. Especially if you are new to yoga and haven't yet developed the kind of bodily awareness that comes with sustained practice, a good teacher will be better than you at judging whether a particular yoga practice is inappropriate.

While classes can be a great form of preventive medicine, many aren't appropriate for someone with a chronic illness or an acute problem. Some teachers, particularly those with many years of experience, are able to adapt what they are teaching to individuals with specific health challenges. Before assuming this is the case and just turning up at class, however, contact the teacher to find out whether the class is right for you.

> **TIP** Yoga injuries often occur during the transitions in and out of postures. It's natural to pay a lot of attention during the pose, but as soon as the teacher says to come out, to proceed in an almost unconscious way. For safety's sake, bring as much, if not more, attention to the transitions as to the poses themselves.

The Safety of Hands-On Adjustments

Yoga students are frequently injured by overly aggressive adjustments, when a teacher—usually one with insufficient experience—attempts to coax or force their body into a yoga pose. I've been hurt myself this way in classes. At greatest risk, once again, are the very flexible. You always have the right to politely refuse if you don't feel comfortable with getting an adjustment. Many teachers will say so up front.

Some adjustments are inherently more dangerous than others. Roger Cole believes that adjustments in Lotus pose (Padmasana) are a particular risk to the knees. He suggests you only allow an adjustment if you're confident that the teacher knows what she is doing. Another common source of injury he says is when "teachers 'help' people by pushing on their backs in forward bend," an adjustment Roger thinks should almost never be done. If you find yourself being adjusted in a forward bend, he suggests you quickly bend your knees, lowering the risk of injury.

The safest kind of adjustments are not really adjustments at all, but rather a laying on of the hands in order to bring the student's awareness to a particular area of the body. Tom Alden describes the first time he worked with B. K. S. Iyengar in India. Iyengar flicked his hand on Tom's outer thigh, and "His touch brought awareness, and the direction of his touch brought the direction of action. It woke up my intelligence." That's a lot different—and a lot safer—than a teacher's wrenching your body deeper into a pose.

Yoga in Hot and Humid Conditions

Partly because heat facilitates muscle relaxation as well as calming the mind and nervous system, yoga is generally done in a warm room. But some styles, most notably Bikram and various classes billed as "hot yoga," heat the room to in excess of one hundred degrees Fahrenheit (thirty-eight Celsius). Since there tend to be many bodies sweating profusely in these classes, it quickly becomes a humid room as well. While the heat and humidity may facilitate going deeper into poses, they also increase the risk of dehydration and heart attacks, and are particularly dangerous for people with MS, epilepsy, chronic fatigue syndrome, fibromyalgia, and inflammatory conditions such as lupus or Crohn's disease, as well as any pregnant woman. Heat may also increase how much ligaments stretch, and that can lead to injury. Luckily, the body acclimates to hot and humid conditions over time. This is most safely accomplished by building up slowly over a matter of several weeks. If you take a break for a month or two from practicing hot yoga, however, you may need to start the process all over again.

> **CAUTION** When it's hot and humid, it's easy to become dehydrated. To prevent this potentially very serious problem, it is necessary not only to drink plenty of fluids during a hot yoga class but also beforehand and afterward. Some hot yoga teachers do not permit students to drink water during class, an unsafe policy in my opinion. Since alcohol can lead to mild dehydration, drinking the night before can increase the risk. A persistently high heart rate is often the first sign of dehydration so you may want to monitor your pulse during and after the class. Unless you are very out of shape (in which case, you should start with a less intense style of yoga), your heart rate should drop to near normal within minutes of stopping exercise if you are getting enough fluids.

If you're fifty or older and haven't been exercising regularly, you may want to get a stress test before beginning hot yoga or any other vigorous style, since the intense workout could conceivably precipitate a heart attack. The more risk factors you have for heart disease—such as smoking, diabetes, high blood pressure, elevated cholesterol, or a strong family history of premature heart attacks—and the stronger the practice you're undertaking, the more important this becomes, and the earlier you should have it. If your practice is a gentle one like Viniyoga or Integral yoga, such testing may not be necessary. For descriptions of the intensity level of different styles of yoga, see chapter 6.

Avoiding Falls

It is possible to fall out of yoga poses, particularly out of balancing poses like Headstand or Tree pose. This is of particular concern for anyone who is frail or who has osteoporosis and could fracture a hip or other bone. People with bleeding disorders or low platelet counts and those taking blood-thinning medications (such as heparin or warfarin) should exhibit caution or avoid balancing poses entirely, as a fall could cause serious internal injuries and bleeding. And, of course, a fall can injure someone near you, too.

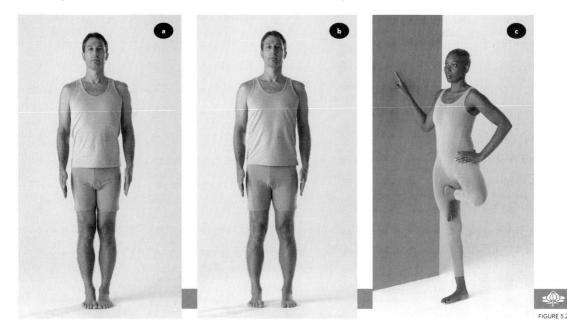

FIGURE 5.2

a) Tadasana b) Tadasana with feet hip's width apart c) Tree pose with fingers touching the wall.

Widening your stance in poses like Tadasana (figure 5.2b) can lessen the risk of a fall. Another strategy is to do balancing poses like Tree with your back close to a wall, or to lightly touch your fingers to the wall, since you can use it to regain your balance (figure 5.2c). If balance is a problem for you, most standing poses can be done in front of a wall or counter. In addition, in standing poses, you will be more stable if you learn to plant your feet squarely and distribute the weight equally between the front and back feet, and on the front, back, inside, and outside surface of the sole of each foot.

Pranayama and Meditation

From a psychological standpoint, breathing practices, done improperly, are among the riskiest yoga tools. Yoga lore includes stories of people who have suffered psychological breakdowns after pursuing vigorous breathing practices without proper supervision, particularly those who attempt to do too much too soon, though how common this is isn't known. According to Aadil Palkhivala, "Pranayama is to the nervous system what the physical asana practice is to the musculoskeletal system." Overly intense asana can damage the muscles and the bones and cartilage, he says, and too intense a pranayama practice can damage the nerves. Except for the simplest practices like basic Ujjayi and Bhramari (see chapter 1), pranayama should only be done under the guidance of an experienced teacher.

> **TIP** If you learn to pay close attention, the quality of the breath is often the best indication of whether a pranayama practice is appropriate. Specifically, pay careful attention to the very next breath after trying a practice. Say, for example, you lengthen your exhalation, which is known for its calming effects. If you end up having to gasp or strain in any way on the subsequent breath, it's a sure sign that you've been too aggressive and need to back off. The other main area of feedback is your mind. If you find yourself feeling agitated or spaced out after an exercise, something is not right. In such instances, most experts would advise you to end your practice for the day and simply relax with a good, long Savasana or other restorative practice. The next day you can try again, reducing the intensity of the practice. If you sleep poorly or feel agitated the next day, you may need to take a longer break. As always, when in doubt consult a seasoned teacher.

Like pranayama, meditation may not be appropriate (or even possible) for people who are very anxious or depressed. There are case histories of people having psychological breakdowns after intense meditation, particularly on long retreats. Anyone with clinical depression, a history of schizophrenia, or other serious psychological problems should consult a mental health professional before beginning a meditation practice. As with pranayama, some people who have difficulty with meditation due to agitation or brooding may have an easier time if they keep their eyes open. Guided meditation exercises may also be easier than self-directed efforts.

Some people who normally aren't prone to anxiety may get anxious if they try to meditate. (It's also not uncommon for students to experience a flood of emotions when in Savasana or other restorative poses, or when performing asana such as backbends, forward bends, or twists.) Meditation is a place where psychological trauma that has been walled off may be released. The results can be extremely uncomfortable, but what you learn during meditation can help you transcend painful events in your life and lead to a degree of happiness and calm you haven't felt before. If problems arise, working with a yoga teacher experienced in meditation and, if necessary, with a psychotherapist can be helpful.

Yoga During Menstruation

Most yoga teachers believe going upside down during your period is contraindicated, but many female students choose to ignore the proscription. Are they risking their health? Some teachers warn that inversion during menstruation could cause blood to leak out the fallopian tubes and result in endometriosis, a painful condition in which small clusters of uterine cells grow in the abdominal cavity. Scientific evidence suggests, however, that this so-called retrograde menstruation occurs in over 90 percent of women—most of whom never develop endometriosis. It simply isn't known if inversions increase the backward flow or the risk of endometriosis.

I believe that it may be best to refrain from inverting when flow is heavy. Aside from any other considerations, this tends to be the time when cramps are painful and energy levels are low. For most women, these symptoms occur predominantly on the first few days of the period, though it varies a lot. Brief inversions, say a minute or less, especially if done later in the period, seem less likely to cause problems than more sustained ones. One alternative to standard inversions are postures that place the head lower than the heart but which keep the pelvis level, like supported Bridge pose (figure 5.3). This pose is also restorative, and can be safely done at other times when your energy is low.

Supported Bridge pose on a bolster can provide the calming effects of Headstand and Shoulderstand without affecting menstrual flow.

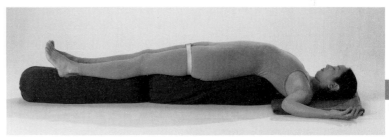

FIGURE 5.3

 TIP Perhaps even more worrisome than inverting during menstruation is insisting on maintaining a vigorous practice no matter how you feel. If you are tired and achy, your body is telling you to take it easy. My advice is to refrain from all strong asana—Sun Salutations, standing poses, unsupported backbends, arm balances, and inversions alike—in favor of a more restorative practice.

If, despite the uncertainty about the risks, you want to do inversions during your period, it seems reasonable to adjust your practice based on your symptoms and your body's reaction to going upside down. Especially if you are a seasoned practitioner or have otherwise developed your inner awareness, notice what happens to your energy level and to your menstrual flow if you invert. If you are tuned in and you don't notice any problems or additional discomfort during the pose or over the next several hours, I doubt you'll be causing any long-term damage. A brief halt in flow followed by normal bleeding doesn't concern me much. If you do notice any symptoms, however, it may be wise to back off.

Yoga During and After Pregnancy

It's best to attend classes (or study privately) with a teacher experienced in working with pregnant women, or attend one of the growing number of specialized pregnancy classes. It's also vital for the health of the fetus to avoid dehydration and overheating. Thus, if a pregnant woman has an established Bikram or "hot yoga" practice before becoming pregnant, she should switch to a milder practice until after delivery.

A major concern with yoga during pregnancy has to do with the increased levels of the hormone relaxin. Relaxin helps loosen the ligaments connecting the pubic bones in order to facilitate delivery, but it also leads to the stretching of other ligaments throughout the body. If you do yoga at this time you may discover new levels of flexibility in your body, but that flexibility can come at a cost—joint instability. This means that it's not safe to push toward your edge in the same way you might have before you became pregnant. Instead, you'll want your practice to be gentle and less goal oriented. Focus on the quality of the experience, keep the breath smooth, and let go of any striving to push yourself. That can be hard for a lot of people, but it's what's best for you and your baby.

While teachers vary in which poses they consider appropriate during pregnancy, here

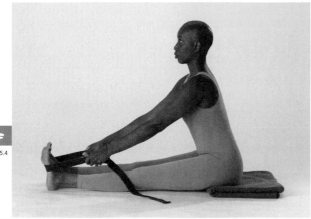

FIGURE 5.4

is some general advice. If risk of miscarriage is high, some teachers recommend avoiding asana in the first trimester. After the first trimester, avoid vigorous twists and forward bends with the legs close together, which could put pressure on the uterus. Forward bends should mostly be done with concave back (figure 5.4) so as to avoid bringing the lower edge of the rib cage toward the uterus. Poses that stretch the abdomen, such as backbends, can also stretch the linea alba, the fibrous structure that separates the rectus muscles in the front of the abdomen, which is already being stretched by pregnancy. Anything more than mild backbends is contraindicated. Avoid jumping into poses or any other jarring movements throughout pregnancy, but especially in third trimester. Most teachers believe women should only do inversions like Headstand and Shoulderstand if they have an established practice with these postures before they become pregnant, and some teachers recommend skipping them entirely. If upside-down poses are done, they may need to be given up in the latter stages of the third trimester.

TIP Don't lie flat on your back or belly after the first trimester. Savasana can be done on your left side (figure 5.5a) so as not to impair the return of blood to the heart through the vena cava, the large vein that runs along the right side near the midline of the body. Other poses normally done supine can be done on an inclined bolster (figure 5.5b).

a) Side Savasana. This alternative to Savasana is more restful and safer than the standard pose when you are pregnant. A blanket or bolster placed between the knees makes it more comfortable.
b) An inclined arrangement of bolsters and blankets prevents compression of the vena cava in poses normally done supine.

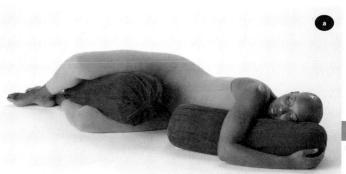

FIGURE 5.5

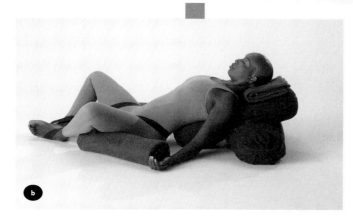

Gentle pranayama is appropriate at all stages of pregnancy. Judith Hanson Lasater recommends against any retention of the breath or any forcing whatsoever. She also advises against rapid breathing practices like Kapalabhati and Bhastrika. Meditation is fine during all three trimesters.

TIP Women need to reintroduce asana practice slowly after delivery, since they may not be as fit as they were before the pregnancy. Although the levels of the hormone relaxin drop quickly after delivery, the ligament-loosening effects linger for about three months. Thus women need to be careful not to push too hard or they risk injury. Women who have had a C-section need to restart their yoga practice even more gingerly, especially poses like twists and backbends, which can put pressure on the surgical scar. Breath work, meditation, and gentle asana may be more appropriate.

CHAPTER 6

CHOOSING A STYLE OF YOGA AND A TEACHER

As one practice cannot suit everyone, various methods will be advanced, and everyone by actual experience will find out that which helps him most.

—SWAMI VIVEKANANDA

 Deedee Eisenberg was a PhD student in environmental science at the University of Wisconsin when she first learned about yoga. She was walking by a storefront in the Madison neighborhood she had just moved to, when through the plate-glass window, "I saw people hanging upside down from ropes. I was completely blown away. I was so curious. I walked in, and I interviewed the teacher, Roger Eischen." She must have liked what she heard because she was soon a regular in his classes.

At the time, Deedee was in the middle of writing her dissertation, working on a computer for many hours a day, and it was taking a toll on her body. "I had headaches all the time, because of chronic upper body strain." What she learned in class "really transformed my life. I was in my thirties and I began to become athletic, which I hadn't ever been before." Her arms and legs grew stronger and so did her confidence. She joined a bike club, and on weekends went on long outings.

When Deedee moved to Seattle to do a postdoctoral fellowship, she found another Iyengar teacher there, Felicity Green, and once again found herself applying yoga in a therapeutic fashion—this time for the effects of a low-grade seasonal affective disorder (SAD), a type of depression linked to low light exposure, which she developed because of Seattle's many overcast days. Deedee was so interested in learning more that she went to the Iyengar Institute in Pune, India, and spent four months studying there, primarily with Geeta Iyengar, the daughter of B. K. S., and now the principal teacher at the Institute.

After Deedee returned from studying yoga in India, she discovered that her priorities were different. "When I came back, I changed my whole life. I moved to the East Coast, and I decided to give up my research career and just teach yoga and Feldenkrais" (an alternative healing modality she had begun to study in Seattle). The change in life direction, she says, "was really in response to the intensity of the experience in Pune." She began commuting to New York City to study with Mary Dunn, a senior Iyengar teacher, whom Deedee revered. Then, without warning, her entire world changed.

In a freak accident at a gym, she was struck in the temple by a piece of exercise equipment. At first she simply felt a little out of it, but over the next few weeks her condition got worse. "When I went to the supermarket, I felt as though there were ten television sets tuned to different channels blasting simultaneously, and it was impossible." She realized the only thing she could do was rest. "I remember one of the doctors I saw said, 'Well, you walked in here. Unless you have a bullet in your head, there's nothing we can do.' In other words, I wasn't getting any answers from there."

Frightened and disoriented, Deedee wasn't able to do any formal yoga practice. When she returned to her usual practice some months later, she discovered that the tools that had served her so well up to that time weren't useful. "Unfortunately," she says, "I didn't have enough maturity to recognize that I needed to do something different, or I needed to ask for a different kind of help. Because I was so scared, I was in denial, so I wasn't very open to getting the kind of help I needed at the time." Out of stubbornness, she was trying to do what she used to do. She now says, "It was completely inappropriate. In fact, I was harming myself."

Nonetheless she kept it up for more than a year, although she'd added other treatments, including acupuncture, homeopathy, and craniosacral therapy. Finally she gave up her yoga practice altogether, though she did improve enough to resume her Feldenkrais training. Another yoga teacher in that program recommended Deedee read *The Heart of Yoga*, by T. K. V. Desikachar (whose teachings form the basis of Viniyoga). Before she read the book, she says, "I had been so stubborn, I had never believed that anything but Iyengar yoga was worth investigating." She ended up writing Desikachar a brief letter. To her surprise, he wrote back, suggesting that she study with one of his senior teachers in the States, Sonia Nelson.

At first, Sonia's work with viniyoga was completely foreign to Deedee. Deedee would show her Downward-Facing Dog pose the way she'd been doing it and Sonia would say, "We don't do things that way. We move in and out with the breath. We don't stay in one position, except if we have a particular reason for doing that." Despite her doubts, Deedee persisted with the extremely gentle, flowing practice Sonia prescribed. She found the focus on the breath so precise that it was like doing pranayama and asana simultaneously. "Slowly, slowly, with my great resistance, it began to seep in," Deedee says.

"When I was first exposed to the Viniyoga, really to moving in and out of poses with the breath, I found that I could do yoga again and there was no ill effect." Any time she had tried her old way of practicing, she says, "it would harm me." This experience led her to fully embrace Viniyoga, becoming a true believer in that system, and reject her former allegiance to Iyengar yoga. (In fairness, had she been able to reach out for assistance, it's likely that approach, with its vast therapeutic toolbox, including restorative poses and pranayama, could have helped her, too.)

Sticking with Viniyoga, Deedee continued to slowly improve. Over the next several years, she got stronger and was able to function more and more normally. Now more than a decade after the head injury, she says, "Sonia still can't believe how much better I am. Every time she sees me I'm better." Indeed, in just the last few months, Deedee has been able to reincorporate inversions like Headstand and Shoulderstand into her practice.

With time and growing maturity, Deedee has also come to realize that there's more than one good approach to yoga and yoga therapy. She feels grateful to have studied with wonderful teachers in more than one tradition. "I don't feel that I have to reject any of them," she says. Depending on her students' needs, she'll sometimes teach a Viniyoga practice and sometimes bring in elements of the Iyengar method. "So now in my practice and in my teaching I can be very creative. I don't need to worry about breaking rules."

Different styles of yoga vary enormously and thus one of your central tasks in beginning a yoga practice, whether you want to use it for therapeutic purposes or to enlarge your approach to well-being, is to figure out what kind of yoga to do. The number of choices available is bewildering and there is no reliable way to determine which yoga systems are the best. Although dozens of studies have examined the effects of yoga, almost none have compared different styles of yoga or different sets of practices within one style. What is best for one person may not be for another, and as Deedee experienced, what is best may change with your circumstances. In my experience, there is healing to be found in every style of yoga I've looked at, though as we'll see, it's not just the style of yoga that has to be considered but the quality of the teacher, which can make an enormous difference.

That said, some styles come out of deeper traditions than others and some train their teachers more thoroughly. Some systems routinely include practices that may not be appropriate for people with serious medical conditions (see chapter 5). In order to try to help you sort through this, I will share my subjective impressions of the many systems I've both observed and tried. Please consider that any judgments I make reflect my own tastes and experience, and yours may be different.

I'll outline some of the major approaches below. To learn more, I suggest you turn to part 3 of this book, to see how teachers from a variety of traditions work. If a particular style is attractive to you, you may want to read a chapter featuring a teacher from that tradition in part 3—even if you don't have the particular condition they're covering. If Anusara interests you, you might check out the infertility chapter featuring John Friend. If the Viniyoga approach sounds appealing, read the chapter on chronic fatigue syndrome featuring Gary Kraftsow.

Even though I favor some styles over others, I strongly believe you can find good teachers in every yoga tradition. If your goal is healing, then committing yourself to daily practice—going on the inward journey to awareness that any good yoga system can facilitate—is more important than the style you choose.

Different Styles of Yoga and Yoga Therapy

Yoga includes an ever-growing number of styles, schools, and traditions, as well as the innovations of countless yogis over the centuries. Yoga has continually incorporated new influences. Rather than thinking of yoga as being ancient, it's probably more accurate to view it as something with ancient roots.

What the ancients were doing and what modern yogis do differ a lot. Although meditation techniques and sitting postures like the Lotus pose are age-old, many of today's widely practiced poses appear to be fairly recent inventions. Some elements of British gymnastics, for example, found their way into modern asana practice in the nineteenth and twentieth centuries when India was a British colony. These days, there is frequent hand-wringing about whether current incarnations are true to the ancient spirit of yoga. My take is that one of the deepest traditions in yoga is constant innovation. Some new approaches appear to be useful and some are probably not so valuable. Some innovations will endure and others will fade away. That's the way it's always been.

In judging the various systems, I incorporate my perspective as a physician. I am particularly concerned about the possibility of yoga injuries, the potential of causing more harm than good. When I evaluate different styles of yoga and make recommendations about what seems most appropriate, I compare the risks and the potential benefit. Some types of yoga, for example, may do enormous good but with a significant number of casualties along the way. This suggests there may be better choices for people whose health is already compromised.

IYENGAR

Named after yoga master B. K. S. Iyengar, Iyengar yoga strives for precise anatomical alignment in poses, which serves as the primary meditative focus for the practice. Breath is given less attention, particularly with beginning students and in therapeutic settings, though some teachers talk about it more than others. Pranayama practices are taught only after the student has attained proficiency in asana, generally after at least two years of study. The attention to precise anatomical detail makes Iyengar yoga particularly well suited for problems like carpal tunnel syndrome, back pain, and arthritis, in which dysfunctional alignment may be either contributing to or causing the problem. That said, Iyengar yoga teachers treat the full gamut of disease, from depression to heart disease to Parkinson's.

Iyengar pioneered the use of various props like blocks, bolsters, straps, benches of different sizes and shapes, as well as ropes mounted to either the wall or the ceiling to achieve various effects. One of the main uses is to allow students who lack sufficient flexibility or strength to do the poses with good alignment and with a minimal risk of injury. Although the poses can be modified for some students, more often props are used to guide the individual into the posture. Props are also essential to another of Iyengar's innovations—and perhaps his greatest for therapeutic purposes—restorative yoga (see chapter 3). Restoratives are particularly useful for students who are weak or tired from disease or as a consequence of treatment. They are also useful when otherwise healthy students are menstruating, tired, or feeling stressed.

Therapy in this system is only done by teachers with many years of experience. The strictest in terms of teacher training and certification, Iyengar yoga requires any teacher offering therapy to be certified at the Junior Intermediate II level or above (see their website for a list of teachers worldwide and their level of certification). These strict requirements mean, unfortunately, that this very effective form of therapy is difficult to find in most areas. Where it is available, Iyengar therapy tends to be taught in group classes, although the presence of many assistants ensures that each student gets personalized attention. It is possible to take "medical classes" at the Iyengar Institute in Pune, India, working with the guru and senior teachers, but it is difficult to get a spot and the waiting list is long. (If you are interested in pursuing this option, it's generally best to speak to an Iyengar teacher in the West, who can advise you.) Recently, simple pranayama exercises were added to medical classes in Pune.

As the Beatles have influenced every subsequent pop group, so has Iyengar had an impact on the majority of Western yoga teachers, specifically through his emphasis on anatomical alignment—whether they know it or not. Iyengar is much more influential in the West than he is among other yoga gurus in India, however, and for this reason the awareness of alignment in Western yoga is generally much more precise than in the vast majority of yoga I've seen in India.

VINIYOGA

Viniyoga, as the system is generally referred to in the West, was propagated by T. K. V. Desikachar, the son of Krishnamacharya (who was also the guru of Iyengar and Pattabhi Jois). It focuses intensely on the breath, and incorporates pranayama techniques and chanting into asana practice, although both pranayama and chanting are also done in their own right. The postures are gentle, and students flow in and out of the poses, sometimes holding them, but only briefly. Because the movements are never forced and the poses are not held for long periods of time, the risk of injury is extremely low, making this style particularly well suited for students with chronic disease. Students and teachers of Viniyoga often dress in street clothes and leave their socks on when they practice.

Therapy is always done one-on-one, though there are some group classes taught in the West. This insistence on individualized attention has to do with the belief that the program must be tailored to the character and life circumstances of the person. In their assessment of patients at the Krishnamacharya Yoga Mandiram (KYM), teachers perform Ayurvedic pulse diagnosis to establish the student's constitution and help formulate the treatment plan (see chapter 4). Perhaps their most important reason for teaching only private lessons is their conviction that the relationship between student and teacher is - vital to healing.

Until recently, it has been hard to find Viniyoga teachers in many geographic areas. Gary Kraftsow, another of Desikachar's senior US teachers, is now training large groups of teachers. Many of these teachers go on to train as therapists, so this deep system of therapeutic yoga will soon be more available. It is also possible to travel to Chennai (Madras), India, to study with teachers at the KYM, though students should understand that they may only get one or two lessons a week, and will otherwise be expected to work on their own. Desikachar and his son Kausthub frequently teach workshops throughout the world. A. G. Mohan, another disciple of Krishnamacharya, and his wife, Indra, do similar work just outside of Chennai and take on some Western students. In addition to his decades of yoga experience, Mohan has trained extensively in Ayurveda.

ASHTANGA/POWER YOGA

Ashtanga, based on the teachings of K. Pattabhi Jois of Mysore, India, is one of the most vigorous styles of hatha yoga. Its practitioners perform fixed series of postures that flow rapidly and continuously, often jumping from one posture to the next. The entire practice is done while breathing loudly in the style of Ujjayi pranayama (see chapter 1), which is said to energize the body and focus the mind. Also characteristic of Ashtanga practice is the attention paid to engaging the root lock (mula bandha) and solar plexus lock (uddiyana bandha) as well as to the direction of gaze (drishti) during asana practice. Pranayama is generally only taught to students who have studied for several years. Many students enjoy the energetic workout, but Ashtanga is probably not for people who are less fit or less flexible, those with serious medical conditions, or those with back, knee, or shoulder problems.

Some Ashtanga teachers do yoga therapy but it is a minor part of the tradition. If you seek therapeutic help from an Ashtanga teacher, it should be done either in a "Mysore style" class, in which students practice at their own pace, or in a private session. Power yoga, Jivamukti, and "vinyasa flow," which include a vigorous workout with repeated Sun Salutations in every class but usually not the rigidly defined set of poses found in most Ashtanga classes, are variations of the Ashtanga theme. As with Ashtanga, these styles may have therapeutic benefits for their practitioners but the intense workouts, lack of personalization, and risk of injury make them less appropriate options for most people seeking yoga as medicine.

BIKRAM/HOT YOGA

Bikram yoga is a vigorous style done in a room often heated to over one hundred degrees. The classes invariably involve doing the same twenty-six practices in sequence twice, including standing poses, one-legged balancing postures, floor exercises, and pranayama. Students hold each pose for thirty to sixty seconds. The classes are standardized, with teachers often reciting the instructions more or less verbatim. Choudhury Bikram, the inventor of this system, is currently trying to patent his sequence of practices down to the very words of the instructors' banter, which accounts for the near total uniformity of the classes. As with Ashtanga yoga, many Bikram students enjoy the predictability of the sequence of poses because they know what to expect and can easily chart their progress week to week.

While therapy is generally not part of Bikram yoga, its proponents believe that the practice can be helpful for a wide variety of medical conditions. A demanding routine, done in hot and humid conditions, however, means that these classes are too challenging for most people who are of advanced age or seriously ill (see chapter 5). In particular, anyone with multiple sclerosis, chronic fatigue syndrome, fibromyalgia, epilepsy, an inflammatory condition of any kind, or who is pregnant should avoid working out in the heat. (Bikram instructors recommend that pregnant women do a modified routine.) Despite these safety considerations, taking on the discipline required to do this practice can be life transforming. I have received email testimonials from students who report amazing recoveries from illness from this style of yoga—but also one that told of a man who had a heart attack in the parking lot coming out of class.

KRIPALU

This system is perhaps the most New Age in feel of the yoga styles common in the West. Kripalu teachers stress the importance of creating an emotionally safe space for students to practice, and encourage their students to go into and "process" their feelings, reflecting Kripalu's conscious integration of insights from Western psychotherapy with Eastern wisdom. There is an emphasis on emotional release, spiritual growth, and self-acceptance. Rather than being the creation of one person, modern Kripalu yoga represents the collective efforts of the group of disciples who gathered around yogi Amrit Desai starting in the 1970s. With the guru now gone, the continuing evolution of the path is powered by the community and an influential group of senior teachers. Since there is no one central authority in the system, however, it is also one of the most variable styles, with different teachers taking very different approaches.

Kripalu yoga tends to start out gently, incorporating some chanting, pranayama, and meditation with asana practice. The stress is on coordinating all movement with the breath, feeling the movement of energy, or prana, and working to your "edge." In more advanced classes, poses are held longer and the practice can be quite vigorous. Toward the end of some classes, students are encouraged to embark on free-form improvisation of whatever postures they feel drawn to, a practice they call "meditation in motion." Some teachers include strong Kundalini practices, designed to raise energy quickly, in their classes. You might, for example, hold Bridge pose for one minute, breathing in rapid Kapalabhati fashion (with a forced exhalation and passive inhalation) the entire time.

Such practices may be too intense for some people with serious medical conditions. But the methodology of Kripalu yoga continues to be refined. A few years ago, for example, there was very little focus on anatomical alignment in asana, but teachers seem to be stressing it more now (though to nothing like the degree you would find in Iyengar or Anusara classes).

The Kripalu Center for Yoga and Health in Lenox, Massachusetts, runs residential programs lasting from a few days to a month or longer, and features both Kripalu teachers and those from a wide variety of yoga and holistic health disciplines. Therapy has not been a major feature of Kripalu yoga in the past, though it seems to be growing. Many of the residential programs offered at the center have a therapeutic focus (though most of these are taught by teachers from other traditions). One thing that the Kripalu Center has consciously set out to do—and is succeeding at—is making people of color feel welcome and comfortable, which has not always been the case in the yoga world, unfortunately.

PHOENIX RISING YOGA THERAPY

Phoenix Rising Yoga Therapy (PRYT) is a specifically therapeutic approach developed by Michael Lee, an Australian who comes out of the Kripalu tradition. There are similarities in the approaches, particularly in the integration of yoga and Western psychology, but there are also significant differences. In PRYT, the therapist moves your body through a number of yoga postures while you remain passive (for example, in a supine position) and encourages you to verbalize any responses to the intervention in a manner analogous to psychotherapy. You are asked to focus on any thoughts, sensations, or emotions that arise as part of this inward journey. Invariably, people start to hit "a recurring theme," Michael says, "and it usually has some deep connection to what's going on in their life." Meditation, journaling, and other awareness exercises are also emphasized.

Although the system comes out of yoga, it is different from most of the yoga therapy approaches described in this book because of the emphasis on passive movement and psychology. PRYT might more appropriately be considered a hybrid of yoga, bodywork, and psychotherapy, though the PRYT therapist, unlike a traditional psychotherapist, does not attempt to offer psychological insights. While potentially very helpful for stress-related and psychological conditions, PRYT is generally not used for structural problems. I once asked a well-known PRYT instructor what he would suggest for someone with knee pain. His answer: "I'd tell them to see a doctor." The gentle nature of the exercises makes the risk of injury low.

(PRYT is differentiated from Phoenix Rising yoga, which is a gentle style where you do the postures without assistance.)

ANUSARA

Anusara yoga is a system developed by John Friend, a longtime student of Iyengar yoga. Anusara yoga combines the precision of alignment found in Iyengar yoga with a warm, playful teaching environment that is, they like to say, "heart centered." While the focus of classes is on asana, some chanting, pranayama, meditation, and discussion of Tantric philosophy may be incorporated.

Though not yet studied in scientific experiments, in my experience the Anusara approach to therapy is powerful and effective. Its focus on alignment is heavily influenced by Iyengar, but John has developed his own approach to therapy shaped by years of working with clients. Hands-on manipulation of muscles and joints is a major part of what an Anusara yoga therapist does in a one-on-one setting. But the key to making any changes last, Anusara teachers stress, is to practice fifteen to twenty minutes daily at home, so the students always leave with homework to do after the session.

It should be noted that regular Anusara yoga classes can be quite vigorous and may not be appropriate for many people with serious disease. Therapy sessions are personalized, however, and thus are fine even for those with serious illness. As many teachers are being trained, in coming years we are likely to see Anusara yoga therapy become much more available than it currently is.

KUNDALINI

To me, Kundalini yoga in the style of Yogi Bhajan has a more religious feel than most Western schools of yoga, though its practitioners might dispute this. Some of its followers convert to a form of Sikhism, with many of the top teachers wearing white clothes and turbans, and taking the last name Khalsa, meaning "pure." (Never once, though, have I seen any indications of proselytizing.) A number of strong breathing techniques are used along with asana, chanting, and meditation. General Kundalini classes can be very intense, however, potentially stimulating the sympathetic nervous system to a degree that may not be appropriate for some people with medical conditions. Kundalini therapists, like Shanti Shanti Kaur Khalsa, however, personalize the approach for the client, starting with gentler practices as appropriate. Preliminary scientific evidence is validating the therapeutic efficacy of this style.

"Kundalini yoga is characterized by movement with the breath," says Shanti Shanti Kaur. According to her, there are some kriyas, by which they mean a sequence, in which the poses are held, but she says that's rare. You might do a repetitive movement, for example, accompanied by vigorous breathing while you repeat a mantra in your mind. "Almost everything we do has movement in it. The concept is that it works for the lymphatic system, it works for the pranic body, it works for releasing toxicity, it works for circulation, it works for deepening the lung capacity. It's a hallmark of Kundalini yoga." Anatomical alignment is not the central concern of this practice. "If the person doesn't do a practice correctly, and we demonstrate it, and we model it out, and we use our voice to tell them about it, we let it go. We are actually instructed not to touch people, which is very different from how most hatha yoga instructors are trained."

INTEGRAL

Integral yoga is a gentle style that includes asana, pranayama, chanting, and meditation as well as discussions of philosophy and ancient yoga texts. This multifaceted approach, using several different yogic tools, is taught from the first class. Founded by the late Swami Satchidananda, Integral yoga is similar to Sivananda yoga, which is better known in Europe than in the US. Swami Sivananda was Satchidananda's guru. In both systems a standard sequence of poses is taught in most classes. Reflecting Sivananda's influence, Integral yoga encourages a commitment to selfless service (karma yoga) among its followers, and this focus is central to the approach.

Therapy is a major feature of Integral yoga. While lacking the anatomical precision that might be useful for some structural problems, it has been successfully used for people with serious conditions, including cancer and heart disease. A yoga program designed and implemented by Nischala Joy Devi, based on the basic Integral class, was a crucial element in Dr. Dean Ornish's scientifically documented program for reversing heart disease (see chapter 19). Ornish, himself a longtime disciple of Satchidananda, is now applying a similar approach to men with prostate cancer, and early results are encouraging. The gentle approach and the lack of hands-on adjustments make this form of yoga very safe. Residential therapeutic programs, taught by Integral teachers as well as by some from other disciplines, are offered regularly at Yogaville, their ashram, outside of Charlottesville, Virginia.

TANTRA

At one time, yoga was only taught to the elite of Indian society, male Brahmins, and then only to those who dedicated their life to it. The teachings and practice of yoga were kept secret from the rest of the world. This changed around the tenth century C.E. with the flowering of Tantra, one branch on the tree of yoga. Most of what we know of as yoga in the West, particularly the physical practices of hatha yoga, owes much to this tradition.

Tantra views the body as a manifestation of the divine and a vehicle for self-transformation, not something to be transcended as quickly as possible. This was a radical departure from some classical yoga approaches, which viewed the body as filthy and vile. Tantra was radical in another way, too: it explicitly offered its wisdom to women, and welcomed people of all social castes as well as so-called householders, people who lived in the community, married, had children, and held regular jobs.

Tantra is a relentlessly pragmatic yogic tradition that uses the widest possible array of yogic tools. In the West and even in India, Tantra has acquired a bad reputation based largely on misunderstandings of what it is, and on the practices of some fringe Tantric cults. The use of Tantra as a healing modality has little or nothing to do with the Tantric sexuality seminars you may have heard about. At the Himalayan Institute, an ashram in Pennsylvania with branches in other cities, the approach is Tantric. They offer numerous educational programs, including some with a therapeutic bent, with a few programs taught by teachers from other schools of yoga. According to Rolf Sovik, in addition to asana and pranayama, the yoga at the Institute incorporates mantra, visualization, and focused meditation practice. Tantric approaches also include cleansing practices (kriyas), as well as Ayurvedic herbs and dietary advice. Tantra is generally very safe but should be learned under the guidance of a good teacher. The visualization exercise, the smile meditation as taught by Rod Stryker, in chapter 3, is an example of a Tantric practice.

GYM YOGA

One of the most common places for people to study yoga in the United States is in health clubs. The classes come in a multitude of styles. In my experience, the classes tend to be vigorous, since they are often trying to appeal to people who might otherwise take step aerobics or kickboxing. Though there are many exceptions, most health club yoga classes are taught by young, relatively green teachers who don't necessarily have the training or experience to work safely with people with significant medical problems. In the hundreds of classes I've taken at health clubs over the years, I've almost never seen a teacher even ask about potential contraindications before putting the entire class into a potentially risky pose. It's been a few years since I've taken a class at a gym, though, and I hope this is changing.

OTHER STYLES

With the boom in yoga in the past decade or so has come a proliferation of styles of yoga and yoga therapy. As teachers continue to innovate and combine insights from disciplines inside and outside of yoga, expect this trend to continue. Many of the top teachers in the West are no longer the formal students of any one guru or school of yoga. They are influenced by various traditions and combinations of traditions and teachers they have worked with. Some teachers give what they do its own name and new brand names are being coined at a fairly rapid pace. In addition to those named above, some of the styles that can be used therapeutically include Forrest yoga, Svaroopa yoga, Structural yoga therapy, and

Integrative yoga therapy. Sam Dworkis, featured in the fibromyalgia chapter, teaches what he calls Recovery yoga. Aadil Palkhivala, the consultant for the high blood pressure chapter, has recently dubbed his work Purna yoga, and has started an accredited college to teach it in suburban Seattle. Other prominent teachers, such as Barbara Benagh, the expert for the asthma chapter, just give workshops without branding their work with a name other than their own.

HOW—AND WHETHER—TO CHOOSE ONE STYLE OF YOGA

While most yoga teachers encourage their students to stick with a single style of yoga, it's certainly a viable alternative to take from more than one tradition. Indeed, frowned on as this is by some, that's what millions of yoga students and teachers are currently doing. Even though they know their primary teachers wouldn't necessarily approve, many people discreetly attend classes and workshops taught by teachers of other disciplines. It's also possible to remain basically loyal to a particular style and yet add a few practices from other sources. For example, because meditation is not taught in some styles of yoga, many practitioners have looked elsewhere within the yoga world or have studied Buddhist techniques (which originally sprang from the soil of yoga). Similarly, practitioners of any style of yoga might add Iyengar-based restoratives or tantric visualizations like Yoga Nidra to their home practice without any loss of fidelity to their teachers. If you make this choice, and feel your teacher might disapprove, you do not have to advertise it. One caveat: superficial sampling of many systems of yoga without going deeply into any of them can be a mistake (except when you are brand-new and are trying to figure out which style is right for you).

How to Find a Yoga Teacher or Therapist

Wandering into a local yoga studio as Deedee first did is one way to find a yoga teacher or therapist, though not necessarily the best one. Studios are certainly a lot easier to find than they were in the mid 1980s, when she happened upon Roger's studio in Madison. While there are many more places to do yoga than there used to be, given the rapid growth of yoga in the last several years, many of those now teaching are relatively inexperienced, meaning it really pays to do your homework when deciding who to study with, especially if you are looking for someone who can help you with a medical condition.

It may be tempting to do yoga therapy on your own, by trying to learn from books or videos. Some people have no choice, of course, but in the beginning especially, it's far better to have a teacher who can observe you and offer feedback. Without guidance, you could choose practices that aren't right for you or do appropriate practices incorrectly and even dangerously. While yoga done properly is extremely safe, serious problems can occur when it's not done right. These are powerful practices and have the ability to affect the body and mind profoundly—for better or worse.

If you are looking for someone to help you with a health condition, call yoga studios in your area for leads. Some disease advocacy groups can also provide leads on finding appropriate yoga teachers. The local chapter of the MS Society, for example, may know about classes in the area where other people with the condition study.

If you can afford them, private lessons can be the best way to start. Alternatively, for somewhat less money, some therapists teach small groups, say two to four people. Whether this is a good choice for you depends on how much attention you need; this in turn is based on how much yoga you already know and how sick you are. Even if you can only have a few private sessions, it may be worthwhile. Shanti Shanti Kaur Khalsa suggests "people start out with an individual class for maybe a couple of weeks, so the teacher and the student learn, they assess, and then the student can decide whether to go to a group class, and if so, which one, and taught by whom."

SIX THINGS TO LOOK FOR IN A TEACHER

1. Training. There are no universal standards or accreditation for either yoga teachers or yoga therapists. Many systems now require teachers to complete either two hundred or five hundred hours of training to be certified (and one organization, the nonprofit Yoga Alliance, registers teachers and training programs that meet its standards, though not all choose to participate). In addition to such training, most teachers will require ongoing study and years of apprenticeship to gain competence as yoga therapists. The less training they have had, the less likely they are to know which techniques could benefit (or harm) people with medical problems, and the fewer their opportunities to develop the ability to detect problems that could result in injury. Yoga teachers at gyms are particularly likely to have had minimal training. There are widely advertised programs that train people to be yoga teachers in two weeks and others in which personal trainers and aerobics instructors become "certified" as yoga teachers with a single weekend course. One outfit offers online certification for $49.99. Of course, people with such minimal training are not qualified to do yoga therapy (and probably not even to teach yoga). Before setting up an appointment, be sure to inquire where the teacher has trained and for how long. Since yoga therapy for problems like arthritis, heart disease, and cancer requires considerable knowledge—of anatomy, physiology, the effects of medications, and contraindications to various aspects of the practice—look for someone who has received additional training in those areas or who by virtue of prior training in a health care profession already has it. As it turns out, many people doing yoga therapy have such training.

> **CAUTION** Yoga teachers, even very experienced ones, shouldn't be relied on to diagnose the cause of your symptoms. This is not their area of expertise and could lead to some very serious problems if a misdiagnosis gets in the way of necessary treatment. Another concern is that some yoga teachers confidently dole out health advice they are not qualified to offer. Because the teachers are in a position of authority and respected for their yoga expertise, students may assume that they really know what they are talking about even when they don't. My advice is to listen respectfully but take their recommendations with a grain of salt and see your doctor about any potentially serious condition.

2. Experience. There can be no hard and fast rules for how much experience a yoga therapist should have but in general the more, the better. Someone who's been doing it for ten years will likely know a lot more than someone at it for five, and both of them will probably pale in comparison to those with twenty years of experience. It's no coincidence that most of the teachers I've chosen for part 3 of this book have more than twenty-five years in the field. That's part of what puts them at the top of their profession. Of course, some people with much less experience do excellent work, particularly if they have expertise in other areas like Feldenkrais, the Alexander Technique, or physical therapy. Often, these people make some of the best therapists because of their extensive understanding of anatomy and kinesiology (human movement). Moreover, there's often a trade-off between the greater expertise of a master teacher and the greater availability and personal attention you'd get from a less-experienced one. Many of the most senior teachers, including a number featured in this book, no longer give private lessons, and spend most of their time training other yoga teachers.

3. Reputation. Part of what makes a good teacher good can't be entirely explained by looking at who they trained with or how long they've been at it. Some people seem to be particularly talented at teaching, or at making students feel comfortable emotionally, or at reading bodies, or any number of the other skills that great therapists possess. Word of mouth remains one of the best ways to find a great teacher. There are good and not-so-good teachers in all styles, so you shouldn't just choose by label alone (e.g., Iyengar or Viniyoga). If you are able to attend classes, you may learn a lot about which teachers are most highly regarded by talking to your fellow students.

4. Flexibility of Approach. No yoga therapist should impose a template for practice that was formulated without seeing you and learning the particulars of your situation. The best teachers are careful observers who adjust to your individual needs, preferences, circumstances, and responses. "Good teachers look at what you're doing and teach from what they see, not just what they know," says Mary Dunn, a senior Iyengar teacher. Five people may all have back pain but a skilled teacher will see differences among them and choose different approaches accordingly. The teacher's ability to adapt and shape treatment to the individual is one of the hallmarks of high-quality yoga therapy. Though standardized approaches can work—as numerous scientific studies have documented—and some people find that instructional yoga videos can help motivate them to practice, they are just not the best that yoga has to offer.

5. They Practice What They Preach. Real yogic understanding, the kind that can help transform a student, is most likely to come from teachers who themselves walk the path of yoga. You understand yoga by doing it, and doing it consistently for years. That's how you develop the ability to sense in yourself and see in others. And that's how you have the depth of understanding to teach it to others. When you are evaluating a teacher or therapist, be sure to ask the nature of their own practice. Find out what they do and how much they do it. A dedicated daily practice, even a short one, is ideal (practicing alongside students while teaching is not enough, in my opinion). While some teachers may only do asana practice, committed practitioners will likely also have a pranayama and meditation practice. The best teachers are also lifelong students, so try to find out what they do to advance their understanding, whether it's reading, studying anatomy, attending workshops, or working in an ongoing way with a guru or more senior teacher.

6. They Motivate You to Practice. The biggest determinant of success in yoga therapy is steady practice. Regardless of his or her technical skills, any teacher who can motivate you to get on your mat and keep up your practice is doing something right. Shanti Shanti Kaur says that people tend to believe that the technique is all you need, but she finds that the student-teacher relationship is critical. You want to feel listened to and respected, even if you're not a "natural" at yoga. Teachers who themselves are inspired by the practice can motivate students to take the kind of leap of faith I spoke about in the book's introduction. If they have confidence from their own experience and from having helped other students, it can be infectious.

What to Expect in Your First Yoga Therapy Session

When a skilled yoga therapist is helping you in a one-on-one setting, you can expect a thorough evaluation of your body. The teacher will assess you for symmetry, strength, flexibility, postural patterns and tics, muscle and tissue tone, as well as mood and motivation. Experienced teachers can gather much of this data so quickly that you may not even know it happened.

Based on the evaluation, the teacher will typically choose certain practices that seem as though they may be helpful to you and will then watch you try out the recommended practices. You will be monitored to ensure that you are doing the poses and other practices safely and that you understand how to practice them on your own. In asana, expect the therapist to look closely at what you are doing and offer suggestions, adjustments, props, or modifications. Based on what therapists see as you practice, they may realize that what they thought would work doesn't. As Judith Hanson Lasater puts it, "It doesn't matter whether something is supposed to be good for you. It only matters if it actually is."

Expect to leave your appointment with a prescription for what you can do at home. Almost anyone can do some form of yoga practice on their own, even if it's something as simple as breath awareness. In future classes and treatment sessions your teacher will modify and refine that plan as your body and medical condition change.

When You Can't Find a Yoga Therapist

It's not always possible to work with a yoga therapist. You may not be able to afford it right now. You may live in a place where there are none, or be unable to travel due to illness or other circumstances. Thus you may need to cobble together what you can learn from local teachers who may not be experienced in therapy with what you learn in books, articles, and videos. Another possibility is that you may be able to find restorative and gentle classes that are appropriate for some people with serious illnesses. Introductory-level classes in Integral yoga, Viniyoga, Kripalu, and some classes billed as gentle hatha yoga may be fine for many people who are ill, but be sure to speak with the teacher in advance to find out if it would be appropriate for you. Styles like Anusara, Iyengar, and Kundalini are all useful therapeutically when personalized, but general classes in these styles may be too strenuous for anyone with a serious illness. However, one advantage of Iyengar yoga is that even junior teachers learn how to use props to adapt the routine to the individual, as Roger Eischen did with Deedee. The ability to do this effectively grows with teaching experience.

If you are interested in jump-starting your journey into yoga and can afford the time and money, a yoga workshop or a trip to a center that specializes in residential retreats may be ideal. These workshops provide a means to study for an extended period of time with some of the most seasoned teachers. The best of these workshops can be downright transformational. Because the teacher or teachers get to know you over the course of days or even weeks, depending on the length of the program and the number of participants, they may be able to personalize a practice designed just for you or at least offer some guidance. The goal should not only be to make progress while you're there, but to come away from the workshop with a plan for a practice that you can do on your own.

In the US, such centers include The Kripalu Center for Yoga and Health in Western Massachusetts, the Feathered Pipe Ranch in Montana, and Inner Harmony in California. For Westerners who are open to it, study in India is another possibility. Residential centers I have personally visited and can recommend include Kabir Baug in Pune, the Vivekananda ashram outside of Bangalore (a physician oversees the therapy at both of these centers), and the Yoga Institute, located in Santacruz in suburban Mumbai (Bombay).

One thing that was striking about the various yoga therapy clinics and teachers I consulted in India was how different their recommendations were for dealing with the nerve condition affecting my right arm. At the Vivekananda center, the physician in charge, Dr. Nagaratha, suggested breathing exercises during which I was to imagine bringing prana, or life force, into the area of my right upper chest where the nerve blockage was. Mr. D. K. Shridar at the Krishnamacharya Yoga Mandiram (who now runs his own clinic in Chennai) and Dr. A. G. Mohan, a disciple of Krishnamacharya's who also practices in Chennai, recommended similar, though not identical, sets of gentle asana coordinated with breathing exercises to open my shoulders and upper spine. Dr. Karandikar, who runs Kabir Baug in Pune, prescribed a series of poses in which ropes and belts put traction on my spine, and others which taught me to use my shoulder blades to open my upper back. Although the practices were on the surface very different, I found all of them useful.

Dr. Karandikar worked as a family-practice doctor for years before dedicating his life to yoga therapy. His work now combines yoga with medical diagnostic tools, and he was the first person to suggest an X-ray of my spine. Considering how long I'd been doing yoga and how much I practiced, he thought my spinal movements were abnormally restricted. His medical intuition proved to be correct: the X-ray revealed significant calcification along the lower thoracic spine, what doctors call ankylosing. (Although my condition on X-ray resembles the autoimmune disease ankylosing spondylitis, I came to realize that it was most likely the result of a serious injury I'd suffered as an eleven-year-old, when I fell out of a second-story window.)

When I returned to Boston, I completely transformed my yoga practice to correct this restriction in spinal movement and heal the nerve condition in my arm, which I felt was at least indirectly related to it. In addition to what I'd learned in India, both Patricia Walden and Tom Alden in Boston gave me very helpful suggestions. I also worked regularly with a physical therapist, Rachel Berger, trained in various bodywork modalities including craniosacral therapy as well as with a master traditional Japanese medical practitioner, Dr. Akira Naoi, who used shiatsu, moxibustion (the burning of medicinal herbs over acupuncture points), and other modalities.

Over the next several months, the numbness and tingling in my arm gradually disappeared. By early 2005, three years from the time I developed thoracic outlet syndrome, I was able to gently reintroduce Shoulderstand, then Headstand a few months later, and, finally, Plow pose. By that time, my body had changed so much that these formerly contraindicated asana had become not only possible, but a pleasure to do.

On my next trip to India in 2005–2006, I combined a mostly restorative yoga practice with various Ayurvedic treatments, which included rest, a low-fat vegetarian diet, herbal concoctions, and daily massages using medicated oils at two different Ayurvedic centers in the southern state of Kerala. One treatment I found particularly effective involved placing a reservoir of heated oil infused with medicinal herbs directly onto my back over the vertebrae. The oil was continually reheated and allowed to soak in over forty-five minutes on fourteen consecutive days. These measures brought still further opening to my spine, and I left the clinic more relaxed than I'd felt in years.

The oil reservoir was prescribed by a traditional Ayurvedic physician, A.C. Chandukkutty Vaidhyar, a wise, curious, spry seventy-six-year-old with a gleam in his eye, whose father and grandfather began training him at the age of four (and who in turn trained his own son). Watching him practice during a return visit I made to India in 2006–2007, I was deeply impressed with his diagnostic and therapeutic abilities. Using strong massage with medicated oils, herbal concoctions, poultices, steam baths, and more oil reservoirs—on my upper spine as well as on my breast bone—his therapists were able, in their words, "to bring my spine into my body," reversing the way the bones were protruding at the skin surface. The result was the best alignment of my spine since childhood, though Chandukkutty says it will take one more forty-one day course to correct the last of my calcified C-shaped slump. I left Kerala feeling grounded and balanced. And in what seems like more than a coincidence, for the first time returning from India—twenty hours in the air and more than a dozen time zones away—I had no jet lag and from the first night was able to sleep soundly.

Given all that I've done, it's impossible for me to know for sure which treatments (or combination of treatments) were the most important to my recovery. Ultimately in yoga, you learn to let your personal experience and intuition guide you—and the more you practice the more you can rely on them. Given the multitude of good choices, almost everyone can find a teacher and style of yoga that will work for them. I have found many.

GETTING STARTED AND KEEPING IT GOING

In stages, the impossible becomes possible.

—T. K. V. DESIKACHAR

 Yoga is a systematic methodology for achieving greater health and contentment. The key to yoga as medicine is to establish a regular practice. This is what forges new grooves of thought and action, new samskaras, to help you overcome the bad habits you have formed over time.

Establishing a Personal Practice

As discussed in chapter 1, I believe that a home yoga practice is generally the most efficient way to build your yoga groove. In my experience, class is where I learn, but my personal practice is where I make what I learn in class my own. As useful and healing as a relationship with a great yoga teacher can be, ultimately what you do in your own practice is the most important determinant of success in yoga therapy. If you are taking yoga classes but not practicing at home, you may be missing the best—and potentially most therapeutic—part of yoga. Your personal practice is where the deepest work happens, when you go inward, and go at your own pace.

There's no denying, however, that for those who find it difficult to practice by themselves, classes can be an invaluable means of finding the discipline to practice. Some people also really benefit from the feeling of community that can arise in a class. Ultimately, whatever best motivates you is what you should do. As Nischala Joy Devi says: "Better to do it the way you like it than not do it."

WHAT YOU'LL NEED TO GET STARTED

The props you'll need will depend on the style of yoga you end up doing. Most people these days practice on a sticky mat on the floor, which provides a tacky surface so that your hands and feet won't slip. In many Indian settings and some classes in the West, students practice on a small rug instead. Most beginners also need a pillow or folded blanket to put under their head when they lie down, and to prop themselves up when they sit cross-legged.

At first you may just want to get a mat. (Following the principle of ahimsa, many yogis choose to buy ecologically nonharming yoga mats, avoiding ones made with PVC plastics and other potentially harmful chemicals.) You can buy other props later on, as needed. If you are willing to invest a bit more you could buy one or two blocks and a strap, in addition to the mat. They're easy to find separately, or you can buy all of these as part of a starter kit, available in some stores and catalogues, though often the items in a kit are lower quality than those purchased separately. It's entirely possible to start doing yoga without buying a thing. In a pinch, you can practice on the bare floor or a carpet. If you need props, you can use chairs, pillows, books, and old ties lying around your house to improvise what you need. You can allow your practice to convince you when and if it's time to upgrade.

If you plan on making restorative poses part of your home regimen—and I highly recommend that you do—consider buying two blocks, one six- to ten-foot strap (depending on how tall and broad you are), three yoga blankets, and a cylindrical bolster (ideally with

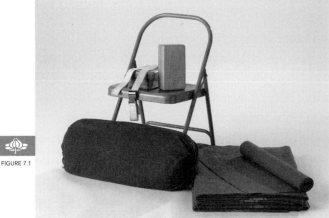

FIGURE 7.1

a firm filling like cotton batting). For some supported poses taught in part 3 of this book, you'll need a metal office chair that has had the back removed (figure 7.1). These are available from a number of yoga equipment suppliers (see appendix 1), but you can simply buy a standard metal office chair and have the back removed. An eyebag may also be worthwhile, to increase your ability to go inward when you relax.

These props will run over a hundred dollars, but once you experience what restoratives can do, you'll likely consider them an excellent investment. Think of what a single month of most prescription medications costs.

WHAT TO WEAR

The proper clothes for yoga depend on where you will be studying. If you will be attending a class where adjustments are made or proper anatomical alignment is stressed, I recommend formfitting clothes, so that the teacher can see your body well enough to check your alignment. You may be compressing your spine when you bend backward, but if you are wearing a baggy sweatshirt the teacher may be hard-pressed to detect it. You should also learn to be an observer of yourself. Rodney Yee says he tells all the teachers he trains to wear as little as possible when they do yoga at home. "You've got to be able to read when your knee is aligned, and you've got to see the skin, where it's white, where it's flushed." He thinks being able to see your body helps you do what you're doing more accurately. In India and in some ashram settings, however, modesty is considered paramount. People favor baggy clothes and generally do not wear shorts or sleeveless shirts.

Although in some yoga classes people wear socks, unless you have a good reason to do so, I strongly encourage you to do yoga postures with bare feet. A major component of asana practice is going deeper and deeper into the fine sensations of your body, and you simply get a better feel with bare feet than you can through socks. One exception is Savasana and restorative poses, in which it's vital to stay warm to sink into deep relaxation. In the fall and winter, you might do the active part of your practice in bare feet and then put on socks before doing Savasana or other relaxation poses.

WHEN TO PRACTICE

The short answer is: whenever you can. For many people, first thing in the morning is an ideal time to practice—before the phone starts to ring, the interruptions start piling on, and you get caught up in your day. Also, since yoga is best done on an empty stomach, particularly if you will be doing twisting postures, forward bends, or inversions, a prebreakfast yoga session is ideal. If you do need a morning snack, most teachers recommend eating something light no less than ninety minutes before you practice.

Afternoon or early evening may be better if morning stiffness is a problem (though a hot shower first can help you feel more limber). In the late afternoon, the body tends to be more flexible and you may find yourself able to go more deeply into the poses. Afternoons may be the best time for people with fibromyalgia; those with asthma may find breathing a bit easier then.

If you have days that are so busy that you can't find time to practice, try to fit in a few poses or a couple of minutes of breathing exercises. While walking through a doorway, for example, you could grasp the sides and lean forward into a gentle energizing stretch of the chest, shoulders, and arms. Standing in front of a desk or countertop, fold forward into a simple spinal stretch for a few breaths (figure 7a). While sitting in a chair, you could twist to one side and then the other (figure 7b). If you are under the weather or ill or injured, do a simple breathing exercise or lie on a bolster in a supported pose.

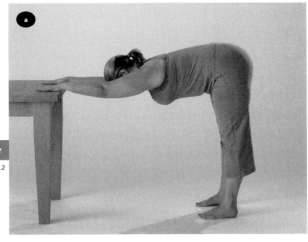

FIGURE 7.2

Quick yoga poses. a) Countertop stretch b) Chair twist

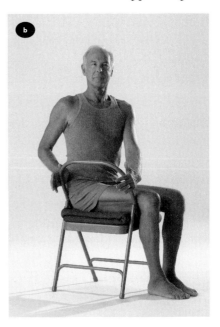

Here are a few more possibilities. Before you get out of bed in the morning, why not lie there and do yogic breathing for a couple of minutes? Later in the day, could you take a minute or two while sitting in your chair at work to tune in to your breath, notice your posture, and sit up a little straighter? If you are in line at the store and find yourself feeling a little stressed, could you gently lengthen your exhalation or notice the way your feet are pressing into the ground? Once you get into the spirit of exploration, you'll find you can fit many little yoga moments into your day.

Try to find a place to practice that is as quiet as possible and where you are unlikely to be disturbed. Turn off the TV and the phone. Make sure the temperature is warm enough that you can relax. Dim the lights if possible during the quiet parts of your practice, as partial darkness can lessen the stimulation of the nervous system and facilitate deeper relaxation.

One way of honoring your yoga practice, if you can spare the room, is to set aside a dedicated place for yoga. If you practice again and again in the same spot, you deepen the samskara. Creating a little shrine with photographs, religious icons, candles, incense, or fresh flowers helps create the right mood for some people. Anything that increases your odds of sticking with a regular practice is worth doing.

The Yoga of Action Applied

Chapter 1 outlined Patanjali's Kriya yoga, the yoga of action, which consists of tapas (discipline), svadhyaya (self-study), and Ishvara pranidhana (giving up the illusion of being in control). Tapas can also be thought of as what you do, svadhyaya as noticing what happens as a result, and Ishvara pranidhana as accepting reality, whether it's what you'd like it to be or not. These three combined with the yogic tool of intention, sankalpa, provide a road map for building a yogic groove and with it transforming your life (figure 7.3). As you cycle through these four steps again and again, you steadily deepen healthy samskaras.

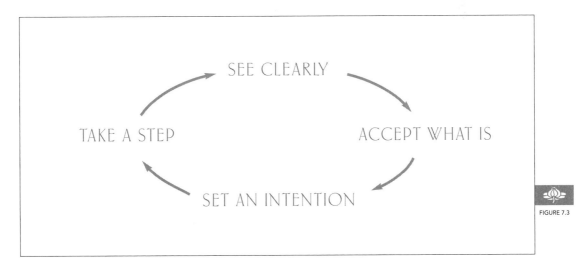

FIGURE 7.3

To effect change in your life, the yogic prescription is to cycle repeatedly through the four stages of noticing, accepting, planning, and acting.

SEE CLEARLY

To change dysfunctional patterns of behavior or thought that may be undermining your health and well-being, you first need to be aware of them. Future suffering, Patanjali taught, can be avoided. The key is to begin with accurate perception, or what yogis call "seeing what is."

> **TIP** Part of seeing clearly is to notice the way your mind resists establishing a consistent yoga practice. You'll find yourself coming up with a million reasons why you don't need to practice today, how you don't have the time, or really should do something else instead. Observe your mind as it attempts to bargain, but unless there is a truly compelling reason not to, practice anyway. One of the most powerful ways to establish tapas and to overcome bad habits is to do what's good for you even when you don't feel like it.

ACCEPT WHAT IS

You may not like what you see when you turn the spotlight on yourself and your patterns. That's okay. A willingness to acknowledge an uncomfortable reality is a huge step toward changing it. Your reality may be that you are stressed beyond the breaking point, your diet isn't good, you've got a self-defeating attitude, or you are seriously ill.

If you are ill, a fundamental reality you must confront is that you cannot control if you are going to get better—though you may well be able to improve your chances. When you accept that you cannot control what happens, it can relieve you of the tremendous burden of trying to control the uncontrollable, allowing your mind and nervous system to relax in a way that can actually increase your odds of recovery.

SET AN INTENTION

Sankalpa is the yogic tool of intention. Setting your mind on doing something, yogis believe, greatly increases the chances that it will happen. There is a subtle distinction between sankalpa, what you intend to do, and what you want to happen as a result. Thus "I intend to lose ten pounds this week," "I'm going to beat this cancer," and "I plan to be able to do Lotus pose" are desired outcomes, not intentions. They are what you hope will happen in the future, and yoga says you can't control that. What you have much more influence over is what you do.

To get off automatic pilot and get out of the ruts worn by powerful old samskaras, it helps to make a promise to yourself about what you plan to do, and keep reminding yourself of your pledge. Sankalpa is about planning, with as much specificity as possible, a course of action. Your intention might be to practice yoga for twenty minutes a day. It might be to cut down on junk food or spend more time with your kids. If you combine your intention with imagery, visualizing yourself doing what you intend, you may further increase the likelihood that it happens.

TAKE A STEP

There's a saying, "No farmer has ever hoed a field by turning it over in his mind." Yoga is not about theory. It's about what you do. To make progress, you must practice steadily. There is no other way. Regularity is more important than the length of each session. The more you can keep the practice up, the greater the fire you'll generate to strengthen your body and mind. That's tapas. It's the force that helps you overcome the samskaras that keep you stuck where you are.

 TIP Just as the journey of a thousand miles begins with a single step, so does yoga. B. K. S. Iyengar says, "Take a step, no matter how small." The only step you may be able to take today might be to get your yoga mat out and spread it on the floor. It might be a single Dog pose. Once you've really established your yoga groove, however, just taking these initial steps—even if you don't really feel like practicing—will probably be enough to get you going. I sit every morning for an hour of pranayama and meditation. Some days when I get up, I have no idea how I'm going to be able to make it for that long. But if I simply begin, I'm almost always able to complete the entire practice.

A Plan for Yoga for Life

Unless your health precludes practicing on your own, I suggest an experiment: commit to practice every day for one week and see what happens. Decide in advance how much time you intend to practice and write your intention in a notebook, which you can also use to record your observations about the effects of the practice.

Don't be too ambitious in your commitment. If you promise yourself that you're going to practice two hours a day and you don't, your failure to live up to your intention could end up being counterproductive. Better to start small and work your way up. For most people fifteen to twenty minutes a day is a realistic place to begin.

If you don't have a teacher guiding you when planning your practice, look over the practices described in this book and try to include some exercises that build tapas, such as

Dog pose or Sun Salutations, along with others that allow you to relax and experience calmness of the mind. When you set your intention, imagine exactly which practices you are going to do, the order you'll do them in, where you'll practice, and at what time of day.

If you are a complete novice at yoga and want to study with a teacher before getting started on a home practice—which is not a bad idea—start asking around for recommendations. Since finding a suitable teacher and getting an appointment could take a while, you could perhaps start out with few simple practices from this book and then modify what you're doing after you've had a professional evaluation.

At the end of your first week, I suggest you take stock. How did your experiment go? How often and for how long were you able to practice and how does that compare with your intention? If you've kept brief notes during the week, they can help jog your memory. Ask yourself whether you feel more relaxed after your yoga practice. More peaceful? Energized? Any other changes? If you weren't successful in practicing some days, what obstacles got in the way? Is there a way that you could anticipate such problems in the future and work around them?

Decide for yourself whether what you have seen so far is promising enough that you are ready to commit to the next step: establishing a daily practice for another predetermined span of time. My guess is that after one week, you'll notice enough change that you'll decide that committing to a month is worth it. If so, I suggest you go through a similar process and set an intention for how much time you'd be willing to commit to for the month. Perhaps you've seen enough benefit already that you want to increase your time to half an hour a day. Whatever feels right to you. Once again, though, be as specific as you can in setting your intention, and write it in your notebook. Keep building from there— week by week, month by month, setting your intention, recording the results, evaluating whether to continue.

At the end of a year, look back through what you've written, noting the regularity and amount of time you were able to practice, and any changes in symptoms or outlook you've experienced. Do you have lower levels of stress? Fewer headaches? Less stiffness? More patience with your kids? Almost everyone who gives yoga a serious try with a year of steady practice will stick with it. They find that life is so much better that no matter why they came to the practice, they don't want to give it up.

After a year of steady practice, your yoga groove will be well dug. With the yoga habit established, you may find other less beneficial grooves beginning to fade away. You may be eating a little better, taking more walks, or not getting as worked up if you get cut off in traffic. In all likelihood, you will continue to do yoga in some form or other for the rest of your life. If you give it up for a while, you'll probably find yourself missing it and coming back.

TIP Well-known in the yoga world are the students who come to yoga because of a health concern, take on the practice, get better, decide it's okay to stop practicing, and then have a relapse of symptoms. When patients ask Dr. Karandikar, who runs a huge yoga therapy center in Pune, how long they need to keep up their yoga practice, he responds with a question of his own: "How long do you need to keep brushing your teeth?" To avoid losing what you've gained, whenever possible, continue your yoga no matter how bad or how good you are feeling.

If the plan laid out above is more than you can commit to right now, that's okay. If you can only give five minutes a day to practice, do that. If all you can do right now is read a little of this book, okay, that's where you are. Maybe next week you'll do a couple of doorway stretches and maybe the month after that you'll start doing a five-minute Savasana a few times a week. Take the first step into yoga and it could take you on a much longer journey.

The path of yoga can transform your life. Yoga can improve your health, reduce bothersome symptoms, and as part of a broader plan, even reverse some medical conditions entirely. It can bring calmness of mind, help you discover a sense of purpose and a connection to the world around you, and improve the quality of your life in many, many ways— whether you are cured of what ails you or not. Establishing the kind of steady practice that can bring these benefits begins with a single step from wherever you are right now. Are you ready to take it?

PART THREE

YOGA THERAPY IN ACTION

The land of healing lies within, radiant with the happiness
that is blindly sought in a thousand outer directions.

—SWAMI VIVEKANANDA

ANXIETY AND PANIC ATTACKS

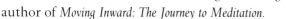 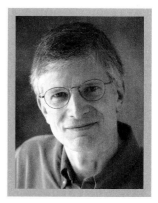

ROLF SOVIK began studying yoga with Swami Rama in the early 1970s. At his guru's suggestion, he pursued a doctorate in clinical psychology, writing a master's thesis comparing cognitive therapy to yoga, and completing a research project on the use of breathing in the treatment of anxiety. Rolf practices as a psychotherapist, teaches yoga, and with his wife, Mary Gail, is codirector of the Himalayan Institute of Buffalo, New York. He is the coauthor with Sandra Anderson of the book *Yoga: Mastering the Basics,* and author of *Moving Inward: The Journey to Meditation.*

Just over ten years ago, Graciella Rodriguez (not her real name) turned up in Rolf Sovik's class at the Himalayan Institute in search of relief from panic attacks and "a lot of anxiety." At that time, she was having panic attacks every couple of days, for no apparent reason. "I would feel a terrible sense of doom. I would break into a sweat, and I would think I was going to die because my heart would really hurt. I had terrible chest pain. It felt like a building was on me."

At one point, Graciella thought she was having a heart attack. She underwent a series of tests including a cardiac angiogram, in which a catheter is threaded into the small coronary arteries to check for blockages. Once the test showed her heart was fine, Graciella says, "I sort of thought to myself, this could be because I overthink." It was then that she decided to find out what yoga could offer.

Overview of Anxiety

Anxiety is a pervasive emotional problem. There is no one who doesn't have the feeling of anxiety at some point in their life. Says Rolf, "There is a 100 percent incidence." As inevitable as anxiety is for most of us, some people experience it with an intensity that can seriously undermine their health. Rolf alludes to stress management guru Robert Eliot's take on anger: "He used to say, 'Why become enraged when a little irritability will do?' You could say the same thing about anxiety: why become terrified when a little nervousness will do?"

When anxiety spirals out of control and becomes more than "a little nervousness," it can cause debilitating symptoms, including obsessive thinking, insomnia, migraines, intestinal problems, dizziness, nausea, shortness of breath, and heart palpitations. Full-fledged panic attacks like Graciella's are an extreme form of anxiety. As you can see, anxiety experienced with that much intensity can drastically undermine your quality of life—and your health and well-being.

For example, excessive worry appears to undermine the ability to heal. A recent study showed that people suffering from the autoimmune skin condition psoriasis, which causes large scaly red plaques on the skin, took twice as long—an additional nineteen days—to respond to ultraviolet light therapy if they worried a lot. Conversely, another study found that when psoriasis patients listened to guided meditation tapes while undergoing UV treatments they improved much more quickly.

Another problem, according to Rolf, is that anxiety can be so consuming that you focus only on the symptoms of anxiety but lose sight of the root cause. If you lose track of what's causing your anxiety, it becomes much more difficult to take action to alleviate it. Of course, there are some sources of anxiety over which you have no control. So yes, an asteroid could indeed strike the planet and wipe out humankind—but worrying about the possibility can only make you miserable, and there is absolutely nothing you can do about it.

Other times, anxiety can actually serve a function. If there is a genuine danger, then thinking about it and how you might either avoid it or respond to it could save your life. Anxiety is a useful emotion insofar as it helps you make better choices for how to live. Thinking obsessively about the same problem when it doesn't bring any further insight and makes you more miserable serves no purpose.

How Yoga Fits In

Yoga can help with anxiety in a number of ways. It offers specific techniques that can reduce symptoms, both in the short and longer term. Because of its focus on tuning in to inward states, yoga can also help you get beneath the surface of anxiety to figure out what might be triggering it, such as unresolved conflicts or habitual thought patterns.

One of the key yogic techniques used to counter anxiety is to focus on the breath. Perhaps nowhere is the connection between the mind and the breath more obvious than in anxiety. During anxious or fearful moments, breathing is disturbed in a wide variety of ways. It may become quick and choppy, rigid and constricted, or even stop altogether for periods of time. When you are calm, on the other hand, breathing tends to be smooth and rhythmic.

 TIP Some people who are anxious or depressed have the sense that they can't take a full breath. Yoga teaches that one way to improve the inhalation is to focus on the exhalation. By learning to engage the abdominal muscles to gently squeeze a little more air out with each exhalation, you will be able to take in a deeper, more satisfying breath.

Anxious breathing occurs disproportionately in the upper chest, and doesn't fully engage the diaphragm, the large sheet of muscle separating the chest cavity from the abdominal organs. When the diaphragm contracts, it descends, creating more space in the chest and lowering the pressure in the lungs so that they can draw in more air (see chapter 3). Yogis sometimes use the shorthand "chest breathing" to describe rapid, shallow breaths and "abdominal breathing" to indicate the slower, deeper breaths in which the diaphragm moves more freely.

If you have been predominantly a chest breather, you will benefit from yoga's emphasis on breathing in a deeper, slower, more relaxed manner, although it may prove challenging at first. Rolf believes that in most cases, including Graciella's, people with anxiety have developed a chronic form of muscle restriction affecting the abdominal muscles that encircle the belly. When these muscles tighten from tension (or from the habit of holding in the belly to look thinner), the belly can't move freely and breathing is impaired. Another area of chronic tightness in people with anxiety that restricts breathing is in the intercostal muscles, which lie between the ribs. Whatever the cause of muscular tension, it may take a while to learn to release it and enjoy the benefits of fuller breath, but the practices designed by Rolf for Graciella show how that can be done.

From a yogic point of view, optimal breathing is deep, smooth, quiet, and even, without significant pauses. The diaphragm should be engaged, while so-called accessory muscles of respiration, such as those in the neck and chest, should remain quiet, except when you bring in a larger-than-usual volume of air. In general, both the inhalation and exhalation should be through the nose.

The breath is the one automatic function of the body that you can readily take over with conscious effort. And controlling the breath turns out to be the entry point to calming down an overactive stress response system. By breathing through the nose on exhalation, the exhalation is lengthened and the respiratory rate is slowed (because the nasal passages are narrower than the mouth and offer more resistance to airflow), both actions that tend to promote calmness of mind. Rapid, anxious breathing, on the other hand, serves to further activate the sympathetic nervous system, causing the release of stress hormones, increasing agitation (see chapter 3). When you breathe quickly, you expel more carbon dioxide from the system, and this, too, tends to put you more on edge, thus contributing to the vicious cycle of agitation, rapid breathing, and more agitation. One of the major fruits of sustained yoga practice is a spontaneous reduction in the breathing rate, even during periods where you are making no conscious effort to control the breath. While twelve to twenty breaths per minute is considered normal, experienced yoga practitioners often breathe at half that rate. The longer you practice, the more ingrained yogic breathing becomes and the calmer your mind.

 TIP If you have trouble breathing through your nose due to nasal congestion, try using a neti pot once or twice per day to rinse your nasal passages with warm salt water. While the idea may be anxiety provoking at first, once mastered, the technique (see pp. 80–81) becomes pleasant and soothing.

Beyond awareness of your breath, yoga also teaches awareness of thought patterns. You may, for example, be able to recognize the first glimmers of anxiety that could turn into a full-fledged panic attack, and detect them early enough that you could intervene with a relaxing breathing technique. Another useful technique when troubling thoughts crop up, recommended by Patanjali in the *Yoga Sutras,* is to cultivate the opposite thought. This might mean turning your focus from your anxieties to what you are grateful for or what you can do for others. But yoga, like cognitive therapy, also asks you to acknowledge such negative thoughts and look honestly at what is, so that you can understand whether you are contributing to a bad situation through your behavior or thought patterns. This kind of reality testing is what differentiates yoga from mere "positive thinking."

Part of what yoga can do for anxiety has to do with slowing down the rush of thoughts, the so-called monkey mind we discussed in chapter 3. When you do yogic relaxation—which uses a variety of tools including asana, breathing, and heightened awareness of internal and external states—it facilitates detaching from those thoughts long enough to begin to see them more clearly. Your mind becomes relaxed but not dull, tuned in yet disengaged from your normal relationship to the outer world. Rolf finds that achieving this kind of relaxation is far from easy at first, but that over time it becomes "the insulator that changes the character of anxiety altogether."

Yoga's inherently holistic approach teaches that a multitude of factors can affect anxiety levels. To summarize very briefly: Poor breathing is both a cause and a result of stress, and there are many breathing practices within yoga that can deepen and improve the breath. If poor breathing is partly the result of a slouching posture or tension in the lower abdominal muscles then, of course, various yoga postures can help correct those problems. Gratitude, a quality that tends to arise spontaneously with the regular practice of yoga, helps diminish anxiety. The yogic principle of Ishvara pranidhana, surrendering to the universe or, as I like to think of it, giving up the illusion of control, another by-product of yoga practice, is also calming. The heightened awareness your body gains through yoga may allow you to make connections between your emotional state and the foods you eat, the music you listen to, the books you read, and the people with whom you share your life. Yoga helps you learn to trust the messages from the body and mind, and fuels the tapas (discipline, fire) to act on them when necessary.

Finally, engaging in a yoga practice can also provide a sense of hope, according to Rolf, because you discover that there is a technology you can employ to change your situation. The hope created by your practice can grow over time as you continue the practice, because just as anxious thoughts can dig deep grooves (samskaras), a steady practice and the change in attitude that accompany it can also deepen with repetition. This ancient yogic idea of samskaras is now finding confirmation in the latest findings of neuroscience, but instead of expressing this idea in terms of grooves, scientists talk about how repeated firings of neurons change the wiring of the brain. Change your wiring and you change your mind.

The Scientific Evidence

Rolf Sovik points to a number of studies to show that yogic breathing is an effective method of combating anxiety. Voluntarily slowing the breathing during a period of stress counters a number of physiological components of stress while reducing feelings of anxiety. Increasing the length of exhalation relative to inhalation has similar effects. Training in relaxed, diaphragmatic breathing reduces the frequency of panic attacks.

A 1973 double-blind controlled study, published in the *American Journal of Psychotherapy*, was conducted by N. Vahia and colleagues on twenty-seven psychiatric patients aged fifteen to fifty years old who suffered anxiety and who had not responded to earlier treatments. The results showed that a combination of asana, pranayama, and meditation significantly reduced anxiety as measured by the Taylor Manifest Anxiety Scale. Of note, the combination of asana and pranayama was even more effective when concentration exercises and meditation were also included. Another small study by the same authors found that yoga was significantly more effective in relieving anxiety than tranquilizers.

In a 1991 study done as part of a doctoral dissertation for Penn State University, J. M. Harrigan compared yoga postures with and without diaphragmatic breathing exercises to breathing exercises alone. The subjects took a thirty-minute class twice a week for six weeks and were asked to practice half an hour per day on their own. When the postures were done without attention to the breath (which many yogis consider essential), there was no significant reduction in anxiety as compared to a control group which only heard lectures. The group who only did diaphragmatic breathing had a significant reduction in anxiety. The best response was seen in the group that did the postures combined with diaphragmatic breathing. As in the study cited above, this points out the synergistic effects of different aspects of yoga practice.

In a study of forty children and adolescents hospitalized in psychiatric wards, researchers from the University of Miami and Duke University Medical Schools found that a single hour-long session of relaxation therapy reduced anxiety. The intervention, which included asana and guided meditation, resulted in significant reductions in self-reported anxiety as well as in such anxious behavior as fidgeting. Reductions in cortisol levels in the saliva were also noted in most subjects. No reduction in anxiety was seen among a control group of twenty subjects who watched a relaxing video.

In Germany, Dr. Andreas Michalsen of the University of Duisburg-Essen and colleagues studied twenty-four women with anxiety, comparing a three-month program of Iyengar yoga to a control group placed on a waiting list. The two weekly ninety-minute classes emphasized backbends, forward bends, standing poses, and inversions. Compared to the eight controls, the sixteen women in the yoga group demonstrated "pronounced and significant improvements" in perceived stress, anxiety, well-being, vigor, fatigue, and depression. Of note, those in the yoga group who reported headaches or back pain noted "marked pain relief." Salivary cortisol decreased significantly after taking a yoga class.

A study by Dr. Jon Kabat-Zinn, founder of the Stress Reduction Clinic at the University of Massachusetts Medical Center, and colleagues found that an eight-week mindfulness meditation-based stress-reduction program that included yoga asanas significantly reduced feelings of anxiety, depression, and panic in twenty of twenty-two patients diagnosed with generalized anxiety disorder and panic disorder. These results were maintained in the eighteen patients the researchers were able to recheck three years after completion of the program, the majority of whom were still practicing on their own.

It's worth noting that another study by Kabat-Zinn found that patients whose anxiety manifested mainly in mental symptoms like constant worrying tended to find hatha yoga preferable to mindfulness meditation, whereas those whose symptoms of anxiety tended to manifest mainly in the body preferred the less body-oriented meditation. As Jon says, "people need different doors to come into the room, so to speak, of self-awareness and self-knowing. Some people just can't go through the mind door. They get the body door instantly." For others the opposite is true.

Rolf Sovik's Approach

While the practice described below was developed specifically for Graciella, many of its elements have proved useful to other students who have come to Rolf with anxiety and other stress-related health conditions.

When Graciella first began classes it was apparent to Rolf that she was having difficulty with breath awareness and relaxation. She was restless during the relaxation, and her breathing was not smooth. More important, restrictions in her breathing seemed to remain outside her awareness. Although she was not particularly symptomatic at that time, Graciella also had a long history of asthma, which was another reason she had sought out yoga instruction.

Rolf felt that good breathing was key to dealing with Graciella's anxiety problem. But during her initial exposure to the breathing practices that Rolf gave her, she told him that trying to shift attention to her breathing frustrated her and made her even more anxious. So Rolf created an approach designed to take the emphasis off the mechanics of breathing and instead teach her to undo the muscle tensions that block a smooth respiratory rhythm. He also wanted to strengthen her diaphragm which, he believes, the first exercise below is particularly good at doing.

Here is the sequence of the practices and instructions that Rolf provided for Graciella:

EXERCISE #1. **SANDBAG BREATHING, five to ten minutes.** Set up for Deep Relaxation pose (Savasana) by placing a blanket or cushion under your head so that it supports the arch of your neck more than the back of your head (figure 8.1). When you are settled, begin to focus on your breathing. Soften your abdomen, and feel it rise with your inhalation and descend with your exhalation. Then, when the flow of your breath is well established, place a ten-pound sandbag or another item (such as bag of rice or beans) of the same weight on your upper abdomen. This provides what Rolf calls "weight training for the abdomen." As you breathe in, gently lift the bag using your diaphragm, not by pushing your abdominal muscles out. As you exhale, the weight of the sandbag will tend to push the air quickly out of your lungs. So consciously slow down your exhalation, trying to make it equal in length to your inhalation. After completing the exercise, remove the sandbag but remain where you are for another minute or two, observing any differences in your experience of breathing.

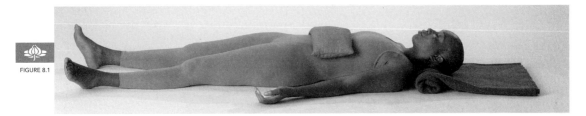

FIGURE 8.1

Rolf asked Graciella to practice sandbag breathing for five minutes and gradually increase the time to ten minutes. He recommends practicing it for three days on, one day off, for one month, and then stopping for good. Once you've done this exercise for a month, according to Rolf, you can maintain the strength gains simply by including twists and mild inversions, such as the ones below, in your regular yoga practice.

EXERCISE #2. **CROCODILE BREATHING (Makrasana), six to ten minutes.** Lie on your belly with your legs a comfortable distance apart. Turn your toes either in or out, whichever is more comfortable. Fold your arms, placing each hand on the opposite elbow, and rest your forehead on your forearms (figure 8.2).

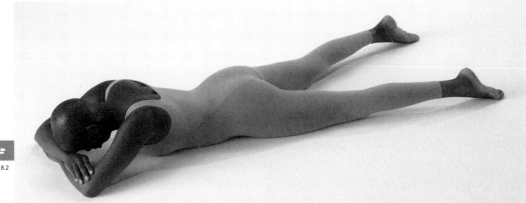

FIGURE 8.2

Rolf's five-step approach to Crocodile Breathing is:

Step 1: Bring your awareness to your breath as it flows out and in. As your breath flows out, feel how your breath empties, how the exhalation cleanses and releases tension. As your breath flows in, feel how your breath fills you, how the inhalation nourishes you and restores fresh energy. Continue watching the flow of your breath, feeling it empty and then fill you again.

Step 2: While you're feeling the flow of your breath, gently soften your navel region, allowing your abdomen to relax.

Step 3: Notice that as you inhale, your abdomen gently expands, and as you exhale, your abdomen slowly contracts.

Step 4: When you come to the end of your inhalation, simply relax and exhale. In the same way, when you come to the end of your exhalation, simply relax and inhale. Let each breath flow slowly and smoothly into the next, without a conscious pause.

Step 5: Observe the smooth and unbroken flow of your breathing. Like a wheel turning over and over, the breath flows out and in, and you are the witness of your own breath.

OTHER YOGIC IDEAS

A number of breathing practices, taught in a variety of yogic traditions, can help calm the mind. Among the simplest and most useful is a 1:2 ratio of inhalation to exhalation. If you normally inhale for three seconds, for example, see if you can slow the exhale to six seconds while inhaling at your usual pace. As with all yogic breathing exercises, you should never feel any shortness of breath or discomfort while prolonging the exhalation. If you do, immediately return to your normal rate of breathing.

EXERCISE #3. **SIDE STRETCHES.** For the first stage, stand with your feet a little wider than hips' width apart, hands on your hips, and gently tip the pelvis from side to side. See if you can feel the stretch down through the inner thigh muscles (the adductors). For the

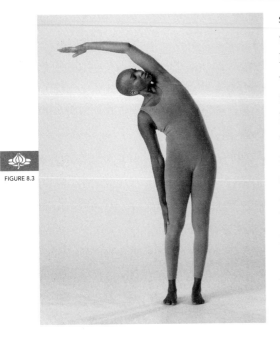

FIGURE 8.3

second stage, try to deepen the stretch through the torso as you bend more deeply to each side. If you are bending to the right, the right hand will end up somewhere near the right knee. In the third stage, lengthen the opposite arm and bring it up and alongside the head, allowing the weight of the arm to increase the stretch a bit more (figure 8.3). Inhale as you lift and exhale as you lower, moving from side to side and coordinating the movement with the feeling of breathing. This stretches the sides of the torso, including the intercostal muscles between the ribs, which need to open for the fullest expression of the breath. After moving side to side, stay on one side for four to ten breaths, then repeat on the other side.

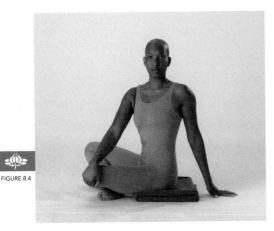

FIGURE 8.4

EXERCISE #4. **CROSS-LEGGED TWIST (Parsvasukhasana).** Start by sitting in a simple cross-legged posture, with a cushion or folded blanket underneath your hips to lift your pelvis off the floor. Exhale and twist to the left, taking your right hand to the left knee and your left arm behind (see figure 8.4). Inhale and return to center. Repeat on the other side, and go back and forth several times, moving with your breath. Keep your spine erect and your breath flowing smoothly throughout the repetitions.

CAUTION Twisting asana restrict the movement of the breath into the abdomen and make it a little more difficult to breathe, which can increase feelings of anxiety. However, if you can learn to do these poses with equanimity, an example of what Rolf calls "breathing in a tight spot," it can be part of the remedy for anxious feelings in other situations.

After warming up the spine with this exercise, hold the pose for four to eight breaths on each side. Rolf suggests placing a block under the back hand to help your arm relax. Use your arms to help stabilize the pose and encourage spinal lengthening, not to artificially pull you deeper into the twist (which could cause injury).

EXERCISE #5. **HALF SPINAL TWIST (Ardha Matsyendrasana), six to twelve breaths.** Start by sitting in a simple cross-legged posture. Bend your right leg over the left thigh and place the right heel alongside the left hip. Wrap your left arm around the bent knee and rest your right hand on the floor or a block behind you. Before twisting, Rolf believes that it's helpful to inhale and contract the pelvic floor then exhale and relax it, getting a

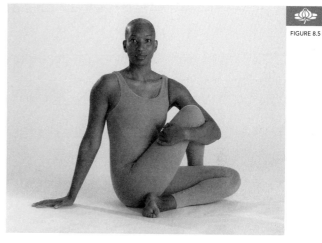
FIGURE 8.5

sense that these muscles are going to be involved in the twist and helping to create stability at the base of the pelvis. As you move into the pose, imagine that the twisting movement starts from the pelvic floor. After twisting the abdomen, rib cage, and shoulders, in that order, gently turn the neck and head. Hold the pose on each side for six to twelve breaths, softening your gaze and trying to relax into the pose (figure 8.5).

EXERCISE #6. **SUPPORTED LEGS-UP-THE-WALL POSE (Viparita Karani), thirty to ninety seconds.** Set up for the pose by placing a bolster, a cushion, or a stack of two folded blankets about six inches away from a wall. To come into the pose, sit toward one end of the bolster with your side facing the wall, press your hands down onto the bolster to hold it in place (a folded sticky mat placed underneath the bolster will also help keep it from moving), and swing your legs up and onto the wall. Once you're up, scoot your pelvis into place on the bolster so that just the bottom of your tailbone is hanging off the bolster (your pelvis

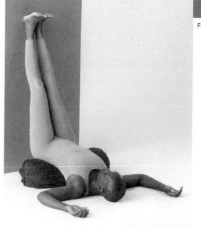
FIGURE 8.6

will be in a slight backbend). Make sure that your weight is on your shoulders and your hips, and that your head and neck are soft and relaxed (figure 8.6). Rolf says that because this pose is a mild inversion, it allows you to get used to the idea of being upside down, and to the resulting changes in blood pressure and breath dynamics. It normally takes a little more effort to breathe in inversions. Rolf asked Graciella to start out holding this pose for thirty seconds and over time slowly work up to ninety seconds.

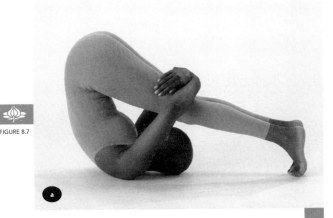

FIGURE 8.7

EXERCISE #7. ROCKING CHAIR POSE, ten to twenty repetitions. Start by sitting up straight, with your knees bent and your hands underneath your thighs. On an inhalation, round your lower back, rock back onto your shoulders (not onto your neck), and straighten your legs (figure 8.7a). On your exhalation, keeping your lower back rounded, rock forward and bend your knees (figure 8.7b). Repeat ten to twenty times, maintaining the roundness of your lower back while using your legs to bring you backward and forward. Rolf says that this pose helps you to invert your body without any support, and is a good massage for your spine.

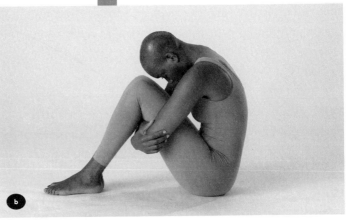

EXERCISE #8. SUPPORTED SHOULDERSTAND (Salamba Sarvangasana), with feet on the wall, thirty to ninety seconds. Set up for the pose by placing a folded blanket near the wall for your shoulders to rest on. To come into the pose, sit on the floor, facing the wall, and move your hips close to the wall. Raise your legs onto the wall, bend your knees, and place the soles of your feet on the wall. Using your feet to bear your weight, press down into your back, rock your pelvis, and come up onto your shoulders, with your feet on the wall and your weight resting on your feet and the backs of your shoulders. Your head and neck should be soft and bearing no weight. Release your arms underneath your torso. In this version of Shoulderstand, your torso is not completely vertical; it's tilted fifteen to twenty degrees (figure 8.8). Start by holding this pose for thirty seconds and over time slowly work up to ninety seconds.

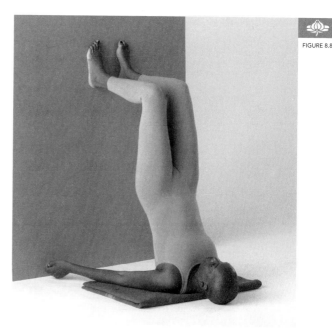

FIGURE 8.8

EXERCISE #9. **STANDING BALANCING.** Start by standing with your arms out to the sides as if you were walking a tightrope. Shift your weight to one leg and lift your other foot off the ground, just far enough that you are balancing (figure 8.9). If you need to, you can bring your toes back down to find your balance. The purpose here is to get a sense of the wobbling that occurs in your ankle joint when you try to balance that enables you to do so. Once you've got the feeling for how that shifting back and forth leads to balance, it's easier to move into the next balancing pose, and the many other yoga poses that rely on balance. Stay in the pose long enough to balance but not so long that you are likely to lose your balance. If you do, come right back into the pose so that you can practice coming down in a more controlled fashion. Repeat on the other side.

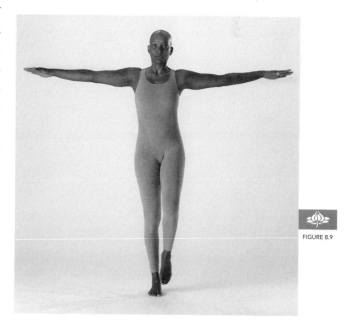

FIGURE 8.9

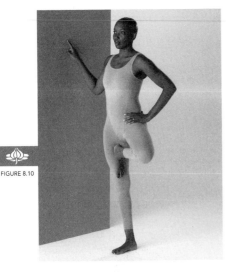

FIGURE 8.10

EXERCISE #10. **TREE POSE (Vrksasana).** Start by standing with your right side near a wall and one of the fingers of your right hand touching the wall. Next bend your left leg and press your left foot against the inside of your right thigh (and your right thigh against your left foot). If you can't press your right foot against your thigh, try pressing it against your shin, just above the ankle (it's hard to hold the leg up halfway). As soon as you feel balanced and confident, try taking your finger away from the wall, knowing you can put it back at any moment. As much as possible, keep your hips square to the front, allowing your hips and knees to open (figure 8.10). Repeat on the other side.

EXERCISE #11. **DEEP RELAXATION POSE (Savasana), five to ten minutes.** Set up for the pose by placing a folded blanket or cushion underneath your head to support your head and neck (figure 8.11). Lie back with your head on the support, so your chin tilts toward your chest. Roll your legs open and turn your palms up, with your arms a comfortable distance from your body. If you like, you can cover yourself with a blanket to keep you warm while you relax. Some people who are anxious may feel vulnerable and exposed in this pose, and being covered can be comforting. When you are comfortable, begin to observe your breath. (For an in-depth discussion of Savasana, see pp. 59–61.)

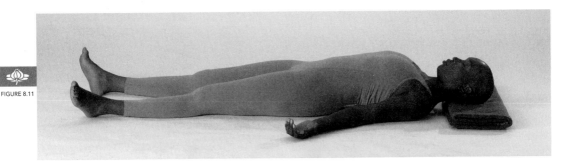

FIGURE 8.11

"For someone experiencing anxiety, relaxation is like aspirin," says Rolf, "a pill that you can take regularly." He's had people with panic attacks practice Deep Relaxation pose up to six times a day. Every two or three hours they lie down for five to ten minutes in Savasana, just observing the flow of the breath.

After several months Rolf added a seated meditation practice to Graciella's regimen.

EXERCISE #12. **SITTING MEDITATION, ten minutes.** Sit in any comfortable seated position. If your legs, hips, or back are tight, use plenty of cushioning. For example, if you sit in a cross-legged position on the floor, place cushions or folded blankets under your hips as well as your legs (figure 8.12). If you prefer to kneel on a bench, to sit up in a straight-backed chair, or even to lean back in a soft reclining chair, that's fine. What is important is that there is no anxiety or discomfort caused by your posture, so that your focus can remain internal. When you are comfortably seated, bring your awareness to the feeling of the breath touching inside your nostrils, and focus on this sensation.

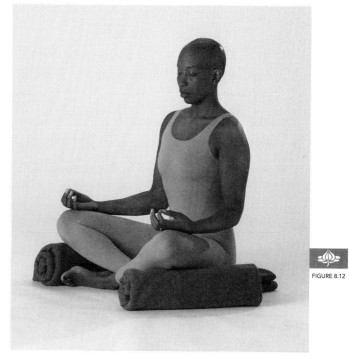

FIGURE 8.12

After some time, you can add the mantra "so ham" ("so" is said silently with the inhalation and "ham"—pronounced "hum"—is said silently with the exhalation). "The intent," Rolf says, "is not to drown other thoughts in a tumult of mantra repetitions, but to rest in the sound of the mantra while being aware of other thoughts as they travel through your mind."

He usually suggests starting with a six- to eight-minute relaxation lying down, followed by at least ten minutes of seated meditation. It's ideal to practice twice a day for eighteen to twenty minutes, he believes, but he also realizes not everyone can manage this.

> **TIP** Some people quit meditation before giving it a real chance to work because they believe they aren't good at it. The biggest problem, Rolf says, is that people believe that the goal of meditation is to make the mind empty. They have the impression that their minds should become blank in some way and that their worries should be replaced by that blankness. But, Rolf says, "It will never happen. The process of meditating is a process of replacing anxiety and distractions with a relaxed focus. Inevitably, distractions and anxiety coexist with that relaxed focus." But relatively quickly, he says, the person who is meditating gains distance from the anxiety and distracted thoughts and will relax even more deeply.

A Holistic Approach to Anxiety and Panic Attacks

* Depression, alcohol abuse, diabetes, and thyroid disease, among other conditions, can cause anxiety and should be ruled out or treated.

* If significant anger or a low level of self-esteem is part of your symptoms, you may have an underlying depression and may benefit from consulting with a physician or psychotherapist.

* Psychotherapy can be an important tool for anxiety. The combination of therapy and drugs or therapy and yoga is likely to be more effective than either alone.

* Although tranquilizers in the Valium family are often prescribed for anxiety, due to side effects including drowsiness and addiction, when drugs are needed, most experts favor antidepressants such as Prozac (fluoxetine) or Zoloft (sertraline).

* News reports, particularly television news, can fuel anxiety. Instead of watching the news for half an hour a day, do yoga instead and see if you feel better.

* Rolf suggests cutting back on processed foods, junk food, and chemicals that increase the activation of your nervous system. In particular, he advises reducing or eliminating caffeine, sugar, alcohol, and nicotine. Rolf also favors well-cooked as opposed to raw foods in people with anxiety, advice in line with Ayurvedic thinking (see chapter 4).

* The omega-3 fatty acids found in some deepwater fish and in flaxseed oil appear to reduce anxiety.

* German chamomile, tincture of passion flower, supplemental B vitamins, and magnesium are safe remedies that appear to have antianxiety properties. Aromatherapy with such fragrances as lavender has been shown to be calming.

* Other measures to combat anxiety include acupuncture and regular aerobic exercise.

Contraindications, Special Considerations, and Modifications

People who have been in prolonged states of anxiety can reach a state of vital exhaustion. These people may only become more depleted if they take on an overly strenuous yoga practice too soon. Vigorous Sun Salutations, intense standing poses with long holds, and working in a hot and humid room may all be inappropriate. The rule of thumb is first recharge your batteries, then ramp up the intensity of your practice. Standard restorative postures are not always appropriate at first either. "Someone who comes in who's extremely anxious may not respond very well to rejuvenating and propped poses," says Rolf. "They lie there wired with their eyes wide open, waiting for you to give them some sort of instruction."

Active relaxation, such as Yoga Nidra (see chapter 3), where a teacher or a recording guides the student, may keep the roaming mind quieter and more focused than complete silence. Inversions can also play an important role in calming the mind, but there are some special considerations for people with anxiety. Rolf says that when people first attempt inverted poses of almost any kind, they will experience a feeling of pressure in the head. Some people with anxiety, he says, don't respond well to that sensation. If that's the case, he suggests starting with less intense inversions like Bridge pose or Legs-Up-the-Wall which don't lift the body as high, and as a result generate less head pressure. He also tries to reassure anxious students that if they allow themselves to be in the pose for a little while, the pressure will turn into a feeling of fullness which they will find enjoyable. "But if you're resisting the pose out of anxiety," he says, "your fixation on the pressure may mean it won't change."

Some asana and pranayama practices may not work well for those with anxiety. Backbends, which tend to be energizing, will sometimes make people with anxiety even more anxious. However, learning to do backbends with gentle breathing and a sattvic, or balanced and peaceful, state of mind can be an effective tool to combat anxiety. Including a number of quieting practices after backbends to calm the nervous system is also useful. Similarly, any practice which prolongs inhalation or which focuses on breathing through the right nostril may prompt agitation (see p. 62). Generally it's better to focus on lengthening the exhalation or keeping inhalation and exhalation even. For people who tend to slip into an overly anxious or dark state when attempting pranayama, meditation, or even Savasana, one solution is to keep the eyes open throughout the entire practice.

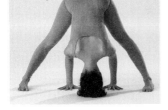

OTHER YOGIC IDEAS

In Iyengar yoga, a number of poses are used as part of the treatment of anxiety. Postures in which the head is gently supported, such as Wide-Legged Standing Forward Bend (Prasarita Padottanasana), are considered particularly calming. If your head does not reach the ground when bending forward, use a block, blanket, bolster, or other prop to support the crown of your head or you may lose the "brain-quieting" effects.

Yoga has proved to be tremendously helpful to Graciella. "If it wasn't for yoga, for breath awareness, and being able to quell my anxieties," she says, "I don't know where I would be." On medication, she assumes.

The practice also appears to have helped her asthma. Over the years, Graciella had needed various drugs for her asthma, including theophylline, albuterol, and steroid inhalers. In the time since she's been doing yoga regularly her asthma symptoms have all but disappeared and she currently takes no medication for it.

Some of the benefits of yoga were less expected. After Graciella began to practice regularly, she says, her body felt more fluid. "In doing the asanas I felt that finally some sort of grace was coming my way." She also noted a major improvement in her posture. Now her family tells her that she's got a completely new body.

It hasn't all been easy. At first she felt claustrophobic facedown in Makrasana. Meditation was a particular challenge but she now believes meditating has helped her more than anything to deal with the emotional issues that may have fueled her anxiety.

Graciella does about an hour a day of asana and another half hour of meditation and breathwork. Although she tries to practice every day, she is not always successful. When she misses even a single day, though, she notices a huge difference in her energy level and her mental clarity.

Yoga has also given her the courage to tackle new challenges. In an attempt to make the best of a climate far harsher than her native South America, just after beginning her yoga studies with Rolf, Graciella learned to ski. In the beginning, she would get mild panic attacks on the slopes. She was fortunate to have an instructor who recognized what was going on. Graciella laughs when she tells the story. "He would say to me, 'Can we do some breathing, please?' If it wasn't for the yoga, I don't think I would have been able to do it."

ARTHRITIS

MARIAN GARFINKEL first met her teacher, B. K. S. Iyengar, in 1974, and has been traveling to India annually to study with him ever since. She was so impressed with the master's work with people suffering from a variety of health conditions that she was inspired to conduct scientific studies of his approach. Marian is best known for her randomized controlled trial, published in the *Journal of the American Medical Association (JAMA)* in 1998, which showed the benefits of the specifically adapted program of Iyengar yoga that she created for people with carpal tunnel syndrome (see p. 230). Eight years before that, for her doctoral thesis in health education at Temple University, she conducted a study demonstrating the effectiveness of Iyengar yoga for arthritis of the hands and finger joints, which was later published in the *Journal of Rheumatology*. She continues to teach, research, lecture, and perform and publish clinical trials at the University of Pennsylvania Medical School and at Temple University. She is also the founder and director of, and teaches at, the B. K. S. Iyengar Yoga Studio of Philadelphia.

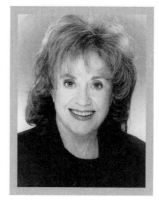

Liz McDonough (not her real name) came to see Marian Garfinkel because of problems she was having with her knees. She'd been taking yoga classes for several years, but the pain in her knees, which had been worsening even after she had surgery to correct it, led her to seek treatment in private session with Marian. Liz had been a competitive runner for most of her life and now, in her early fifties, it appeared to be catching up with her. Three years earlier she'd been diagnosed with degenerative arthritis (osteoarthritis) of both knees. A year earlier, she'd undergone arthroscopic surgery on her right knee, which had reduced her pain, but only for a while. Most of the time, even everyday activities such as walking pained her. Liz had particular trouble going up and down steps.

Overview of Arthritis

There are many varieties of arthritis. By far the most common form is osteoarthritis (OA), the wear-and-tear kind that often affects the joints in the back, neck, hips, fingers, or, as in Liz's case, the knees. In a healthy joint, a well-lubricated lining of cartilage covers the ends of bones, allowing them to slide smoothly over one another. In a joint affected by osteoarthritis, the protective cartilage is damaged and worn down, allowing bone to rub painfully on bone. Genetic factors, old sports injuries, bad postural habits, the kind of work you do—all can play a role in damaging the cartilage. Among the elderly, OA of the knee leads to more chronic disability than any other medical condition.

Less common but potentially more serious is rheumatoid arthritis (RA), an auto-immune inflammatory disease that leads to redness and swelling of joints, and if left unchecked can result in major joint deformities. Whereas degenerative arthritis affects men and women more or less equally, women are far more likely to develop RA, and it often comes on at a far earlier age. There are several other inflammatory forms of arthritis, such as those associated with lupus and with the skin disease psoriasis, in which the joint damage more closely resembles that in RA than OA.

How Yoga Fits In

Yoga is particularly well suited to help prevent or minimize the erosion of cartilage that causes the joint pain of osteoarthritis, and to create greater ease of movement and decrease pain within joints that have already sustained such damage. From a yogic perspective, most of the factors that are responsible for the damage to cartilage are related to how the body sits, stands, and moves through space. Misalignment of bones, dysfunctional movement patterns, lack of body awareness, poor posture—all of these overlapping and interconnected factors can cause wear and tear on the cartilage, and all of them are problems that yoga can help correct. Yoga is also ideally suited to deal with stress, which is believed to be a factor in the worsening of symptoms in both OA and RA. And for those people whose arthritis is severe, yoga can teach them how to cope better with pain that they cannot eliminate entirely. Experienced meditators, for example, appear to be able to modulate their reaction to pain. They may still have the discomfort, but are less bothered by it.

The painful rubbing of bone on bone that occurs when cartilage wears down is often the result of misalignment that the average doctor has little idea how to correct. Such misalignments can be the result of unconsciously holding in some muscles, the failure to engage other muscles, dysfunctional patterns of use, and unusually shaped bones. (Two of these misalignments are so well known, and so obvious, that the names for them are part of colloquial speech: bowlegged and knock-kneed.) An experienced yoga teacher can help deal with misalignments, first by being knowledgeable and observant enough to identify them, and then by being skillful enough to help the student readjust so that there is less stress on the joints. In therapeutic yoga you learn to actively engage the muscles that can help realign the bony parts of the joints. Marian Garfinkel describes what she does to help students with arthritis as "trying to create space in the joint, so the bones can move more readily."

Yogis like to say that everything is connected, and nowhere is this more obvious than in the case of anatomy. The hip bone really is connected to the thigh bone, which is in turn connected to the knee joint, so it's no surprise that how you move your hips will ultimately affect what happens in your knee. A skilled yoga therapist sees these connections and understands how movement in one joint might affect movement in another. If you have a knee problem, a yoga therapist might focus on increasing the range of motion in your hips. And because even seemingly distant areas of the body are linked, you might also be taught to open up the spaces between your toes and ground the feet more fully during standing poses, as a way of helping not just with knee pain but with back and neck problems, too.

Yoga can also help you become aware of habitual misalignments and patterns of movement that may contribute to problems in the future, or worsen problems you already have. Unless you have a background in dance or some other discipline that builds body awareness, you probably have little sense of what your knees are doing when you walk, sit, or stand—how, for example, the kneecaps track when you bend and straighten your knee joint along a certain axis of movement. If you don't realize you are moving in a potentially injurious way, you could continue to do so for many years, digging deeper behavioral grooves, samskaras, which manifest on the cartilage and ultimately on the bones themselves. A good asana practice can help you become aware of maladaptive patterns and start to change them. Yoga can get you out of an unhealthy groove, literally and figuratively.

While it may not seem obvious, poor posture is another samskara that can contribute greatly to knee problems like Liz's, to degeneration of the vertebral joints in the lower back and neck, and to many other problems from the head to the toes, quite literally. Yoga is, of course, one of the most effective ways to improve posture ever invented. If, for example, you normally stand with your shoulders slumped and your head held several inches in front of your spine—a postural habit common to most people who sit at a desk all day—you are putting excessive pressure on the joints in the lower body (see pp. 32–35). Postural changes and chest-opening poses like backbends can slowly correct the problem.

Yoga exercises its effects on posture partly through bringing awareness to formerly unconscious postural habits and to their consequences. Yoga practitioners may notice, for example, that even standing with the phone cradled to their neck puts pressure on the knee joint. (If this seems far-fetched, try it out and see if you notice any sensation of compression on the outside surface of the knee on the side you're leaning toward.) Such awareness allows you to make corrections before more significant damage is done.

Another way yoga can help arthritis is by keeping people moving. Although people with arthritis tend to avoid using sore joints because of the pain involved, evidence suggests that inactivity weakens muscles and further reduces movement in the joints (causing what doctors refer to as "decreased range of motion"), so that a vicious cycle is set in motion: pain leads to restricted movement; lack of movement causes the muscles to become both weak and tight, leading to further misalignment of the joint surfaces and more pain. Gentle movement under the supervision of a skilled yoga therapist can put a stop to this cycle.

Asana is also great preventive medicine. Most people who aren't actively working to maintain flexibility in their muscles and other tissues, and range of motion in their joints, become more restricted in their movements as they age. Asana takes your joints through a wide range of motion, inscribing new and healthier movement "grooves" in your body. Movement distributes lubricating synovial fluid, continually secreted into the joint by its synovial lining, over the surface of the cartilage that caps the bones. When the cartilage is well lubricated, the joint surfaces glide more easily across each other, reducing wear and tear. Joint movement also helps bring nutrients into cartilage, which lacks its own blood supply. You can think of cartilage as a sponge that gets squeezed by movement. Stale synovial fluid, depleted of nutrients, leaves, allowing a fresh supply to soak in from the joint when the compression is released. Areas of the joint surface that rarely get used because they are outside the normal grooves of movement fail to get the nutrients they need and over time tend to degenerate—an example of "use it or lose it."

Yogis believe that stress may play a role in worsening symptoms of OA, and contribute to flare-ups of inflammation in RA. This belief is now being confirmed by pain experts who increasingly recognize that tight muscles (characteristic of people under stress) are often a major cause of pain in arthritis. Another cycle may ensue, as constant pain can itself be very stressful, causing further tightening and tension of the muscles. With measures that both reduce stress and relax muscles, yoga can interrupt this feedback loop.

The Scientific Evidence

When I visited various yoga therapy clinics in India, I heard several dramatic stories of the relief people with arthritis had obtained from practicing yoga. These stories are just anecdotes, of course, but they suggest what may be possible, and yoga's efficacy is beginning to be borne out by studies (though much more research is needed).

Marian Garfinkel's doctoral dissertation, later published in the *Journal of Rheumatology*, was a randomized controlled study of twenty-five patients with degenerative arthritis (OA) of the hands. She found that a program of adapted Iyengar yoga and relaxation resulted in significant reductions in pain and an increase in range of motion. Beyond these objective measures, Marian believes the students also experienced improvements in their mood and energy levels.

More recently, Marian and several colleagues from the Division of Rheumatology at the University of Pennsylvania School of Medicine published a small pilot study evaluating an eight-week program of adapted Iyengar yoga for OA of the knee. Marian designed and taught the yoga intervention. Seven women, all obese and over fifty, none of whom had done yoga before, completed the protocol by attending at least five of eight weekly, one- to one-and-a-half-hour sessions. No home practice between lessons was required. After eight weeks, the women averaged a 47 percent reduction in pain, a 39 percent improvement in physical function, and a 39 percent reduction in stiffness. The women also experienced a statistically significant improvement in their mood compared to before the trial began. There were no injuries or other adverse reactions to the yoga protocol.

A small controlled trial, published in the *British Journal of Rheumatology*, found that a three-month program of gentle asana and breathing techniques resulted in improved grip strength in patients with rheumatoid arthritis. The study's authors included Robin Monro, PhD, of the London-based Yoga Biomedical Trust, along with researchers from the Swami Vivekananda Yoga Research Foundation near Bangalore. While the effect was small, it is noteworthy that all the patients who tried yoga wished to continue it after the study was completed. Another study at Vivekananda found that a more intense fifteen-day program resulted in large increases in grip strength in twenty patients with rheumatoid arthritis, especially among the women (who on average were quite weak prior to starting the program).

Dr. Jon Kabat-Zinn, founder of the Stress Reduction Clinic at the University of Massachusetts Medical Center, evaluated a ten-week program teaching mindfulness meditation and hatha yoga to fifty-one people with chronic pain who had failed to improve with conventional medical care. The most common types of pain in the group included low back, neck, and shoulder pain. Half of the patients experienced a 50 percent reduction in pain and

65 percent had a one-third reduction in pain scores. There were large improvements in mood and other symptoms. The response was similar for all types of pain. The majority of patients in mindfulness-based stress-reduction programs appear to continue their practice when the program is over, demonstrating long-term improvements in function.

Marian Garfinkel's Approach

Marian made the following observations about Liz when she walked in for her first appointment. "She appeared to be carrying all the weight in her knees, and was hunched over and had very little body awareness. Her head was going forward and her knees were more prominent than normal." Marian deduced that Liz probably had some calcification in the joints. Liz was also bowlegged, her knees angling out to the sides.

On the right side, where Liz had had her knee surgery, Marian says, "the shin bone was totally different. It was projecting toward me, and it was not aligned with the femur" (the thigh bone). Marian suspected that some of this abnormality may have been the result of the operation. The right foot looked contracted. The toes were bunched together, particularly toward the outside of the foot. Standing, Liz couldn't lift her toes at all, a reflection of tightness in the muscles of the sole of the foot, which should be soft. She also found that Liz had a great deal of tightness in some of the muscles in her arms and back, and she believed this tension was causing a chain effect that was adversely affecting Liz's knees.

When Marian asked Liz to show her the asana she had been doing, she saw that Liz was doing the postures incorrectly. "She had almost no awareness of her alignment. What she was doing was really not helping her. If you have OA of the knee, you need to modify the pose to work the leg differently so that you place less weight on the knee. If poses are done incorrectly, it could cause other injuries." Marian also believes that there are specific modifications that need to be made for bowlegs.

Here are the poses and instructions that Marian provided for Liz in each of their three lessons together:

LESSON 1

Marian began their first lesson with a restorative pose, a passive chest opener, due to her suspicion that Liz was both tired and mildly depressed. When people are in pain, Marian stresses, it is necessary to proceed slowly. "The first thing I have to do is manage their pain to give them the confidence to want to continue. You need to be certain not to make their condition worse."

EXERCISE #1. **RECLINING COBBLER'S POSE (Supta Baddha Konasana), on a platform or table, five to ten minutes.** Start by sitting on a platform or strong table in Cobbler's pose, approximately six inches in front of a cylindrical bolster. Place folded or

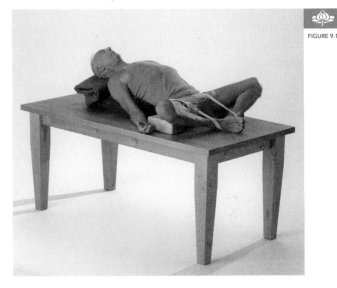

FIGURE 9.1

rolled blankets or yoga blocks under your thighs and calves so that your legs are supported and you feel no tension in your groin. Next, loosely fasten a yoga strap around your buttocks and the tops of your feet. Then, lie back over the bolster and tighten the strap (no more than is comfortable). If your chin is higher than your forehead, place a folded blanket under your head (figure 9.1). Stay in the pose for several minutes, breathing gently in and out through your nose.

 TIP Marian Garfinkel has a platform in her yoga studio, about the height of a high table, on which students with arthritis and other problems that restrict mobility can practice their poses. Not having to get up and down from the floor makes practicing easier, less painful, and safer. If you don't have a platform, she suggests that you use a strong rectangular table, which you can make even more secure by pushing it against a wall. Start by standing with your back to the table, move your pelvis back onto the table (left), and then swing your legs up (right).

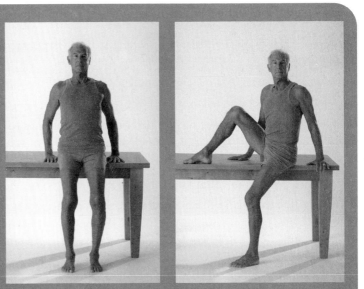

EXERCISE #2. **HALF STANDING FORWARD BEND** (Ardha Uttanasana), **with hands on the wall, one minute.** Start by facing a bare wall, standing approximately two feet from it, with your feet parallel to each other. Place both your hands on the wall, a bit lower than shoulder height. Step back one foot at a time until you are far enough away from the wall to bend at your hips and stretch your arms straight in front of you (figure 9.2). Keep your feet directly under your hips and elongate your legs. Try not to round your lower back. Rather, allow your lower back to retain its natural inward curve.

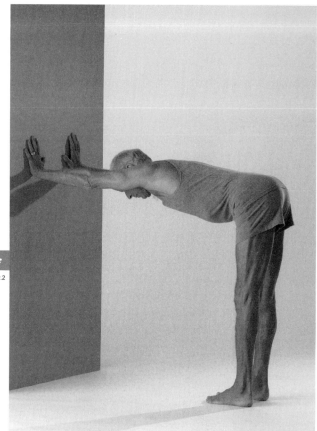

FIGURE 9.2

Marian used this pose both as a diagnostic tool and to teach Liz proper alignment of the legs, with the ankles, knees, and hips stacked evenly. Normally in this pose, the hips should be even, but Liz's left hip was higher than the right, in part due to all the muscular tightness in her right leg. As is common in runners, Liz was putting most of her weight on the ball of the foot and less on the heel, especially on the right side. An additional benefit of this pose is that it gives traction to the spine, which helps take the pressure off the knees.

Because Marian felt that Liz had not yet learned to use her legs properly in asana, she asked her not to do any other yoga until their next lesson, out of concern she'd end up doing more harm than good. Marian says that getting alignment right is vital for a condition like arthritis, so the only homework she gave Liz was to be aware of how she walked and how she sat, observing precisely what she was doing with her knees and legs. Marian's goal with these self-study exercises was to help put Liz more in touch with her body, to begin to cultivate awareness in her everyday life. To avoid further knee damage, Marian asked Liz not to cross her legs when she sat.

Liz returned the following week for her second lesson. She'd had some improvement in knee pain, and Marian felt she was now ready to begin more difficult standing poses.

EXERCISE #3. **WARRIOR II POSE (Virabhadrasana II), with back to a platform, fifteen seconds.** (At home Marian suggested that Liz use a high table, kitchen counter, or any other sturdy surface about that height.) Start by standing with your back to the platform, and place your hands on the surface behind you. Separate your feet three or three-and-a-half feet apart. Turn your right foot out ninety degrees and your back foot in fifteen to thirty degrees. Next, keeping your hands on the surface behind you, bend your front knee so that it is directly over your ankle (figure 9.3) and your thigh is as close to parallel to the floor as possible. Stay briefly in the pose and then come out by reversing your steps. Repeat on the other side.

The purpose of putting your hands on a platform is to give you stability and to take some of the weight off your legs.

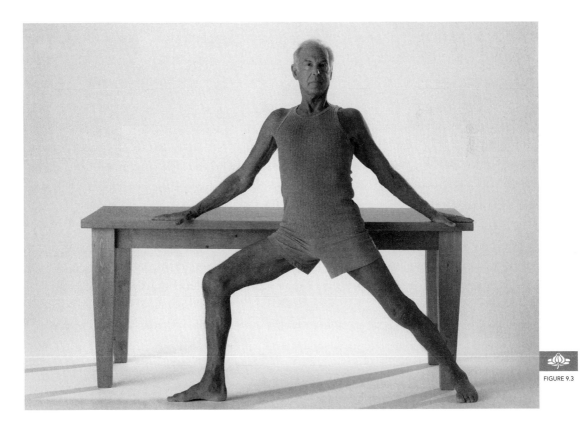

FIGURE 9.3

EXERCISE #4. **TRIANGLE POSE (Trikonasana), against a platform, with right foot propped on a slant board, thirty seconds.** Start by standing on a yoga mat with your back against a platform (or high table, kitchen counter, etc.). The yoga mat will help keep the prop under the ball of your front foot from slipping. Place your hands on the surface behind you. Separate your feet to three or three-and-a-half feet apart (wider, if you have longer legs). Turn your right foot out to ninety degrees and place a slant board (a wedge-shaped yoga prop) under the ball of your front foot (figure 9.4b). If you don't have a slant board, you can use a piece of two-by-four, a book, or any

FIGURE 9.4

other object that lifts the ball of your foot. Sliding your right arm along the platform, lengthen the sides of your body and move your torso to the right to come into the pose (figure 9.4a). To come out of the pose, reverse your steps. Repeat the pose on your left side, propping the left foot. Do twice on each side for thirty seconds.

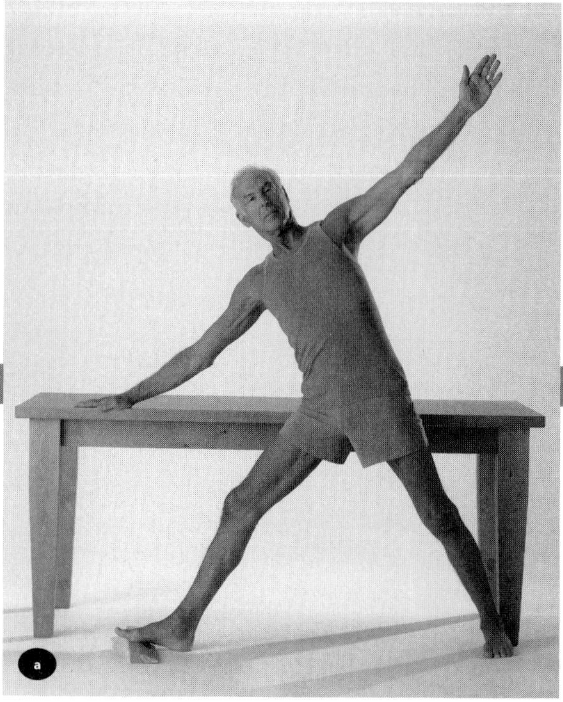

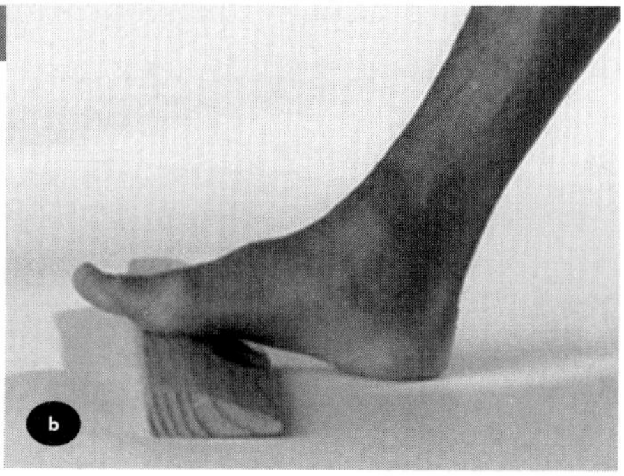

Because Liz's adductor muscles (in her inner thighs) were tight, probably from all the running she had done, using the prop under her foot gave her more opening in the hip and greater freedom to move into the pose without risking compression of her knee.

> **TIP** Marian stresses that in Triangle pose the most important part of the pose is having a straight back leg. In other words, if you are doing the pose to the left, be sure to fully straighten the right leg. To straighten the leg, press strongly into your back heel while keeping the knee soft (so it does not lock or hyperextend). The work of the back leg is the element of the pose that Marian believes is most beneficial for knee osteoarthritis.

Although Liz had made good progress, Marian did not assign her these poses as homework because she wasn't yet convinced that Liz could do them well enough to gain benefit and not risk harm. Instead, Marian asked her to continue her awareness training as before. She also asked her to simply sit in a chair and align her knees and ankles. From this position, she asked Liz to raise and lower her hands a few times, to try to release some of the tightness in her arms and back (figure 9.5).

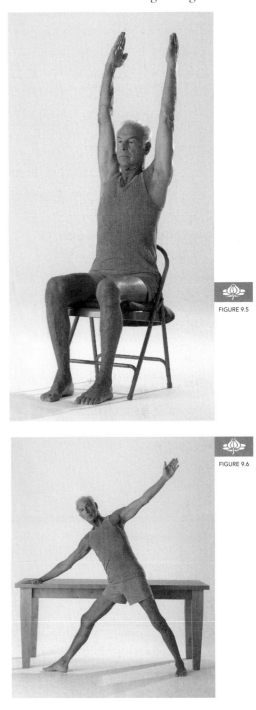

FIGURE 9.5

LESSON 3

Three weeks later, Liz returned for her third lesson, already noticing an improvement in her symptoms. Marian says that she was able to do the poses with better alignment, more flexibility in the foot, and no compression in the knee joint. Marian therefore modified the way she had Liz do Triangle pose, removing the prop under her foot, and instead, having her turn her front foot out slightly more than the standard ninety degrees. Increasing the angle of the foot reduces compression of the knee, though not to the same degree as the slant board does. Eventually, as Liz gained flexibility and strength, Marian would have her do the pose in the usual way: without a prop and with her foot turned out just to ninety degrees.

FIGURE 9.6

EXERCISE #5: **TRIANGLE POSE (Trikonasana), against a platform, with front foot turned out, thirty seconds, twice on each side.** Follow the instructions for Triangle pose in exercise #4, placing your front foot directly on the floor (rather than on a prop) and turning it out to slightly more than ninety degrees (figure 9.6). Stay in the pose for thirty seconds, then repeat on the other side.

Because of the progress Liz had made in alignment and flexibility, Marian felt it was appropriate to add the hamstring stretches described below. They wouldn't have been good for Liz when she first came in, because she was in pain then and Marian felt these stretches would have increased her pain, to the point where she wouldn't have been able to walk the next day.

EXERCISE #6. **SUPINE HAND TO FOOT POSE, TO THE SIDE (Supta Padangusthasana II), using a strap, fifteen to twenty seconds, two times on each side.** Start by lying on your back, with your knees bent and the soles of your feet on the floor. Next, bring your right leg into your chest, wrap a cotton yoga strap around the arch of the foot, straighten your leg until it is perpendicular to the floor, and then transfer both ends of the strap to your right hand. Hold the strap with a light grip. Straighten your left leg

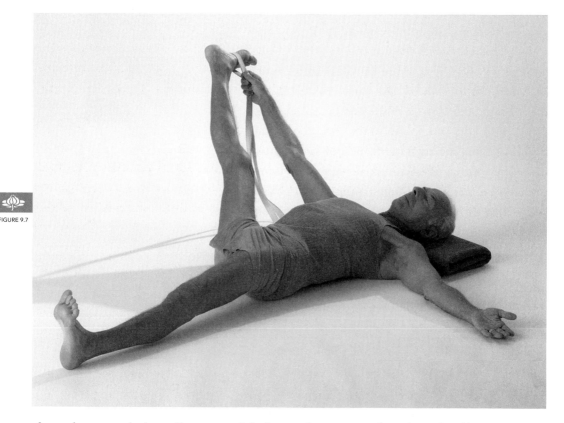

FIGURE 9.7

along the ground, then allow your right leg to drop out to the side and pull it up toward your shoulder (figure 9.7). Keep your shoulders dropped and your hips level. Breathe through your nose, keeping your breath soft, and relax your temples and your throat. Hold the pose for approximately fifteen to twenty seconds. Repeat on the other side.

EXERCISE #7. **SUPINE HAND TO FOOT POSE (Supta Padangusthasana I), using a strap, fifteen to twenty seconds, two times on each side.** Start by lying on your back,

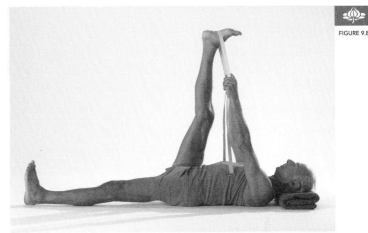

FIGURE 9.8

with your knees bent and the soles of your feet on the floor. Next, bring your right leg into your chest, wrap a cotton yoga strap around the ball of your right foot, and hold the ends of the straps in both hands. Straighten your right leg and lift it up toward the ceiling and straighten your left leg along the ground. Press the ball of your right foot into the strap while creating resistance with your hands. The more you press your foot into the strap, the more you pull the belt toward you. Pull the outside of the belt a little more strongly than the inside (this helps open up the little toe side of the foot). Do twice on each side (figure 9.8).

EXERCISE #8. **SUPPORTED RELAXATION POSE (Savasana), with chest elevated and support for the legs (figure 9.9), ten minutes.** Marian suggests using blankets under the head and neck, and under the back from the waist up, both for elevation and the softness they provide. Set up for the pose by folding a blanket and placing it lengthwise on your mat to support your entire torso and head. Then sit in front of the folded blanket (but

not on it) and lean back so the bottom of the folded blanket hits you at the waist. Place a second folded blanket on top of the first blanket under your head to support your head and neck. Place a rolled blanket with a diameter of three to four inches under the top of the thighs to support them, which takes the pressure off the knees.

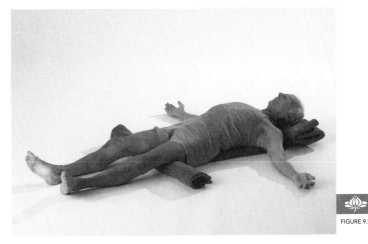

FIGURE 9.9

Yogic Tool: **VISUALIZATION.** One of the common postural problems that teacher Joan Arnold, trained in both Anusara yoga and the Alexander Technique, sees in people with knee pain is the habit of pushing the pelvis down into the legs, which puts pressure on the knees. "When we think about the pelvis going up, it creates more space in the hip joints and frees the action of the legs," she says. "The most efficient, effortless way to achieve this is to use our capacity to visualize." To do the exercise, stand in Mountain pose (Tadasana) with your feet hips' width apart. Once you settle into the pose, imagine a pure, central core of energy flowing evenly from the middle of the pelvis, midway between the pubic bone and the tailbone, up toward the head. Think of lightness in the pelvis and spaciousness in the hip joints. This helps you tap into the torso's internal suspension system, which includes the pelvis. Try not to do anything muscularly to lift or push yourself up, though your muscles will probably make subtle adjustments in response to the visualization. Then return to your normal posture, and see whether you notice a difference between what you are used to and what you've just achieved. Your feet may feel heavier and more grounded.

Contraindications, Special Considerations, and Modifications

If you have arthritis, it's generally better to move in and out of poses rather than hold them. The transitions should be slow and smooth, always coordinated with the breath. Don't jump into poses, even if you're in a class and that's what everyone else is doing. If there is evidence of muscle fatigue, such as shakiness or increasing discomfort, it's best to

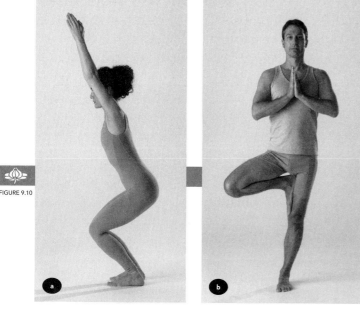

FIGURE 9.10

come out of the pose, as tired muscles may not be able to hold good alignment and the result can be further damage to the joint. If necessary, rest in Savasana between poses until you've regained your strength.

Squatting poses like Chair pose (Utkatasana, figure 9.10a) and Garland pose (Malasana) may be inappropriate for those with arthritis of the hips, knees, or ankles. One-legged balancing poses like Tree pose (Vrksasana) may put too much pressure on the joints of the standing leg (figure 9.10b).

In deciding whether a pose or series of poses is appropriate, it is important to evaluate both how you feel while doing the pose and how you feel afterward. More than your usual level of stiffness a couple of hours after practice, or the next morning, may be a sign that you need to scale back your practice, build up more slowly, or eliminate some poses entirely.

> **TIP** If you use pain medication for arthritis, try to take it long enough in advance of your practice to allow it to be absorbed into your system. This may require a couple of hours. Some "time-release" drugs should be taken several hours ahead of time. Check with your doctor or pharmacist. Over time, as you gain internal awareness from your practice, you'll be able to fine-tune when to take your medication for optimal results.

The yogic approach for rheumatoid arthritis and other inflammatory types of arthritis needs to be different from that used in osteoarthritis, because there tends to be much more swelling of joints. "I would not ever start with standing poses with rheumatoid arthritis," Marian says. She uses lots of props to provide support, suggests doing the poses briefly two or three times on each side, and builds up the duration of the practice very slowly to avoid a flare-up. When a joint is acutely inflamed—marked by warmth, redness, swelling, and/or increased pain—it may be necessary to rest the joint and concentrate on other yogic practices until the inflammation settles down. Practices such as breath work, chanting, and meditation are almost always appropriate. Simple restorative yoga poses which work the joints more passively may also be appropriate until you get to the stage where you can cautiously increase the activity.

Students who have had hip- or knee-replacement surgery need to take special precautions when doing yoga in the first several months after the operation. Even after the tissue is well healed, some yoga poses risk causing a dislocation or other injury. In general, you don't want to push the joint that's been operated on through its most extreme range of motion. Instead, focus on building functional strength in the surrounding muscles, and consciously limit the range of motion. Since there are a number of possible surgical approaches to hip replacement, and the movement contraindications vary depending on what exactly was done, it's best to consult with the surgeon who performed the operation and the physical therapist involved in your postoperative rehabilitation before embarking on or resuming a yoga program. Twisting poses, forward bends, backbends, or asanas, which require extreme external or internal rotation of the hips (see appendix 1, "Avoiding Common Yoga Injuries") may be off limits to you. If you've had knee replacements you should avoid one-legged balancing poses and asanas in which you squat, as this places the joint in a vulnerable position.

A Holistic Approach to Arthritis

* Walking, swimming, or another form of aerobic exercise is advisable.

* Topical medications like capsaicin, derived from red peppers, appear to be effective for arthritic joints near the surface of the body, such as the knees, but are less useful for joints like the hips.

* Directly applying either heat to reduce stiffness or cold to cut pain can be surprisingly helpful.

* Nonsteroidal anti-inflammatory drugs (NSAIDs, pronounced EN-seds) like ibuprofen, commonly prescribed for arthritis, have pain-relieving and—if used consistently in high-enough doses—anti-inflammatory properties, but may also cause serious side effects. Check with your doctor or pharmacist.

* Some patients with osteoarthritis get good pain relief from the drug acetaminophen (Tylenol), which is a cheaper and generally safer option than NSAIDs.

* Acupuncture is safe and can relieve pain.

* Cognitive/behavioral therapy to learn coping strategies and to change self-defeating attitudes can be useful.

* Even a few pounds of weight loss can lessen symptoms, especially for arthritis involving the legs or lower back.

* High heels put most of the body's weight on the ball of the foot, reducing its ability to absorb shock and putting strain on the knees.

* Working with someone who understands functional anatomy, such as a good physical therapist or a teacher of the Alexander Technique or the Feldenkrais Method, can be very useful.

* Two dietary supplements often combined in one pill, glucosamine and chondroitin, appear to be safe and effective in treatment of OA. More recently they have been combined in a topical salve.

* S-Adenosylmethionine, or SAMe, appears to be safe and effective though is quite expensive. MSM (methylsulfonylmethane) may also be useful.

* Vitamin D, which you can get from either a few minutes of sunlight a day (without wearing sunscreen) or via supplements, may lessen the progression of arthritic symptoms.

* Oils rich in arachidonic acid, such as peanut and corn oil, may promote inflammation while omega-3 fatty acids, found in flaxseeds, flaxseed oil, and such fish as herring, mackerel, salmon, tuna, and sardines, tend to reduce it. Canola oil is a better choice for cooking. Fried foods, red meat, refined sugars, and trans fats can fuel inflammation.

* A diet low in harmful fats and rich in whole foods such as grains, beans, fruit, nuts, and vegetables of a variety of colors, contains lots of vitamins and natural anti-oxidants, and can reduce arthritic symptoms. Bioflavonoids, found in berries and other fruit, appear to reduce inflammation in joints. Healthy nuts include almonds and walnuts.

* Some alternative healers believe that nightshade vegetables, such as eggplants, peppers, tomatoes, and potatoes, may exacerbate arthritic symptoms and contribute to flare-ups of rheumatoid arthritis. Most conventional doctors disagree. The yogic approach would be to let your own experience guide you. If you suspect nightshades could be contributing to your symptoms, cut them out of your diet for a couple of weeks, and then see what happens when you add them back.

* Ginger, a traditional Ayurvedic arthritis remedy, can be used in cooking or made into tea. Turmeric also has anti-inflammatory properties.

* Dehydration can dry out the fluid in the joints, so drink plenty of water and other liquids.

* For some with marked symptoms of pain and loss of motion, joint-replacement surgery is the best alternative.

Over the time Marian worked with her, Liz's strength, flexibility, and alignment all improved. She was able to do more asana, and gradually reduced her need for props. More important, she experienced much less knee pain in the course of her everyday activities. The right knee never improved as much as the other, however, which Marian thinks was probably due to complications from the surgery. Liz was still doing well three years later when Marian bumped into her.

Marian had stressed to Liz the importance of consistent and mindful practice. "Even if you do ten minutes a day, that's an hour a week," she had told her. "What's important is the regularity of it, not that you do an hour one day and nothing the next." Liz got the message and has been good about keeping up a daily practice, however brief the practice often is.

Beyond giving her more mobility and less pain, the regular practice appears to have helped Liz reap psychological benefits. Marian says Liz seems more hopeful than she had been when they first met, even though she never did get back to running. Much of her improvement is likely a consequence of having found in her yoga practice concrete steps she could take to improve her condition. When you feel you've accomplished something, says Marian, it gives you a sense of empowerment, which can have a big impact on mood. Marian sees herself only as "a messenger." The yoga practice does the rest.

ASTHMA

BARBARA BENAGH'S influences are diverse. She studied Iyengar yoga in the 1970s and 1980s, and later trained intensively with yoga teacher Angela Farmer. Her interest in using yoga for asthma was sparked by her own problems with the disease, including frequent pneumonias and many hospital stays, including a near-fatal incident requiring admission to intensive care. It was after that ICU stay that she dedicated herself to learning all she could about breathing. She was inspired by the work of Dr. Gay Hendricks, author of *Conscious Breathing,* and Dr. Konstantin Buteyko, a pioneer in the use of breath retraining for people with asthma. Her experience with yoga told her that "If I persevere, and I continue to work, I will eventually find things to help me." After much 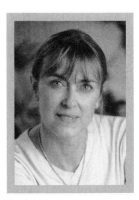 trial and error she hit upon a series of exercises that slowly transformed her entire relationship with breathing. By a few years ago, she'd improved so much that she was even able to return to a passion she'd had to drop ten years earlier: long-distance bicycling. Barbara has been teaching yoga in the Boston area and internationally for more than thirty years.

Ken Paul figures he's been an asthmatic for fifty-four years, ever since he was about two. Because his doctors misread his symptoms for years, however, he didn't know what was wrong with him until sometime in his twenties, when he visited family in Ireland. By that time, Ken had already had pneumonia five times, and had been hospitalized on several occasions. His brother-in-law, a pulmonary specialist there, told him he clearly had asthma and introduced Ken to Cromolyn, an inhaler that was not yet available in the US. Back in Boston his doctors eventually put him on Azmacort, an inhaled steroid, which he remained on for years. Even though inhaled steroids kept his condition under control, and his doctors had no qualms about prescribing them, Ken was concerned about the effects of the medication being absorbed into his system, and he wanted to learn about possible alternatives, including yoga.

Ken began to study yoga twelve years ago, and has had a daily home practice for the last ten. At a friend's suggestion, he also started taking a regular class with a Kripalu teacher, which he enjoys. While helpful in many ways, however, his asana practice hadn't resolved his breathing troubles. He got more serious about wanting to address his asthma after reading an article Barbara Benagh had written in *Yoga Journal* about her path to recovery after having almost died of asthma. He identified closely with the experience. "I've had some episodes, especially with the pneumonias and some of the bronchitises, when I wasn't sure I was going to make it." He figured that trying out the breathing exercises and other ideas Barbara wrote about in the article was worth doing, since she had made such remarkable progress.

Overview of Asthma

Asthma is a condition in which the bronchial tubes in the lungs become swollen, constricted, and blocked with mucus secretions, causing the characteristic symptoms of wheezing, chest tightness, cough, and shortness of breath. It has been linked to genetic factors, allergies, and environmental conditions, though its causes vary from person to person. Asthma often begins in childhood, but can occur at any age. While some children seem to outgrow their asthma, if it begins in adulthood, it tends to be more persistent. For reasons that are not completely understood, the incidence and death rates from asthma have been rising dramatically in recent years. Air pollution, rising stress levels, and a lack of exposure to germs during childhood that may render the immune system hypervigilant have all been suggested as possible reasons.

The rising incidence of fatal asthma attacks may also be linked with bronchodilating medications. These bronchodilators—called beta-agonists because they stimulate the beta-receptors in the lungs—dilate constricted bronchial tubes, and when inhaled, can calm down asthma symptoms within minutes. It's possible, however, to use these inhalers too often (when what is needed is stronger medication), temporarily suppressing symptoms that inevitably rebound. Worse, the bronchodilators may also mask an impending asthmatic crisis, causing a delay in getting emergency treatments, sometimes until it's too late. Due to these problems and the increasing understanding of the role that inflammation plays in asthma (which beta-agonists do nothing to reverse), anti-inflammatory cortisone drugs (steroids), inhaled or in more severe cases oral, have become the gold standard of conventional treatment in all but the mildest cases.

How Yoga Fits In

From a yogic perspective, many people—and not just asthmatics—breathe in a dysfunctional and inefficient way (see chapter 3). Improving their breathing patterns can increase oxygen supply to the tissues, lower stress levels, and induce muscular relaxation, good for everyone but potentially lifesaving for someone with asthma. Barbara Benagh sees a half dozen dysfunctional breathing habits in people with asthma (see box). Despite years of yoga, Barbara realized she had had almost all of these habits herself. "I wasn't a diaphragmatic breather. I was a mouth breather, a breath holder, high-chest breather. I was like an asthma person waiting to happen. All it took was for me to catch pneumonia for it to be the final straw. I had everything already set up to go, and a lot of people do."

COMMON DYSFUNCTIONAL BREATHING HABITS IN PEOPLE WITH ASTHMA

1. Chest Breathing
2. Inhalations Stronger Than Exhalations
3. Breath Holding
4. Mouth Breathing
5. "Reverse" Breathing
6. Overbreathing

Chest breathing means that most of the air goes into the upper and middle chest, and less goes to the lower portions of the lungs. Stress is one reason for chest breathing, and yogis believe further stress can be the result of breathing this way. Think of the way you breathe if you are startled—with a quick, shallow inhalation you can feel just below your collarbones. Some people with asthma breathe like this most of the time, and if you try it for a few breaths, you'll see that doing so is agitating to the mind. Another result of chest breathing is that the lower areas of the lungs, richly supplied with blood vessels, don't get enough oxygen to fully replenish the blood passing through those vessels.

A slumping posture, common in modern society (see pp. 32–35), also contributes to chest breathing by pushing the lower ribs into the upper abdomen. This limits the movement of the diaphragm, the large dome-shaped sheet of muscle beneath the lungs, which ought to be the primary muscle of respiration, so the chest (and sometimes the neck) muscles take over. With chronic chest breathing, the diaphragm can become weak, just like any other muscle that doesn't get enough exercise, exacerbating the problem. Chronic poor postural habits also can lead to tightness in such muscles as the pectoralis in the chest and the intercostals between the ribs, as well as in ligaments and connective tissue in the chest, all of which can limit the ability of the rib cage to fully expand and contract (see p. 228).

Most people with asthma have much more difficulty exhaling than inhaling, and the wheezing characteristic of the disease happens primarily on the out breath. Difficulty exhaling reflects the narrowing of small bronchial tubes due to inflammation, swelling, and bronchospasm (constriction of the bronchial tubes), as well as the accumulation of mucus in the airways. As the lungs expand on inhalation, traction is exerted on the airways, which opens them, but they tend to collapse as the lungs recoil on exhalation. Since the lungs take in too much air relative to the amount of air that is exhaled, stale air stays in the lungs, leaving less room for new oxygen-rich air to come in, thus compromising the oxygen supply to the rest of the body. In response, the breathing becomes quicker, and as we've seen, quick, small-volume breathing is both inefficient and stressful (see chapter 3). From a yogic perspective, weakness of the abdominal muscles—and failure to engage them with exhalation—is an additional factor in difficulty breathing out.

Breath holding is the usually unconscious tendency to hold the breath after the inhalation. Pressure builds up, making it even harder to exhale in a relaxed fashion. This is stressful, and if done chronically, may put additional strain on the heart and lungs.

Mouth breathers inhale and exhale almost exclusively through the mouth. They tend to breathe more quickly, since the mouth offers less resistance to airflow than the nasal passages, and they lose the benefits of the nose's warming, filtering, and humidifying of incoming air. (Cold air can be shocking to lungs, triggering bronchospasm, and fueling any inflammation that is already going on.) Mouth breathing also tends to dry out the mouth and throat, which can lead to further irritation in the airways.

In reverse breathing (paradoxical breathing), the diaphragm rises with inhalation and drops with exhalation, the opposite of normal. This reduces the efficiency of respiration and contributes to chest breathing, with all its disadvantages.

Overbreathing is the tendency to hyperventilate. Asthmatics often have abnormally high respiratory rates. If normal is twelve breaths per minute, they might breathe at two or more times that rate. They may take in plenty of oxygen, but at the expense of exhaling more carbon dioxide (CO_2) than is healthy. With low levels of CO_2 in the system, the pH of the blood rises (becomes more alkaline), and as a result, hemoglobin holds on to oxygen molecules more tightly than usual and the cells can't get as much oxygen as they need. This can lead to a vicious cycle where the asthmatic breathes even faster to bring in more oxygen, blowing off even more CO_2. Rapid breathing also tends to cool and dry out the respiratory passages, which can cause bronchospasm.

A number of yogic practices specifically address the six common breathing problems that Barbara outlined above. A number of breathing exercises, for example, strengthen the diaphragm and encourage its full excursion as it descends to bring air into the lungs. This so-called abdominal breathing is the opposite of chest breathing. A number of yogic practices, especially asana, systematically improve posture and with it the breath.

In yoga, you learn to engage the abdominal muscles as you exhale, squeezing additional air out of the lungs. This and improved posture allow more air to be taken in on the subsequent breath. Studies show that yoga can both increase lung capacity and the volume and efficiency of the exhalation (see pp. 175–176).

By bringing awareness to your breathing through yoga, you learn to reduce unconscious breath holding. This new habit comes first during your yoga practice, but after you've practiced long enough, this and other beneficial breathing patterns tend to become your default mode, even when you are not thinking about it. Similarly, bad habits like mouth breathing and reverse breathing can be reduced and eventually eliminated by bringing awareness to the breathing process. The more dedicated and regular your yoga practice, the more effectively you'll be able to replace dysfunctional breathing habits with the healthier ones you are practicing. For those who have difficulty breathing through the nose due to nasal allergies or a buildup of mucus, rinsing the nasal passages with salt water using a neti pot can open the passageways and remove allergens and inflammatory immune cells that can contribute to asthmatic symptoms (see pp. 80–81).

Yoga counters the tendency to overbreathe by cultivating slow, deep, regular breaths. Once you've practiced yoga long enough, you start to realize that you can get more air in and out of your lungs with slow, mindful breaths, using as little effort as possible to move air, than by breathing rapidly. When your breath becomes labored, slow respirations calm your nervous system and help keep your mind less agitated. As some yogis with asthma will testify, sometimes the only way to move air during an attack is to breathe slowly and smoothly. Getting agitated will only worsen symptoms, causing a vicious cycle in which poor breathing leads to agitation, which makes the breathing even faster and more erratic.

Yoga can also help people with asthma by increasing their sensitivity to the state of their breathing. Many patients I've seen with asthma have gotten so accustomed to their limited breath capacity that they hardly notice it. Most are also completely unaware of their dysfunctional breathing patterns. As in all yoga therapy, recognizing the problem is the first step toward changing it. By tuning your awareness of your breathing in yoga you learn to become what Barbara calls a "breath detective." One concrete advantage of greater sensitivity is that you may detect a flare-up of your asthma earlier in the process, when it's easier to remedy and interventions are more effective.

Studying yourself—svadhyaya—can be facilitated by keeping a notebook where you track your asthmatic episodes, what foods you had eaten, how much sleep and exercise you had had, and any other factors that might have a bearing on your breathing. If your doctor has you measuring your peak flow rate (by using a small handheld device designed for that purpose) to monitor your breathing, or using other tests of your lung function, you should write those numbers down as well. Studies suggest, however, that monitoring symptoms may be just as valuable as monitoring peak flow rates. Yoga, because it sensitizes people to their breathing patterns, helps them become very good at gauging their symptoms.

Many yogis (and even some doctors) feel that stress plays a role in asthma, too. In addition to writing in a journal, talking to a psychotherapist or simply becoming more mindful of emotions as they arise—which a dedicated yoga practice helps you do—are also forms of svadhyaya.

A study published in the *Journal of the American Medical Association* demonstrated the usefulness of writing about emotional issues. Patients with chronic asthma were asked to write about the most stressful event of their lives for twenty minutes on three consecutive days. Patients in the control group were asked to write about an emotionally neutral topic, such as their plans for the coming day. Four months later, those who had written about the emotionally charged events showed a 20 percent improvement in their FEV_1 (the maximum amount of air you can exhale in one second). There was no change in the lung function of the asthmatics who wrote about their plans.

 I advocate writing in a stream-of-consciousness fashion for a short while every morning. Combined with yogic awareness, journal writing can be a wonderful complement to psychotherapy. And unlike therapy, which insurers don't generally like to pay for anyway, the only expense is for the pen and paper. I particularly like a style of journaling known as "morning pages," described in the book *The Artist's Way* by Julia Cameron.

Yogic Tool: **MEDITATION.** Perhaps more than any other yogic tool, meditation puts you in touch with subconscious thoughts and feelings that could be affecting your breathing. Stephen Cope, a psychotherapist and Kripalu yoga teacher, says, "I've noticed on long meditation retreats that almost all of my asthma symptoms resolve."

The Scientific Evidence

A number of studies have examined the effectiveness of yoga for people with asthma. In 1967, the first clinical trial on yoga for asthma ever published was done by Dr. Mukund Bhole at the birthplace of the scientific investigation of yoga, the Kaivalyadhama ashram in Lonavla, India. In a later study there, Bhole and colleagues investigated the effects of a two-month program of various asana, breathing techniques, and yogic cleansing techniques (kriya) on fifty-five patients with asthma. They found that 40 percent had a good response, 33 percent a fair response, and 16 percent a slight response. It should be noted that their criteria were tough. A "good response" meant no attacks in the subsequent six months and no use of asthma medications for at least two months. A "fair response" was at least a 50 percent reduction in attacks with use of medication. A "slight response" meant the rate of attacks was reduced by 25 percent. When I met with Dr. Bhole, who is now semiretired, at his home in Lonavla, he told me that many of the patients they treated eventually relapsed, because once they felt better they stopped their yoga practice.

Dr. Virendra Singh and colleagues from the Nottingham City Hospital in England, in a study published in *The Lancet,* examined the effects of simulated pranayama in eighteen mildly asthmatic patients. The research subjects breathed through a device that slowed exhalation to twice the duration of inhalation (note the similarity of this procedure to the 1:2 breathing technique taught by Barbara later in the chapter). The control group used a similar device that did not restrict exhalation. The most significant finding was that it proved harder to provoke an asthmatic attack in the group who did the simulated pranayama when they were exposed to a chemical that can constrict the airways.

S. C. Jain and B. Talukdar, of India's Central Research Institute for Yoga, studied forty-six adult asthmatics who took part in a forty-day residential program that included asana, pranayama, kriyas, and a vegetarian diet. Yoga training was associated with significant increases in FEV_1, peak flow rates during exhalation, the amount of oxygen in the blood (both at rest and after exercise), and exercise capacity. Follow-up one year later was reported on thirty-one of forty-two patients who continued to practice fifteen to thirty minutes daily. Of these thirty-one, eighteen whose asthma was initially rated moderate to severe remained asymptomatic without medication.

A randomized controlled study, published in the *British Medical Journal* and conducted at the Swami Vivekananda Yoga Research Foundation near Bangalore, assessed the effects of an integrated yoga program which included asana, pranayama, yogic philosophy lectures, kriyas, and meditation. Drs. R. Nagarathna and H. R. Nagendra compared 53 asthmatics, ages nine to forty-seven, who underwent yoga training with 53 matched controls. Follow-up at fifty-four months included only the 28 patients who had continued to practice yoga at home at least sixteen times per month. These individuals showed significant improvement in peak flow, fewer attacks per week, and less need for medication. The same authors tracked 570 asthma patients who followed the same program over three to fifty-four months and found that approximately two-thirds were able to get off steroid drugs and other medications while demonstrating highly significant improvements in a number of measures of lung function and general health. Of note, those patients who continued to practice regularly showed the greatest improvements.

Not all yoga studies on asthma have shown clear-cut benefits. One showed small improvements in lung function that did not reach the level of statistical significance. Another found that a yoga group and a control group that did stretching exercises had improvements in symptoms and lung function, with no significant difference between the groups. A third study found no improvement in lung function, but showed a trend toward decreased use of bronchodilators in the yoga group. The authors of this study also reported that "the yoga group reported a better sense of well-being overall with more positive attitude and enthusiasm based on the Weekly Questionnaire" but this result was not quantified.

Barbara Benagh's Approach

Before beginning exercises specifically designed to help people with asthma, Barbara typically does a kind of diagnostic test—a test you can do yourself to get some idea of what kind of condition your lungs are in. The idea is to inhale for two seconds, exhale for three seconds, and then hold your breath as long you comfortably can. The normal hold is more than thirty seconds, something Barbara says she can rarely do. She suggests that if you have asthma, you do this test every day. If your result is much below thirty seconds, you probably need to modify your breathing habits, or if your numbers start to go down from what they usually are, a flare-up may be in process and you might need medical attention.

Fundamental to Barbara's approach to asthma is educating yourself. "The first thing is to learn what is a normal breath: mouth closed, twelve breaths or fewer a minute." If you're relaxed or doing Savasana, the exhalation should naturally be longer than the inhalation. "That's the nature of a relaxed breath," she says, but some people find it very hard to do.

The following program is Barbara's updated version of the program that appeared in the *Yoga Journal* article that Ken read. Ken never worked with Barbara personally, but he based his own program on what she wrote and on his perception of what was working for him. He also consulted regularly with the yoga teacher whose classes he attended.

EXERCISE #1. **DEEP RELAXATION POSE (Savasana), with relaxed breathing, mouth closed, five to ten minutes.** This exercise allows you to watch your breathing, but does not involve doing anything to change it. Start by lying down in Deep Relaxation pose with your arms and legs splayed to the sides (figure 10.1a). Barbara says that this

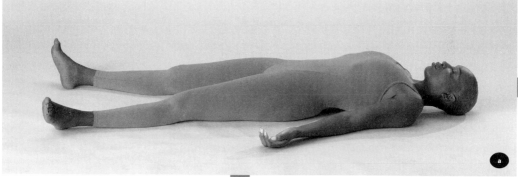

FIGURE 10.1

is the easiest position for diaphragmatic breathing. Sitting upright requires that you work against gravity when you exhale, and a big problem for someone with asthma is not being able to exhale. This is also why inversions, such as Shoulderstand, are helpful, a topic covered below. If lying down is uncomfortable, as it is for some people with asthma, Barbara recommends sitting in a chair and leaning forward over a table, resting your head on your folded arms, and turning your face to one side (figure 10.1b).

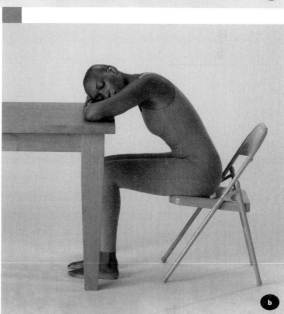

FIGURE 10.2

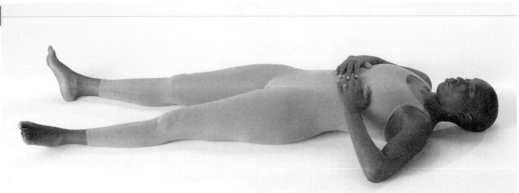

Once you are comfortable, begin breathing with your mouth closed. Next, tune into your exhalation; simply paying attention is the key. As you continue breathing, place your hands half on your ribs and half on your upper abdomen (figure 10.2), which will allow you to feel the movement of your rib cage and upper abdomen without interfering with that movement in any way. On your inhalation, you should feel the expansion in every direction except up (toward your head), and on your exhalation, you should feel relaxation everywhere except down. However, Barbara says that in an asthmatic the ribs may contract on the inhalation and expand on the exhalation. This is what she calls "reverse breathing."

> **TIP** Some yoga students are taught to push the belly out on inhalation, but in Barbara's experience, doing so does not guarantee that the diaphragm is working properly. She says that if you watch a sleeping baby or someone who is very relaxed, you'll see the belly expand on the inhalation and retract on the exhalation, which has led to the conclusion that you're supposed to push the belly out on the inhalation and draw it in on the exhalation. But this shouldn't be a willed movement; rather it is caused by the diaphragm's rise and fall during normal breathing. However, if you *push* your abdomen out, you don't have to use your diaphragm at all.

Once you have observed your breathing pattern, you can use the following exercises to teach yourself diaphragmatic breathing. They will heighten your awareness of when you are engaging your diaphragm and help you to strengthen it and use it more fully during breathing. Barbara suggests that you start with three to five breath cycles each of exercises two through six. Over time, as your symptoms allow, build up to ten to fifteen breath cycles of each exercise. Barbara says that with any of these exercises, it is fine to take several breaths between cycles of the exercise. Remember, do not force.

EXERCISE #2. **THE WAVE.** Start by lying on your back, with your knees bent, and your hands on your knees (figure 10.3a). As you exhale, gently bring your upper thighs toward your lower abdomen (figure 10.3b). As you inhale, let your feet drop toward the floor, arching your lower back. Keep your hips on the floor for the entire exercise, and allow your hands to remain on your knees as you move back and forth. The movement of your legs and abdominal muscles mimics the piston effect of natural breathing, which is different from the way most people with asthma breathe. Barbara stresses that the movements need not be large, though they may expand as you settle into the exercise.

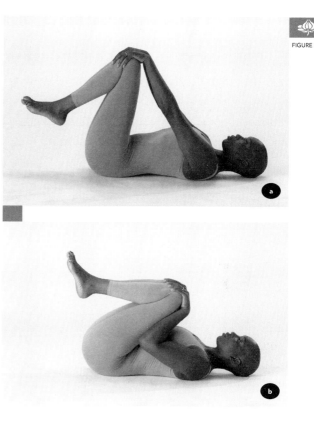

FIGURE 10.3

EXERCISE #3. **PURSED-LIP EXHALING.** Start by lying in Deep Relaxation pose (Savasana). When you are comfortable, purse your lips so that there is only a tiny opening for your exhalation (figure 10.4). Pursing your lips during the exhalation will engage the abdominals, causing a stronger exhalation than if you don't use these muscles. Can you feel the abdominal muscles help to squeeze the air out? On your subsequent inhalation, you should be able to feel air being drawn down effortlessly into the bottom portion of your lungs. Barbara says that the ideal position for this exercise is sitting, but begin by lying down and practice that way until you are completely comfortable sitting up.

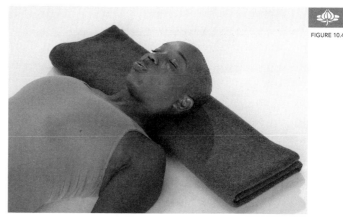

FIGURE 10.4

EXERCISE #4. **1:2 BREATHING.** You can do this exercise either lying down in Deep Relaxation pose (Savasana) or sitting up. Start by softening the effort you use to inhale, and gradually decrease the length of your inhalation until it is half as long as your exhalation. For example, if you usually exhale for four seconds, you'll end up inhaling for two seconds and exhaling for your usual four seconds. Don't struggle to lengthen your exhalation, simply shorten your inhalation. If you feel anxious or short of breath at any time, take a few normal breaths before resuming the practice.

EXERCISE #5. **1:2 BREATHING, PAUSING AFTER THE EXHALATION.** Repeat the last exercise but this time try to add a pause after your exhalation (but not after your inhalation). Gradually increase the length of the pause until it is as long as your exhalation.

EXERCISE #6. **1:1 BREATHING, WITH AN EXTENDED PAUSE AFTER THE EXHALATION.** In this exercise, keep your inhalation equal in length to your exhalation, but add a pause after your exhalation (but not after your inhalation). Eventually, make your pause two to four times as long as your inhalation and exhalation. Barbara refers to this exercise as "Nature's bronchodilator," because she has found that it can effectively lessen an asthma flare.

CAUTION While these exercises can be useful as "first aid," if you are tempted to do them more than once an hour for symptom control, you probably should seek medical care instead. Barbara also advises against skipping asthma medications when doing these exercises, as some students try to do.

In addition to the exercises above, Barbara recommends inverted poses for asthmatics. When your body is upside down, your diaphragm moves with gravity on the exhalation, not against it as it does when you are upright. Barbara says, "That's why Headstand and Shoulderstand—Headstand in particular—are so good." When she has problems with her breathing, she'll do supported Shoulderstand over a chair, and Legs-Up-the-Wall pose (Viparita Karani). However, if like Ken, you have problems with dizziness when doing inverted poses, you may not be able to do these poses. See appendix 1, "Avoiding Common Yoga Injuries," for more on doing inversions safely, and pp. 275–76 for instructions on how to do Chair Shoulderstand.

Besides breathing exercises and inversions, there are no yoga poses or practices that Barbara sees as specifically therapeutic for asthma. But she feels strongly a regular asana practice will be beneficial. She suspects the reason so many people with asthma feel so much better from their asana practice "is the fact that you have made the transformative decision to spend some time on your mat every day. That, even of itself, is so life changing, that you're going to feel better for it." She expands on her philosophy: "To me, what yoga is above all else is a behavioral modification. If you stop doing these things that you normally do, and instead you do yoga exercise, meditation, and breathing exercises every day, that's going to make you feel better, and you're going to be generally more healthy."

> **TIP** Dysfunctional breathing habits can be entrenched; particularly for those with long-standing asthma, it can take a while to change. In the meantime, a fake-it-till-you-make-it approach can be useful. Barbara recommends mimicking healthy breathing until your body and your nervous system get reprogrammed. She sees changing your breathing as being the same kind of challenge as making any other change—losing weight, becoming a vegetarian, etc. "At first it's difficult. But eventually it becomes second nature. It becomes a habit." When people hear of Barbara's prescription for asthma, some tell her that it can't be that simple. Her reply is that the exercises are simple. What is not simple is doing them every single day. "You don't even have to do them lying down," she says. "I've done them sitting in my car. I've done them sitting in a plane. I do them any time my situation tells me I should. To me, it's like brushing my teeth."

Contraindications, Special Considerations, and Modifications

Shortness of breath, coughing, or wheezing may indicate poor control of asthma, in which case you may want to avoid an active asana practice. Cough is sometimes the only asthma symptom and may not be recognized for what it is. A decline in peak flow readings can signal an impending attack, and the need to refrain from an active practice. Colds, even if they are otherwise only mild, can exacerbate breathing problems and may necessitate caution.

Any exercise, including yoga, can bring on asthma attacks in susceptible individuals. If you use an inhaled bronchodilator, take two puffs fifteen minutes before starting your practice (a steroid inhaler won't help if used this way). Since cold air also can trigger wheezing, a warm room is probably the best environment to practice in. It's also useful to warm up and cool down slowly, as happens in most yoga classes. Be careful about working out in hot and humid rooms without replacing fluids, as dehydration can worsen asthma symptoms (see p. 96).

Barbara finds that a lot of the standard advice she's heard about asthma in yoga circles didn't work well for her. The rapid breathing technique known as Skull Shining Breath

OTHER YOGIC IDEAS

To help students suffering an asthma attack, Iyengar teachers often recommend supported forward bends. For example, the student might sit in a simple cross-legged position resting the chest and head on a bolster or stack of blankets placed on the floor (left). A student who is tight in the hips could lean

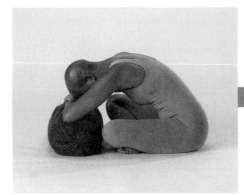

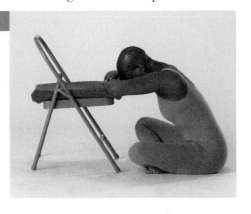

forward resting the forehead on a chair (right). Students who are able to do so comfortably would be encouraged to stay ten minutes or longer in each pose.

(Kapalabhati), which some teachers advocate for asthma, disagreed with her, particularly anytime she was having a flare-up of symptoms. Similarly, some teachers recommend backbends. "I would say, no, no, no, not backbends," unless you're totally asymptomatic.

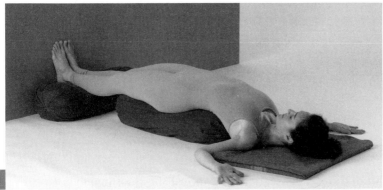

"When you're symptomatic, backbends are virtually impossible to do. Your chest is so tight. It makes you start to cough and gasp." She finds backbends take too much out of you if your energy is low, a

FIGURE 10.5

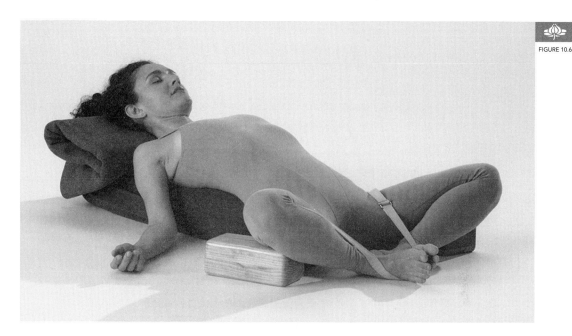

FIGURE 10.6

common predicament among people with asthma. Backbends can also be overstimulating if you're already anxious, also common in the condition. If, however, you are asymptomatic, Barbara believes that backbends, especially when supported and done as part of a regular practice, can be very useful to help open tight intercostals. Examples of restorative chest openers include Supported Bridge (Setu Bandha Sarvangasana) (figure 10.5) and Supported Cobbler's pose (Supta Baddha Konasana) (figure 10.6).

Barbara advises that people with asthma refrain from any pranayama practices in which you extend the inhalation or retain the breath after inhaling. She worries that strong Ujjayi breathing may constrict the throat too much and contribute to breathing problems. If using a milder Ujjayi, she stresses not forcing it and making sure that the exhalation stays equal to the inhalation. Pranayama techniques like Sithali (see p. 454), where you inhale through the mouth, may also be inadvisable, since the cooled air could trigger bronchospasm, impeding the flow of air.

In many flowing classes including Ashtanga and power yoga, you are supposed to change from one posture to the next during a single inhalation or exhalation, a real strain for many people with asthma. Barbara believes that asthmatics should avoid such rapid-paced vinyasa flows. If you take such classes, Viniyoga teacher Leslie Kaminoff suggests that you never force the breathing. If your system isn't accepting the prescribed breathing pattern, Leslie says, "it's for a reason." Whenever necessary, he suggests you take a catch-up breath, an extra breath in between, so your breathing is never strained.

A Holistic Approach to Asthma

✳ People who engage in regular aerobic exercise have fewer asthma flare-ups, use less medication, and miss fewer days of school and work.

✳ Weight loss can be helpful because people who are overweight tend to breath more shallowly and that can make the airways more likely to go into bronchospasm.

✳ Coughing, wheezing, or shortness of breath at night may signal a need for medication or a change in the time you take it.

✳ Oral steroids like Prednisone can be necessary and even lifesaving for some patients—as Barbara and Ken can both attest. But they should be avoided when possible or used at the minimum effective dose and for the shortest possible time, because if used for a long period of time they can cause devastating side effects, including suppression of immunity, weight gain, high blood pressure, serious mood disturbances, as well as osteoporosis and other bone problems.

✳ Inhaled steroids are much safer than oral steroids but may thin bones, among other side effects. One simple way to reduce the amount that gets absorbed into your system is to rinse out your mouth after each dose.

✳ The inhaled medication Cromolyn, while not as effective as inhaled steroids, appears to be extremely safe. If steroids still prove necessary, using Cromolyn might allow you to get away with a lower dose.

✳ Pneumonia vaccines and annual flu shots are advisable.

✳ Take steps to lower your exposure to polluted air, both indoors and outdoors (see pp. 79–81).

✳ The overwhelming majority of people with asthma have environmental allergies that can trigger inflammation and reduced lung function. Avoidance is key.

✳ If you have pets, keep them out of your bedroom since you probably spend more time there than in any other room. Also avoid wool, which acts as a magnet for dander. Try cotton instead.

✳ Dehumidifiers eliminate excess moisture that can lead to the buildup of mold and dust mites.

* On-the-job exposures to chemicals, molds, and other irritants and allergy-inducing substances can play an unrecognized role in exacerbating, even causing, asthma. Wearing protective equipment, limiting exposures, and if necessary, getting a different job or different job assignment may be advisable.

* Food allergies are an underrecognized trigger of asthma attacks, particularly life-threatening ones. Nuts, wheat, soy, and eggs can be problematic for some. An "elimination diet" (see p. 76) can help sort out what's okay and what's not.

* Diet can play a role in either fueling or cooling down inflammation (see "A Holistic Approach to Arthritis," p. 167).

* The spices ginger and tumeric have anti-inflammatory properties and can be used in cooking or taken as supplements.

Ken feels his yoga practice helped him to understand "that there's a whole lot more to the way you breathe than simply something that's mechanical and keeps you alive," and he became much more conscious of the entire process. Besides keeping up his yoga practice and doing the exercises in Barbara's article, he found a recording of breathing practices by Dr. Andrew Weil and started doing them. "I would try Barbara's techniques, and then sometimes I would try Andy Weil's techniques. I kind of came to my own method, I guess." He also does supported backbends lying down over bolsters at the beginning and end of his yoga practice, because he finds they help open his chest.

This kind of pragmatic approach is completely in line with Barbara's philosophy. "It doesn't matter what the problem is, no one method works for everybody. If something doesn't work, I throw it out. If it does work, I keep it in." Her suggestion for customizing your own program: "Attention, trial and error, persevering until you come up with something that reliably works."

Just over two years ago, with his doctor's blessing, Ken was able to get off steroids and he's been steroid-free ever since (although he does still occasionally need to use Albuterol, the bronchodilator). In addition, Ken is still working on becoming a full-time nose breather. Barbara's article had made him aware he was a mouth breather, and he understands why that's a problem, but finds it a challenge to change such an ingrained habit.

As a result of the practices, Ken's awareness of his breathing and his ability to regulate it extend beyond his yoga mat. "I used to breathe very shallowly. I definitely breathe more deeply and more slowly now. I'm very conscious about the exhale, so I spend a lot of time measuring. Am I exhaling at least twice as long as I'm inhaling? Am I pausing after the exhale? Am I making sure I'm not pausing after the inhale? It's a very conscious thing, when I'm walking, when I'm on the subway, whatever." Ken has found the 1:2 breath practice so useful that he does it during the course of his day as often as he can, and is trying to make it his normal way of breathing.

Beyond improving his asthma, the exercises have made breathing more pleasurable, Ken says. "Breathing always used to be a struggle for me, even in the best of times." Now, he says, "breathing feels good, emotionally as well as physically."

From a yogic point of view, of course, breath is intimately connected to your emotions and to your spirit. Indeed, yogis like to point out that the roots of the words *spirit* and *respiration* are the same. In Sanskrit the word *prana* means both breath and life force. Bring awareness to your breath, yogic philosophy teaches, and you can calm the mind and get closer to the source of wisdom inside you, the calm inner witness that some people call spirit.

The changes Ken has experienced have been so profound that they've transformed his relationships to the people around him, too. "I'm much calmer," he says. "I used to be very high stress. I was a nightmare to work for. I would just get people all excited and running around. That is gone from my life. Even the people at work say, 'It's really nice to be around you now.' My kids have said it, my friends have said it, so it must be true."

BACK PAIN

 JUDITH HANSON LASATER calls herself a yoga teacher who also happens to be a physical therapist. She was already teaching yoga when one day, some thirty-five years ago, it occurred to her she should become a PT, "because I wanted to be a better yoga teacher. My husband asked me, 'Have you ever been to one?' No. 'Do you know what they do?' No. 'Do you know anything about it?' No. But I literally woke up and knew that was what I wanted to do." This intuition proved to be a good one. Her PT training gave her a much deeper understanding of human anatomy and kinesiology and has allowed her to take what she's learned back to other yoga teachers to help them to become more professional and better at communicating with doctors. Judith herself regularly gets referrals from MDs, some of whom she's never even met. Judith also holds a doctorate in East-West psychology, and is the author of six books on yoga, including *Relax and Renew: Restful Yoga for Stressful Times,* on the practice and therapeutic aspects of restorative yoga. She teaches in the San Francisco Bay Area and worldwide.

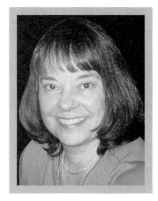

The first time Bonnie Willdorf's back "went out" was in 1980 when she was lifting an infant out of a car. "I had sciatica, with pain going down my right leg all the way to the foot. For two or three years in a row, I was flat on my back for a few months at a time." Another long flare-up of back pain a few years later prompted a trip to a surgeon, who as surgeons are wont to do, recommended an operation. "He said, 'Maybe we should schedule you,' and then the next day I got better."

Drawing the obvious conclusion that there was a psychological component to her pain, Bonnie recalls a month-long trip to the Southwest that started with so much pain she didn't think she could continue. "By the second day it was gone, because I was on vacation." When she continued over the years to have flare-ups, she consulted various orthopedists and tried physical therapy, but other than soaking in a hot tub nothing seemed to help much.

Besides stress, Bonnie felt her back problems were probably related to "bad body mechanics. I've always had bad posture. I tend to hunch my shoulders over and stick my head forward. I was not an athletic person growing up. I grew up in a family where the only muscle you were supposed to exercise was the one in your head. We did poetry readings on Sundays, we didn't take hikes." She thought perhaps yoga could help. At a friend's suggestion, she began to study with Judith.

When she started with Judith in 1993, Bonnie couldn't do a lot of the asana in class because the poses hurt her lower back. But Judith always has a "hospital row" in the back of her classes, and a "hospital row assistant" who puts people in restorative positions, under Judith's direction. Gradually Bonnie was able to move out of hospital row, and then decided to study privately with Judith to work more intensively on a solution to her back pain.

Overview of Back Pain

Nearly everyone experiences low back pain at one time or another. Current estimates rate back problems as the second most common reason for visiting MDs, the top reason for visiting a chiropractor, and the leading cause of disability of people under forty-five. The most common malady is referred to as low back strain, a catch-all phrase that includes minor muscle, ligament, and joint problems in the lumbar spine and surrounding tissues. While a seemingly trivial event such as sneezing or getting out of a chair can trigger a bout of back pain, doctors recognize that the pain is usually the culmination of years of subtle injuries and trauma to the back. Generally more severe is sciatica, a condition most commonly caused when the shock-absorbing disk that separates two spinal vertebrae bulges out and compresses a nerve root exiting the spinal cord, causing pain which radiates down the leg, sometimes all the way to the foot. A few people have sciatic leg pain but no pain in the back.

The medical profession's approach to back pain has shifted a lot in recent years. When I was in medical training, bed rest was the standard approach, and that's what was recommended to Bonnie early on. Doctors now realize that lying around is actually counterproductive, leading to a decrease in conditioning and an increase in pain. The longer you stay in bed the more muscle mass you lose (up to 3 percent per day, according to some authorities), and the resulting loss of strength can interfere with your rehabilitation, and force you to overwork other muscles to compensate. Rather than babying a back injury, doctors now recommend people start gentle activities the first day.

How Yoga Fits In

Though physicians tend to take a one-size-fits-all approach to low back strain, from a yogic perspective this doesn't make a lot of sense. There are dozens of possible causes of back pain other than sciatica. Ligaments can be strained. Arthritis can develop in the small facet joints that link one vertebra to the next. Due to postural problems, scoliosis, or injuries, the vertebrae and the ribs may be poorly aligned with one another. Whatever the underlying cause, the result may be muscle spasms in a variety of locations that can be more painful than the original problem. Given all the possibilities, it's extremely unlikely that the same set of exercises, the same medications, or the same operations will help everyone.

Despite the ubiquity of low back pain, it is one of the conditions that modern medicine does the worst job of treating. Partly due to the imprecision of diagnosis and relative ineffectiveness of most conventional treatments, many people with back pain end up on the conveyor belt that sooner or later leads to surgery. These operations are often not terribly effective, usually fail to address major underlying factors, cause their own problems, and in the vast majority of cases can be avoided. While there are instances when surgery is required—sometimes on an emergency basis—back operations continue to be one of the most commonly performed unnecessary surgeries. Keep in mind when evaluating your therapeutic options that most cases resolve in six to eight weeks, pretty much no matter what you do. Even with herniated disks, the overwhelming majority of people recover without an operation. Above all, you do not want to rush into surgery, when other, safer, less invasive methods are available—methods that are in the long run more effective and less likely to cause problems. If you are scheduled for elective surgery, you might consider canceling the operation and seeking the opinion of the best yoga therapist or bodyworker you can find to make sure you're not about to make a huge mistake. They may be able to figure out what set you up for back trouble in the first place, by examining factors like posture, your emotions, and your work and living environment. Failure to address these issues is another reason back surgery is less successful than it might be, and why many surgical patients wind up needing a second or third operation to address problems that develop at another level of the spine.

Although conventional physicians tend not to examine the role of stress in back pain, many people, like Bonnie, see a connection between their back problems and psychological tension. When the body's stress-response system is activated, tension in muscles increases, which by itself can cause pain. Some experts outside of the mainstream, most notably physician John Sarno, the author of *Healing Back Pain: The Mind-Body Connection,* argue the cause is usually entirely psychological. Dr. Sarno believes that back muscles go into spasm and cause pain because of mental tension, and that if you can get to the root cause of the tension the pain will disappear.

Yoga teacher Aadil Palkhivala also sees the connection between emotional difficulties and back pain, which is reflected in the expression "unable to bear the burden." He suggests writing in a journal to find relief. "Burden the page with your burden," he says. As someone who has dealt with his own significant back injuries, Aadil reports that he "can feel the nerves starting to relax as I write." When the nerves relax, when the balance in the autonomic nervous system is shifted to the restorative parasympathetic side, the deep muscles that may be the source of the pain start to let go.

From a yogic perspective, other factors are important, too. Beyond stress, and emotions like anger and dissatisfaction, yoga links back pain to posture, muscle tightness, and muscle weakness, as well as to a lack of body awareness—all issues that yoga is very effective in addressing.

Posture is a critical factor. A person with good posture has a spine that curves gently forward in the lower back and backward in the upper back. This S-shaped curve acts like a shock absorber for the pressures placed on the spine. When these healthy curves either flatten or arch too much, it can compress the vertebrae and the spinal disks between them, causing pain or irritation of the nerves coming out of the spine.

The sloped shoulders, forward head position, and C-shaped slump of the upper back so typical of modern life can lead to chronic neck and back pain. In some people, partly due to tightness in the hamstrings, the pelvis tips backward and the lower back rounds, reversing its normal inward curve. This position puts enormous strain on the spinal disks in the lumbar region and can lead to herniation and sciatica. For more on the yogic approach to improving slouching posture, see chapters 2 and 13.

Doctors often prescribe abdominal exercises like stomach crunches to people who have had back pain, to prevent recurrences once they are out of the acute phase. Such advice reflects the notion that most back pain is related to weak abdominal muscles. From a yogic perspective, abdominal weakness is often part of the problem, but that approach is imprecise. Indeed, too many crunches or other abdominal exercises can increase the tightness in hip flexors like the psoas (a large muscle deep in the abdomen that connects the lower spine to the top of the leg bone), potentially exacerbating some back problems. Besides tight hamstrings, many people with back pain have tight hip rotators in the pelvis. Yogis also realize that often the back extensors, the muscles that run on either side of the spine and keep you from slumping, are weak. The yogic approach is to determine which

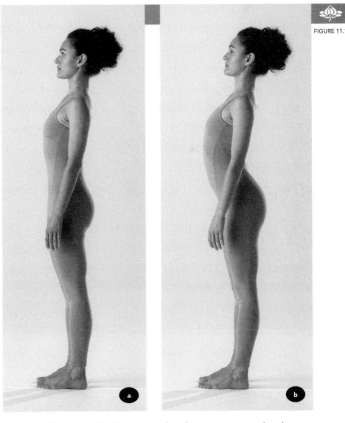

FIGURE 11.1

specific muscles need strengthening and which ones need stretching, and design a program to address those needs. This individually tailored yoga approach is much more likely to be effective than the kind of blanket recommendation to strengthen your abdominal muscles typically issued by MDs.

Some people get back pain because of excessive flexibility in their joints. Pain can be the result, for example, of arching the lumbar spine too much, exaggerating the normal lower back curve. This situation, known as swayback (figures 11.1a & b) is more seen in women, and can be exacerbated due to the hormonal changes during pregnancy (and the weight of the

a) Normal posture b) Excessive lumbar curve, swayback

baby). Weakness of the lower abdominal muscles can contribute to swayback. By learning to engage these muscles (move your navel toward your spine is the instruction yoga teachers often give), students can learn to flatten out some of the excess in the lower back curve. While sit-ups may be useful in this situation, a number of asana systematically address weakness, as well as lack of flexibility, in the four different layers of muscles in the abdomen, in ways that exercises like stomach crunches don't.

Independent of the effect on individual muscles, asana movements help back pain by improving the circulation that brings nutrients to the intervertebral disks while removing toxins. Gelatinous shock absorbers that cushion vertebrae that are adjacent to each other, the disks don't have their own independent blood supply, and thus depend on movement of surrounding structures to aid in the delivery of nutrients. Movement causes the disks to be compressed, which squeezes out stale disk fluid, and then to expand, bringing a fresh supply. Yogis believe that asanas, with their systematic stretching, bending, wringing, and soaking of the disks are particularly effective at delivering the oxygen and other nutrients the disks need to remain healthy and pain free.

Attention to breath, as always, is part of the yogic prescription for back pain. Slow, deep breaths help ratchet down an overactive stress-response system, which can lead to muscle relaxation. With the fuller exhalations that occur when the abdominal muscles assist in pushing the air out, more oxygen is brought into the body on the subsequent breath. In addition, the undulations of deep inhalations and exhalations gently massage the spinal column, which also helps bring nutrients to spinal disks.

Awareness is crucial to the yogic approach to back pain. Many people with bad postural habits may simply not notice what they are doing. It becomes natural to bring the awareness of alignment learned during asana practice to your everyday life. You may notice, for example, your habit of slumping in an office chair, on a couch, or even standing in line. Again and again, says Judith, you may need to remind yourself to be attentive to how you are using your body when you wash dishes, pick up the laundry, watch TV, or engage in any of the routine activities that are part of everyday life.

Awareness and the focus on breathing differentiate some yoga stretches from similar-looking exercises you might get in conventional physical therapy. In yoga asana, your attention is focused on what you are doing and on how it affects sensations in your body and mind. Most PT exercises, in contrast, are usually done fairly mindlessly and mechanically, perhaps even while watching television. When you do PT exercises without awareness, without tuning in, they are exactly the same thing every day—rote and uninteresting. No wonder so many people stop doing them.

Yoga done right gets more interesting over time. Good yoga asanas don't just improve the functioning of the physical body, they engage your mind. Bringing your attention to what you are doing, and precisely how you are doing it, builds the ability to feel your body's signals. Bring yogic awareness and conscious breathing to standard PT exercises and my guess is that they, too, will be more effective. This greater proprioceptive awareness (your felt sense of your body position) also allows you to notice subtle changes that would once have eluded you—serving as an early warning system when stress, poor posture, or other factors may be leading to back pain.

The Scientific Evidence

A program of mindfulness-based stress reduction, which includes mindfulness meditation and hatha yoga, proved effective for patients with chronic pain, including back pain sufferers. There is also evidence that McKenzie physical therapy exercises, which use gentle backbends resembling yoga poses, can help with back pain. The large survey of yoga practitioners mentioned in chapter 1 found that 98 percent of more than one thousand people with back pain found yoga helpful.

Another survey supporting yoga's effectiveness in back pain comes from an out-of-print book called *Backache Relief,* coauthored by Dava Sobel, author of *Longitude* and *Galileo's Daughter.* The authors polled almost five hundred back pain sufferers to try to find out what had worked for them, asking about care from orthopedic surgeons, osteopaths, chiropractors, acupuncturists, Rolfers, and Feldenkrais practitioners, as well as the use of muscle relaxants, anti-inflammatory drugs, hot packs, ice packs, shoe orthotics, TENS nerve-stimulation units, and even marijuana. Overall, yoga was judged the "most successful of all approaches to backache relief for nonincapacitated backache sufferers—with twenty-three out of twenty-four survey participants [who did yoga] reporting significant long-term improvement." Of note, the survey respondents who tried yoga through books, articles, and tapes got some relief but much less than those who worked with a yoga teacher (whether in a class or private session was not specified). Several participants recommended simple abdominal breathing (for instructions, see pp. 55–56), up to five minutes a day, to reduce stress and build abdominal muscle tone.

A recent randomized controlled study of twenty-two people, published in *Alternative Therapies in Health and Medicine,* studied hatha yoga for people with chronic low back pain that had not responded to at least two modalities such as physical therapy and chiropractic. The six-week intervention included twice-weekly one-hour classes for six weeks consisting of gentle asanas, meditation, and relaxation. As compared to controls, the yoga group showed improvements in balance and flexibility, disability, and mood, though none of these reached the level of statistical significance. Three months later, eight of the eleven people in the yoga group completed a survey. Six of eight reported improvement in back pain since the completion of the study. Seven of eight reported ongoing benefit from the yoga intervention. All eight believed that yoga facilitated relaxation and greater awareness, and recommended yoga to other people with chronic low back pain.

A randomized controlled trial led by Kimberly Williams of West Virginia University School of Medicine compared the effects of an adapted regimen of Iyengar yoga on patients with chronic low back pain to a group that received a weekly informational newsletter. Of sixty subjects enrolled at the beginning of the study, forty-two completed the study. The yoga group attended sixteen weekly classes. Compared to controls, the yoga group experienced a 64 percent reduction in pain, a 77 percent reduction in "functional disability" (problems with accomplishing everyday tasks), and a 25 percent improvement in perceived control over pain. They also gained significantly in hip flexibility. Of those patients taking pain medication at the beginning of the study, 88 percent of the yoga group either reduced their dose or eliminated medication entirely as compared to 35 percent of controls.

A randomized controlled trial, published in the *Annals of Internal Medicine,* compared Viniyoga to conventional therapeutic exercise to a self-care book in 101 people with chronic low back pain. Patients in both the yoga and exercise groups had a seventy-five-minute class weekly for twelve weeks, while the third group received a booklet about strategies for coping with back pain. The yoga and exercise groups were encouraged to practice at home between sessions. At the twelve-week mark, the yoga group had a small but statistically significant improvement compared to the exercise group, and a large improvement compared to the booklet group. Between twelve and twenty-six weeks, only the yoga group continued to improve; the other groups worsened. When the participants were questioned twenty-six weeks after starting the protocol, 12 percent in the yoga group had sought back-related treatment from a health care professional, compared with 19 percent in the exercise group and 31 percent in the group given the booklet. In the yoga group, 21 percent had taken medication for back pain in the twenty-sixth week, compared to 50 percent of the exercise group and 59 percent in the booklet group.

Judith Hanson Lasater's Approach

"There are many causes of back pain and many different ways it manifests and many different ways to approach it," says Judith. "Some people just need a lot of stress reduction and posture education. Other people need stretching and strengthening." While it sometimes seems like an inevitable part of aging, Judith feels that "in the overwhelming majority of cases, back pain can be prevented. Some problems are congenital, some are the result of accidents, but the majority have to do with how we use our bodies." Her approach is to look for the simplest cause first. "I would look first at standing posture, sitting and driving posture, and sleeping posture." She finds that "almost no one stands well," a problem she suspects is related to "spending all of our time in chairs, which puts the maximum pressure on the disks and weakens the abdominal muscles."

Like many of the back-pain students Judith sees, Bonnie had a sedentary job and the postural problems that typically accompany long periods spent in a chair. She tended to flatten her lower back, her head was held forward of her spine with her chin tipped up, and her shoulders were rounded forward, suggesting the interscapular muscles, the ones that hold your shoulder blades upright, weren't doing their job.

TIP Dr. Galen Cranz, a professor of architecture at the University of California at Berkeley and the author of *The Chair: Rethinking Culture, Body, and Design*, as well as a yoga practitioner and a teacher of the Alexander Technique, thinks that most chairs are poorly designed for spinal health, particularly for anyone under five foot six inches. She suggests sitting whenever possible with the feet flat on the floor and the sit bones (the bony prominence in each buttock) higher than the knees. This position allows the lumbar spine to maintain its normal, healthy inward curve. Ideally, the angle between the legs and the trunk, she says, should be around 120 degrees, but anything greater than 90 degrees is helpful. If your chair can't be adjusted to this angle, you can place a book or cushion on the seat of the chair to raise the level of the hips, and another book on the floor if your feet don't reach the ground. Otherwise she suggests scooting forward to perch on the edge of the chair, keeping your spine straight and maintaining a healthy angle between the legs and torso (this may not sound inviting but is a surprisingly comfortable position) (see p. 229).

Judith pays particular attention when people have radiating pain, because that indicates there is an impingement of the nerve, whether it's coming from a herniated disk or from a tight piriformis muscle pressing on the sciatic nerve in the buttocks (which is often missed by doctors). In Bonnie's case, the pain radiated down her leg all the way to the foot and suggested disk herniation in the lumbar region.

After taking a history, the first thing Judith often does in a private session with a student with back pain is ask to see a position in which the student is pain free. Often it's lying on the back with the knees bent, which eliminates all the stress of gravity. Judith tells the rare students who can find no position of comfort that they need to seek a medical evaluation before she can work with them. She wants to be sure there isn't something that is beyond her area of expertise at the root of the problem.

While serious or even potentially life-threatening causes of back pain are a lot less common than poor posture and stress, sometimes a trip to the doctor is definitely in order. The older you are, the more you should consider seeing a doctor before you consult a yoga therapist. Four major medical conditions that can cause pain similar to what accompanies run-of-the-mill low back strain include:

1. Infection. Rarely, the spinal bones themselves become infected, but more commonly back pain can be caused by a kidney infection. Suggestive symptoms include fever, and for kidney infections, frequent and uncomfortable urination.

2. Cancer. Multiple myeloma is a bone marrow cancer that can take up residence in the spine. Other cancers, notably breast and prostate, can spread to bones of the spine.

3. Spinal Fracture. Both cancer and osteoporosis can predispose to spinal fractures. Unrelenting pain not relieved by changing positions may be an indicator.

4. Neurological Problems. Several back conditions can cause loss of sensation in the legs or difficulty with urination or bowel control. These symptoms should prompt an immediate medical evaluation.

Because Bonnie had already had a number of medical evaluations and Judith could see a clear relationship between her symptoms and her posture as well as her stress levels, she felt comfortable proceeding, and confident that yoga could help. Judith lists a number of goals the following yoga routine was designed to address for Bonnie: "I was looking for abdominal strength, more lumbar curve, greater strength in the interscapular [between the shoulder blades] muscles, and a better head position."

Here is the sequence of the poses and instructions that Judith provided for Bonnie:

FIGURE 11.2

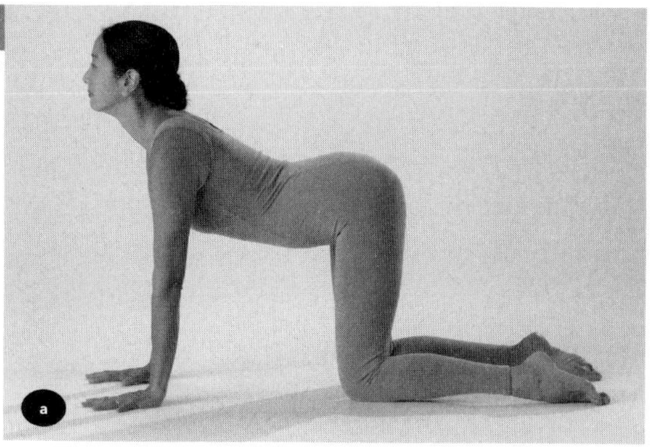

EXERCISE #1. **CAT/COW, ten to twenty times.** Start by kneeling on all fours, with your spine in neutral position, your knees directly beneath your hips, and your hands beneath your

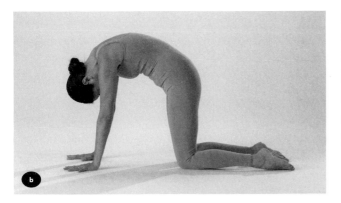

shoulders. Exhale and gently arch your spine (figure 11.2a), then inhale and round your back (figure 11.2b). Move slowly between the two positions, coordinating the movements with your breath.

EXERCISE #2. **CAT/COW, turning the head and looking back, five times to each side.** Start on all fours as before, in neutral position. As you exhale, turn your head and look back at your right foot. Let your trunk bend on the right side and stretch on the left side as you look back. As you inhale, return to the starting position. Then, exhale and look toward your left foot, feeling the response in your spine.

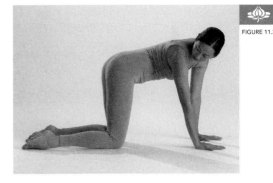

FIGURE 11.3

EXERCISE #3. **CAT/COW, lifting arm toward ceiling and following it with your eyes, three to five times on each side.** From the same all-fours position, inhale, rotate your trunk, and lift your right hand up toward the ceiling and follow it with your eyes. On the exhalation lower your hand. Repeat on the other side. Do the entire exercise three to five times, alternating sides. "This is a rotational movement," Judith says, "but it's in a different relationship to gravity than a seated twist and so often feels better than sitting and twisting." All these Cat/Cow exercises create mobility in your spine.

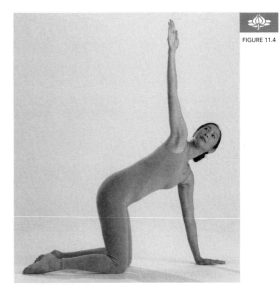

FIGURE 11.4

EXERCISE #4. **COBRA VARIATION, with arms at your sides, three times.** Lie face-down on your mat. Keeping your legs on the floor at least hips' width apart and your knees turned inward toward each other, raise your hands slightly and lift your upper body into

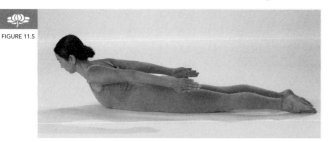

FIGURE 11.5

a slight backward arch as you exhale. Hold for several breaths and then lower yourself down as you exhale. Turn your head to one side and rest. This is strengthening for the lower-back muscles and mobilizes the middle back area, which often becomes stiff from sitting and bending forward at a desk for hours. Try this three times if it feels good, alternating the direction in which you turn your head when you come down.

EXERCISE #5. **COBRA VARIATION, with arms bent, three times.** Lie facedown on your mat. Move your arms out to the sides, so your body is in the shape of the letter T, and then bend the elbows to 90 degrees. From this position, exhale as you come into a gentle

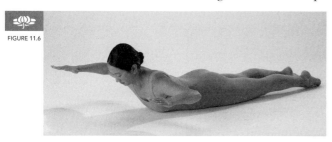

FIGURE 11.6

backbend. Be sure to keep your legs on the floor and your chin slightly dropped so as not to compress your neck. Stay for several breaths and come down as you exhale. Rest, turning your head to one side. When you repeat, turn your head the other way.

EXERCISE #6. **COBRA VARIATION, with arms extended in front of body, two times.** Repeat Cobra pose as in the previous exercise, using the same breathing, this time

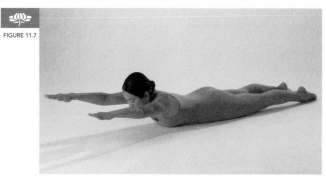

FIGURE 11.7

with your arms forward, like Superman, over your head. You'll be tempted to lift your legs, but be sure to keep your legs on the floor. Judith says that this exercise uses the intrinsic back muscles to lift you instead of the arms and is quite strengthening. Try this two times, exhaling as you lift.

EXERCISE #7. **SUPINE HIP ROTATOR STRETCH, three times on each side.** Start by lying on your back with your knees bent. As you exhale, tilt your pelvis slightly backward and bring your lower back to the floor and your right knee halfway in toward your chest. Take your left foot and cross it over your right knee, and with your right hand, reach around the outside of your right leg and hold the back of your right thigh just above the bend of the knee. Place your left hand on the inside of your left knee. On an exhalation, simultaneously bring your right knee toward you as you gently push your left knee away. Feel the stretch in your outer left hip (figure 11.8). Hold for several breaths. To come out of the pose, exhale and place your right foot and then your left on the floor with your knees bent. Repeat on the other side. Be sure to keep breathing as you practice.

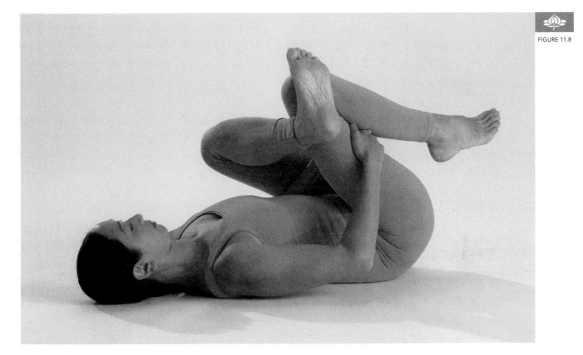

FIGURE 11.8

Judith says that this exercise is a good stretch of the external rotators of the hip. If people are really tight in their rotator muscles, it interferes with the ability of the pelvis to move in normal daily activities like walking. When the rotators hold the pelvis too much, the biomechanical forces of movement are transferred up to the next movable segment in the kinetic chain, which is the lumbar spine.

For people with back pain, the standing poses, such as those below, are very important because of the loosening effect they have on the hip joints. They stretch all the major muscle groups around the hip joints: the adductors, the quads, the rotators, and the hamstrings. Judith says that if you stop doing them for a week, you will feel the difference.

EXERCISE #8. TRIANGLE POSE (Trikonasana), three to five breaths on each side, twice. Stand with your feet three and a half feet to four feet apart. Turn your right foot out 90 degrees and your left foot in 15 to 30 degrees. Raise your arms to your sides with the

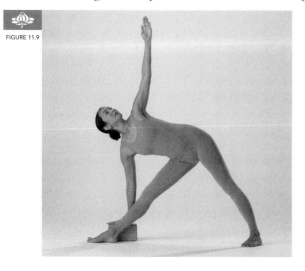

FIGURE 11.9

palms down. On an exhalation, bend at the hips and bring your right arm down onto a block placed outside and just behind your right foot (figure 11.9). Judith suggests allowing the top of your pelvis in the back to slightly rotate forward to stretch the rotators on your back hip. Slightly rotate the chest up toward the ceiling. Be sure to allow a normal inward curve in your lower back. In other words, don't tuck your pelvis. Hold for three to five breaths and come up on an exhalation. Repeat on the other side, and then do both sides again.

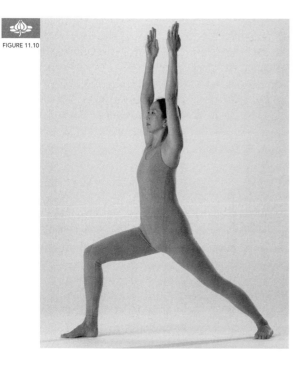

FIGURE 11.10

EXERCISE #9. WARRIOR I (Virabhadrasana I), three breaths on each side. Stand with your feet three to four feet apart. Turn your right foot out 90 degrees and your left foot in 30 to 40 degrees. Bring your hips around so they are square with your front foot. Raise your arms over your head and bend your front leg to 90 degrees to come into the pose, being careful not to allow the knee to extend beyond the ankle or drift inward. Judith says this pose stretches the hip flexors and the quadriceps (the big muscles in the front of the thighs). It is not only strengthening but also empowering. Hold for three breaths, and repeat on the other side. Keep breathing as you move.

EXERCISE #10. **REVOLVED TRIANGLE POSE (Parivrtta Trikonasana), three breaths on each side, twice.** Stand with your feet as in Warrior I. Raise your left arm and

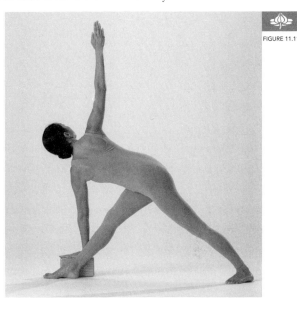

FIGURE 11.11

on an exhalation twist your spine, place your left hand on a block placed on the outside of your right foot, and lift your right arm toward the ceiling (figure 11.11). Move slowly so you can pay attention to how the pose feels for your lower back. Inhale as you come out of the pose. Repeat on the other side, again moving into the pose on your exhalation and coming out on your inhalation. Judith says this pose is a strong weightbearing stretch of the rotators, and is only for those who feel okay in the lower back area and are not in an acute phase. Stay for three breaths. Do the pose twice on each side.

TIP Using a block under the lower hand in poses like Triangle and Revolved Triangle maximizes the therapeutic benefit by creating more stability and allowing you to ground yourself more completely in your legs, which in turn creates more freedom in the lower spine and allows you to rotate your rib cage more easily. The added height also allows greater movement of your spine and ribs.

EXERCISE #11. **CHILD'S POSE (Balasana).** Sit with your toes together and your knees separated to a comfortable degree. Then fold forward between your knees and stretch your arms out behind you, palms up, along your sides. Place your forehead on the floor, and keep your lower back rounded. Stay in the pose for thirty seconds to two minutes if it feels good. Keep your breathing soft.

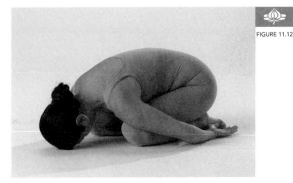

FIGURE 11.12

Yogic Tool: **HANDS-ON ADJUSTMENTS.** When Bonnie did Child's pose in class, Judith or one of her assistants would typically give Bonnie an assist. Judith would stand behind Bonnie, and put her hands with her fingers pointing toward her own body over Bonnie's sacroiliac joint area, where the spine and the pelvis meet, pressing diagonally back and down. She doesn't just press down toward the floor or back toward the student's feet. Pressing diagonally down and back, she says, relieves all the erectors by stretching them and the connective tissue in the area. The lower back erectors often get tight, in part because of our sitting and standing posture.

OTHER YOGIC IDEAS

David Coulter, former anatomy professor, yoga teacher in the tradition of the Himalayan Institute, and author of *Anatomy of Hatha Yoga,* has found that a supine

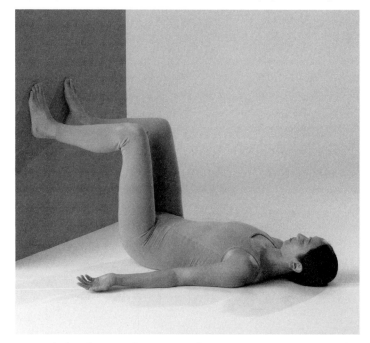

position with the knees bent and the soles of the feet against a wall allows you to do a gentle motion of the lower back (the lumbar spine) that most people find soothing. Feel the small curve in your lower back. Then, as you exhale, press your feet into the wall to coax your lumbar spine to flatten toward the floor. Release your foot pressure as you inhale to allow the curve to return to your lower spine. Repeating this several times allows you to begin moving your spine in a safe and controlled way.

EXERCISE #12. **RELAXATION POSE (Savasana).** Lie on the floor with your head supported, your eyes covered with a soft cloth, and your arms and legs at a comfortable distance from your body (figure 11.13). You may find the pose easier on your back if you place a bolster or a rolled blanket under your knees. Many students also appreciate a smaller roll under their Achilles tendons at the back of their ankles. When you are comfortable,

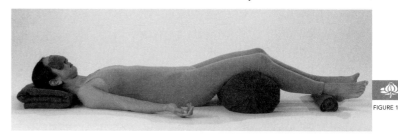

FIGURE 11.13

breathe slowly and allow yourself to sink into the floor, letting go of all tension and allowing your mind to focus on the sensation of your breath. To come out of the pose, bend your knees and roll slowly to your right side. Rest a moment, then use your arms to push yourself to a sitting position (see pp. 60–61). Remain quiet for a few more moments before getting up. Judith always recommends this pose for people with lower back pain. She says, "This is the most important pose we can practice."

Contraindications, Special Considerations, and Modifications

Forward bends, particularly if there is also an element of twisting involved as in Head-to-Knee pose (Janu Sirsasana), can compress nerve roots and aggravate sciatica (figure 11.14). People with lumbar disk problems generally shouldn't be doing seated twists or forward bends. Seated forward bends are harder on the lumbar spine than standing forward bends because it is more difficult to tip the pelvis forward when it's on the ground. Although standing forward bends cause less pressure in the spinal disks than seated versions, the pressure can still be too high to make these poses safe for people with acute back injuries. The safest forward bends for the low back are those done lying on your back, as when you bring your knees to your chest. In the acute stage avoid Boat pose (Navasana), straight leg raises, Staff pose (Dandasana), and Lotus pose (Padmasana).

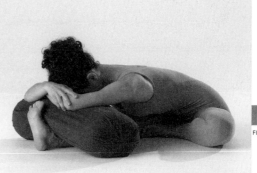

FIGURE 11.14

Head-to-Knee pose (Janu Sirsasana) can be trouble with back pain.

Backbends are sometimes part of the therapy for back problems, but in other cases are not appropriate. They can be dangerous for anyone with spondylolisthesis, a condition in which one vertebra slips forward relative to its neighbors. A backbend could worsen the slippage, potentially compressing nerve roots in the spinal canal.

There are so many causes of back trouble that what's appropriate for back pain will vary widely. In general, the best approach is to have an experienced teacher look at you and come up with a personalized evaluation of what's safe. The better you develop your body awareness, the more you will be able to make these determinations yourself.

Working through mild discomfort appears to be appropriate for people with back pain. Studies suggest that the speediest recoveries are made by back pain sufferers who began physical therapy the day of the injury or the day after, and the same is likely to be true of yoga. Avoid any sudden changes of position, and step rather than jump into poses. Even when symptom free, take special care coming in and out of asana, as it is often during transitions—when attention tends to flag—that back injuries occur.

A Holistic Approach to Back Pain

* Frequent changes of position are natural and healthy. At work, try to take regular breaks and set up your office so that you have to get up to file or answer the phone.

* When lifting heavy objects, use your legs as much as possible. If you need to bend forward, don't bend at the waist. Fold forward from the hips without allowing your lower back to round. Try to maintain a normal curvature in the lower and upper spine and avoid twisting and bending simultaneously, as this is a common mechanism of back injury.

* Wear the right shoes. Narrow-toed shoes lead to tension in the legs and back. High heels shorten the calf muscles and hamstrings and can contribute to back strain.

* Topical creams containing capsaicin or arnica and liniments based on methyl-salicylate, menthol, and camphor are soothing and very safe.

* Many people find applications of ice helpful and, once the injury is starting to heal, switch to moist heat, either alone or alternating with ice. Heat can also be useful to reduce stiffness before attempting to exercise.

* Willow bark tea (which contains the active ingredient of aspirin) may be useful.

* If your pain is severe and does not respond to over-the-counter or prescription anti-inflammatory pain relievers, ask your doctor about prescribing opioids. They are generally more effective and safer than many other pain medications, but due to exaggerated fear of addiction, they aren't used as often as they ought to be.

* The evidence on acupuncture for back pain is mixed, but it is very safe and worth considering.

* Hands-on bodywork approaches, such as chiropractic, physical therapy, therapeutic massage, and osteopathy can help you through a flare-up of back pain (though not all osteopaths do spinal manipulation, so ask before making an appointment).

* Judith finds many people with back pain get better results if they combine their yoga with bodywork such as myofascial release designed to iron out the kinks in muscles and connective tissue, and free up scar tissue and other residuals of past injuries.

* I have found the Alexander Technique, which stresses postural education, particularly effective for back problems, both as prevention and treatment. The Feldenkrais Method may be similarly valuable.

Working with Judith helped Bonnie's back a lot. "I started having fewer flare-ups, and felt like my back was getting strengthened." She also acquired tools that could help her ward off trouble. "I had poses and relaxation practices that I could do when I felt like things were going to start up." Originally, if she didn't feel good, she wouldn't go to class. "Then I came to a point where I realized if I didn't feel good and I went, I'd feel better. That was a revelation for me."

She adds, "I just got more confident about being physical. For years, I wouldn't do any yoga at home, because I was so afraid that I would do it wrong, and then I would get hurt. But five years ago, I got to the point where I felt I can do some poses, and if I'm not doing them perfectly, it doesn't matter. It just matters that I'm doing them. I can lie down and do Savasana, and I can put my legs up the wall, and I can do things that feel good, and that will be helpful."

Judith says, "Her posture has definitely improved and she's gotten much stronger—more of an inner strength, a certain comfortableness in her body." When Bonnie was having so much back pain, she wasn't able to engage in life as she likes to. She seems happier now, Judith says. "I think that she feels empowered now that she has a tool that can help her control her pain. That's one of the things that leads to depression, when people feel powerless in their life."

"When I've been doing yoga regularly," Bonnie says, "I stand better and I'm more aware of my body, my posture, and my movement." Although she hasn't practiced as regularly as she'd like, what Bonnie has consistently done is attend an annual week-long retreat that Judith teaches at the Feathered Pipe Ranch in Montana. Last summer at the workshop, Judith asked Bonnie how her back was, a subject that hadn't come up all week. Surprised at first, Bonnie said, "My back? Oh yeah, my back!" They both laughed. "As long as I do my yoga," Bonnie told her, "it's fine."

"There was a time when I thought I was destined for back surgery," Bonnie says. "In fact, I made tapes of the entire season of *Upstairs, Downstairs,* because I figured that's what I would do when I was recovering." Those tapes have been collecting dust for more than a decade.

CANCER

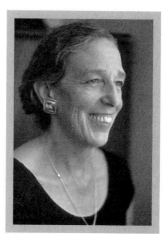

JNANI CHAPMAN is a registered nurse who teaches yoga for the Osher Center for Integrative Medicine at the University of California, San Francisco, to people with cancer, heart disease, and other chronic illness. Her style of teaching and yoga therapy is based on the Integral yoga of Swami Satchidananda, with a strong influence from her time with T. K. V. Desikachar and his students. As an integrative medicine specialist, Jnani also practices acupressure and massage at UCSF, at the Commonweal Cancer Help Program in Bolinas, California, and the Smith Farm Center in Washington, DC. She worked for Dr. Dean Ornish's Program for Reversing Heart Disease as a yoga/stress-management specialist from 1986 to 1999, and was the executive director of the International Association of Yoga Therapists from 1994 to 1997. Jnani certifies yoga teachers in adaptive yoga therapy for people with cancer and chronic illness through Yogaville, the Satchidananda ashram and teaching academy in Virginia.

In the summer of 2002, when she was thirty-nine, Erin Brand noticed a lump in her breast about the size of a hazelnut. "I found it," she remembers, "because there was actually pain. I sometimes sleep on my stomach and I noticed that I was kind of sore." She wasn't at all nervous about it because she knew that lumps that are tender are unlikely to be cancer, and because there was no history of breast cancer in her family. The fact that she'd had a baby at a relatively young age eliminated another known risk factor. She figured it was probably just a fibroid cyst, which are common and noncancerous.

Two weeks later, when she went to see her gynecologist, she had a needle aspiration of the lump just to be sure, though the doctor agreed it was probably just a cyst. Within a few days the call came, saying that they had found cancer cells. "They wanted me to meet with a surgeon the next morning," Erin says. "It was pretty shocking."

Three weeks later she had surgery to remove the lump. They also removed a so-called sentinel lymph node from under her arm but found no signs of cancer in it—an indicator that all the nodes are likely cancer free. The cancer turned out to be "an invasive tumor" less than an inch in size, surrounded in some of the nearby tissue by a less dangerous cancer, known as a ductal carcinoma in situ, or DCIS. With a small tumor and no involvement in the lymph nodes, Erin was surprised when her doctors recommended chemotherapy and radiation as well as the drug tamoxifen to block the female hormone estrogen from stimulating the cancer, but they felt that "because it was a high-grade, aggressive tumor, that was the best treatment to ensure that I wouldn't have a recurrence." Erin soon started the first of five rounds of chemotherapy.

In the middle of her second round of chemo, Erin began yoga. She'd never done it before but the hospital offered a gentle beginning yoga class for cancer patients, taught by Jnani.

Overview of Cancer

Cancer is probably the most feared disease in the modern world, although heart disease still comes first in the number of fatalities (approximately ten times as many women as from breast cancer, for example). Cancer of various varieties can be related to dietary, genetic, and environmental factors (see chapter 4), and often more than one precipitating factor must be present for the disease to manifest. Subtle abnormalities in the immune system may also play a role in the disease. Abnormal cells with the potential for uncontrolled growth—the hallmark of cancer—form in everyone's bodies with some regularity, but a healthy immune system normally gets rid of them before a tumor develops. While many members of the general public believe that stress can cause cancer, there is little scientific evidence to back this notion.

While the incidence of cancer continues to rise, survival rates have improved. Recent research published in *The Lancet* found that twenty-year survival rates were almost 90 percent for thyroid and testicular cancer, better than 80 percent for melanomas and prostate cancer, about 80 percent for endometrial cancer, and almost 70 percent for bladder cancer and Hodgkin's disease. The study estimated a twenty-year survival rate of 65 percent for breast cancer, 60 percent for cervical cancer, and about 50 percent for colorectal, ovarian, and kidney cancers. These numbers are all considerably better than in the past, at least in part due to improvements in treatment. Even in cancers where the survival odds are lower, some individuals beat the odds, and are either cured or live far longer than doctors might guess.

How Yoga Fits In

A number of yogic practices may be helpful for people with cancer in reducing stress and managing side effects, both during chemotherapy and medical procedures and after. Although people being treated for cancer usually do not have enough strength to do a vigorous asana practice, the poses can be adapted to meet almost anyone's needs. Restorative postures and simple pranayama exercises can be both energizing and relaxing, and require almost no physical effort. Meditation and guided imagery (such as found in Yoga Nidra) can be deeply relaxing and reduce anxiety. Some cancer survivors, once they are in recovery and have regained their strength, find volunteer work or other forms of service (karma yoga) to be useful in providing a sense of purpose and meaning.

Other yogic tools can help with pain, a frequent cancer symptom, particularly in its later stages, including relaxation, meditation, and breathing practices. The slower, deeper, more regular breathing that yoga facilitates can help you feel calmer and more energetic during the stressful period of being diagnosed with cancer and enduring treatment for it. Learning to cope with that stress can help you get through the ordeal, and may even improve your odds of survival.

Yoga philosophy has very practical implications for people with cancer. Yoga encourages you to listen to messages from your body (physical, emotional, and otherwise) and adjust your practice accordingly. This lesson can be extended to the rest of your life, too. If you tire after less work than you're accustomed to, yoga would say honor that. Do less. Ask friends and family to step in to help out.

Yogic Tool: **SANGHA.** Yoga stresses the value of community (sangha), and a good cancer support group can provide this. There is evidence that involvement in a group may even increase your odds of survival, though follow-up studies have not confirmed the initial very positive findings. If you are interested, the key is finding one that meets your needs. Some are geared to providing information, others focus more on addressing emotional issues. Keep looking for a group that feels right to you, even if the first one you try doesn't. If you aren't drawn to support groups, however, please don't think you need to be in one to give yourself the best shot at a cure.

· · ·

At the time of a cancer diagnosis, many people find themselves taking stock of their lives. This is a form of self-study, or svadhyaya. People tend to ask themselves if they are spending their time and energy in ways that feel good to them. This line of inquiry helps in the yogic process of finding your dharma, figuring out why you are here, taking advantage of your strengths and interests to do something meaningful to you. This is something anyone can benefit from, but sometimes it takes a life-threatening diagnosis to slow you down enough to do this work. The silence facilitated by such practices as meditation often allows the inner wisdom that lies deep inside you to surface.

Since cancer inevitably brings up fears and worries about death, for those who are willing, spirituality is an important element of yoga as medicine. Jnani suggests that you simply try to "open a spiritual space," to see things exactly as they are without trying to fix anything. "We are all intolerant of uncertainty," she says. "Spirituality opens us to whatever happens. This paradoxically increases hope and faith," which all by themselves have therapeutic benefit and can definitely improve the quality of your life. Jnani finds that an openness to spirituality can also improve the dying process.

Perhaps more than any other condition, cancer makes people feel like victims of a medical system over which they have no control. Things are done to them, often with very unpleasant side effects. Feelings of powerlessness are natural. By providing concrete steps you can take to feel better right now, and quite possibly increase your chance of long-term survival, yoga can change the whole psychology of the experience. In addition, people who feel betrayed by their bodies learn that they can still find relaxation and even joy in the body. In this space, yoga teaches, true healing can occur.

The Scientific Evidence

So far there are no scientific studies on whether yoga can improve the survival rate of people with cancer. But suggestive evidence comes from Dr. Dean Ornish, best known for his work using a comprehensive lifestyle program that included yoga for heart disease (see chapter 19). Dr. Ornish has recently begun to study a similar approach for prostate cancer. The yoga portion of the program includes gentle asana, breathing techniques, and meditation. Early results are encouraging: When the blood serum of patients following the Ornish program was added to a line of prostate cancer cells in the laboratory, the serum inhibited their growth by 67 percent, compared to only 12 percent for controls. Prostate Specific Antigen (PSA) levels, a marker of prostate cancer, decreased 3 percent in the patients following his program, while increasing 7 percent in subjects in the control group.

Dean says they found a direct correlation between the degree of change in diet and lifestyle and the change in PSAs. In other words, just as in his earlier work on heart disease, the better people followed the plan, the better their results. "This may be the first randomized controlled trial showing that the progression of not only prostate cancer, but any cancer, may be affected through diet and lifestyle alone," he says. "If it was true for prostate cancer, there's a chance that it may be true for breast cancer as well."

Researchers from the University of Calgary in Canada studied the effects of a seven-week program of Iyengar yoga on cancer survivors, primarily women treated for breast cancer. Once a week, the students took a seventy-five-minute yoga class, which consisted of gentle breathing in the pose Viparita Karani (Legs-Up-the-Wall), followed by fifty minutes of gentle asana modified to their needs and fifteen minutes of the Deep Relaxation pose Savasana (see chapter 3). The students were encouraged to practice at home between classes. Compared to those in the control group, the yoga group had significantly less tension, anxiety, depression, confusion, anger, fatigue, diarrhea, and emotional irritability. The yoga group also showed improvements over the course of the seven weeks in their physical fitness and their heart rate, both when resting and after exercise. One surprising negative finding was the yoga students reported more pain, which the researchers speculated might be related to increased body awareness as a result of their practice, though this question needs to be researched more.

Preliminary findings are encouraging from a pilot study of Iyengar yoga for breast cancer survivors with marked fatigue conducted at UCLA. Eleven women with little or no prior yoga experience completed twice-weekly ninety-minute classes of poses thought to alleviate fatigue and depression, including restorative chest openers (see chapters 3 and 15). The women showed what researchers call "strikingly large" improvements in fatigue going from 6.3 on a 10-point scale to 2.7. The women went from feeling fatigued 7 days per week to 4.6. These changes were still present on follow-up testing three months later. The women reported less pain, though the degree of improvement did not reach statistical significance. In addition, the women had significant improvements in depressive symptoms and in overall health.

A randomized controlled study conducted at the M. D. Anderson Cancer Center in Texas looked at the effects of a seven-week program of Tibetan yoga, a style not widely available in the West, on people with Hodgkin's disease and non-Hodgkin's lymphoma. The regular practice of gentle physical movements and deep, mindful breathing resulted in significantly improved duration and quality of sleep, and less use of sleeping pills. The effects were still present three months after the program was completed. There were no significant improvements noted, however, in anxiety, depression, or fatigue.

Studies of mindfulness-based stress reduction, which includes mindfulness meditation and hatha yoga, have found that it can improve mood, fatigue, and feelings of stress in people with a variety of types of cancer. Guided imagery and relaxation have been found to result in potentially beneficial changes on measures of immune system function in women with breast cancer. A program of cognitive-behavioral therapy which included group support and instruction in relaxation techniques resulted in significantly lower levels of fatigue, depression, and confusion, and improved activity of cancer-fighting natural killer cells in patients with malignant melanoma, the most serious form of skin cancer. When the researchers followed up on the melanoma patients six years later, they discovered that only three out of thirty-four patients who had done the program had died, as compared to ten out of thirty-four in the control group.

A recent randomized controlled study done by Dr. Raghavendra Rao and colleagues at the Swami Vivekananda Yoga Research Foundation in conjunction with doctors at the Bangalore Institute of Oncology looked at the effects of yoga on ninety-eight women with stage II or III breast cancer who were undergoing conventional medical care including chemotherapy, radiation, and surgery. The yoga group did asana, pranayama, meditation, and chanting, among other practices. In addition to taking regular classes, they were asked to practice an hour a day at home. The control group received supportive counseling sessions. The researchers found large and statistically significant reductions in anxiety, depression, distress, severity and number of treatment-related symptoms, and toxicity of treatments, as well as major improvements in quality of life among the yoga group. The reduced toxicity of treatments may be particularly important since when side effects are too great doctors sometimes need to stop treatment or reduce doses in ways that may diminish its effectiveness. The same authors have collected sophisticated measures of immune function in both groups, but these results have not yet been published.

Jnani Chapman's Approach

Jnani's classes for cancer patients are gentle. Some students like Erin are relatively strong but are still feeling the effects of their cancer treatment. Others are weakened by the disease. Others, having completed their treatment and gone into remission, have the strength and endurance to take on a vigorous practice. So as not to exclude anyone, Jnani teaches practices that everyone in the room will be able to do, though some students will need to modify the poses to do them safely. In choosing asanas for people with cancer or with other major illness, Jnani places a premium on safety, in line with her training as a nurse.

Most of the practices are done sitting in a chair or on a mat on the floor next to the chair, but all of them, with the exception of tuning in at the beginning and meditation and

Yoga Nidra at the end, involve movement. Usually, Jnani says, "We think the body will relax only when it is still, but I've found that slow, regular, and mindful movement of the body can induce a release of tension." In the beginning stages she stresses this continual slow movement. If students hold poses at all, they are instructed to tune in to their bodies and to come out of the hold at the first sign of any tension. Her thinking in this regard has been heavily influenced by the approach of T. K. V. Desikachar (see chapter 6).

When students are first learning the practice, Jnani errs on the side of being too gentle. She quotes Nischala Joy Devi: "If you give your students too much, you will give them indigestion. If you give them small morsels, you will increase their appetite." To keep the level of fatigue down, Jnani stresses a model of "exert, rest, exert, rest." Only when you've recovered from one pose should you move on to the next.

Here is a typical sequence of the poses and instructions Jnani teaches in cancer classes like the ones Erin attended.

Jnani begins each class with a "tuning in" process that she calls the Witness Practice, a step-by-step tour through the body. The idea is to check in with your physical body, with your mind and your thoughts, with your feelings and emotions. "Yoga teaches that by heightening your awareness—even of something painful—you can lessen its impact," Jnani says. She encourages her students to include this kind of tuning in process at the beginning of their home practices as well.

EXERCISE #1. **TUNING IN.** Start sitting up straight in your chair, getting as comfortable as you can. If your feet don't touch the floor, place a bolster beneath them so your legs can be passive and soft (figure 12.1). Let yourself relax as much as possible. When you are comfortable, begin the tuning in process:

1. Bring your awareness to the crown of your head and notice any physical sensations present in your scalp, in your face muscles, in your whole head. Whatever you notice, let it just be. In a similar fashion, draw your awareness to your neck, to your shoulders, and progressively through every part of your body. Jnani says, "You're simply saying hello, as if you are taking inventory as a completely disinterested party."

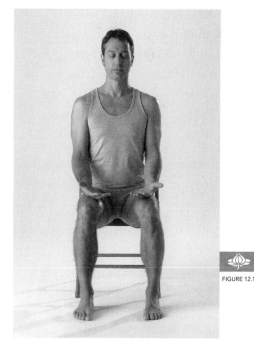

FIGURE 12.1

2. Bring your awareness to your emotional level. Notice if there are any feelings bubbling up for you that want to be acknowledged. Whatever's present, let it be.

3. Bring your awareness to your thinking level. Begin to become aware of each thought that pops into consciousness. Notice any habitual patterns of thinking, any recurrent themes.

4. Bring your awareness to your energy level, noticing whether you are feeling tired or restless or some combination of the two, or if you are feeling completely relaxed and peaceful.

5. Bring your awareness to your breath, without trying to control it. How many seconds does a natural breath take to come in? How many seconds does a natural breath take to go out?

6. Bring your awareness back to your physical body, noticing, for example, which parts of your body are pressing against each other or the chair.

Next Jnani teaches a series of seated postures for the head, neck, shoulders, and upper back. She introduces this head and neck series because most people have tension, if not pain, and some range-of-motion limitation in their neck and shoulders.

EXERCISE #2. **VERTICAL HEAD MOVEMENT.** Start with your head in a neutral position. As you exhale, let your chin drop down toward your chest (figure 12.2a). Then as you inhale, extend your chin gently up toward the ceiling (figure 12.2b). Continue at your own pace, using your breath, deeply and completely, and coordinating each steady movement with each inhalation or exhalation. Take long, slow exhalations and full, deep inhalations. Jnani stresses that how far you can go is less important than the attention you bring to each point along the way. Repeat this action several times.

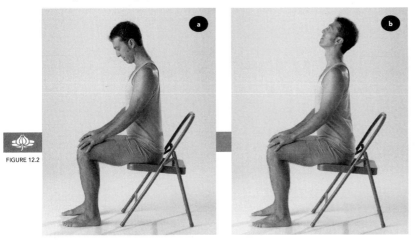

FIGURE 12.2

EXERCISE #3. **HORIZONTAL HEAD MOVEMENT.** Start with your head in a neutral position. As you exhale, turn your chin toward one shoulder in a horizontal line, for the full length of your exhalation (figure 12.3). As you inhale, bring your head to center. As you exhale, turn your head toward the opposite shoulder for the full length of your exhalation. Turn your head to each side a number of times, moving with your breath, and then return to center.

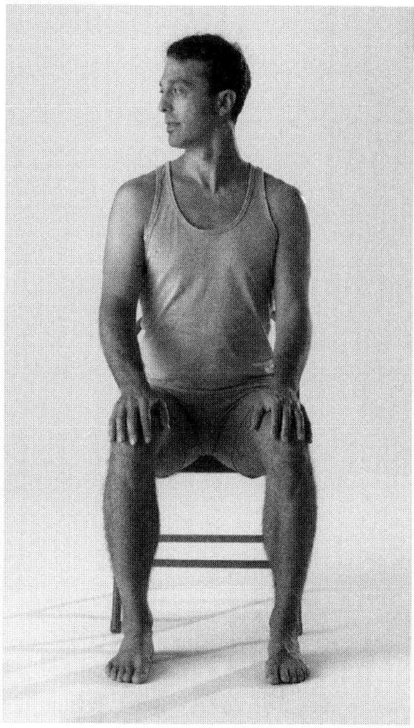

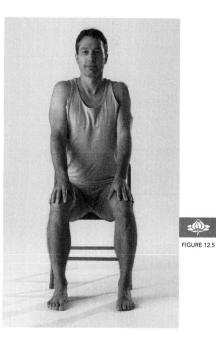

FIGURE 12.3

EXERCISE #4. **HEAD TILTING.** As you exhale, without rotating your head, drop your right ear down in the direction of your right shoulder for the full length of your exhalation (figure 12.4). Then inhale back up to center. As you exhale, drop your left ear down toward your left shoulder for the full length of your exhalation. Jnani says, "Even if the head only tilts a quarter of an inch to each side, that's where the benefit is. So accept what is, and just witness it and the breath."

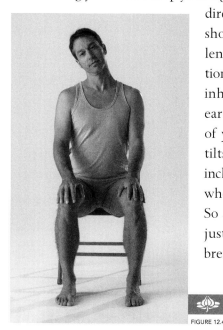

FIGURE 12.4

EXERCISE #5. **SHOULDER SHRUGS.** As you inhale, shrug your shoulders up to your ears, for the full length of the inhalation (figure 12.5). As you exhale, press your shoulders down toward your feet. Continue at your own pace.

FIGURE 12.5

EXERCISE #6. **FULL CIRCULAR ROTATION OF SHOULDERS.** As you inhale, bring your shoulders forward in front of your chest (figure 12.6a), and continue inhaling as you raise them up toward your ears (figure 12.6b). As you exhale, bring your shoulders back behind your chest (figure 12.6c), and continue exhaling as they come all the way back down, making a full circle.

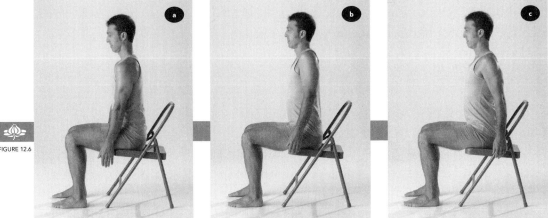

FIGURE 12.6

When you have finished these movements, begin to move your head, shoulders, and neck any which way, exploring their range of motion. Shake out your arms, and notice whether your shoulders feel different. Do you feel that you have more range of motion? If your shoulders feel tighter, you may have been trying too hard and should back off a bit next time.

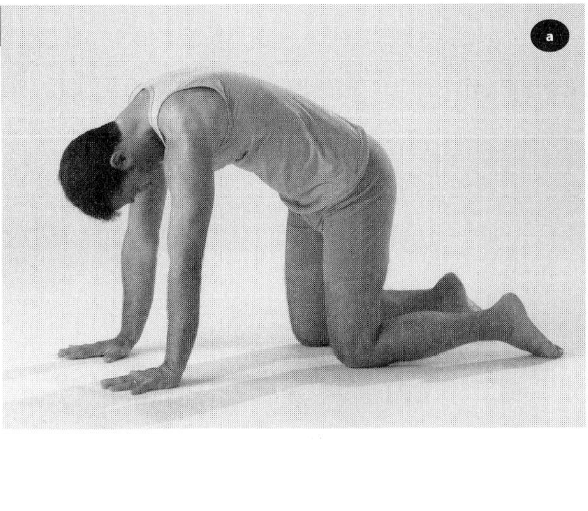

FIGURE 12.7

EXERCISE #7. **CAT/TABLE.** Kneel on all fours on a padded mat or a rug to protect your knees. Place your knees directly below your hips and your wrists directly below your shoulders. As you exhale, tuck your tailbone in and under and round your back, lifting it as you draw your abdomen up and in. Tuck your chin in toward your chest (figure 12.7a). Then as you inhale, flatten your

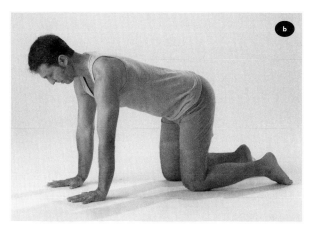

back, extending your tailbone and the crown of your head in opposite directions (figure 12.7b). Repeat these actions several times, moving with your breath.

EXERCISE #8. **MODIFIED SHOULDERSTAND.** This pose gradually teaches the body to be upside down, and helps create strength and flexibility in the spine. Before doing the pose, be sure to remove any jewelry or clothing from around your neck. To set up for the pose, place a chair so that its back is against a wall. To come into the pose, lie on your back in front of the chair with your buttocks as close to the chair as comfortable and place your calves on the seat of the chair. Rest there with your arms alongside your body for at least a minute (figure 12.8a). Then, when you are ready, turn your palms down as close to the body as is comfortable and bring your feet to the front edge of the chair. Push off with your feet as you press down on your palms and lift your buttocks off the floor. Place the palms of your hands on your buttocks for support (figure 12.8b). Never strain, and be sure your breath stays smooth and regular. Begin by holding the pose for ten seconds, eventually working toward thirty seconds.

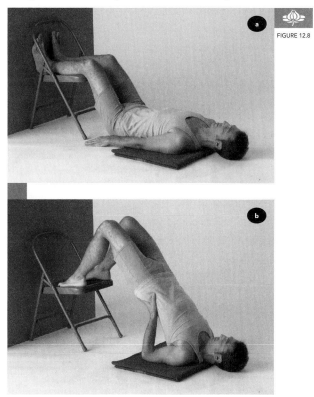

FIGURE 12.8

EXERCISE #9. **EXTENDED EXHALATION BREATH.** Start by coming to an erect position on your chair, as you did for the tuning in process that began this practice. When you are settled, think back to the Witness Practice when you noticed the length of your inhalations and exhalations. In Jnani's experience, most people who haven't done yoga inhale for one to three seconds and exhale for one to two seconds (though you may be different). The idea behind this practice is to make the exhalation twice as long as the inhalation. Now place your hands on your belly. On your exhalation, draw your belly in toward the back of the chair, pushing out all the air, in a steady, even, controlled way for four seconds if possible. On your inhalation, expand your abdomen, and try to fill your lungs in two seconds. Depending on your comfort level in this exercise, you can raise or lower the amount of time you inhale and exhale, but try to keep the 1:2 ratio (figure 12.1).

EXERCISE #10. **MEDITATION.** Sitting in an erect position on your chair, close your eyes and let yourself settle in. Then either find a focus (see below) or simply watch your breath. Let the breath come and go without trying to control it, and draw your awareness to the in breath and the out breath. After a few minutes, very slowly begin to bring your focus back into the room. As you feel ready, let your eyes open (figure 12.1).

> **TIP** One question you may have about meditating is where to place your focus. With beginning students, Jnani often suggests following the breath as it moves in and out. For people who are more visual, focusing on an image such as a candle or a star may feel better. People who respond more to sounds may want to concentrate on a mantra, a syllable or phrase to repeat silently. The mantra could be in Sanskrit, or it could be an English word like "one," "love," or "peace." If you are religious, repeating a phrase from your faith works well, as Harvard Medical School's Dr. Herbert Benson recommends.
>
> Jnani says that what is commonly called meditation is really an exercise in concentration. With focus, the mind may sometimes drop into a state of meditation. However, it is the nature of the mind to wander, so don't beat yourself up if you continually lose your focus and need to bring your mind back. That happens to everybody. Jnani cites Dr. Benson's research on meditation, which found that the physiological benefits of the practice come even to people whose subjective experiences were that they weren't doing a good job of it.

EXERCISE #11. **YOGA NIDRA.** Following is a relatively short version of this yogic form of guided imagery, which Jnani based on the teachings of Swami Satchidananda. Yoga Nidra (see pp. 67–68) can be useful to cancer patients, especially those feeling a lot of stress, because, as Jnani puts it, "It's moving a person from the physical level of reality to deeper and deeper levels." Jnani recommends that you practice Yoga Nidra lying on your back, either with soft pillows under your knees, or if it is more comfortable for your back, with your feet and calves resting on the seat of a padded chair.

Lie on your back and allow your legs to rest comfortably on the prop. Use a neck roll or pillow under your head if needed for comfort. Extend your arms out to the sides, with your palms up. You can rest the hands on small pillows if that feels better. Then settle in to let your body relax as much as possible.

Inhale deeply, hold the inhalation, and lift your limbs an inch or so off the ground, and squeeze all of the muscles in your body, including your face muscles, buttocks, and abdominal muscles. When you need to exhale, drop your limbs back to the beginning position and relax all of your muscles. Repeat this sequence two or three more times.

Allow your body to settle into the most relaxed position possible. When you are ready, begin the guided imagery portion of Yoga Nidra:

1. Bring your awareness through your body systematically, from your feet and legs up through your torso and trunk, your hands and arms, and your neck and head. Suggest to each part of your body that it relax and soften completely. Picture or feel a flow of relaxation moving upward. Practice this body scan for one minute.

2. Bring your awareness to the breath in its natural flow. Watch it come and go, without trying to change it. Continue observing your breath for one minute.

3. Bring your awareness to your mind and observe the thoughts that bubble into consciousness. When you notice a thought, simply let it come and let it go. Continue observing your thoughts for one minute.

4. Allow your awareness to rest in the center of your being, that center of radiant light, deepest peace, and fullest joy that yoga says is your own true nature. Rest there in stillness for five minutes.

When you are ready to come out of Yoga Nidra, please be slow and mindful. Begin by bringing the awareness back to your breath in its natural flow. Use your imagination to invite any quality of healing you desire to come in with the breath and to radiate to every cell in the body. Invite harmony and balance, patience and perseverance, peace and joy to every cell, every muscle, every tissue, every organ, and every system in your body. Slowly begin to wiggle your fingers and toes, roll and stretch your arms and legs, and gently help yourself up to a seated position.

In addition to the practices described above, Jnani often teaches her students with cancer such postures as modified Sun Salutations and gentle spinal twists. Alternative nostril breathing is a relaxing pranayama that she also finds very helpful. Jnani also teaches the Humming Bee Breath, Bhramari (see p. 16). Realizing that not all elements of the yoga program she teaches will appeal to all students, Jnani suggests her students follow their intuition in deciding which practices to stay with. She quotes her late guru, Swami Satchidananda: "Be unwilling to let go of your peace for anything. If something doesn't resonate with your experience, let it go."

Contraindications, Special Considerations, and Modifications

Both cancer itself and its treatment can lead to profound fatigue. It is therefore essential not to overdo your yoga practice. For patients undergoing chemo, Jnani believes that quick changes in posture are not advisable. Her experience is that most injuries happen when people combine movements such as lifting and twisting at the same time. She will only add more complicated poses that combine different movements once she is sure the student has gained awareness and ease with the simpler actions. Some asana practices could lead to fractures in people whose cancer has spread to the bones and weakened them in the process. Since Jnani's approach is gentle and places the highest priority on injury prevention, fractures have not been an issue, but they could be in more vigorous styles of yoga. While not opposed to the kind of strenuous classes that have become the norm in health clubs, Jnani urges caution, even for those whose bones are strong. "These classes can help improve strength, muscle tone, flexibility, and cardiovascular conditioning," she says, "but for people who are already somewhat depleted by their medical condition, these classes could make things worse."

In addition, for anyone at risk of lymphedema, vigorous asana practice—particularly "hot yoga" often done in rooms heated to more than 100 degrees Fahrenheit—is contraindicated. Lymphedema is a frequent complication of treatment for breast cancer, especially if the lymph nodes under the arm are removed. Symptoms include pain and swelling of the affected arm, though in other cancers the problem can be in the legs. There is a high risk of infection, and wounds may be slow to heal. In women with breast cancer and lymphedema, it may be necessary to prop up the arm during asana practice and wear a supportive wrap to prevent swelling. Caution should be the rule. Sudha Carolyn Lundeen, a Kripalu yoga teacher and three-time breast cancer survivor, recommends no stretching for a week after surgery and stresses that the rule of thumb should be to "do less." She recommends when moving the arms keeping the elbows bent, to shorten the lever of the arms and exert less pressure at the fulcrum of the shoulder. Jnani suggests that when doing poses like Cat/Table, it's best to keep the arm on the affected side elevated to

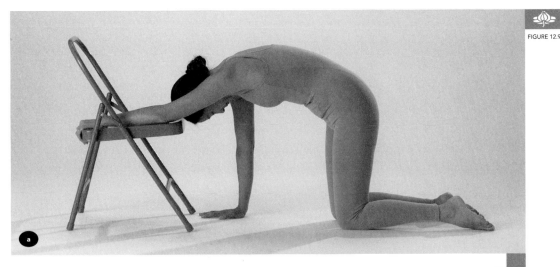

FIGURE 12.9

avoid the swelling that can result from the force of gravity. To modify Cat/Table, put a chair in front of your body so you can place the arm on the affected side on the seat of the chair during the whole pose (figure 12.9a). To modify Downward-Facing Dog, you could substitute Standing Half Forward Bend (Ardha Uttanasana) with the arms on the wall (figure 12.9b) or on the back of a chair. Women with or at risk of lymphedema should consult a yoga teacher who has experience with this problem. It is much better to take steps to prevent lymphedema than to have to deal with it once the swelling has begun.

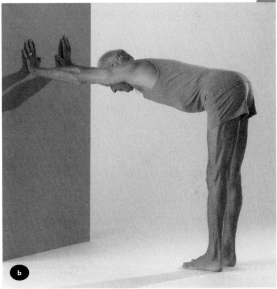

a) Cat/Table with affected arm on the seat of a chair
b) Standing Half Forward Bend against a wall

Because of her belief in the healing power of the improved oxygenation that comes with yogic breathing, Jnani does not teach breath retentions to her clients with cancer. "They need the oxygen," she says. Jnani stresses that deep diaphragmatic breathing can help move lymph and theoretically improve immune functioning, but she warns that Skull Shining Breath (Kapalabhati) and Bellows Breath (Bhastrika) can increase fatigue and may not be appropriate for those who are seriously ill, already depleted, or taking multiple medications.

A Holistic Approach to Cancer

❋ Dietary measures may be helpful in both preventing and treating cancer (see chapter 4). For example, recent evidence suggests that it is the olive oil in the Mediterranean diet that helps protect women in that region from breast cancer, and women living in countries like Japan, where the diet includes a lot of soy products, also tend to have a much lower incidence of the disease.

❋ Depression is a common complication in people with cancer. Psychotherapy and antidepressant medication, in addition to measures like yoga and meditation, can improve mood and perhaps the prognosis (see Chapter 15).

❋ Even though cancer pain can be controlled in nine out of ten patients, one study found that more than half fail to get relief. One reason is that doctors sometimes don't prescribe narcotics—the most effective pain relievers—out of the usually groundless fear that their patients will become addicts. Ask for them if you need them. According to pain experts, there is no such thing as a standard dose for narcotics. The doctor should keep increasing the dose until the patient is comfortable, as long as side effects such as nausea, constipation, and sedation don't become unbearable. You (or your loved ones) may have to be assertive to get what you need.

❋ Controlled experiments have found that acupuncture can diminish pain after surgery for breast cancer.

❋ Acupuncture or acupressure on the point P6—located three finger breadths up from the wrist crease in the center of the wrist, between the two rope-like tendons palpable just beneath the skin—has been demonstrated to reduce chemotherapy-induced nausea and vomiting.

❋ Massage can be a useful addition to treatment of cancer because it can reduce both pain and anxiety, and induce relaxation.

❋ Lymph drainage massage may be particularly useful to both prevent and treat lymphedema associated with breast cancer and other forms of cancer. It's best to try this approach as early as possible in your recovery.

❋ Modalities such as therapeutic touch, healing touch, and Reiki appear to improve quality of life in cancer patients.

* Although antioxidant vitamins might be useful in preventing some cancers (the jury is still out on this), it's probably prudent to discontinue use while actively undergoing treatment, as they could interfere with the effectiveness of conventional radiation and chemotherapy. Fruits and vegetables and other foods high in antioxidants are fine.

* Herbal medicine can help control side effects due to therapy. Ginger, in the form of capsules, tea, or the fresh root, can relieve nausea. Marijuana is also effective for this purpose in people undergoing chemotherapy, as well as to stimulate appetite, but cannot be used legally in most places. Valerian can help with insomnia and anxiety, particularly when taken regularly. With her oncologist's approval, Erin took Chinese medicinal herbs throughout her course of chemotherapy.

Erin started taking Jnani's class when she was already two infusions into her chemotherapy, and "I just took to it right away." Erin thinks her yoga practice played a major role in helping her go through chemotherapy with relatively few side effects. She lost all her hair, but she never experienced nausea, one of chemo's most common and unpleasant side effects. Erin says, "I'm kind of my oncologist's poster child, the shining star example of someone who was able to get through chemotherapy, pretty heavy-duty, and not suffer greatly."

Now, even when Erin doesn't do the stretching exercises, she does the breathing practice every day, usually when she first wakes up, and typically while still lying in bed. When time allows, she'll go straight from that into meditation, which she also does lying in Savasana position (though Jnani recommends it be done sitting). When she does an asana practice at home, she does it to a gentle yoga tape that lasts twenty-five minutes. In addition, she often does a half dozen Sun Salutations before she leaves for her morning radiation treatment. The Sun Salutations are modified as Jnani had shown her, for example, bringing the knees down to the mat in Plank Position or Chaturanga (see p. 238).

Erin feels she has gained a lot of awareness of her body from her yoga practice. "It helped me learn to relax specific muscles in my body." Her growing awareness extends to her breathing. "I would say that it crosses my mind at least twenty times a day. How am I breathing? Am I sitting in a way that I'm keeping a space open to take deep breaths? Am I breathing slowly? Certainly it's become almost like a reflex that if something stressful is going on, I just start doing the deep breathing. I haven't had too much trouble with insomnia, but the few times I've woken up in the middle of the night and couldn't sleep,

I did that, and it helped me get to a place where I could fall back asleep." She adds that "the breathing really came in handy when I was getting the different procedures for the needle localization, prior to the surgery."

Getting diagnosed and treated for cancer has involved a lot of emotional ups and downs. The practice that Erin finds most useful in this regard is meditation, which has helped her observe and move through her emotions. Just after being diagnosed, Erin had started doing "a little bit of guided imagery and meditation." Erin says her hypnotherapist taught her to find a place of sanctuary in her own mind, a restful place, to be and feel safe, which she found very useful. Deep relaxation has also been important. "It really creates a place where you can go inward and kind of clear your mind and relax. Afterward my sense of well-being is so improved. I just feel relaxed, like everything is all right—a really calm, wonderful feeling."

Erin feels that the many modalities she used during and after her cancer experience have worked synergistically to help her heal. She includes not just asana practice, the guided imagery taught to her by her hypnotherapist, and deep relaxation, but also acupuncture, Chinese medicinal herbs, and an art therapy workshop which functions much like a support group for her.

She's also made changes in her diet, moving away from what she calls "'white foods'—white rice, pasta, all those heavy carbs"—and including more fruits, vegetables, and whole grains in her meals. "I eat for the most part as though I'm vegetarian, although I don't totally restrict myself." It's made a big difference, she says. She's lost 20 pounds, down from 170 to 150, "and I feel really good."

Indeed, Erin says she now feels better than she did before she got cancer. "I know it's odd, but that's absolutely true. I personally believe that you can turn it around to make it a positive experience—but you do have to stop and deal with this in a very direct way. Two days after I got the original phone call from my gynecologist saying that they found cancer cells, I woke up at home, alone, in my room, and I had this epiphany. I had this real will to do whatever it took."

Before her cancer diagnosis, Erin had never been particularly drawn to alternative healing practices like acupuncture and yoga. What Erin particularly likes about yoga is that it can be tailored to the individual. If some practices don't interest you, or are beyond your current capabilities, yoga still has plenty to offer. Even if all you can do is imagine a particular asana, Erin says, you're going to benefit from it. "You only have to do what you can do."

CARPAL TUNNEL SYNDROME

 More than thirty years ago, TOM ALDEN was a serious yoga student who wanted to learn more about anatomy. After considering the options, he decided to become a chiropractor. His yoga study has been primarily with Iyengar teachers. Over the years, he has combined what he learned about functional anatomy from both his yoga practice and his clinical work as a chiropractor "to teach people to take care of themselves through yoga." He teaches yoga and anatomy workshops and runs a private chiropractic practice from his office in the Boston area.

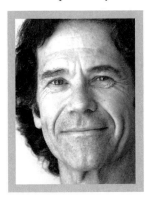

Gwyneth Catlin first met Tom Alden years ago, after a friend referred her to him for a stubborn leg problem related to running. Tom diagnosed it as piriformis syndrome, caused by a tight muscle in the back of the hip. She'd already seen eight or ten other bodyworkers before him, a couple of whom had actually made things worse. Tom worked with her and told her she'd make a rapid recovery. His prediction came true. As Gwyneth recalls, "I was running in a week after hobbling around for months."

Gwyneth had sampled numerous styles of yoga prior to studying with Tom, including power yoga, Jivamukti, and Bikram. In subsequent years, she continued her practice, which became increasingly influenced by Tom's teaching. She also consulted him when other problems arose, including the wrist condition described below.

Gwyneth had just started working as a technical writer for a leading high-tech firm in an extremely stressful situation. After a few weeks she began to notice wrist pain. "It hurt on the inner forearm, and then going to the wrist, and then there was a sensation of burning in my palms. It was uncomfortable to type." She was putting in fifty-five-hour work weeks, including weekends, and estimates she spent five hours a day at her laptop. She'd worked at similar jobs at other companies where ergonomic experts would help people arrange their workspace for their particular needs, but this job didn't offer that kind of help.

Gwyneth found the job emotionally toxic. Her boss had the reputation of being a tyrant. "I was terrified," she says. Making matters worse, Gwyneth found very little emotional support among her coworkers. "In most of the jobs that I've been in, I've been able to make really good connections with people, which would keep me going in the job. I mean, tech writing is meaningless to me." At this job, she remembers sitting at her desk and not speaking to a single person all day.

The wrist problem required her to make some changes in her yoga practice. Poses like Downward-Facing Dog, in which a substantial portion of the body weight lands on the wrist, for example, were painful, so she skipped them. But she kept up her practice as well as her running, because she felt they were what was keeping her sane in a time of great stress.

Overview of Carpal Tunnel Syndrome

The carpal tunnel is a narrow passageway in the wrist formed by ligaments and the eight small carpal bones. These bones are arranged in two rows of four, and lie on either side of the crease between the hand and forearm. Carpal tunnel syndrome (CTS) is caused when the median nerve to the hand gets compressed in this tunnel. CTS has become a near epidemic among computer users, musicians, and others in recent years, particularly those whose work or hobbies include some kind of repetitive hand movements or the use of vibrating tools.

The problem, however, is not always caused by repetitive motion. Anything that decreases the space in the wrist joint and compresses the median nerve can lead to CTS. Fluid retention due to pregnancy or thyroid disease, for example, can narrow the carpal tunnel, as can cysts, old fractures, or arthritic changes in the bones. One reason women are so much more likely to get CTS is that their wrists tend to be smaller than men's, with less room to spare.

The characteristic symptoms of CTS include intermittent numbness and tingling in the hands, which often wake people up at night. The abnormal sensations typically occur in a characteristic pattern (figure 13.1), in the area of the palm served by the median nerve, though some people get pain in the arm and shoulder. Left unchecked, compression in the wrist can progress to permanent nerve damage and muscle weakness in the hands.

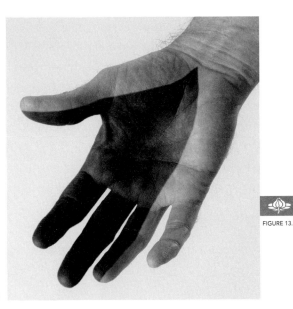

FIGURE 13.1

Darkened area indicates typical area of numbness and tingling in carpal tunnel syndrome

How Yoga Fits In

During my medical training, the entire conversation about carpal tunnel syndrome focused on about one inch of anatomy, the canal in the wrist through which tendons and the median nerve pass. There is some validity to this perspective. Tom explains that compression of the carpal tunnel often happens when people engage in activities like typing which require that they pronate the forearms, that is rotate them so that the palm faces down. The pronation can cause flattening of the normal arch made by the carpal bones. Cocking the wrists up, as many people do at the keyboard, can intensify this flattening of the carpal tunnel arch, putting further pressure on the tendons and the median nerve. But from a yogic point of view the failure to consider other factors beyond compression in the carpal tunnel is shortsighted. It is precisely this myopic approach that results in surgeries to open up that space before other options have been thoroughly explored.

While the medical profession tends to view carpal tunnel syndrome primarily as a problem involving the wrists, the yogic approach is to look at the whole body. Senior Iyengar yoga teacher Mary Dunn explains, "Posture has a huge impact on this condition. It's not just the position of the wrists. It's the position of the head on the shoulders, whether the chest is sunken, how tense the person is," etc. Medical textbooks mention that posture can play a role in CTS, but in my experience, physicians rarely address the issue in clinical practice.

Like Mary Dunn, many yogis believe that the disruption of nerve impulses to the median nerve in the wrist can begin upstream in the neck, shoulders, and chest. If you adopt the common postural habit of rounding your back into a C-shaped slump, nerves and blood vessels can be compressed on their way to the arm (figure 13.2). If this bad posture is habitual, muscles, ligaments, tendons, and fascia (the connective tissue that wraps muscles and organs) in the chest and neck can shorten, potentially further compromising nerve function. Yoga also teaches that if your alignment is bad in one area it can cause ripple effects. Tom finds that collapse in the upper body can lead to collapse of structures in the wrist, intensifying the compromise of nerve function.

FIGURE 13.2

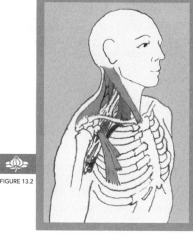

A. Healthy upright posture

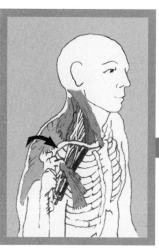

B. Slight slumping, shoulders rolling forward

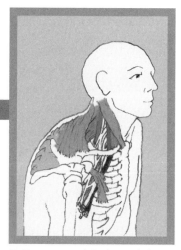

C. Pronounced C-shaped slump

The C-shaped slump can compress nerves and blood vessels
going into the arm, shoulder, and chest.

TIP Plush office chairs or cushy car interiors can contribute to poor posture and worsening of CTS symptoms. Yoga teaches that in order to lift your chest and shoulders up, you must be able to push down. When sitting in a chair, that means being able to press your sitting bones onto a relatively firm surface, and ideally, your feet onto the floor. If the seat of your chair is too soft, get a firmer one, or in a pinch, put something firm between you and the too-soft cushion. If your feet do not reach the ground, try placing a phone book or a stack of them on the floor in front of your chair. Set up your desk so that your keyboard is just slightly lower than your elbows, and your elbows, wrists, and fingers are roughly in a straight line. If you can get used to them, ergonomic keyboards with split keys for the left and right hands can help reduce symptoms. Experts recommend typing with the tips of your fingers and not the pads.

Yogis find that breathing is also an issue in CTS. Tom says that most people in the modern world don't know how to breathe effectively. He finds that those who have arm or wrist problems almost always have constricted breathing, too. Typically, they sit slumped forward, so that the back ribs—essential for deep breathing—can't move much, and the chest doesn't expand or contract enough when they breathe.

Tom has also observed that those with CTS have isolated the movement of their wrists from movement of the arms and the shoulder blades. "The wrists become sort of disengaged." In other words, the shoulders aren't sharing in the work of the forearm and the wrist. When one area is underutilized, another area has to compensate by working too hard and "the area that is overused becomes problematic." While CTS often gets lumped into the category of repetitive stress, Tom views it as being, more typically, "a holding injury." He differentiates repetitive stress from sustained stress. "The over-holder keeps one position for a long time. The repetitive stress person is doing something over and over again."

Bringing yogic awareness to your daily habits can reduce the likelihood of wrist problems. When typing, for example, many people strike the keys with much more force than necessary. It's also common to slouch at the keyboard, thus potentially contributing to problems at the wrist. Similarly, when driving, many people hold the wheel with a death grip. If you find yourself doing this, keep reminding yourself to lighten your touch, as you actually have better control of the wheel with a less forceful grip. Kripalu yoga teacher and bodyworker Lee Albert recommends holding the wheel at four and eight o'clock, rather than the more usual ten and two o'clock, to lessen muscular tightness in the arms and shoulders. Try it both ways and see which is more relaxing for you. Also tune in to your breath while driving or typing to see if rapid or irregular breathing could be contributing to increased stress levels.

Yoga's focus goes beyond posture, breathing, and usage recommendations, to the broader question of what's going on in your life. Tom says you need to examine "the state of mind that you're in when you're typing, the way you're holding your tension, how often you take breaks, and how much you care about your own well-being."

If your job is stressful, if you lack autonomy, if your boss is a jerk, if you are asked to do more than you reasonably can—a good description of Gwyneth's job—you are more likely to develop pain. Yoga would predict that marital problems or anything else that added stress or took joy out of life might have an impact. Factors like depression or anxiety can make just about anything worse, and CTS is no exception. Tom says, "Many of the people who have carpal tunnel put their emotional tension into their forearms." Many of his CTS patients are people who have been forced for financial reasons to do a clerical job they hate.

> **CAUTION** Wrist rests for the keyboard and mouse are often recommended for CTS but I believe they can be counterproductive. Many people who use them lean into them, directly compressing their wrists. Wrist rests can also lead to the kind of disconnect that Tom speaks of, where the shoulders aren't moving much and the wrists and forearms do all the work—and pay the price. If you try a wrist rest and compare it to typing without one, you will probably notice that your forearms are tighter when your wrists are pressing down into it than when they are lightly poised above the keyboard. This is an example of using yogic awareness to determine whether common ergonomic advice makes sense for you or not. As Tom puts it, "Ergonomics is not a substitute for awareness."

The Scientific Evidence

Although yoga teachers have been using yoga to successfully treat carpal tunnel syndrome for years, the first scientific evidence of its effectiveness came in a 1998 article in the *Journal of the American Medical Association* (*JAMA*). In a randomized trial of forty-two patients conducted at the Medical College of Pennsylvania, half of the patients took part in an eight-week program of Iyengar yoga while the control group received wrist splints. Marian Garfinkel, the study's lead author and a senior teacher of the Iyengar method of yoga, taught the subjects in the yoga group eleven yoga postures designed to strengthen and stretch each joint in the upper body, along with Savasana. After the intervention, the people who had done yoga had less pain and a significant improvement in grip strength as compared to the controls. While the group studied was small, and a longer-range study might be more revealing, the results were encouraging.

Tom Alden's Approach

Gwyneth went to see Tom soon after developing wrist symptoms. He observed that rather than slouching, she was very driven and hyperalert, holding herself in one position for long periods of time, "the classic sustained stress, positional fatigue, contraction pattern that people on keyboards get." While examining Gwyneth, Tom observed muscular holding in both the forearm flexors, which bend your wrists forward, and the forearm extensors, which bend the wrist backward, as well as in a muscle called pronator teres, which pronates the forearm. He also saw that she had a pattern of mild flattening of the natural arch of the carpals; she was collapsing and compressing the area of the carpal tunnel not only when she typed but even when she sat with her arms in neutral alignment (see below).

The exercises he gave her were designed to increase her bodily awareness, adjust her alignment, and help her let go of tension. In keeping with his emphasis on self-care, he also taught her bodywork techniques that enabled her to self-administer the kind of first aid work he did on her when she came in with the problem.

Here is the sequence of poses and instructions that Tom provided for Gwyneth.

EXERCISE #1. **ESTABLISHING NEUTRAL ALIGNMENT.** Sitting with your elbows bent, position your forearms in neutral alignment with your thumbs pointing in the same

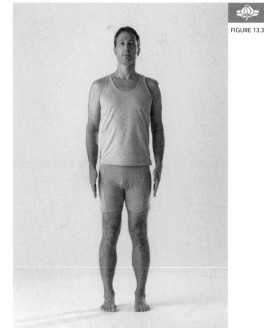

FIGURE 13.3

direction as your biceps, that is, with your forearm neither supinated (palm up in this position) nor pronated (palm down in this position). Alternately, you can find neutral alignment of the arms in Mountain pose (Tadasana). When you stand in Mountain pose, your biceps and thumbs face forward and your palms face your thighs (figure 13.3). From neutral alignment, you can feel the muscles that flex your wrist (bend it forward) on the palm side of your forearm and the muscles that extend your wrist (bend it back) on the outside part of your forearm. Neutral alignment of the wrists is the position least likely to cause compression in the carpal tunnel (though in Gwyneth's case the compression was present to some degree even in neutral alignment).

EXERCISE #2. **PUMPING THE WRIST.** Sit with your elbows bent and your arms in neutral alignment, as described above. Now bend your right wrist forward and then cock it back, keeping the forearm muscles relaxed. You can help this action by using your left

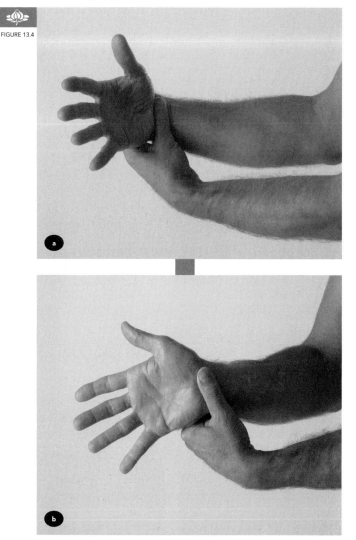

FIGURE 13.4

thumb, placed on the palm side of the right wrist, to lift and open the wrist joint as you bend the wrist forward (figures 13.4a & b). Repeat this wrist "pumping action" half a dozen times on each side. Tom says the pumping action releases tension in forearm muscles which are short and tight. When you move the wrist into the forward bend, you are lengthening the extensors, and when you move the wrist into the backbend you are shortening the extensors. This exercise teaches the extensor muscles that just because they are in a shortened position doesn't mean they need to hold the grip of tension.

Tom also uses hands-on work to facilitate muscle relaxation and the person's awareness of it. He does this through myofascial release, a massage technique designed to increase the circulation and relaxation in the contracted muscle. The pressure from his hands helps direct the student's attention into the problem area. With awareness comes a greater ability to let go of the tension. "That's the yoga of it," he says.

As part of his strategy of encouraging self-care, Tom demonstrated the bodywork on himself so Gwyneth could learn how to do it to herself. Press the four fingers of your left hand into the belly of the tight extensor forearm muscle on the right arm, and move your

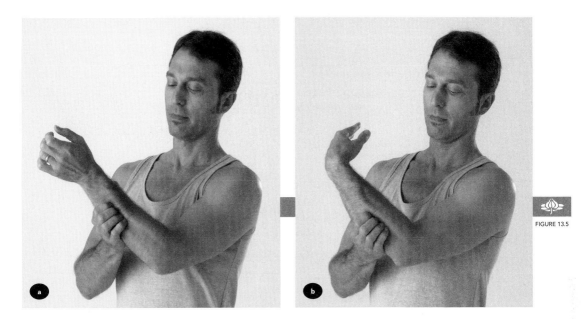

FIGURE 13.5

fingers along the length of your extensor muscle from elbow to wrist, all the while gently flexing and extending your right wrist back and forth (figures 13.5a & b). Repeat on the other arm. You can do the same massage on your wrist flexor muscles.

EXERCISE #3. **PRAYER POSE (Namaste).** From either a standing or sitting position, begin with your hands in Prayer position (Namaste) in front of your chest. Lightly touching the skin of your hands together, note the warmth, moisture, and other sensations (figure 13.6a). Then slightly increase the pressure until you are aware of the muscles underneath the skin. From there, bring your elbows up to a 90-degree angle with the wrist joint, and press still harder until you can feel the bones underneath the muscles (figure 13.6b). This exercise is designed to bring awareness of the different layers of tissue and to build subtlety in your ability to feel them.

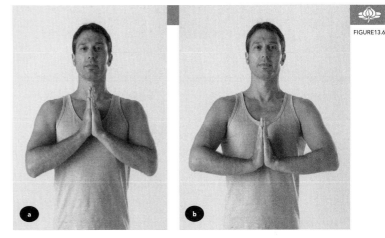

FIGURE13.6

In Tom's experience, one of the reasons for compression in the carpal tunnel is that many people bend the wrist backward at the wrong place. When you fold your hand forward at the wrist, the movement takes place primarily between the radius (one of the two bones in the forearm) and the wrist bones. When you arch your hand back, as you might if you were signaling someone to stop, the movement should take place between the two rows of wrist bones, about half an inch closer to the fingers. Most people have two creases on the palm side of their wrist. The joint between the two rows of carpal bones is below the deeper crease, closer to the hand. The joint between the radius and the first row of carpal bones is beneath the first, lighter crease. You can feel the difference between correct and incorrect movement as you bend your wrist back by holding your wrist with the pad of your thumb as you did in exercise #1, and moving your wrist up and down. You should notice that cocking the wrist back happens right beneath the deeper wrist crease. If it doesn't, use the fingers of your opposite hand to place gentle traction on the wrist, stretching the creased skin over the carpal bones as the wrist bends back. Use your opposite thumb behind the wrist as a lever to facilitate the opening.

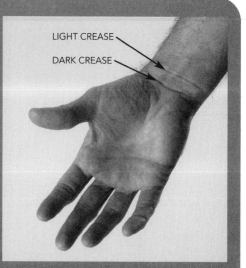

LIGHT CREASE

DARK CREASE

EXERCISE #4. **ALTERNATING FLEXION AND EXTENSION OF WRISTS, with arms in neutral anatomical alignment (palms facing down).** While seated, turn your hands palms down and move your elbows out to the sides so that your forearms are in anatomical neutral (the thumbs and biceps point in the same direction). Interlace your fingers and begin to gently pull your wrists apart (figure 13.7a). You should feel a mild traction in your wrist, creating space in the joint. Maintaining that traction, raise your right arm and lower the left, bringing the right wrist into a forward bend and the left wrist into a backbend (figure 13.7b).

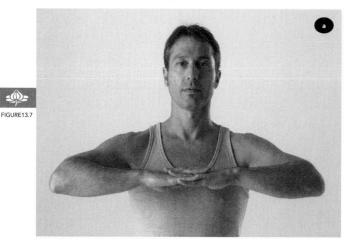

FIGURE13.7

a

Allow your right arm to do all the work while your left arm is passive. This way, the right arm, which is in the forward bend, can grip the fingers of the left hand and pull the left wrist more into a backbend, releasing tension in the left wrist flexors and encouraging backbending in the left side carpals. Be sure that when the wrists bend back, the movement comes primarily from the area between the two rows of carpal bones, not from between the wrist

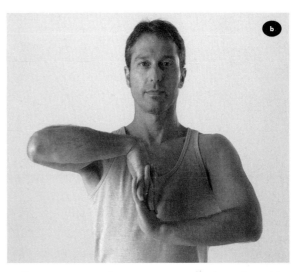

and arm. Maintaining the interlace of your fingers, repeat the movement on the other side, using your left hand to open the right wrist, which now passively receives the action. Go back and forth a number of times.

EXERCISE #5. **ALTERNATING FLEXION AND EXTENSION OF WRISTS, with arms in supination (palms facing toward you).** Start in the same position as in exercise #4 and turn your palms to face toward you. Interlace your fingers and begin to gently pull your wrists apart. Repeat the arm movements in exercise #4, keeping your palms facing toward you.

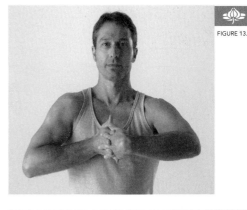

FIGURE 13.8

EXERCISE #6. **ALTERNATING FLEXION AND EXTENSION OF WRISTS, with arms in pronation (palms facing away from you).** Start in the same position as in exercise #4 and turn your palms to face away from you. Interlace your fingers and begin to gently pull your wrists apart. Repeat the arm movements in exercise #4, keeping your palms facing away from you.

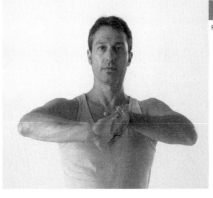

FIGURE 13.9

Tom calls the last three exercises "the typists' equivalent of flossing." Gwyneth says that they feel so good, she could do them all day.

After Gwyneth had spent a few weeks on these basic exercises, Tom added a few more exercises to her regimen. The following exercise was designed to help correct a muscular holding pattern he thought was contributing to her wrist condition. Because Gwyneth did so much typing every day, the internal rotators in her shoulders (in particular her subscapularis muscle) had become so tight that if she tried to relax into neutral alignment, her upper body collapsed in on itself. In other words, in normal typing position, her upper arm bones (the humeri) tended to internally rotate, the shoulders tended to roll forward, her elbows flared out, and her wrists turned in.

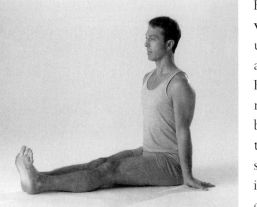

FIGURE 13.10

EXERCISE #7. **STAFF POSE (Dandasana), with fingers facing toward back.** Sit upright on your mat or on a folded blanket and straighten your legs in front of you. Place your hands on the floor or on blocks next to your hips, with your fingers facing backward. This position externally rotates the humerus (upper arm bone) and stretches the area in the front of the chest, including the pectoralis (upper chest) muscles, releasing the muscles that get tight when you type. Bring the same sensitivity to feeling the way your hands meet the floor in this pose as you did to feeling your hands in the Prayer pose exercise above.

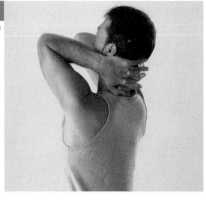

FIGURE 13.11

EXERCISE #8. **CERVICAL CRADLE (seated backbend with fingers interlaced behind neck).** Sit in any comfortable position on your yoga mat or in a chair. Interlace your fingers and cradle the back of your neck with your fingers. Do not increase the curvature of the cervical spine (the back of your neck), but pull forward with your elbows and root your shoulder blades down and out (away from your spine) so that you're creating a backbend in your upper back.

EXERCISE #9. **MEDITATION.** Sit in any comfortable seated position on the floor or in a chair. When you are settled, begin to focus on feeling your inhalation, observing the movement of air through your nose, throat, and into your lungs. On your exhalation, simply relax and spread your awareness throughout your body. As you continue to meditate, focus on the inhalation and relax with the exhalation.

Tom suggests that people with CTS breathe in meditation by expanding the rib cage while the abdomen stays fairly still. This differs from the common instruction to allow the belly to expand with the inhalation and move toward the spine on exhalation. Tom feels this latter method of breathing also has value, but doesn't address the habit of not expanding the ribs when they breathe common to people with CTS. He told Gwyneth, "Take a slow, steady inhalation through your nose and throat into your lungs. As you breathe in, feel your lower ribs widen and lift, your back ribs fill, and your upper ribs rise."

Tom sees CTS and many of the other symptoms that bring patients to him as a doorway into yoga and self-examination, because his way of dealing with the symptoms requires the development of self-awareness, an understanding of what's going on anatomically, and the use of specific yogic techniques designed to address the problems. Although many people come in to tackle a particular problem, his patients end up viewing their injuries in a much more holistic way.

Contraindications, Special Considerations, and Modifications

The asanas that are hardest on the wrists are those that combine bending the wrists back with putting weight on the hands. Among the worst are Handstand, various arm balancing poses, Upward-Facing Dog, low push-up position (Chaturanga Dandasana), Side Plank (Vasisthasana), and full backbend (Urdhva Dhanurasana). If you are having symptoms of CTS, it may be advisable to avoid these poses entirely, at least for a while. If you can learn to do these postures, however, without flattening the carpal tunnel, placing more weight on the knuckles and less on the wrists, they may be fine and even therapeutic (see "Wrist Injuries" in appendix 1 for more on this topic). Learning to engage your legs more can take some of the burden off the hands as well.

Yoga teacher Ana Forrest suggests students with wrist problems try a few exercises to warm up and stretch out the hands and wrists before their usual yoga practice. First, stretch each finger open one at a time, by grasping the finger and pulling it back for one breath. You should feel the stretch in the fingers and across the palm and a little into the forearm. Next, place all of the fingers on the floor or a table, with the fingertips facing toward your torso. Stretch the fingers, but not the palm of the hand, down toward the surface. From that position, see if you can stretch the whole palm down, though you may not make it the whole way. Finally, extend the arms straight out from your shoulders, parallel to the floor. Curl the fingers one by one into the palm, starting with the little finger and ending with the thumb, forming a fist. First curl the fist in toward the underside of the wrist and then stretch it out. Repeat this exercise a few times before you put weight on your hands.

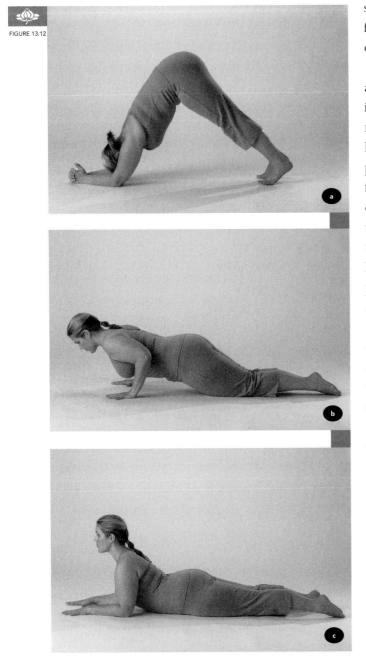

FIGURE 13.12

Tom's emphasis on neutral alignment can be useful in avoiding compression of the carpal tunnel in various yoga poses. In Downward-Facing Dog, for example, if your biceps are turned to face the midline, in the same direction as your thumbs, it tends to be easier on the wrists than if the biceps rotate to face upward. In that position, there's more pronation of the forearm and this can compress the carpal tunnel.

If symptoms are marked, then even Down Dog with good alignment may be too much on the wrists. Ana Forrest recommends substituting Dolphin pose (figure 13.12a), which is precisely what Gwyneth had come to on her own. Ana suggests Chaturanga be modified so the knees are down (figure 13.12b), taking weight off the wrists. She suggests substituting Cobra pose with your forearms on the ground (figure 13.12c) for Upward Dog. If even these modified poses cause numbness or tingling, however, you shouldn't do them.

A Holistic Approach to Carpal Tunnel Syndrome

＊ If you feel pain, tingling, or numbness at night, wrist splints can help you avoid sleeping with your wrists angled (which can precipitate symptoms).

＊ Anti-inflammatory drugs like ibuprofen and naproxen can relieve the pain of CTS but do little to get at the underlying causes.

＊ Ice bags placed over the wrist can reduce pain and inflammation.

＊ Cortisone injections can reduce symptoms enough to enable you to start doing yoga and take other measures designed to help you avoid surgery.

＊ Deep tissue massage, Rolfing, myofascial release, and other bodywork techniques can be helpful for people with tight muscles or adhesions in the connective tissue that surrounds muscle.

＊ The Alexander Technique and the Feldenkrais Method are useful to improve posture and dysfunctional movement patterns that may contribute to CTS.

＊ Acupuncture may be helpful and is very safe.

＊ Dietary measures appear to be of some use in CTS. Emphasize foods that tend to reduce inflammation and avoid those that promote it (see p. 167).

＊ A trial of vitamin B_6 seems to help some sufferers, though it is toxic in large doses. Be sure to discuss this with your doctor. Although the scientific data is mixed, I have had two students report remarkable recoveries in long-standing symptoms after starting B_6. If after several months on the vitamin your symptoms aren't improved, it's probably not worth continuing.

＊ Once symptoms have progressed to a certain point, your best option is surgery. Muscular weakness not caused by pain can be irreversible. If the muscles of the thenar eminence, the fleshy hillock on the palm just beneath the base of the thumb, are atrophied, that is an indication that you've already waited too long. The operation, which is usually done in a doctor's office under local anesthesia, has a very high success rate, especially if not delayed too long. Do all you can to avoid the operation, but if it's clear you're going to need one, it's better to have it sooner than later.

OTHER YOGIC IDEAS

Eleanor Williams, an Iyengar yoga teacher who has had CTS, offers two exercises that can be done in yoga practice as well as during the course of the day, in order to correct the chronic forward roll of the shoulders that is typical of people with CTS. The first she calls "hitchhiker thumbs." Standing or sitting with your arms at your sides, bend your fingers into your palms and stick out your thumbs as if you are trying to hitch a ride. Notice the external rotation of the upper arm bone (the humerus) and the openness of the chest that results. Eleanor also finds simply grasping your elbows behind your back results in similar opening in the shoulders and chest. Rather than standing around with your arms crossed in front of your chest as many people often do, she suggests getting in the habit of holding your arms behind your back instead. If you can't reach your elbows, simply hold one wrist in the opposite hand. The doorway stretch mentioned in chapter 7 similarly opens the shoulders and chest. The "rope jacket" described in chapter 2 and shown here is also useful in this regard.

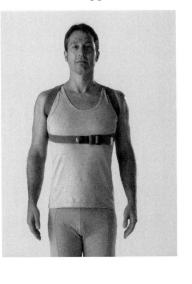

Gwyneth says that she experienced almost immediate relief from the exercises that Tom recommended, and has continued to do them. Before starting her asana practice, she meditates, then does the whole sequence of wrist stretches and openers. Gwyneth also works the breathing meditation into the cracks of her day, even if it's just for a few seconds or a minute. "I do it all the time."

When Gwyneth was able to change how she bends her wrist to allow the movement to come between the two rows of carpal bones, she also noticed a difference in Down Dog. "There's more of a feeling of lift, and it allows you to extend the weight through your hands more." When she does it her old way, she can feel the row of carpal bones at the bottom of her wrist (between the creases) pressing uncomfortably into the floor.

The increasing awareness that came to Gwyneth with her yoga practice had other effects as well. The contrast between the calm and serenity she found in her meditation and yoga practice, and the feelings she had at work made her realize that although technical writing was lucrative, it was not what she wanted to do with her life.

Years ago, Gwyneth had begun training in shiatsu, a Japanese bodywork technique also known as acupressure, but stopped for a variety of reasons. As part of her life change, she decided to finish that program. Reflecting on the shift she made from technical writing to the healing work she does with Shiatsu, Tom says, "Over the course of five, six, seven years, she has actually used her injury patterns as an opportunity to self-reflect and steer her life choices." In yogic terms, you could say that Gwyneth allowed her experiences to help her find her dharma, her life work, or a sense of purpose and direction. She has now finished her Shiatsu training and has begun to see patients.

The exercises that Tom taught her have allowed Gwyneth to keep up her growing Shiatsu practice with almost no wrist problems. She found the idea of the neutral alignment of the arm to be particularly helpful for her massage work. Though she has occasionally forgotten and wound up with a mild recurrence of CTS symptoms, her heightened awareness proved useful. As soon as she began to feel even the slightest symptoms, she reminded herself to correct her alignment, and it worked.

Gwyneth has even been able to teach her wrist exercises to some of her clients, including a woodworker who was very worried about whether he would be able to keep doing his job. "I found he had the exact same thing I did, the extreme muscle gripping in the flexors, and I did for him what I do on myself, and it was almost immediately effective for him." To see that she can take what she's learned and use it to help others, Gwyneth says, "feels really good."

CHRONIC FATIGUE SYNDROME

 GARY KRAFTSOW began his study of yoga in India with T. K. V. Desikachar, son of the legendary Krishnamacharya, in 1974, while still a college student. Although Gary holds a master's degree in psychology and religion, his desire is to demystify yoga and make it relevant to people in the modern world, including those who come to yoga because of a medical condition. The viniyoga approach he teaches is gentle, with slow, flowing movements always coordinated with the breath. The emphasis is on home practice with short sessions, say, twenty to thirty minutes a day, that most people can fit into their busy lives. Gary developed a twelve-week practice series for a study that found yoga an effective treatment for back pain, recently published in the *Annals of Internal Medicine* (see chapter 11). He is the founder and director of the American Viniyoga Institute in Maui, Hawaii, the author of *Yoga for Wellness* and *Yoga for Transformation,* and conducts workshops and teacher trainings around the US and internationally.

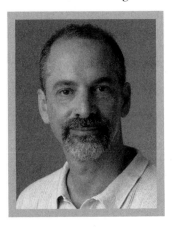

Janice Oldenberg (a composite of different students Gary has taught) was in her mid-thirties when she noted a gradual loss of energy. She described it to Gary Kraftsow as coming on after a two-week, low-grade fever and flulike illness that she couldn't seem to shake. After many months of symptoms, her doctor ruled out other causes and she was finally diagnosed as having chronic fatigue syndrome (CFS). A friend at work had been a student of Gary's for years, knew he'd had success with others suffering from CFS, and recommended Janice give it a try. Although she'd done some yoga at her gym in the past and liked it, she hadn't stuck with it.

Janice holds a fairly high-level job, in an environment that is competitive, political, and mainly male. Because the office is understaffed, she works long hours. When she began her sessions with Gary, she ate mainly in restaurants, grabbing things on the run, and rarely cooking at home. She didn't get much sleep, drank a lot of coffee, and sometimes went to her twenty-four-hour gym late at night to work out because she wanted to lose a few pounds. Gary describes her as being "mildly depressed, not having a lot of fun, and working too much."

Janice's home reflected how overworked she was. She admitted to Gary that there were piles everywhere, including research for work. To Gary, this reflected her state of mind. "There's a psychological thing about not cleaning, or not being able to let go of things that accumulate, holding on," which he links to the Ayurvedic concept of kapha, the constitutional type associated with inertia (see chapter 4).

Overview of Chronic Fatigue Syndrome

Chronic fatigue syndrome, which is also sometimes referred to as chronic fatigue immune deficiency syndrome (CFIDS), is a potentially debilitating disorder of unknown cause. CFS appears to affect multiple systems in the body including the nervous system, the immune system, and the hormonal system. When it first started getting public attention in the 1980s, some people felt it was related to infection with the Epstein-Barr virus, the same one that causes mononucleosis, but this theory has not been borne out by subsequent research; attempts to tie the disorder to other viruses or toxic exposures have also been inconclusive.

> **CAUTION** Because fatigue can be caused by a wide range of medical conditions, be sure to have a thorough evaluation by a physician before assuming your fatigue is related to CFS. Conditions like anemia, hypothyroidism, sleep apnea, and even cancer can cause fatigue, so doctors will often conduct a number of tests to rule these out. In women and the elderly, so-called vital exhaustion may be the only symptom of an impending heart attack (see chapter 19).

The most prominent symptom of CFS is overwhelming fatigue, often after even minimal exertion. The syndrome often strikes previously healthy individuals in the prime of their lives and typically starts with viral-like symptoms that just don't seem to go away.

Other common symptoms include low-grade fever, sore muscles, problems with sleep, difficulty thinking straight (sometimes dubbed "brain fog"), headaches, and sore throat. Because of the substantial overlap between these symptoms and those experienced by people with fibromyalgia, some speculate that the disorders may be related. The official criteria for the diagnosis from the Centers for Disease Control require severe fatigue that is not otherwise explained by another medical condition like cancer or depression, lasting for at least six straight months. Also required to make the diagnosis is the presence of four or more of the common symptoms mentioned above. It's important to remember, however, that this definition was formulated for research purposes and that people may have the condition even if they don't meet all the criteria.

Because there are no lab tests to definitively confirm CFS, some doctors doubt whether it's a real illness. Many people have essentially been told it's all in their head, that the real problem is anxiety or depression. While depression is common among people with CFS, being sick (and not being acknowledged as sick) may have made them depressed, and not the other way around. Indeed, the depression that characterizes CFS usually differs from that of clinical depression (see chapter 15). People with the latter may feel tired but also often lack motivation, while people with CFS are often highly motivated and frustrated by the inability to do what they want. People with CFS find other activities they are still able to do pleasurable, whereas those suffering from clinical depression tend to find little pleasure in anything. Despite these differences, anyone with CFS who has signs of serious depression should seek professional help, and may benefit from psychotherapy and antidepressant medication.

> **TIP** One common cause of fatigue that doctors sometimes forget to consider is medications. Hundreds of drugs, from antidepressants to blood pressure medication, can cause fatigue, so be sure your doctor is aware of all the drugs you take, both prescription and over-the-counter. Sometimes reducing the dosage, substituting a different drug, or cutting out the medication entirely can solve the problem.

How Yoga Fits In

Yoga can be helpful in CFS for a number of reasons. First of all, gentle asana practice stretches muscles and keep joints limber without straining the body the way that overly vigorous aerobic exercise can. Restorative yoga, breathing exercises, and other relaxation practices can usually be done no matter how tired you are, and can help rejuvenate you.

Although the cause of CFS may turn out to be infectious in nature, stress appears to play a role. Anecdotally, many people with the syndrome report burning the candle at both ends right up until the moment they crashed. These people may have been living with their stress-response system turned on most of the time, until their bodies finally said "enough." Research shows that people with CFS often have abnormalities in what's known as the HPA axis, which stands for the hypothalamus, the pituitary, and the adrenals, three organs that coordinate the release of stress hormones, including cortisol. Many, though not all, people with CFS have abnormally low levels of this stress hormone, as if their adrenal glands have weakened after years of working on overdrive. Yogis believe these people need restorative practices and deep relaxation before their strength can be built back up.

Whether or not stress plays a role in causing or predisposing you to CFS, having the condition can be very stressful, and stress can make matters worse. Since yoga is perhaps the best stress-reduction measure ever invented, it's likely to provide benefit regardless of what causes CFS. And since the effectiveness of yoga tends to increase the longer you stay with it, yoga offers a path to steady, albeit gradual, improvement.

To keep up the hectic pace that may have contributed to their burnout, many people with CFS have become accustomed to ignoring their body's messages about the need to slow down and rest. Like Janice, they may use caffeine or other stimulants to help override the body's objections to their lifestyle. For people who are not used to listening to their bodies, the heightened internal sensitivity that the regular practice of yoga brings can be of particular benefit. The better you can assess your internal states and correlate them to how you feel later on, the better you'll be able to gauge how your activities are affecting you (and feel justified in saying no to demands that you can reasonably predict will be too much). This applies to your yoga practice as well. As you gain awareness, you can recognize when you need to shift your practice away from what you usually do to something more restorative.

Specific yoga practices can be helpful for the sleep problems that are often an important contributor to CFS symptoms. CFS sufferers seem to have difficulty going into deep sleep, which scientists believe is when a number of restorative functions occur. Studies of longtime meditators have found that while meditating they exhibit brain wave activity which may serve some of the same restorative functions as deep sleep, and their ability to function does not appear to be as affected by the loss of a night's sleep as nonmeditators are. Yogic practices such as asana and breathwork can also improve sleep (see chapter 23).

Gary Kraftsow believes pranayama can play an especially important role in CFS. Speaking from his experience using pranayama, Gary says, "It seems to make the whole metabolic system function better, with increased immunity, better digestion, better sleep, more energy, more vitality, and the regulation of hormones. It seems to be a homeostatic equalizer, to balance everything, and make people feel better."

Like meditation, many pranayama practices require little physical exertion. Gary tries to keep the pranayama practices he teaches fairly simple. "I don't ask most people to do tremendous gymnastics with breath control. That's for people who have time and interest, to go deeper into it. But for most people who are living in the world, it's an adjunct to a healthy lifestyle, and fifteen minutes of conscious breathwork once or twice a day is enough. It doesn't have to be complex ratios and fancy techniques." The benefits, he stresses, come with repeated practice and consistency over time.

Some people with CFS believe their prognosis for a return to a more normal life is bleak, that there is little they can do to improve their situation. The self-examination that yoga encourages can help you be alert to that kind of negative and self-defeating thinking. Self-study, or svadhyaya, extends to examining your lifestyle, too. Are you living in a way that promotes health? Are you sleeping enough? Do you eat meals at regular times? Is your food nutritious? Do you balance work with play?

Yogis believe that finding your dharma, knowing what you should be doing with your life, can be vital to recovery from CFS. With self-study and greater sensitivity, you may come to realize that your job, relationship, or living situation isn't right for you. The quieting of the mind that yoga facilitates helps you tune in to messages you may previously have been unable to hear due to the high level of background noise. What you do with that information is for you to decide. Yoga simply helps put you in touch with it.

Finally, there is the social aspect of yoga. Due to their exhaustion, many people with CFS may give up previously enjoyable activities, focusing whatever energy they have left on their job. Being with people, making new friends, and forging a relationship with a teacher can all help alleviate isolation. This is what yogis call sangha, community, and it can be a powerful tool for healing.

The Scientific Evidence

So far no controlled studies have examined the effectiveness of yoga for CFS. The best evidence to date comes from a two-year prospective study published in the *Journal of Clinical Psychiatry*. Dr. Arthur Hartz and colleagues at the University of Iowa asked 155 people with unexplained chronic fatigue which measures, both alternative and conventional, they were using to deal with their symptoms. The researchers then correlated the answers with changes in self-reported levels of fatigue, depression, and other symptoms after 6 and 24 months. Subjects had suffered from fatigue for an average of 6.7 years at the beginning of the study. Among the approaches the people tried during the 2 years the study lasted were herbs, dietary supplements, prescription drugs, lifestyle changes, and yoga. Much to the researchers' surprise, when the subjects were quizzed at the end of the study, yoga proved to be the most effective approach of all, and the only one with statistically significant benefits. Of those practicing yoga, at both 6 and 24 months, 25 percent reported "substantial" improvement in fatigue compared to an average of only 8 percent of those who tried other interventions. Only 5 percent of those doing yoga noted a significant worsening in fatigue at 2 years, as compared with 10 percent of those who didn't do yoga. Similarly, the only treatment that predicted an improvement in depressive symptoms at the end of 2 years was yoga.

Gary Kraftsow's Approach

In evaluating clients, Gary says, "I draw heavily on what I call the Pancha Maya model which comes from the Taittriyha Upanishad." Gary is referring to the yogic model that views each person as being made up of five layers or sheaths (see table 14.1), starting on the outside, with the body, and moving progressively inward to the layer of bliss.

TABLE 14.1 THE PANCHA MAYA MODEL, THE FIVE LAYERS OF THE HUMAN BEING DESCRIBED IN THE UPANISHADS. SOME YOGIS CALL THE LAYERS KOSHAS.

ENGLISH	SANSKRIT
The body	Annamaya
Energy	Pranamaya
The lower mind	Manomaya
The higher mind	Vijnanamaya
Bliss	Anandamaya

Beginning with the body, the Annamaya, Gary finds that some people with CFS have neck, shoulder, or back problems, and these structural problems influence which asana he recommends. In Janice's case, he designed an asana sequence to deal with his finding that she "had a hip problem, a chronic sacral strain that seemed like a congenital hip imbalance. Her left hip was hypermobile, and she had a lot of nonspecific hip pain." Gary also tends to make a lot of lifestyle suggestions. With Janice, he recommended that she drink less coffee and get more sleep. He also suggested she modify the way she was exercising, and do her cardiovascular exercise in the mornings, when she was better rested, rather than after a full day's work. He also suggested a more consistent schedule, since her gym workouts were rather erratic.

To address the layer of energy, the Pranamaya, Gary asks his patients questions related to their energy levels in the morning and the afternoon, and how restorative their sleep feels. "After that," he says, "I go into Manomaya. One of the things I've noticed with chronic fatigue patients is that there's often something that's not happy about their lives. What I try to do is find things they're interested in that will stimulate their interest, their motivation." Janice, Gary discovered, loves to throw pots. "It's very good for her, but she hardly ever had time to do it, so I encouraged that." Since the Manomaya layer is related to education, he encourages his patients to learn as much as they can about their condition, and the relationship between their lifestyle and their condition. He wants them to understand how much exercise is good and how much is too much. If they have digestive problems, he tries to explain possible connections to their diet.

> **TIP** You may think you don't have time to pursue interests that do nothing more than give you joy, but yoga teacher Ana Forrest finds they can be essential to healing. One of her students with CFS "desperately wanted to be a painter," but she had children, and a husband who didn't have a regular source of income. Before she collapsed she'd been the main breadwinner, so she had put her needs aside. Ana told her that painting every day was "part of your rehab. So it's not like you do it only if you have time and everybody's fed." Although Ana felt it would be crucial to her eventual recovery, she says, "It was almost like she needed my adamancy around in order to have permission to do something as 'unimportant' as her dreams."

The next level Gary addresses, Vijnanamaya, "has to do with people's values and direction in life, what's important for them." He tries to understand his students' emotional makeup, in particular their patterns. Janice, he says, was overwhelmed with work. Quitting was always at the back of her mind. "When you're in a job that you don't like, and you are overworked, and you're always thinking about quitting, it's not embracing your life as it is. It's the same thing if you are in a relationship, but always thinking about getting out."

Finally, Gary tries to help his patients address the Anandamaya dimension. "I try to help them reconnect with sources of joy or nourishment, which may or may not have a spiritual flavor. Many people in our society don't have a church or God, but everybody can find something that is joyful to them. I try to help them reconnect to that."

Obviously, Gary's therapeutic prescription goes far beyond asana and Pranayama. Knowing how busy Janice was, Gary tried to give her a home yoga practice that was doable, dividing it into two different short practices of about fifteen to twenty minutes. The first one, done in the morning right before going to work, was designed to be stimulating. He designed the evening practice to help her relax and unwind from the day, release tension in her neck and shoulders, and improve the quality of her sleep.

Gary used both pranayama and breath control in the asana practice to increase Janice's "threshold capacity," which he believes stimulates immune function. By threshold capacity, he means the duration of the various phases of breath, the inhalation, exhalation, and pauses in between.

Here are the sequences of poses and instructions that Gary provided for Janice.

THE A.M. PRACTICE

EXERCISE #1. **EQUAL STANDING POSE (Samasthiti).** From a standing position (figure 14.1a), inhale and raise your arms above your head (figure 14.1b). Hold your breath for a count of two. Then, on an exhalation, lower your arms slowly. Repeat for one more round. For a third and fourth round, hold your breath for a four count after inhaling. For a fifth and six round, hold your breath for a count of six.

As Janice got stronger, Gary substituted Mountain pose (Tadasana) for Equal Standing pose. In Mountain pose, you lift up on to tiptoes as you inhale and raise your arms overhead. As you exhale, simultaneously lower your arms and heels slowly.

Note that what Gary calls Mountain pose is different from the pose of the same name in other yoga traditions (this is true of many Viniyoga poses).

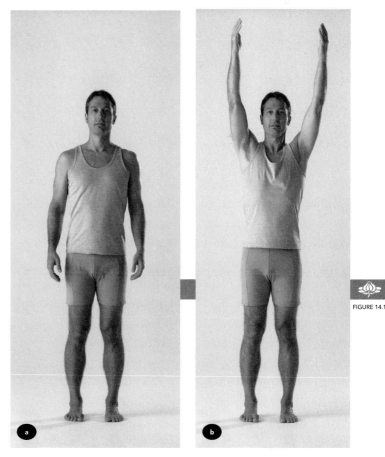

FIGURE 14.1

EXERCISE #2. **STANDING FORWARD BEND (Uttanasana).** Start by standing with your arms at your side. On an inhalation, sweep your arms out and up (figure 14.2a). Then on your next exhalation, lower your arms to the sides and bend forward into Standing Forward Bend, staying down for one complete breath (figure 14.2b). On your next inhalation, sweep your arms to the sides and then overhead as you return to standing. Repeat the round once more, staying in Standing Forward Bend for one breath. For a third and fourth round, take two complete breaths in the forward bend. For a fifth and sixth round, take three breaths in the forward bend. Gary told Janice if she was particularly tired, she should return her hands to her sides between rounds, rather than keeping them overhead.

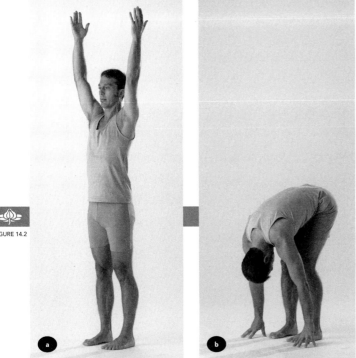

FIGURE 14.2

Because Janice had a slightly kyphotic (rounded) upper back, Gary adapted the traditional pose and asked her to lift her chest and sweep her arms out to the sides when she was inhaling up out of the Standing Forward Bend (figure 14.2c). Having her arms at her sides allows her to use her shoulder blades to help coax more opening in her upper back. He instructed: "On the inhale, lift the chest slightly as if you were lying on your stomach doing Cobra—just slightly. It's not a strong lift, just enough to create some movement in the upper back."

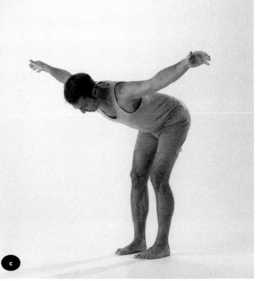

EXERCISE #3. **WARRIOR I POSE (Virabhadrasana I).** From a standing position, step one foot forward and the other back so that your feet are about three feet apart, with your hips square to the front (figure 14.3a). On an inhalation, bend your front knee and raise your arms as if they were the hands of a clock on four and eight, with the palms facing forward (figure 14.3b).

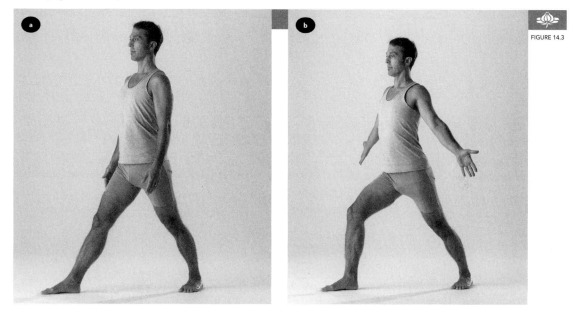

FIGURE 14.3

Hold the pose and your breath for a count of two then exhale back to the starting position. For the next round, inhale and repeat the pose with your arms at two and ten, palms facing forward (figure 14.3c), holding for a count of two, and then exhaling back to the starting position. On your last round, inhale and repeat the pose with your arms at "high noon," palms facing each other (figure 14.3d), holding for two and exhaling back to the starting position.

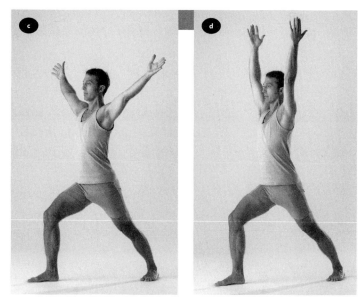

In three versions of the pose, as you bend your knee, allow your shoulders to come forward of your hips, arching in the upper chest, without exaggerating the normal curve of the lower back. The shoulder blades move toward each other. Repeat all three versions holding for a count of four, after the inhalation. Then repeat all three versions of the pose holding for a count of six after the inhalation.

At no point during this sequence of nine repetitions should there be any tension in the breathing. If Gary noticed Janice was having any difficulty with the breath holds, he told her to back off. For example, instead of asking her to hold for a count of two, four, and six, he might make it one, two, and three. If you feel uncomfortable, you can also count a little faster. Just be consistent with the speed from repetition to repetition.

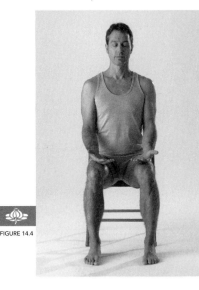

As she bent her front knee and raised her arms, Gary had Janice lean slightly forward from the hips to minimize the compression of the low back and to maximize the opening of the upper spine. To enhance the opening of the upper spine, he also asked her to bring her shoulder blades toward each other when she raised her arms. Both of these instructions were designed to help counter the rounding of her upper back.

FIGURE 14.4

EXERCISE #4. **SEATED REST.** As an alternative to Deep Relaxation pose (Savasana), sit upright in a chair for three to five minutes (figure 14.4). Without making any effort to change it, simply notice your breath as it moves in and out.

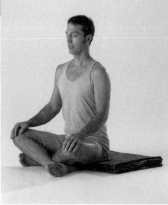

FIGURE 14.5

EXERCISE #5. **TWO-STAGE INHALE (Krama pranayama).** Start by sitting on the floor in any comfortable seated position (figure 14.5). (Less flexible people can do this exercise sitting in a chair.) Stage one: inhale halfway for a count of four, expanding your chest, retaining the breath for a count of four. Stage two: inhale the rest of the way for a count of four, expanding your abdominal cavity, retaining the breath for a count of four. Exhale for twelve counts.

After you become comfortable with the two-stage inhale, you can practice the three stage inhale. Stage one: inhale in the chest for three counts and hold for three counts. Stage two: inhale into the upper abdomen for three counts and hold for three counts. Stage three: inhale into the lower abdomen and the pelvic floor for three counts and hold for three counts, then exhale on a count of twelve. This breathing practice is designed to be both energizing and calming.

THE P.M. PRACTICE

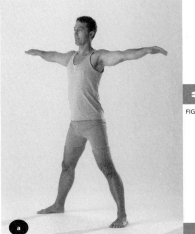

EXERCISE #1. STANDING FORWARD BEND (Uttanasana). Same as in the A.M. practice.

FIGURE 14.6

EXERCISE #2. REVOLVED TRIANGLE POSE (Parivrtta Trikonasana). Start by standing with your feet facing forward and about two and a half feet apart (figure 14.6a). On your exhalation, revolve

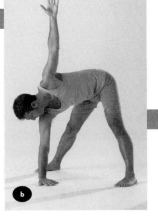

your trunk, placing your right hand on the floor between your feet and extending your left arm straight up. As your arm extends up, turn your head to gaze down toward the floor (figure 14.6b). On your next inhalation, lengthen your left arm alongside your head and turn your gaze upward (figure 14.6c). On your next exhalation, return to your prior position, with the arm lengthening up and head gazing down. Then inhale back to your starting position. Repeat the pose three times on each side, alternating between sides.

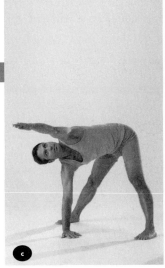

EXERCISE #3. **KNEELING POSE (Vajrasana).** Start by kneeling in an upright position with your arms overhead (figure 14.7a). On your exhalation, bend at the hips and knees to come into Kneeling pose, sweeping your arms behind your back (figure 14.7b). On your inhalation, return to the upright position, lifting your arms back overhead. Repeat six times. Note that this pose resembles what is called Child's pose in other traditions.

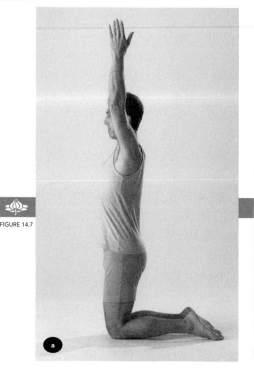
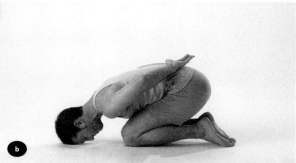

FIGURE 14.7

EXERCISE #4. **SUPINE TWIST (Jathara Parivrtta).** Start by lying on your back, with your knees bent in toward your chest and your arms out to the side along the floor (figure 14.8a). On an exhalation, lower your knees to your right side, toward the floor (figure 14.8b). Stay for one breath, then inhale and return to your starting position. Repeat to the left side. Repeat the entire sequence staying two breaths on each side, and then repeat the sequence again staying for three breaths on each side.

FIGURE 14.8

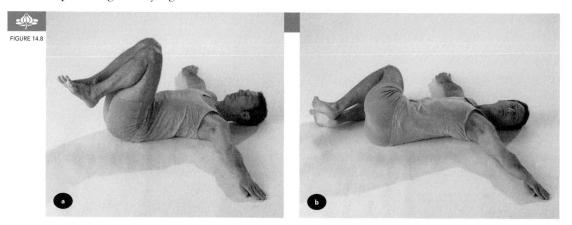

EXERCISE #5. **WIND-RELEASING POSE TO LEG LIFT (Apanasana to Modified Supta Padangusthasana).** Start by lying on your back, with your knees bent in toward your chest and your hands behind your knees (figure 14.9a). On an inhalation, straighten your legs, holding your hands behind the knees (figure 14.9b). Hold the leg lift for one breath, then exhale and release back to your starting position. For a second round, hold the leg lift for two breaths. For a third round, hold the leg lift for three breaths.

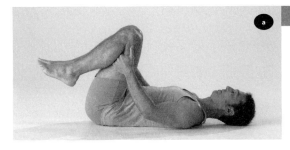 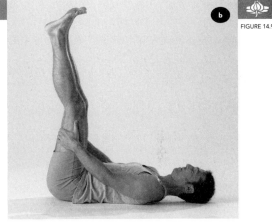

FIGURE 14.9

Note that Apanasana in the Viniyoga tradition resembles what is called Pavanmuktasana in other styles of yoga.

EXERCISE #6. **RELAXATION POSE (Savasana).** Lie on your back, with your hands and feet relaxed to the sides, and your eyes closed for three to five minutes.

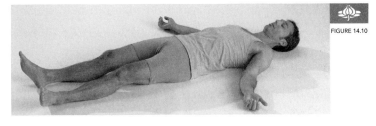

FIGURE 14.10

EXERCISE #7. **SEATED PRANAYAMA, lengthening the exhalation.** Sit in any comfortable seated position. When you are settled, inhale to a count of three and then exhale to a count of eight. Do in this manner three more times. For rounds five to eight, exhale to a count of ten. For rounds nine to twelve, exhale to a count of twelve. This breathing practice, by progressively lengthening the exhalation, is designed to be deeply calming.

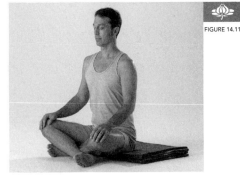

FIGURE 14.11

A practice that Gary often recommends to people with CFS who are also depressed is Chandra Bhedana pranayama. To do it, you inhale through the left nostril, hold the breath, and then slowly exhale through the right nostril. "There's a kind of an emotional lift from the holding after the inhale, and a calming effect with a long exhale," Gary notes. However, proper Chandra Bhedana technique—including the finger positions to partially block the nostril you are breathing in and out of while completely blocking the other nostril—is subtle and is best learned from a well-trained teacher.

In addition to asana and pranayama, Gary thought that yogic chanting would be therapeutic for Janice. But instead of teaching her chants to use in her home practice, he asked her to go to kirtans, public events where groups of people sing mantras in a call-and-response fashion, because he wanted to encourage her to develop her social life.

OTHER YOGIC IDEAS

A number of the restorative practices taught by B. K. S. Iyengar can be useful for fatigue in general and for CFS specifically (see chapter 3). In particular a variation of Supported Bridge pose (Setu Bandha Sarvangasana) also called Cross Bolsters, is a gentle passive backbend than can help relieve fatigue. If you don't have two bolsters, folded blankets or a block can substitute for the lower bolster. You can stay in this pose for five minutes or longer.

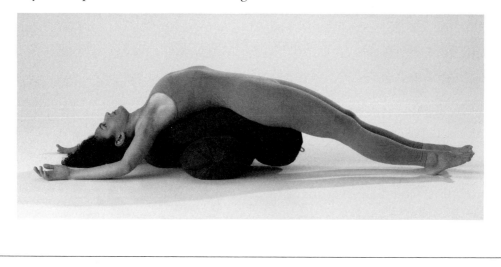

Contraindications, Special Considerations, and Modifications

Gary carefully adapts the intensity of the practice to the energy level of the student. "In an extreme case, the asana is very minimal," he says. "It might be sitting on a chair, doing standing Virabhadrasana, and sitting back down on the chair, and then doing some breathing and then lying down and resting. That could be the whole practice. When they get stronger, the practice can be increased."

In general, people who are fatigued should avoid strenuous postures like full backbends. They should also avoid long holds. It's less tiring to move in and out of poses. Indeed, one reason why a Viniyoga practice may be particularly well suited to someone with CFS is because of its emphasis on constantly moving in and out of the poses, rarely holding a single pose for more than a few breaths. Other ways to modify a practice to minimize exhaustion include adding breaks between poses, interspersing Savasana, and using support like bolsters and blankets to make poses more passive and relaxing.

One of the biggest risks to people with CFS using yoga therapeutically is getting enthusiastic and taking on too much too soon, which can precipitate a flare-up of symptoms. The best plan is to start with modest activity, based on how you feel, then slowly ramp up over a period of weeks to months. It's also wise to adjust how much you do on a daily basis, according to how you feel. If you're feeling more exhausted than usual one day, scale back your practice and do gentler or more restorative exercises. Even some vigorous pranayama techniques may be too much if you are already feeling depleted.

Some people with CFS have a bothersome symptom known medically as postural hypotension; when you sit or stand up quickly, your blood pressure may not adapt fast enough and you may feel light-headed. Drinking plenty of fluids to remain well hydrated can help, as can being careful to make transitions slowly and deliberately both in daily life and in asana practice. If you feel light-headed in a pose, come out of it and relax in Savasana or another comfortable position with the head lower than the heart until you feel better. Gary has students prone to dizziness—including those with CFS, low blood pressure, and hypothyroidism (low thyroid)—avoid poses like Standing Forward Bend (Uttanasana), where the head hangs down, and substitute Utkatasana (Chair pose, see p. 164), moving from a standing position to a half squat. These symptoms may improve over time with steady practice. Some yoga teachers have found that the regular practice of inversions can also help with postural hypotension. For people who have little energy, supported versions of these poses such as Chair Shoulderstand (see p. 327) and Headstand hanging from ropes may offer similar benefits with little exertion.

A Holistic Approach to Chronic Fatigue Syndrome

✳ There is no specific treatment for CFS in conventional medicine, in part because no one has figured out what causes the problem. Various treatments have been tried, including cortisone drugs, but these drugs have significant side effects and the results to date have been mixed at best.

✳ A multipronged approach that includes mild exercise, attention to improving sleep, and cognitive behavioral therapy to learn coping strategies all appear to help to some degree.

✳ People with CFS often find support groups helpful, though if members of the group are pessimistic about the chance of recovery, the experience can be counterproductive.

✳ Exercise can be a two-edged sword. Overdoing can backfire, causing greater fatigue, but doing nothing is even worse, since it leads to a general loss of conditioning, higher levels of depression and anxiety, and lower-quality sleep. To avoid a major flare-up in symptoms, try to carefully adjust your exercise intensity to your energy level in order to build stamina.

✳ Very low doses of tricyclic antidepressants appear to improve restorative sleep (stage 4), even in people with CFS who are not depressed.

✳ Acupuncture is very safe and may reduce symptoms.

✳ Therapeutic massage and other forms of bodywork may reduce stress and alleviate pain.

✳ Hydrotherapy including hot tubs, whirlpools, and gentle water aerobics may have similar benefits.

✳ In traditional medical systems like Ayurveda and traditional Chinese medicine (TCM), there are a variety of herbal tonics said to boost energy levels. Such herbs as ginseng, Siberian ginseng (which isn't really ginseng at all, but an unrelated species), and ashwagandha can boost energy levels and are generally extremely safe. It may take two or three months to assess effectiveness. Rather than self-prescribe these treatments, it's best to consult a practitioner of Ayurveda or TCM.

* The dietary supplement Coenzyme Q10, a natural constituent of the body's cells, is safe and may boost energy.

* Greater regularity in the timing of meals may be beneficial.

* Consumption of essential fatty acids, including the omega-3 fatty acids, found in flaxseeds and some seafood, may help, though the evidence is not consistent.

* Simple carbohydrates may raise insulin levels, quickly leading to a sharp drop in blood sugar and increased fatigue. Complex carbohydrates are a better bet.

* Alcohol can help you fall asleep but should not be used for this purpose because it leads to disrupted, less restful sleep.

* Although it may be tempting to use caffeine for a temporary energy boost, it can make fatigue worse. Some find that a single cup of coffee in the morning doesn't cause problems.

* In general, with these as with any suggested remedies, yoga says trust your own experience to learn what works for you.

Janice enjoyed the asana and pranayama practices Gary taught her, and also found she had an affinity for the Sanskrit devotional chanting he suggested she attend. As Gary had predicted, going to kirtans by performers like Krishna Das became a way for her to expand her social network.

Yoga, as narrowly seen, was only part of Gary's prescription. He often has a lot of lifestyle negotiations with his students. One of the first things he asked Janice to do was to set aside a space in her home for a regular yoga practice. He felt that she needed to clean and organize her house as a way of clearing her mind. He tried to get her to be more consistent in her meal times, more conscious of her food, and more moderate in the quantity she ate. He says, "I also encouraged her to do more exercise in the daytime, rather than at three in the morning." His main lifestyle suggestion was "to work less and have more fun. I encouraged her to create time so that she could do things that she enjoyed," like throwing pots, hiking, and spending time on the beach on weekends. Janice eventually settled into a routine of going to the gym in the morning, instead of doing yoga, and doing an evening yoga practice, which was helpful to her sleep. If she didn't have time to go to the gym in the morning, she did the short asana practice before going to work.

The pranayama work Gary did with Janice made her much more conscious of her breathing, and she eventually brought this awareness to her gym workouts, too. For example, Gary encouraged her to breathe deeply when using the elliptical exercise machine, and to standardize the number of steps she took per breath. This suggestion took hold. Once you start down that path, he says, the breathing really makes everything different, "much stronger and much more effective." This process, of course, also brings yogic awareness to something that most people do mindlessly.

After working with Gary on and off for over two years, Janice is managing her condition much better. She takes better care of herself, and has lost some weight. She also has more friends and is more socially active, and she's spending time out in nature on the weekends. Overall she's less depressed, sleeps better, and has more energy. Although she still works too hard and has a love/hate relationship with her job, "she's valuing her life more."

C H A P T E R   1 5

DEPRESSION

 PATRICIA WALDEN suffered from clinical depression in her twenties and early thirties. She tried private and group psychotherapy, hypnosis, and medication, all of which helped to a degree. "But they left me with a feeling of emptiness, a sense that there must be something more," she says. When she met B. K. S. Iyengar in 1977, "there was something about his method of teaching, from the very first day, that spoke to me directly. His teaching kind of bypassed my brain and went right into my heart. My first class with him, he said, 'If you keep your armpits open, you'll never get depressed.' That made perfect sense to me." She describes her realization about how the body could affect the mind as "a mini-moment of enlightenment for me, actually life changing. From that time on I began to see my yoga practice as a way of helping me deal with my depression, and especially the emptiness that I had felt often throughout my life." Patricia is one of the two senior, advanced teachers of Iyengar yoga in the United States, and is well-known for her best-selling yoga instructional videos. She teaches in the Boston area and internationally.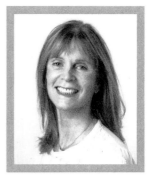

Carrie Benson (not her real name) was first exposed to yoga when she did a program at the Mind/Body Medical Institute at Harvard Medical School to help her deal with stomach pain due to acid reflux. "I did that in 1998, and it was amazing. It changed my life, it introduced me to yoga, which I pursued." Shortly thereafter, she started her first class at Patricia Walden's yoga center. "I had done a lot of dance, so when I started to do yoga it felt familiar in some way," though she found that it included some "elements that were very different, and much more rewarding."

All her life, Carrie had been pushed by her mother to achieve. A single mom and first-generation immigrant, her mother was a big believer in education. Carrie fulfilled her mother's dreams, eventually earning a law degree, and going on to pursue a PhD in anthropology, which she is now finishing. A few years into Carrie's yoga practice, however, a major depression triggered by the movie *Billy Elliot* led her to question her career choices. Seeing the movie—the story of a young boy in a mining town in England enamored of dance, despite the fact that it was completely unacceptable in that cultural milieu—brought back the feelings of loss she had experienced when her ambitious mother made her give up dance, which had been her first love, in favor of a career that would be more practical and lucrative. The boy in the movie persists in becoming a dancer, and his father, ultimately, comes around to be supportive of him. "I saw my own life in this film, with the wrong ending, and it was a real crisis for me."

The resulting depression was not Carrie's first. "Depression first manifested in me when I was in my teens, or postpuberty. It runs in our family. My grandmother clearly suffered from it, but it was undiagnosed and untreated. There was a very strong stigma in my family about acknowledging it. I come from a British background, stiff upper lip, pull yourself up by your bootstraps, and exercise your will to make yourself feel better." But Carrie decided to get help this time. Carrie approached Patricia after class one day and told her about her depression. Patricia felt she could help and they began to work together to address the problem.

Overview of Depression

The term depression, as used by doctors, refers to much more than feeling blue or down in the dumps. Sadness is something all people feel from time to time. Depression must also be differentiated from grief, the natural and healthy reaction to loss, whether it's loss of a beloved person or pet, or a job, or home, or one's health (though normal grief can turn into depression). Clinical depression is a life-threatening medical condition in which sadness and other symptoms can be so overwhelming the person is incapacitated or even suicidal. Doctors look for nine main symptoms in trying to decide whether someone has a clinical depression.

DIAGNOSING DEPRESSION

To meet the criteria for clinical depression, a person needs to have at least five of the following nine symptoms, present for at least two weeks:

1. Depressed mood on most days and for most of each day

2. Loss of pleasure in formerly pleasurable activities

3. Significant increase or decrease in appetite, weight, or both

4. Sleep problems, either insomnia or excessive sleepiness, nearly every day

5. Feelings of agitation or a sense of intense lethargy

6. Loss of energy or excessive fatigue daily

7. A persistent sense of guilt or worthlessness

8. Inability to concentrate, occurring nearly every day

9. Recurrent thoughts of death or suicide

Doctors increasingly have come to view depression as a biochemical problem, related to abnormal levels of neurotransmitters like serotonin, norepinephrine, and dopamine in the brain. Partly due to this belief and partly due to the high cost of psychotherapy, the primary, and often the only, treatment prescribed for depression these days is drugs, most commonly drugs like Prozac and Zoloft, which raise levels of serotonin. These drugs, known collectively as selective serotonin reuptake inhibitors, or SSRIs, are no more effective than older antidepressants, but many patients find the side effects more tolerable. Although not everyone is helped by them, and I feel strongly it's best to use them as part of a multipronged approach, these drugs can be lifesavers. I say this despite the often very negative attitude toward antidepressants found in both the yoga world and among many advocates of alternative medicine.

While antidepressants are far from perfect, some people need to be on them—and stay on them—to function. For others, taking an antidepressant on a temporary basis can give them the energy and strength to engage in the health-promoting activities, like yoga, exercise, and psychotherapy, that could help lift them out of depression. From a yogic perspective, antidepressants are neither good nor bad, they are simply tools. What's crucial is to use them wisely, take them when you truly need them, and avoid them if you don't. As Patricia says, "Thank God we have this option."

Although effective treatments are available, many people with depression are never diagnosed. Some people who are depressed are unaware of it. Men appear more likely than women to fail to recognize when they are depressed. Both men and women may avoid seeking treatment out of a misguided sense of embarrassment, seeing their condition as a sign that they are weak, or believing that there is little to be done for it. But even those who know something is wrong and do seek treatment for it may turn up at their doctor's office with a catalogue of symptoms—including fatigue, headaches, stomach problems, and dizziness—that is hard to diagnose. Primary-care doctors often fail to diagnose depression accurately, especially in men, who are more likely to manifest depression through symptoms like anger and irritability instead of the sadness that women are more prone to. Doctors may also fail to recognize depression in the elderly, whose symptoms may manifest in a primarily physical manner, or in people with conditions like cancer, HIV, and heart disease. Serious illness results in a markedly increased risk of major depression, but doctors understandably tend to focus their treatment on the underlying disease, not the accompanying depression. Unfortunately, failing to recognize and treat depression may undermine therapeutic efforts for these other medical problems, and ultimately contribute to an earlier death.

How Yoga Fits In

Since stress can be a big factor in depression, part of yoga's effectiveness undoubtedly comes from its proven ability to alleviate tension. People who are depressed tend to have persistent activation of the sympathetic nervous system (the fight-or-flight response) and elevations of the stress hormone cortisol (see chapter 3). Indeed, the failure of cortisol levels to go down when they should is the basis of a test sometimes used to diagnose depression (the dexamethasone suppression test). But yoga has been shown repeatedly to lower cortisol levels, which may be a major factor in its ability to lift mood.

From a yogic perspective, there is a connection between your posture and your mood, as Iyengar suggested with his comments on keeping your armpits open. Says Patricia, "A lot of people in the class that day were saying, 'What? What is he talking about, keeping the armpits open?' I think it spoke so clearly to me because my posture was the posture of a depressed person, and my chest was a sunken chest. When he says, 'open the armpits,' he's saying the space between the armpit and the chest grows, becomes wider and more lifted, so the lungs are lifted, the physical heart lifts, you're able to breathe more deeply. Your thoracic spine begins to elongate, and those simple things have an effect on your physiological and mental state. I felt that immediately."

Letting go of muscular tension, yogis believe, can counteract feelings of stress and depression, and may have other beneficial effects. Patricia says, "If you're holding your abdomen tight, and clenching your diaphragm, and your eyebrows are drawn toward each other, people respond differently to you than they would to a person who is standing up straight, with an open chest, a pleasant look on the face, and space between the eyebrows." She also thinks that simply having an expression and a posture like that can cause you to make different decisions than you would with a more relaxed, positive bearing.

The yogic tool of self-study (svadhyaya) may also be useful for dealing with depression. While acknowledging that some depression may have a primarily biological basis, yogis often ask the question: What can you learn from your depression? Beyond simply helping you learn how to modulate your response to stress, which yoga does very well, going to a deeper level involves seeing whether there are areas of your life—your relationships, your work, your ability to set aside time for yourself—that need to be changed. Many people believe that if they feel sad, there is something wrong inside of them. But sometimes a depressed mood can be a healthy reaction to something that's not right in the external world, and dealing with it may be the best means of alleviating the depression. Patricia puts it this way: "Is this dark night of the soul a message that your life needs to be looked at?"

Yogic Tool: **FAITH.** If you have decided on yoga as part of your path out of depression, Patricia suggests having faith, being patient, and committing to the practice. Faith itself, she asserts, can be a healing force. In Patricia's own case, the lift she got from her yoga practice in a time of depression, "would sometimes last for a day and sometimes for an hour. But what did last was the memory of my practice, and that memory was the spark that would help me go to my next practice. Say, for example, I'd had a practice that was very successful, and I felt joyful and calm after. Inevitably those feelings would lessen, but the spark of light that the practice gave me was still in my memory, and that's what brought me to my next practice, to my next session." Faith in yoga is not based on dogma, but comes because you see that what you are doing appears to be working.

— Resistance to opening - why ?? want to keep neg. feelings + stress - holding ??

The Scientific Evidence

A study conducted at Benares Hindu University in Varanasi, India, found that three- and six-month practices of yoga improved the functioning and moods of people with clinical depression. In the study of eighty people, half were treated with the tricyclic antidepressant imipramine and half with yoga. The practice consisted of relaxation poses, inversions and other asana, pranayama, and meditation on various chakras, the energy centers that run along the spine according to yogic teaching. After six months of practice, 60 percent of patients treated with yoga showed improvement in their sleep, digestive symptoms, mood, and social interactions. Improvements in these subjectively rated symptoms were inferior in the drug group, but researchers did not quantify them. Both groups had similar improvements in neurotransmitter levels, with a significant rise in serotonin levels and a decrease in monoamine oxidase levels (lowering MAO levels is the mechanism of action for older and now less commonly used antidepressants like Nardil and Parnate). Cortisol levels in the blood, and levels of other stress hormones in urine declined significantly in both groups. The authors also found that although yoga took a little longer to boost mood, its effects tended to persist longer than those from the antidepressant.

Although not everyone with depression can tolerate Deep Relaxation pose (see p. 277), a controlled study from Punjabi University in India found Savasana an effective treatment for severe depression in female college students. Fifty women aged twenty to twenty-five were divided into two groups. One group did Savasana for thirty minutes every morning for thirty sessions, while the other received no treatment. After fifteen days, the yoga group had significantly improved, and the effect was even greater after thirty days. By the end of the study, eleven of the twenty-five women in the yoga group were no longer depressed, four had mild depression, one moderate depression, and nine had no response. Among the twenty-five controls, at thirty days two were moderately depressed and twenty-three remained severely depressed.

In a randomized controlled trial, Alison Woolery and colleagues at UCLA assessed the effects of Iyengar yoga on women with mild depression. A total of twenty-eight women took part in the study, thirteen of whom went to two yoga classes a week for five weeks, emphasizing asana including backbends, inversions, and vigorous standing poses felt to be beneficial in depression. The control group was placed on a waiting list for yoga classes. Students were not encouraged to practice at home. Even so, halfway into the study, the yoga group showed significantly greater improvements in mood and reductions in anxiety than the control group, and these benefits were maintained on retesting at the end of the study.

Studies of mindfulness-based stress reduction (MBSR), which includes mindfulness meditation and hatha yoga as part of the program, found that it lowers feelings of anxiety and depression. Long-term follow-up shows these results persist three years after the training, with the majority of people still practicing on their own. A randomized controlled trial of a program that combined MBSR with cognitive-behavioral therapy found it cut the recurrence rate for major depression nearly in half. Recent evidence from Dr. Richard Davidson's lab at the University of Wisconsin suggests that MBSR shifts the activation of the front section of the brain, the prefrontal cortex, from the right lobe to the left, a change associated with improved mood and feelings of well-being. This change appears to be greatest among highly experienced practitioners, suggesting that with sustained practice you can shift your emotional baseline toward greater levels of happiness.

Patricia Walden's Approach

Patricia uses concepts found in both yoga and Ayurveda to categorize depression as being either tamasic in nature or rajasic. Tamas is a heavy energy marked by a sense of inertia. Rajas is a hyperaroused, distractible energy (see table 15.1). Sattva is a state of clarity, ease, and balance. Cultivating sattva is one of the major goals of yoga practice.

TABLE 15.1 CHARACTERISTICS OF TWO MAJOR TYPES OF DEPRESSION

TYPE OF DEPRESSION	CONVENTIONAL TERM	SYMPTOMS	TYPICAL BREATH
Rajasic	Agitated Depression	Anxiety, Restlessness, Impulsiveness	Quick and Erratic, Hard to Exhale
Tamasic	Atypical Depression	Inertia, Dullness, Hopelessness	Shallow, Hard to Inhale

Tamasic depression is marked by lethargy, feelings of hopelessness, and melancholia. Crying jags are common. The person may not be able to get out of bed in the morning. Patricia says, "You don't feel your life force, you don't feel powerful, you don't feel hopeful." When Patricia looks at someone suffering tamasic depression, she often sees that the student has slumped shoulders, a collapsed chest, shallow breathing, droopy eyes, an expressionless face, and tension in the abdomen. Patricia likens it to a "deflated balloon. You can barely see them breathing," she says. Bringing breath into that deflated balloon with a deep inhalation is a big part of the yogic remedy. "When you start focusing on your breath, and taking the breath into your chest and breathing deeply, you begin to feel the presence of your breath. What comes with that is a feeling of life returning, a feeling of warmth that percolates throughout your chest at the beginning, but then throughout your entire body."

Patricia's approach to rajasic depression differs. People with this type of depression often manifest high levels of anxiety, a racing mind, anger, and agitation. Patricia refers to this type of depression as "closed fist." She observes that students with rajasic depression often have tightness in their muscles, and a kind of "hardness" in and around the eyes.

These students often can't keep still, their fingers moving nearly continually even when they try to relax in restorative yoga poses. The breath tends to be quick and erratic. To counter the agitation, Patricia asks rajasic students to focus more on the exhalation, trying to make it long and smooth, imagining that the breath allows a relaxing of the chest muscles, and with it a gradual unclenching of the closed fist. "What comes with the space inside your chest is also space in your mental body. You're not holding anymore."

According to Patricia, Carrie alternated between rajasic and tamasic periods but showed more signs of a rajasic depression. "I think that Carrie had a lot of anxiety," Patricia says. "She was tightly wound and could get overstimulated easily. She has a very active brain, very quick." Patricia noticed that Carrie sometimes seemed really driven in class. "She would work too hard in a pose." At other times Patricia thought Carrie seemed lethargic. Although everybody has their high- and low-energy days, Patricia saw the differences in Carrie as more extreme than normal, and even before Carrie approached her correctly intuited that she was going through something difficult in her life.

Following is the sequence Patricia developed while working with Carrie, which was very much a trial-and-error process. For example, Patricia feels that backbends are usually therapeutic for people suffering from depression, in part because the energy required to move into a backbend often overpowers the agitation of the mind, so that they end up feeling calm. But when Carrie did them she often got agitated. Even though Carrie's first instinct as a good type A (see chapter 19) was to fight against doing the restorative poses Patricia recommended, she says she found the sequence "to be an absolute lifesaver."

EXERCISE #1. **RECLINING CROSS-LEGGED POSE (Supta Svastikasana), five minutes.** Set up for the pose by placing a bolster (or folded blankets) on your mat to support your torso and a folded blanket on top of the bolster to support your head so that your forehead is slightly higher than your chin. Sit in front of the bolster (not on it) and lie back. Cross one leg over the other, placing support under your thighs if you feel any tension in your groins (figure 15.1). You can also use a strap around your legs to increase abdominal relaxation. Halfway through the exercise, switch the cross of your legs.

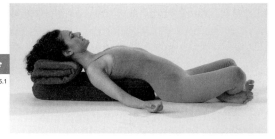

FIGURE 15.1

Patricia says, "Supta Svastikasana is essentially to create space in the body—in the pelvis, in the abdomen, and the chest. Because the chest is supported and opened, it lifts the mind, but also brings the mind into a quiet space. It's both energizing and quieting."

EXERCISE #2. **CROSS BOLSTERS BACKBEND, three minutes.** Set up for the pose by crossing one bolster over another. If you only have one bolster, you can use folded blankets in place of the lower bolster. Then sit on the upper bolster and lie back so the upper bolster runs along the length of your spine, and the back of your head just touches the

floor. Place your arms on the floor overhead, with your elbows bent—sometimes called "cactus" position (figure 15.2).

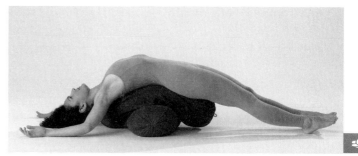

Patricia says this pose opens the chest even more than the first pose. "Because the head is back, it's more stimulating for the nervous system, more enlivening. The chest is open a little bit more with that extra bolster."

EXERCISE #3. **SUPPORTED DOWNWARD-FACING DOG POSE (Adho Mukha Svanasana), three minutes.** Set up for the pose by placing a bolster, folded blanket, or

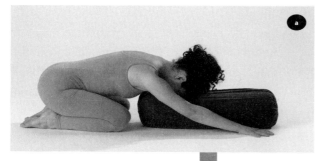

block on your mat to support your head. Come into Child's pose with your big toes together and your knees wide apart, and your head on the bolster or other prop. Extend your arms in front of you and place your palms on the mat with your fingers spread (figure

15.3a). Separate your feet to hips' width apart, and turn your toes under. On an exhalation, straighten your legs to come into the pose. If your forehead does not easily rest on the prop (figure 15.3b), you may either need to move the prop or increase its height.

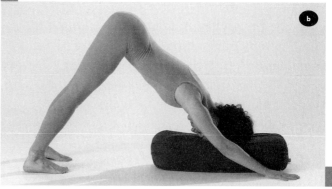

Patricia says this is a very grounding, stabilizing pose for the emotions. Because your hands, feet, arms, and legs are all engaged, it's hard, especially for a beginner, not to stay in the present. She recommends using the head support to counteract the fatigue that often accompanies depression. Patricia had Carrie do this pose for three minutes but might recommend one minute for a less experienced student.

TIP Patricia suggests that if you find yourself brooding during the practice or at other times, exhale slowly and deeply. If you feel your mood sinking, take deep, full inhalations. If negative thoughts keep cropping up, balance them with positive ones. This latter advice is an example of Patanjali's practice, described in the *Yoga Sutras*, of cultivating the opposite.

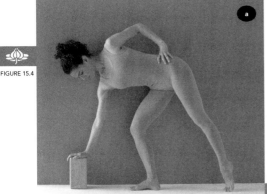

FIGURE 15.4

EXERCISE #4. **HALF MOON POSE (Ardha Chandrasana) at the wall, one minute.** Holding a block in your right hand, stand with your back a few inches away from a wall and your feet about three and a half feet apart. Turn your right foot out 90 degrees and your left foot in slightly. Place the block next to your right foot. Now extend your arms to the side and, on an exhalation, come into Triangle pose, placing your hand on the block (see p. 368). Once there bend your right knee until it extends beyond your ankle, and slide your right hand and the block about a foot in front of your right leg. Come onto the toes of your left foot (figure 15.4a). On an exhalation simultaneously straighten your right knee and raise your left leg parallel to the floor or slightly higher. Raise your left arm to the ceiling and rotate your chest upward (figure 15.4b). Reverse your path to come out of the pose and repeat on the other side.

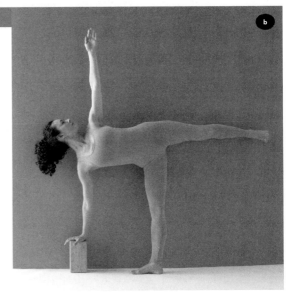

Patricia finds this pose particularly helpful for a tense, constricted mind because of the way it gets you "to focus on the periphery of the body—extending through the fingers, extending through the toes, extending from the center outward. There's a freedom and a liberation in that."

TIP One advantage of working at the wall, even if you can do the pose in the middle of the room, is that you're using minimal muscular effort to keep yourself there. Instead of worrying about balance, you can really just focus on your pelvis, your abdomen, and your chest, and enjoy the spaciousness.

EXERCISE #5. **WIDE-LEGGED STANDING FORWARD BEND** (**Prasarita Padottanasana**), **two minutes.** Stand with your feet parallel, and three and a half to four and a half feet apart. On an exhalation, bend forward at the hips, keeping your trunk extended, and bring your hands under your shoulders, fingers facing forward (figure 15.5a). Inhale, and on the next exhala-

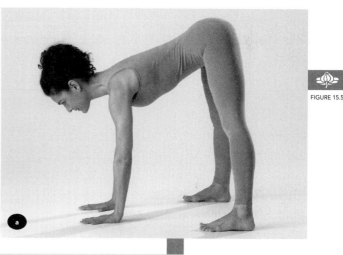

FIGURE 15.5

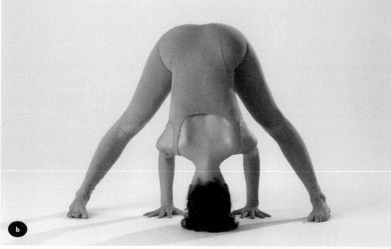

tion bend your elbows and lower the crown of your head to the floor. If you can't reach the floor, use a block under your head. Place your hands in line with your feet, with your fingers facing forward (figure 15.5b).

EXERCISE #6. **HEADSTAND (Sirsasana), three minutes.** Set up for the pose by placing a folded mat or blanket in front of a wall to support your head and forearms. Kneel and place your interlaced hands an inch or two from the wall. Bring the crown of your head to the ground, placing the back of your head inside your palms. Turn your toes under and straighten your legs (figure 15.6a). Bend your knees and bring them over your hips, and then extend your legs into the pose (figure 15.6b). To come out of the pose, reverse the steps. Patricia says this pose makes the brain clear, stabilizes the emotions, and builds confidence.

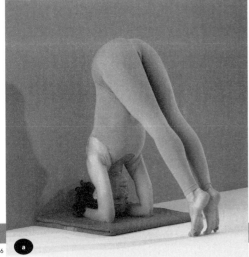

FIGURE 15.6　**a**

From a yogic perspective, active inversions like Headstand and Shoulderstand and restorative inversions like Legs-Up-the-Wall pose are very helpful for cultivating emotional stability. The regular practice of inversions—especially when done for months or years—is thought by yogis to have dramatic effects, calming and quieting the mind and stabilizing moods.

CAUTION For safety reasons, Headstand should be learned under the guidance of an experienced teacher who can evaluate whether you should do this pose, and if any props or modifications are necessary (see appendix 1, "Avoiding Common Yoga Injuries"). Since Wide-Legged Standing Forward Bend (Prasarita Padottanasana) brings many of the same benefits, this sequence can be done without Headstand if you have not already learned to do it.

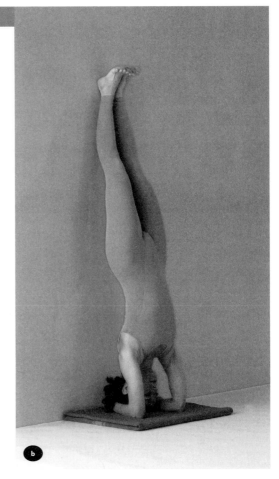

b

EXERCISE #7. **SUPPORTED CAMEL POSE (Ustrasana), one minute.** Set up for the pose by placing bolsters and folded blankets on a chair to support your chest and head. Kneel in front of the chair facing away from it, with your feet and shins under the chair seat. Hold your elbows with your hands and raise your arms above your head. On an exhalation, curve your upper back and come into the pose (figure 15.7). Avoid arching too much from the lower back as this can compress the lumbar (lower) spine. If your spine and head do not rest comfortably against the props, you may need to readjust the props or add more. Patricia says, "Lifting and expanding the chest brings us into a joyful state."

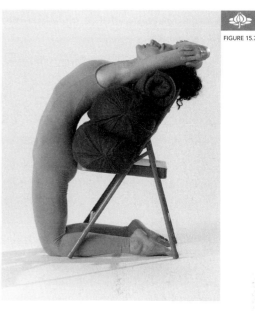

FIGURE 15.7

EXERCISE # 8. **SUPPORTED INVERTED STAFF POSE (Viparita Dandasana), over chair back, one to two minutes.** Set up for the pose by placing a metal office chair on a mat so that the chair will not slip, with a blanket folded over the back for padding. Position the chair approximately three feet from the wall, depending on your height. Stand behind the chair with your knees bent and place your upper spine along the back of the chair (figure 15.8a). From there extend your legs and place your toes up the wall, the soles of your feet on the floor, and clasp your elbows over your head (figure 15.8b). Patricia stresses that

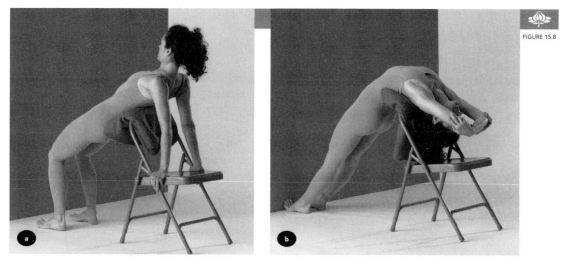

FIGURE 15.8

you're not using a lot of muscular effort in this pose. "When you work with props, you're really working more from the inside out than when you're doing the pose unsupported, when you're really using your arms and your legs strongly."

EXERCISE #9. **SUPPORTED INVERTED STAFF POSE (Viparita Dandasana), over chair seat, three to five minutes.** This pose requires a chair that has had its back removed (available from yoga prop suppliers, see appendix 2). Set up by placing the chair with its back to a wall, approximately two feet away from the wall. Place a folded mat on the chair for cushioning and a bolster or stack of folded blankets in front of the chair to support your head. Sit on the chair facing the back, and slide your legs through the back of the chair, scooting your hips close to the back edge of the seat. Bend your knees, place your feet on the floor, and lean back till your back curves over the front edge of the chair. Thread your arms under the chair and hold on to the rear legs of the chair. Extend your legs until the balls of your feet meet the wall. If the crown of your head does not rest easily on the prop, adjust the height of the prop to accommodate your proportions. If your feet cannot easily reach the floor, you can use a block under your heels (figure 15.9).

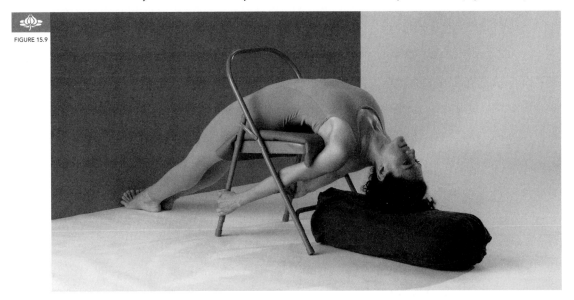

FIGURE 15.9

Patricia says, "In this backbend, you're using your arms and your legs, but not to the degree that you would for the totally unsupported pose. You can see how the edge of the chair is right under the heart, right under the sternum," thus creating opening where it's likely to be most beneficial for depression. She stresses that this is an intermediate pose and should not be attempted by beginners.

EXERCISE #10. DOWNWARD-FACING DOG POSE (Adho Mukha Svanasana), one minute. Repeat this pose, briefly, without the head support. Patricia says that the purpose of this pose at this stage of the sequence is to release the back and spinal muscles after backbending.

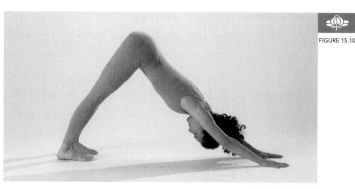

FIGURE 15.10

CAUTION This Shoulderstand variation below requires a chair that will not tip over when you drop back into the pose. Any time you are trying out a new chair, have a friend spot you, ready to keep the chair from tipping over. If the chair isn't stable, immediately slide off and bring your buttocks onto the support on the floor to come down. Although this pose becomes simple once you get the hang of it, it's best to learn it under the guidance of an experienced teacher before you attempt it on your own.

EXERCISE #11. SUPPORTED SHOULDERSTAND (Salamba Sarvangasana), five minutes or longer. Set up for the pose by placing a bolster or two blankets folded into long, thin rectangles on the floor in front of a chair and lean another bolster against the back of the chair. Fold a mat in four and place it on the seat of the chair for padding. Sit facing backward in the chair, grip the sides of the back of the chair with each hand and bring your knees up behind the back of the chair so they straddle the bolster (figure 15.11a). Use

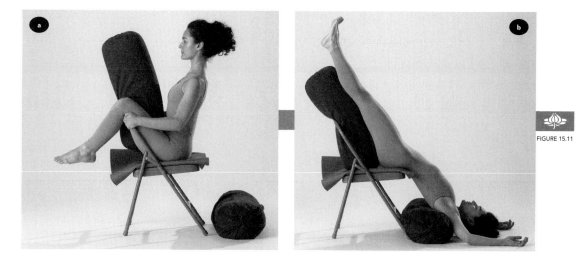

FIGURE 15.11

your knees to hold you up, like a kid on a jungle gym. Keeping your knees on the chair back, release your arms and lean back until your shoulders rest on the support on the floor and your head comes to the ground. Thread your arms under the chair and grasp the rear legs (see p. 327). Then straighten one leg at a time and move them onto the bolster. Place your arms in a cactus shape, with your elbows bent to 90 degrees and the back of your hands on the ground alongside your ears (figure 15.11b).

EXERCISE #12. **SUPPORTED BRIDGE POSE (Setu Bandha Sarvangasana), five minutes or longer.** Set up for the pose by placing a block or bolster against the wall to sup-

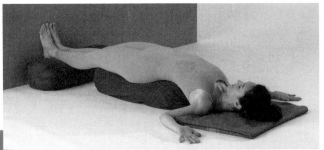

FIGURE 15.12

port your feet, and another bolster perpendicular to the wall to support your spine. Use a folded blanket to support your head. To enter the pose, sit on the center of the bolster with your knees bent, your feet facing the wall and flat on the floor. Next, lie back so your shoulders are resting on the blanket, the edge of the bolster touches the bottoms of your shoulder blades, and your feet are touching the wall with your legs fully extended (you may discover you need to come out and reposition the bolster to get the distance from the wall right for your height). Once you're comfortably in the pose, place your arms in cactus position or rest them by your sides (figure 15.12). For even deeper relaxation, try fastening a belt snugly around your thighs.

EXERCISE #13. **SUPPORTED RELAXATION POSE (Savasana), five to ten minutes.** Set up for the pose by placing a bolster or folded blankets on your mat to support your chest, and a folded blanket on top of the bolster to support your head. Sit in front of the

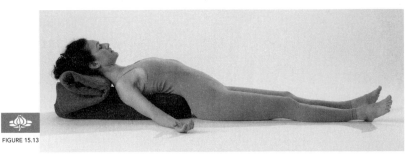

FIGURE 15.13

bolster (not on it) and lie back, arms turned out on the floor, palms up. Lengthen your legs along the ground, feet opening to the sides (figure 15.13).

If you tend to brood when you close your eyes, you can keep your eyes open during Relaxation pose and just enjoy the movement of your breath, focusing on your inhalations. Closing her eyes in Savasana and other restorative poses wasn't a problem for Carrie, though Patricia says she used to see Carrie's eyes moving beneath her eyelids, indicating some kind of mild agitation. For some people Patricia has worked with, however, closing the eyes was terrifying, so she adapted their Savasana. She had them lean back against a bolster angled against the wall. "They were half sitting and half leaning back, so that they were getting the quieting effects, but their chest stayed open, and their eyes stayed open." Patricia says, "Especially for those who are in a really dull, tamasic state, keeping the eyes wide open is really important."

In addition to practicing this sequence, Patricia recommended that Carrie use the yogic tool of chanting. Patricia says, "For many people who are depressed, chanting is really a wonderful practice. Especially when you do it with other people, chanting has the ability to pierce through layers of cloudiness and dullness and bring you into a positive state." She stresses that you shouldn't try to understand these chants with your brain or analyze them, just learn them by heart and use them often.

OTHER YOGIC IDEAS

B. K. S. Iyengar finds that many students with depression hold tension in the outer portion of their eyes. He sometimes asks these students to try to, as he puts it, "move the edge of the eyes toward the temple and ears," while doing a challenging pose.

Contraindications, Special Considerations, and Modifications

Patricia believes that people with tamasic depression may need to begin with more active poses in order to energize the body and overcome the lethargy. She suggests starting with several quick Sun Salutations. Although she normally pays a lot of attention to alignment, she thinks that when you are depressed you shouldn't worry so much about your form. Better to tune in to your breath. For tamasic depression, pranayama techniques that focus on inhalation can also be useful. For those who are able to tolerate them, practices like

OTHER YOGIC IDEAS

Patricia finds that the simple sequence of Mountain pose (Tadasana) to Arms Overhead (Urdhva Hastasana) as described in chapter 1 (see p. 22), done repeatedly, can be very useful for depression. "You can see how people change in a short period of time with just those two poses, synchronizing breath and movement." Another active sequence she likes is to flip back and forth between Plow pose (Halasana) and a Seated Forward Bend (Paschimottanasana). Be careful with this sequence if you have any back or neck problems.

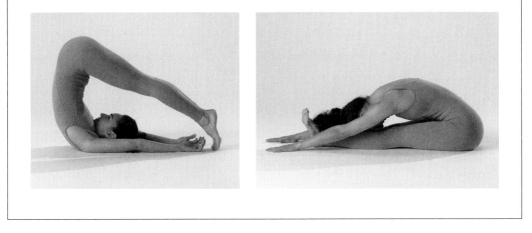

simple Ujjayi breathing, which tends to lengthen both the inhalation and the exhalation, and three-part or interrupted inhalation breathing (sometimes called Viloma) can help.

In using yoga to treat rajasic depression, practices that calm the sympathetic nervous system and thereby relax the hypervigilant state can be useful. Unfortunately, the mind is usually too anxious to benefit directly from simple restorative poses at the beginning (though Carrie was an exception). Instead you may need to first burn off enough of the excess energy with a vigorous practice to settle your mind so that it can respond to inversions and relaxation poses at a later stage. Pranayama practices that focus on the exhalation, which tend to be calming, can be tried at that point as well. However, starting off with a vigorous practice may not be possible for depressed people in a state of nervous exhaustion. They may benefit more from slow, supportive practices that rest their minds without taxing their bodies too much.

A Holistic Approach to Depression

✳ The combination of drugs and therapy is usually more effective than either alone.

✳ Some trial and error may be necessary to find an antidepressant that works.

✳ Regular aerobic exercise is an effective way to elevate mood, and in the long run may prevent relapses of depression better than drugs. Non-aerobic exercise like weight lifting also appears to help.

✳ Omega-3 fatty acids, found in flaxseeds and some deepwater fish, can help lift mood (see p. 167).

✳ Getting enough sleep can keep stress levels down and help prevent downward emotional spirals (see chapter 23). Setting a regular time to get up every day can help stabilize sleep and may be particularly important for people with bipolar disorder (what used to be called manic depression).

✳ The herb St. John's Wort may be as effective as conventional antidepressants (though the evidence is mixed) and less likely to cause side effects. Since this herbal remedy can interact with conventional antidepressants, it's probably better to use one or the other, and to make such decisions with the guidance of a qualified health professional. Due to slow onset of action, give it a couple of months before deciding whether or not it's working.

✳ Supplemental B vitamins appear to have some benefit for depression and are very safe.

✳ The supplement 5-HTP, a metabolite of tryptophan, may help with depression by boosting serotonin levels.

✳ Another supplement, SAM-e, also seems promising, though it is not cheap.

✳ A small pilot study at University of Arizona found that acupuncture treatment was effective in relieving depression in 64 percent of women, a result comparable to medication or psychotherapy.

Carrie's episode of serious depression after watching the movie *Billy Elliot* lasted about six weeks. Ultimately she thinks it may have been a good thing for her because it spurred her to take action, and led her "to a deeper practice in every sense of the word." She says she feels she now has "more tools in [her] tool basket" to help her get out of depressions in the future. "The knowledge that I have these tools, of which yoga is the primary one, is very empowering."

Carrie likes to chant briefly before her daily asana practice using three chants she learned from Patricia. She also plays a recording of a kirtan performer chanting in the background while she practices. She even does Savasana with it playing. While this is not something that Patricia generally recommends, she thinks it's good in this case because it takes Carrie beyond her thoughts. Patricia herself sometimes talks during relaxation if she is working with people who are depressed, turning Savasana into more of a guided meditation along the lines of Yoga Nidra (see pp. 67–68).

Patricia has noticed a definite change in Carrie. She smiles a lot more and seems to approach asana with less striving. Carrie herself says, "It's an absolute transformation. My life previously was characterized by motivating myself to do things through fear." Overall she feels "calmer, more content. And I'm much more aware that what goes on within myself is of paramount importance, and not so much the opinions of others."

Mirroring her teacher's words, Carrie says, "It's not about reading it in a book, it's about doing it and the memory of the experience. Over time you come to rely on those memories of experience, and so I have a great deal of confidence that if I take these actions, nine times out of ten it will make me feel much better, it will pull me out of the cloud."

CHAPTER 16

DIABETES

 More than thirty years ago SANDRA SUMMERFIELD KOZAK was tricked into teaching her first yoga class by someone desperate to have her take over for him. Circumstances notwithstanding, the yoga stuck. Since then, Sandra has had the opportunity to study with many of the field's most eminent masters, including B. K. S. Iyengar, Iyengar's guru Krishnamacharya, Vanda Scaravelli, T. K. V. Desikachar, Sant Keshavadas, Baba Hari Dass, and Swami Muktananda. Hoping to attract physicians to yoga and an understanding of its profound effects on the body, Sandra wrote a master's thesis in the late seventies on the physiological effects of asana, pranayama, and meditation. Still trying to reach out to a broader audience, her current focus is to take "yoga and Ayurveda and translate them into more Western terms." She teaches yoga and yoga therapy in the San Francisco Bay Area and internationally.

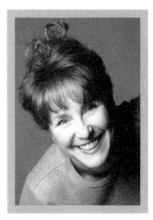

Maggie Solick (not her real name) came to see Sandra Summerfield Kozak for her first yoga lesson after injuring her knee. Maggie had been doing aerobics to try to lose weight. When they met, Maggie was about 150 pounds overweight—a lot of extra weight on a 5'4" frame. She hoped the yoga could help with her knee as well as with her other problems, which included type 2 diabetes, high blood pressure, and asthma.

As the office manager for a small business, Maggie sat at a desk all day and needed exercise both for weight control and for stress reduction. Her hands were full managing her job, her kids, and a long commute to work. A single mother with three kids at home, she didn't have a lot of time to dedicate to either her aerobics or her yoga, but she loved the aerobics while feeling somewhat frightened of the yoga. The one time she'd been in a yoga class, she was very uncomfortable with some of the poses, and Sandra suspects that Maggie might also have been self-conscious about her weight.

Overview of Diabetes

There are two main types of diabetes. Type 1 is what used to be called juvenile-onset diabetes. Due to autoimmune destruction of the islet cells in the pancreas that manufacture insulin, people with type 1 diabetes cannot live long without external sources of this hormone, which regulates blood sugar (glucose) levels. Type 2 diabetes is what used to be called adult-onset diabetes, but due to the recent surge in obesity throughout the population, there are now children developing it as early as grade school. Over 90 percent of people with diabetes have type 2. Their bodies may manufacture normal amounts of insulin, but the body becomes resistant to its effects and as a result the blood sugar rises. Why some people develop insulin resistance isn't known, but overweight and inactivity clearly make the problem worse. While some with type 2 take insulin (usually via injection) to improve blood sugar control, most are treated with oral medication and dietary measures.

> **TIP** Type 1 diabetes doesn't just happen to kids. Doctors now recognize a form of type 1 diabetes that comes on after age twenty-five, and which causes more gradual destruction of islet cells. Doctors believe that perhaps 15 percent of people diagnosed with type 2 diabetes actually have a slowly progressive form of type 1 diabetes, so-called latent autoimmune diabetes of adults, or LADA (also sometimes called type 1.5 diabetes). People with LADA generally are not obese and do not have insulin resistance (though overweight type 1s can develop it). Because of the slow onset of their disease, people with LADA often respond initially to dietary measures and oral drugs, but over time their need for insulin becomes apparent. Some diabetes specialists believe these patients should be treated with insulin from the beginning. If you suspect you might have LADA, ask your doctor for antibody testing.

Although people sometimes think of it as just a "little sugar," a minor illness they don't need to worry much about, type 2 diabetes causes the same potential complications as type 1, including blindness, kidney failure, and amputations. Both forms of diabetes increase the risk of having a heart attack or stroke as much as smoking a pack a day. Diabetes can be thought of as a disease that causes premature aging—and death. People with diabetes die younger and tend to have more years of disability before their deaths.

That's the bad news. The good news is that with type 2 diabetes, more than almost any other condition, what you do can have a tremendous effect on whether you develop it, or if you do have it, on how it progresses. If you are at risk of developing type 2 diabetes due to overweight, a family history of type 2 disease, having had gestational diabetes while pregnant, or already having been diagnosed with insulin resistance as part of the so-called metabolic syndrome—you may be able to prevent it, or at least delay its onset, and minimize its impact by exercising regularly, keeping your weight down, and taking measures to fight stress. Even a few years' delay in getting diabetes can be significant; the later you start the clock, the later the onset of serious complications that often arise decades after diabetes starts. If you start the clock late enough, you may never get complications at all.

Due to the high risk of heart disease and stroke in people with diabetes, many doctors favor much more aggressive attempts to control risk factors like blood pressure and cholesterol with drug treatments in addition to lifestyle changes. Also, the better you control your blood sugar levels via such measures as diet, medication, exercise, and yoga practice, the lower your risk for heart attacks, strokes, and other problems. Once a person develops diabetes, close monitoring of blood glucose levels is key. Experts encourage most diabetes patients to check their blood sugars one or more times per day. Pricking your finger tip to extract a drop of blood, which you put on a test strip, has been the best way to do this, though other methods, some not involving needles, are being developed. Another vital way to monitor how well your diabetes is controlled is by following levels of hemoglobin A1c (aka HbA1c, glycosylated hemoglobin), a blood test that allows doctors to estimate how high your blood sugars have been over the prior three months. The goal should be a level below 7 percent. It is almost impossible to accurately gauge how well your diabetes is controlled unless your doctor is doing this test regularly. Due to the risk of kidney disease, regular screening for microalbuminuria (protein in the urine) with a urine test more sensitive than the standard urinalysis is also recommended.

How Yoga Fits In

"Both yoga and Ayurveda can have a great effect on diabetes," says Sandra. "They can increase willpower, self-confidence, strength, flexibility, contentment, and discipline, which can be a great help with weight loss and other health issues."

Another way yoga can moderate the impact of diabetes is through its effectiveness as a stress-reduction measure. Because high levels of stress hormones like adrenaline and cortisol raise blood sugar levels, and high cortisol levels also tend to promote both overeating and the accumulation of intra-abdominal fat, which contributes to insulin resistance, as well as to the risk of having a heart attack, yoga's impact on stress can ultimately do a lot to promote health and prevent, delay, or minimize the effects of the disease.

Many people with diabetes develop problems with their autonomic nervous system, which controls blood vessels and various organs in the body, with the results that the movement of food through the bowels can be adversely affected, and the body may have trouble regulating the blood pressure when you stand up quickly, leading to light-headedness. Peripheral nerves in the legs can also be damaged, leading to numbness or painful burning sensations, known as diabetic neuropathy. Yoga is known to improve the functioning of the autonomic nervous system and preliminary evidence (see below) suggests it may improve nerve conduction in people with diabetes.

Ulceration of the skin on the feet is a huge problem in diabetes. Given the reduced blood flow and often compromised nerve function of the feet in many people with the disease, even superficial cuts can progress to serious infections requiring amputation. One way yoga can help with this problem is by correcting uneven patterns of weight distribution on the foot. For example, a person who puts most of her weight on the big-toe side of the foot as she walks is placing too much pressure on the ball of the foot (the head of the first metatarsal bone) and would be more likely to develop an ulceration there. The regular practice of standing poses helps in maintaining a more even distribution of weight across the bottom of the foot, lessening the pressure on any one spot.

The Scientific Evidence

A small, early study on yoga for diabetes was published in the *Journal of the Diabetes Association of India* in 1980. Seven people with poorly controlled type 2 diabetes despite taking medication were taught gentle yoga asana (not the type that would burn a lot of calories or raise their metabolic rate), which they did forty minutes per day. No dietary or other changes were made. At the end of six months, all seven subjects had large reductions in their blood sugar, measured in the evening after dinner, from an average of 251 to 169. All seven also had a reduction in the amount of sugar in their urine, meaning better control of their diabetes. Two of the seven had their dose of medication reduced. All seven lost weight, on average more than 11.5 pounds.

As published in *Diabetes Research and Clinical Practice* in 1993, Suresh Jain and colleagues studied 149 subjects with type 2 diabetes in a forty-day residential program that included asana, pranayama, and cleansing techniques (kriyas). The subjects ate a vegetarian diet equal in calories to what they'd been eating before the study. Statistically significant improvements were noted in both the fasting blood sugar and the oral glucose tolerance test. More than one-third of the ninety patients on diabetes drugs at the start of the study were able to discontinue them. Weight loss may have explained some but not all of the improvement as more than two-thirds of patients showed a reduced severity of disease, while only a little more than one-third lost weight.

A small randomized controlled trial of yoga asana and pranayama for type 2 diabetes, led by Robin Monro from London's Yoga Biomedical Trust, found that compared to controls, those who practiced yoga had statistically significant reductions in fasting blood sugar and in hemoglobin A1c. Over the course of the twelve-week program, which included one to two classes per week plus home practice, three of the eleven people in the yoga group had reductions in their doses of diabetes medication. Among the control group, which continued their regular medical care, there were no reductions in medication dosage. In addition, the authors reported the majority of the yoga group "felt better, less anxious, and more in control of themselves."

As part of a Medicare Demonstration Project (discussed in chapter 20), more than two thousand people with heart disease who followed Dr. Dean Ornish's lifestyle program—which includes asana, pranayama, and meditation, as well as a low-fat plant-based diet, walking, and group support—were followed for one year. Those patients who also had diabetes developed statistically significant reductions in fasting blood sugar (FBS) and hemoglobin A1c. After twelve weeks of the program, the FBS dropped from an average of 150 to just under 120. Hemoglobin A1c levels dropped from 7.4 to 6.6 percent on average. At the one year follow-up, the numbers were still improved but less than at twelve weeks.

Researchers from the University College of Medical Sciences in Delhi have conducted several small studies on patients with type 2 diabetes. Daily asana classes of thirty to forty minutes for forty days were found in different studies to result in statistically significant decreases in fasting blood sugars, blood sugar after meals, hemoglobin A1c, systolic and diastolic blood pressure, as well as improved sensitivity to the effects of insulin. One study found increases in measures of lung function. In another, the hemoglobin A1c dropped from 8.8 to 6.4 percent, an enormous improvement. In a third, the yoga group had a significant decrease in waist-to-hip ratio, a reflection of a decrease in abdominal fat, a risk factor for insulin resistance and heart disease. Obese patients in this study also had a significant decrease in their abnormally high insulin levels, likely due to improved insulin sensitivity. A fourth study found that subjects who did yoga had an increase in measures of nerve conduction, while those in the control group who did light physical exercise like walking instead of yoga had a slight worsening in nerve function.

Sandra Summerfield Kozak's Approach

Sandra Summerfield Kozak's approach to yoga therapy is very much shaped by her study of Ayurveda, yoga's sister science. Her treatment recommendations take into account the person's constitution, or prakriti (for a discussion of Ayurvedic concepts, see chapter 4). "It's important to know what combination of vata, pitta, and kapha the patient is." An obese person typically has a preponderance of kapha. She notes that while people of any constitution can develop type 2 diabetes, kaphas with their proclivity for inactivity and weight gain are particularly prone to it. Vatas, in contrast, are less likely to develop type 2 diabetes, she says, because they are "very movement-oriented people, and tend to be thin."

A major pillar of the Ayurvedic approach to disease is dietary, and Sandra's thinking reflects this. She asks her students with diabetes to try to eliminate all processed foods, and as much sugar and salt as possible, and recommends that they balance protein, fat, and carbohydrates at each meal and every snack. Although traditional Ayurvedic doctors often recommend clarified butter (ghee), Sandra advised Maggie to choose olive oil or canola oil.

Yoga, of course, was a central part of Sandra's approach. She designed an asana practice for Maggie that was as energetic as possible, while focusing on safety, taking into particular account the fact that Maggie was carrying a lot of extra weight and that many of the poses needed to be modified accordingly. At first she had Maggie do many repetitions of postures that are held for a short time. Over time, she asked her to increase the duration to build strength. To overcome the kaphic tendency to do too little, Sandra asked Maggie to give "125 percent, and when she felt like she couldn't do any more, to do just a little more anyway"; to stay in the pose ten seconds longer, or do one more repetition. "I know you're tired," Sandra would tell her. "It's okay. Now let's do one more." Sandra finds that if she can get her kapha students to move past their initial feelings of lethargy with fifteen minutes of hard work, they often become "active, lively, and happy." Another thing she finds useful for people of this Ayurvedic constitution is to practice first thing in the morning when energy levels are higher.

Here is the sequence of practices and instructions that Sandra provided for Maggie.

EXERCISE #1. **KAPALABHATI BREATHING.** Start by sitting in any comfortable seated position. Before beginning the exercise, you may wish to blow your nose and keep the tissue nearby. When you are settled, inhale, and then sharply contract your lower abdomen to rapidly expel air from your lungs through your nose. Then passively allow your next inhalation to follow, inhaling through your nose. Try ten to twenty abdominal contractions. Start slowly and find your rhythm, gradually picking up speed. Over time you can work up to fifty contractions if that is comfortable.

Sandra believes that many students incorrectly initiate the abdominal movement for Kapalabhati breathing from around the navel. The correct area is below the navel, midway to the pubic hair. So Sandra asked Maggie to place her right hand on her abdomen with her index finger resting on the area where the inward movement should be initiated. She also began to introduce the concept of the root lock, mula bandha, asking Maggie to subtly lift internally from the area near the anal sphincter as she drew the lower abdomen in.

At first Sandra had Maggie work very slowly, drawing her belly in and releasing it, until Sandra was confident that Maggie's body had learned to initiate the abdominal movement correctly. As Maggie got more proficient, Sandra had her increase the pace of the exhalations (though never exceeding more than fifty breaths).

EXERCISE #2. **ALTERNATE NOSTRIL BREATHING (Nadi Shodhana), six rounds.**
Start by sitting in any comfortable seated position. On your right hand, curl your index and middle fingers inward and extend your thumb, ring finger, and pinky. Rest your thumb and ring fingers on your nose; you will use the pads of the thumb and the tip of the ring finger respectively to close your right and left nostrils. Sandra stresses that you are not pushing the nostrils closed. Instead, find a place on your finger pads that exactly fits your nose without pushing it at all. To begin, inhale through both nostrils. Then place your thumb on your right nostril (figure 16.1a). Exhale slowly and evenly through your left nostril, and then inhale through your left nostril. Change your hand position, releasing your thumb and placing your ring finger over your left nostril (figure 16.1b). Exhale slowly and evenly through your right nostril, and then inhale through your right nostril. This constitutes one round of alternate nostril breathing. Repeat for five more rounds.

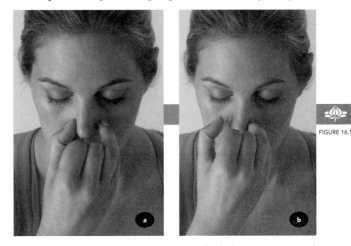

FIGURE 16.1

At the beginning of their work together Sandra didn't have Maggie hold her breath at all during alternate nostril breathing, but later she added brief pauses at the end of the inhalation and at the end of the exhalation. She also asked Maggie to slowly increase the time of the inhalation and exhalation. To be sure Maggie did the practice safely, Sandra asked her to watch that she never ran out of breath and that her heart rate never changed. Sandra says, "It's really important in all pranayama that the heart rate not increase." Sandra is vigilant about this because in her experience students tend to force too much. "I teach my students to hold the breath with their minds, not with their bodies. This avoids the use of muscular force, which is counterproductive in a pranayama practice."

EXERCISE #3. **MINDFULNESS MEDITATION, ten to fifteen minutes.** Start by sitting in any comfortable seated position (figure 16.2). When you are settled in, begin to focus only on your breath. When a thought comes into your mind, notice it. Begin to create cat-

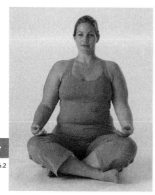

FIGURE 16.2

egories for the thoughts that arise, for example, "animals" if your thought is feeding the dog or "clothing" if you are think-ing about what you are going to wear. The idea is to cultivate mindfulness. After categorizing your thoughts, return to focusing on your breath. Later, when you get comfortable with this practice, you may wish to categorize your thoughts based on any associated emotions. Sandra recommended this technique for Maggie because she sensed there was a strong emotional component to Maggie's difficulties and she wanted to bring her awareness there.

In all of the following poses, you should focus on your breathing, making the evenness of your breath the gauge for how you are doing in the pose. By even, Sandra means that inhalations are the same in length as the other inhalations and the exhalations are the same in length as the other exhalations. Using your breath as your guide, you can deepen your poses as much as possible—"playing the edge"—without going too far. Sandra started Maggie out at ten to fifteen minutes, but encouraged her to do more if she felt comfortable.

EXERCISE #4. **MODIFIED SUN SALUTATIONS.** Use Sun Salutations in the beginning of the practice to excite energy, moving reasonably rapidly between the poses. Repeat the series one or more times, alternating the leg that moves forward in the lunge (for balance).

If you are overweight, you can modify the Sun Salutations as follows:

1. From Mountain pose (Tadasana), bring your arms up overhead but don't do a back-bend (figure 16.3a), as is sometimes done.

2. Move into Standing Forward Bend (Uttanasana) with your knees slightly bent.

3. Rather than the standard lunge, kneel down one knee at a time, and come into Table pose (figure 16.3b).

4. In place of Upward-Facing Dog, use Sphinx pose to avoid putting too much weight on your wrists. To do the pose, kneel down and place your forearms on the mat, with your elbows directly beneath the shoulders (figure 16.3c).

5. Modify Downward-Facing Dog pose (Adho Mukha Svanasana) to protect your wrists and elbows by making the stance shorter than usual (figure 16.3d).

6. After Downward-Facing Dog pose, move back onto your knees, and then move one foot forward (figure 16.3e). Put your weight on your back foot and lift your back knee off the ground, so that now you are in a lunge.

7. From lunge, step forward so you are standing again with bent knees.

8. Round your back to come up (figure 16.3f).

9. Bring your arms overhead, and then back down.

Sandra says that all this movement early on in the practice for Maggie was designed to wake her up and get her feeling energized.

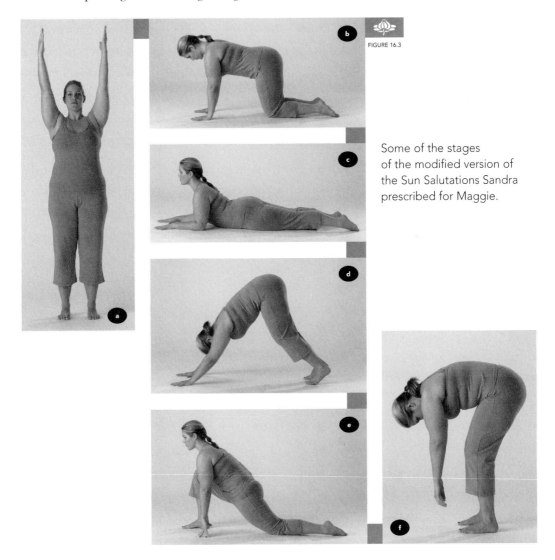

FIGURE 16.3

Some of the stages of the modified version of the Sun Salutations Sandra prescribed for Maggie.

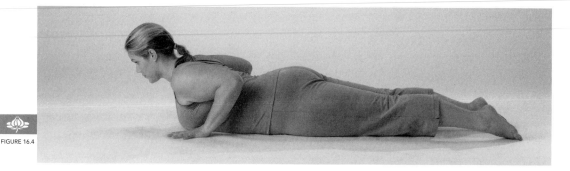

FIGURE 16.4

EXERCISE #5. **COBRA POSE (Bhujangasana), twenty seconds, one to three times.**
Start by lying facedown with your hands flat on the floor beneath your shoulders. Inhale
and raise your head, shoulders, and upper chest off the floor (figure 16.4), without bearing
any weight on your hands. Focus on keeping your buttock muscles as tight as possible and
your lower back meticulously in "neutral" as the foundation for the lift. Sandra says that
if you tighten the buttocks, a strategy she learned from yoga master Vanda Scaravelli, "the
spine just lightly lifts up and extends, growing into the pose."

EXERCISE #6. **LOCUST POSE (Salabasana), one leg at a time, ten to twenty seconds,
on each side.** Start by lying facedown with your hands flat on the floor beneath your
shoulders. Without putting any weight on your hands, lift your chest and upper body as
high as you can and raise your right leg just one inch off the floor. Hold your lower spine
in a neutral position, with your buttocks tightened as much as possible to support your
lumbo-sacral (lower) spine (figure 16.5). Count to ten and then come down with awareness. Repeat with the other leg.

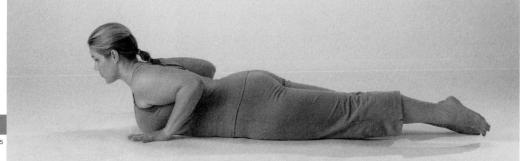

FIGURE 16.5

To make the pose easier in light of Maggie's weight, Sandra placed folded blankets or other
props under her chest and her hips.

EXERCISE #7. **SEATED FORWARD BEND (Paschimottanasana), thirty seconds.**
Start by sitting with your legs stretched out in front of you. Exhale and fold forward from the hips, keeping your spine as straight and elongated as possible. If you cannot easily reach your toes, use a towel or a yoga strap around your feet (figure 16.6). Repeat the pose one or more times if desired.

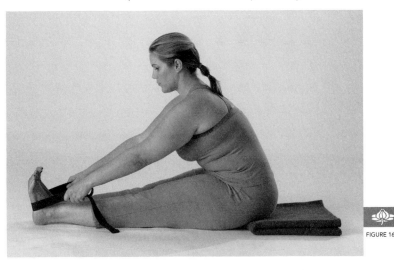
FIGURE 16.6

EXERCISE #8. **TREE POSE (Vrksasana), next to wall, ten to twenty seconds.** Stand with your left side to the wall and place your left hand on the wall. Bring the sole of the right foot as high up on your left thigh as you can with your hips remaining level. Raise your arms up, allowing the back of your left hand to slide up the wall so that your palms face each other, though your arms remain separated. If you are overweight, hold this pose briefly to avoid putting undue pressure on the joints. Repeat on the opposite side (figure 16.7).

In the standing poses that follow (exercise 9 through 12), Sandra initially instructed Maggie to practice in front of a counter for support. After about six weeks of regular practice, Maggie was ready to do these poses with her arms in the traditional positions, which "increases the heat created by the poses, and is beneficial for kaphas," according to Sandra. As her strength increased, Maggie was able to increase the number of times she did each pose, up to three.

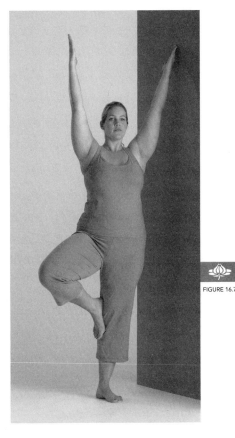
FIGURE 16.7

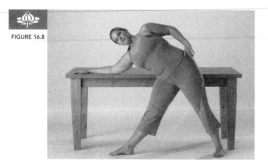

FIGURE 16.8

EXERCISE #9. **TRIANGLE POSE** (Trikonasana), **in front of counter, ten to twenty seconds.** Standing with your back to the counter, step your feet about three feet apart. Turn your right leg out to 90 degrees and turn your back foot slightly in. On an exhalation, slide your right lower arm along the counter and let your torso follow it into the pose (figure 16.8). Repeat on the other side.

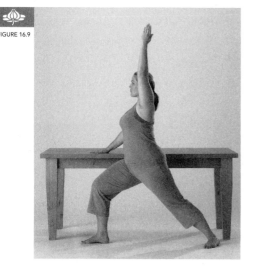

FIGURE 16.9

EXERCISE #10. **WARRIOR I** (Virabhadrasana I), **in front of counter, ten to twenty seconds.** Standing with your back to the counter, step your feet about three and a half feet apart. Turn your right leg out 90 degrees and your back foot in 45 degrees. Square your hips as much as possible so they are facing your front foot and are perpendicular to the counter. Place your right hand on the counter and your left hand on your left hip. With an exhalation, bring your right knee directly over your ankle and, if you are able, raise your left arm overhead (figure 16.9). Reverse your steps to come out of the pose. Repeat on the other side.

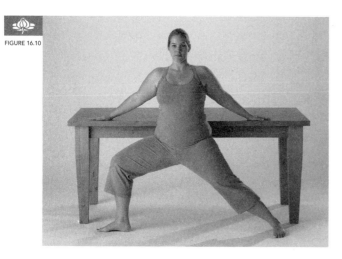

FIGURE 16.10

EXERCISE #11. **WARRIOR II (Virabhadrasana II), in front of counter, ten to twenty seconds.** Standing with your back to the counter, step your feet about three and a half feet apart. Turn your right leg out 90 degrees and your left foot slightly in. With your hands on the counter, keep your upper body as upright as possible and bend your right knee to come into the pose (figure 16.10). Repeat on the other side.

EXERCISE #12. **EXTENDED SIDE ANGLE POSE (Utthita Parsvakonasana), in front of counter, ten to twenty seconds.** Standing with your back to the counter, step your feet four to four and a half feet apart. Place your hands on the counter and allow your front arm to slide along the counter as you bend your right knee and lean your torso toward it to come into the pose. Extend

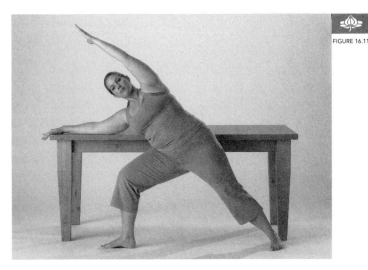

FIGURE 16.11

your left arm alongside your head (figure 16.11). Repeat on the other side.

EXERCISE #13. **STANDING TWIST (Marichyasana), ten to fifteen seconds.** Set up for the pose by standing with your right side next to a wall and a chair positioned directly in front of you. Step your right foot up onto the chair seat and twist gently toward the wall, placing both hands on the wall (figure 16.12). On your inhalation, lengthen down through your standing leg, keeping your standing leg strong and aware of the contact with the floor. On your exhalation, maintaining your awareness of the contact with the floor, lift your spine out of your hips and twist from the bottom to the top, turning the head last. Repeat on the other side.

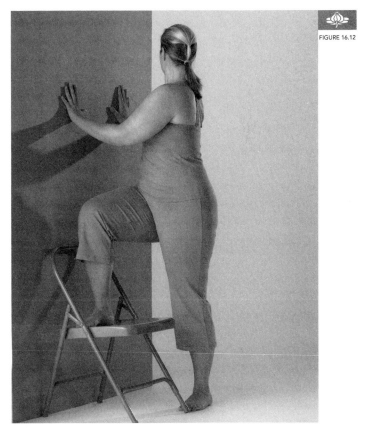

FIGURE 16.12

EXERCISE #14. BRIDGE POSE (Setu Bandha Sarvangasana), fifteen to twenty seconds. Lie on your back, with your knees bent, your feet flat on the floor, and your hands palms down. Step your feet hips' width apart, so they align with your hip bones, not the sides of your hips. Position your feet below your knees, not far from your buttocks. On an exhalation, press your hands and feet into the floor, and lift your hips off the ground as high as you can comfortably go (figure 16.13).

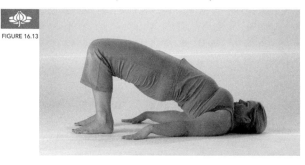

FIGURE 16.13

EXERCISE #15. SEATED TWIST, ten to twenty seconds on each side. Sit on your heels in Thunderbolt pose (Vajrasana), if necessary placing folded blankets between your buttocks and feet to ensure contact. Place your right hand at your breastbone, like one-half of a prayer position, and place your left hand on a block just behind and outside of your left thigh. On an exhalation, gently twist to the left, moving only your spine, and not shifting the weight on your hips at all (figure 16.14). Inhale and return to center, switch your arms, and repeat on the other side. Do the twist on both sides one more time.

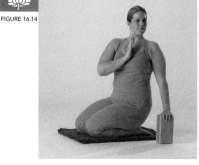

FIGURE 16.14

EXERCISE #16. ALLIGATOR TWIST (Jathara Parivartasana), with one leg bent, ten to twenty second on each side. Start by lying on your back, with your arms in a T position and your palms facing either up, as shown in the photo, or down as Sandra suggested for Maggie. Inhale and place your right foot on your left knee. On an exhalation, turn your hips to the left, arching your upper back a little bit as you turn, and allow your right knee to drop. Don't worry about bringing your knee to the ground (figure 16.15). When you are settled in the pose, if it is comfortable, turn your head to the right. Repeat on the other side. As in the seated twist above, focus your awareness on how much your spine is turning.

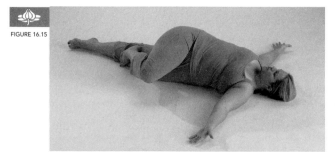

FIGURE 16.15

EXERCISE #17. **RELAXATION POSE (Savasana), modified, up to fifteen minutes.** Set up for the pose by placing two bolsters (or a stack of blankets) on your mat to support your calves (from the knees to the ankles). Sitting with your right side to the props, swing your calves up onto the props. Lie back, relax your legs, and allow your arms to release out to your sides.

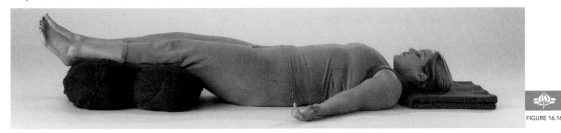

FIGURE 16.16

Elevating your legs will help drain the blood from your legs back toward your heart.

Sandra asked Maggie to stay in Relaxation pose for a maximum of fifteen minutes. She says, "It's her natural state to be in restful positions, so she doesn't need that much. Kaphas tend to go in that direction, and I'm fighting that kapha energy."

Sandra's therapeutic strategy is to see students several times in a brief period at the beginning of her work with them, but then only once a month or less as they grow into the practice. However, she is a strong believer in having one-on-one time with your own teacher. "Students may see their teacher only once a year in a private lesson, but even that small amount of time can expedite their progress down the yogic path."

Yogic Tool: **KARMA YOGA,** the idea of giving service, is part of the yogic path. While it seems that it is others who benefit from your generosity, the evidence suggests the giver benefits as much or more than the recipient. Nischala Joy Devi had a patient who asked to work with her privately. He was a very wealthy man who had diabetes and severe cardiac disease. For months, he did all the asana, pranayama, and meditation she recommended, but he wasn't feeling any better. After contemplating his situation for a while, she asked him if he did any service. He became very indignant and told her he gave a lot of money to various charities. That was laudable, she told him, but she suggested he try one more thing. " I want you to go for one hour a week, until I see you again, to the nearest hospital. Go into the children's ward, find the sickest child there, and sit with that child for an hour." He told her how busy he was and how it would take him forty minutes to drive there. Finally he said he would try, but he was grumpy about it. Three days later he called to tell her he did what she'd suggested, but hadn't stayed for one hour as he'd promised. He stayed for two. He said, "When I sat down with that child, she was so sick, but she reached out for me and she held my hand, I've never felt like that. I made arrangements to go back every week for two hours. And by the way, I just lowered my insulin dose by ten units, and I haven't had angina."

A Holistic Approach to Diabetes

* Keep moving. A recent study found that people with diabetes who walked two hours per week had a death rate in any particular year that was almost 40 percent lower than those who were more sedentary.

* Get enough sleep. There is evidence that sleeping poorly may contribute to both the development of type 2 diabetes and to difficulty controlling blood sugar once you have it. Even people without diabetes have difficulty metabolizing sugar when they are deprived of sleep.

* Take care of your teeth and gums. Studies suggest that marked gum inflammation doubles the likelihood of dying of heart disease or kidney failure if you have diabetes. Good oral hygiene includes regular brushing and flossing and regular dental cleanings. The Ayurvedic practice of daily tongue scraping is also helpful.

* A diet rich in fruits, vegetables, and other complex carbohydrates, and low in simple carbohydrates can help with weight control (see chapter 27) and is less likely to contribute to dental problems.

* A diet low in saturated fat and trans-fatty acids, found in many processed foods, may reduce inflammation, help with weight control, and lower the risk of heart disease.

* The spice cinnamon can improve sensitivity to insulin and lower blood sugars.

* Many healthy foods, including seeds, grains, and leafy, green vegetables are good sources of magnesium, which improves blood sugar control. You may want to supplement your diet with magnesium pills, which should also contain calcium to prevent diarrhea.

* Chromium is another mineral which can help with blood sugar control.

* The supplement CoQ10 may help lower blood pressure, improve blood sugars, and improve the function of blood vessels.

* Both Korean and American ginseng may improve control of diabetes via several mechanisms including improving sensitivity to insulin.

* For those at risk of retinal disease, the herb bilberry appears to be beneficial and has few side effects. Eating blueberries may also help.

Contraindications, Special Considerations, and Modifications

Anyone taking medication to lower their blood sugar levels should carefully monitor their readings in the weeks and months after they begin yoga practice, because glucose levels may sometimes drop dangerously low, causing a hypoglycemic reaction. What once was an appropriate dose of insulin or oral medication may be too much. Do not make any changes in medication without consulting your doctor. You may need to decrease your dose of medication, or in some cases of type 2 diabetes, eliminate it entirely. You should also carefully monitor your sugars any time you greatly increase the intensity of your practice. If you are not taking medication, yoga practice will generally not lead to hypoglycemia.

Although the general recommendation for doing a yoga practice is to avoid eating for several hours before, this may not be a good idea for people on diabetes medication, whose blood sugar may drop precipitously, causing dizziness or even unconsciousness. If you feel any signs of hypoglycemia—dizziness, spaciness, agitation—suck on a piece of hard candy or drink a glass of fruit juice. Doing a vigorous practice, and practicing late in the day or evening, may increase the risk of a hypoglycemic reaction, which can occur during the practice, or later, even in sleep. Do not drink alcohol the night before practicing, because alcohol suppresses the process by which the liver generates extra glucose for about twenty hours.

The risk of hypoglycemia with exertion is greater in type 1 diabetes. Students who inject insulin also need to consider the effects of poses that increase blood flow to the area of the injection, because this can increase the rate of absorption, resulting in a dosage higher than intended. For example, injections in the abdomen could be affected by twisting poses, or stomach churning (Agni Sara). Establishing a regular, predictable practice routine can be very helpful in enabling you to predict how your body will respond. If your routine is variable, you may need to adjust your insulin dose depending on your activity level.

In students with type 1 diabetes (less often with type 2) whose blood sugar is running very high before class, a vigorous practice can precipitate ketoacidosis, a true medical emergency. Marked by sky-high blood sugars (over 300), dehydration, and increased levels of acid in the blood, diabetic ketoacidosis can cause such symptoms as thirst, weakness, lethargy, nausea, and confusion. The best course of action is to call 911.

Retinal detachment and/or bleeding are major risks for people with diabetes. For this reason everyone with the disease—type 1 and type 2—should be getting yearly eye exams. Anyone with diabetes who wishes to do yoga should consult with an eye doctor first. Anyone with established retinal disease should avoid inversions and any other practices which raise pressure in the eyes, unless given clearance by an ophthalmologist. Even poses like Down Dog or standing forward bends are partial inversions that can raise pressure.

Another diabetic complication is peripheral neuropathy, which can cause burning in the lower legs and an inability to feel the feet. Since cuts and minor injuries in those with neuropathy can lead to infections and ultimately to amputations, it's essential to be very careful with the feet. If you practice in bare feet, the floor must be clean. Never jump into poses or make sudden movements that could lead to injuries. Similarly, care must be taken with poses that might lead to falls. Balancing poses like Tree pose can be particularly challenging for those with neuropathy, and can be done near the wall so that you can catch yourself if necessary. Some people with severe nerve or vascular problems may need to avoid these poses entirely. Another complication that affects the nervous system is autonomic neuropathy, which could make you feel light-headed when sitting up or standing up due to a drop in blood pressure. Coming out of poses slowly can prevent falls.

For those with any diabetic complications, experts advise against exercise in extreme heat. Thus hot yoga or Bikram yoga would not be appropriate, though they may be acceptable if you don't have any diabetic complications.

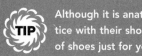 **TIP** Although it is anathema to many yoga teachers, those with neuropathy may want to practice with their shoes on. Viniyoga teacher Leslie Kaminoff suggests having a separate pair of shoes just for yoga, so that you won't track dirt into the studio.

Following Sandra's recommendations to cut down on sugar and other simple carbohydrates was hard for Maggie, but she did it. She lost about thirty pounds during the six months she and Sandra worked together. Although she remained significantly overweight, even a ten-pound weight loss is known to be helpful in controlling type 2 diabetes. Both her asthma and blood pressure also improved. Sandra noticed that over the months, as the pounds came off and her energy levels increased, Maggie seemed happier and more interested in life.

As for the knee problem that brought Maggie to Sandra in the first place: "It just healed itself." Sandra thinks this happened as a result of her practicing asana and stopping the aerobics, because at Maggie's weight, the aerobics were just too hard on her knees.

FIBROMYALGIA

 Sam Dworkis feels a special affinity for people with chronic pain due to his own experience with multiple sclerosis and the fibromyalgia that followed. A yoga teacher since 1975, Sam was diagnosed with MS in 1994. He had so much pain and became so discouraged that he completely gave up his yoga teaching as well as his own practice. But a few years ago, after sharing some yoga concepts with a quadriplegic neighbor and seeing the tremendous progress she made, he reversed course. "When she told me how these exercises had changed her life, I started my yoga up the very next morning after six years of doing nothing." Since then he's lost the twenty pounds he had put on and has regained his ability to do many yoga poses that he thought he'd never do again. "I believe today that I have to do whatever I can to maximize my potential and minimize my liability," he says. "I'm convinced that the practice of yoga moves me in that direction." Sam teaches from his studio near West Palm Beach, Florida. He is the author of two books, *ExTension* and *Recovery Yoga*.

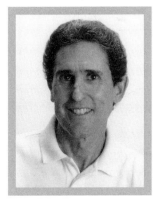

Before Jill Valliere started to study with Sam Dworkis on the recommendation of a friend, she had tried yoga but the results weren't good. She had taken a vigorous power yoga class that involved jumping from pose to pose, and as is common in people with fibromyalgia syndrome (FMS) who do too much, she paid the price. "I was in bed for two days afterward."

For years before seeing Sam, Jill had often felt tired and achy, had sleep problems, and suffered other symptoms suggestive of fibromyalgia, though to date she still hasn't been officially diagnosed by a doctor. When Jill mentioned her symptoms to her physicians and asked about fibromyalgia, she says, "they kind of pooh-poohed it." Another doctor, an "arthritis specialist, who didn't have a great bedside manner, almost insulted me when I mentioned it." A friend told her she would probably get that reaction because some doctors just don't believe in fibromyalgia. Indeed, none of her physicians has ever checked her for "tender points," eighteen specific spots on the upper back, chest, neck, hips, elbows, and knees where tenderness points to a diagnosis of FMS. (She reports that she is still very sensitive to touch in many areas of her body.)

Fibromyalgia is a frustrating disease for doctors and patients alike. Because there is no lab test to diagnose it, many doctors, like Jill's, aren't sure it even exists. Due to this widespread ignorance, many patients bounce from doctor to doctor, enduring a series of unrevealing lab tests and mostly unhelpful drugs, until finally, if they are fortunate, someone hits on the diagnosis. Jill's experience of having her concerns dismissed and even belittled by her physicians is unfortunately quite common. That she could see a string of doctors, including rheumatologists, and never be tested for tender points—a central feature of the condition that any well-informed physician should be aware of—is also unfortunately too common.

During the winter months, Jill raises and trains horses at her stable in Wellington, Florida, which is near Sam's studio. Some of her equestrian friends had been studying with him and recommended that she see if he could help her. The main reason Jill consulted Sam was not FMS, though, but to help with rehabilitation after having undergone neck surgery for ruptured spinal disks. Months later, she was still weak on the left side of her body, particularly in her arm, and was very out of shape from all the inactivity before and after the surgery. When she first saw Sam, she had just started riding again, but it hadn't been easy. "Being forty-eight, unfit, and a little overweight," she says, "I hurt. I ached."

Overview of Fibromyalgia

Fibromyalgia is a painful condition of unknown cause. In addition to numerous tender points, which tend to be located at spots where muscles attach to ligaments or bones, the typical symptoms include widespread pain, fatigue, and poor sleep, all of which Jill had. The sleep is often described as "nonrestorative," meaning the person wakes up in the morning not feeling refreshed. Sleeping troubles are so prominent in this condition that some researchers believe it is the primary cause of the symptoms, and there is some scientific evidence to support this view. While the reality of FMS is likely to be more complex than that, it is clear that poor sleep can exacerbate symptoms and lower quality of life. People with FMS often have other conditions such as irritable bowel syndrome, chronic fatigue syndrome, and restless leg syndrome (marked by itching, numbness, or tingling in the legs, often relieved by walking). For reasons that are not understood, women are about twenty times more likely to develop FMS than men.

While there is no diagnostic lab test for fibromyalgia, the condition is not "all in your head." Researchers have found, for example, dramatically elevated levels of a pain mediator, called substance P, in the spinal fluid in FMS patients. Thus, the problem appears to involve abnormalities in processing pain sensations in the spinal cord and brain that greatly amplify pain. These amplified pain signals cause pain that is real and can be debilitating, even though the sensations of pain are out of proportion to any actual damage or trauma to the muscles and other tissues. While knowing that FMS does not damage joints, bones, or internal organs doesn't necessarily diminish the pain, it can be reassuring. It is also reassuring to know that, despite the pain and the lack of a cure, FMS does not progress or cause death.

> **TIP** Since many doctors are poorly informed about FMS, it's essential to find one who is open-minded, and ideally, has experience treating FMS patients and keeps up on the latest research. Often other people with the condition or consumer groups, such as the Fibromyalgia Network, can provide referrals or leads.

How Yoga Fits In

Yoga, when practiced appropriately, can help people with fibromyalgia in several ways, beginning with the stress response. There is evidence that people with FMS have an overactive sympathetic nervous system (see chapter 3), which is turned on most of the time. A number of yoga practices can ratchet down this stress response and switch the body into the relaxation response, mediated by the parasympathetic nervous system. Learning to modulate your stress response can not only diminish your symptoms, but help you deal with the stress of having a disorder that is poorly understood by both the medical community and the public.

The slow, deep breathing common in yoga practice, which becomes the way long-term practitioners breathe most of the time, is an especially effective way to calm an agitated nervous system. Kristin Thorson of the Fibromyalgia Network, an FMS sufferer herself and patient advocate, says that in her experience deep-breathing exercises (see chapter 8) can help people generate an "inner sense of peace" and create emotional benefits as well, which can be very important for FMS patients, many of whom have been made to feel like "damaged goods" by a medical system that does not acknowledge the reality of what they are going through.

Yoga can improve your ability to sleep and this can be of enormous benefit in FMS. In addition, a number of yoga practices including meditation, Yoga Nidra, and Deep Relaxation (Savasana) appear to provide some of the restorative effects of sleep, even though you are awake (see chapter 3). Yoga asana, as well as practices like pranayama and meditation, can increase energy, improve posture, and create better alignment of the bones, muscles, and other tissues, particularly if they are done regularly over a long period of time.

While asana can help alleviate the pain of FMS, it's easy to overdo (as happened to Jill in her first experience with yoga). This may be why the evidence for the effectiveness of treating FMS with exercise is mixed. While doctors often encourage patients with FMS to exercise, sometimes doing so can be counterproductive. As Sam says, "The harder they try, the worse they get." From a yogic perspective, the problem may be that doctors typically give patients a standardized exercise routine for a certain amount and kind of exercise every day. Such one-size-fits-all approaches are very different from a yoga therapist's personalized and ongoing assessment of what the patient is capable of doing, fine-tuned by the patients' own assessments of their pain and energy levels.

The regular practice of yoga, of course, improves your ability to monitor your body's response to what you do and to judge whether something is benefiting you. Based on what you discover through this cultivated awareness, you can adjust your activity level, and again, notice how your body responds. It's an ongoing process that leads to finer and finer awareness and better choices.

Meditation can play a vital role in helping manage the pain of FMS. Practitioners learn in meditation to tune directly in to their experience and separate painful sensations, which may be bad enough, from their ideas and feelings about the pain, which can be worse, fueling the fire of suffering. By cultivating the ability to selectively focus your awareness, meditation may also help you modulate the pain sensations down to a more manageable level.

Yogic Tool: **SANGHA,** meaning community. The love and support that can come from a community of yoga teachers and practitioners can be therapeutic, especially because FMS sufferers may feel alone and misunderstood because of their illness. Many people with FMS also find it useful to connect with each other, either informally or as part of FMS support groups, in person or via the Internet. Support group members often share information with one another on research developments and recommend supportive physicians and other health care professionals.

The Scientific Evidence

A 1999 study led by Dr. Patrick Randolph, then director of psychology services in the Pain Center at Texas Tech University Health Sciences Center, found that a program of gentle yoga stretches and mindfulness meditation both reduced the pain of fibromyalgia and improved patients' ability to cope with it. The uncontrolled study examined sixty-seven patients who used the mindfulness-based stress-reduction (MBSR) program for as long as seven years, in addition to standard medical and psychological care. Patients attended yoga classes and were also asked to meditate for forty-five minutes a day while listening to an audiotape. Of the participants, the majority of whom were Christians from rural Texas, 78 percent reported an improvement in mood, 80 percent said their ability to handle stress was increased, 86 percent noted better pain management skills, and 98 percent indicated that they had learned something of lasting value. Of note, 90 percent indicated that the program was "moderately" or "highly" consistent with their spiritual beliefs, and a similar percentage found that the program enhanced their spiritual growth.

A study by Kenneth Kaplan and colleagues at the Newton-Wellesley Hospital in Massachusetts found that a ten-week MBSR program for seventy-seven people with FMS resulted in less pain, reduced fatigue, an increase in well-being, more restful sleep, and better mental health. All fifty-nine patients who completed the program improved and more than half showed moderate to marked improvement (there was no control group). In addition to mindfulness meditation, the program included gentle yogic stretching, breathing exercises, and guided imagery. Other studies of MBSR led by Dr. Jon Kabat-Zinn have found that the program reduces pain and improves mood in patients with chronic pain. For more details on Kabat-Zinn's studies, see pp. 155–56.

Sam Dworkis's Approach

As the ancient yogis knew, Sam says, "controlling the breath is the precursor to controlling everything about your life—the physical body, the emotions, and the spirit," and breathing is key to Sam's approach. Used appropriately to calm an overtaxed nervous system and induce relaxation, it can be "the fundamental key that unlocks the tightness of the body." He emphasizes breathing gently and evenly throughout the exercises, never forcing the breath. Although the goal is to breathe entirely through the nose, he tells those students who find nose breathing uncomfortable at first to breathe through the mouth for the time being, and soon all of their yoga breathing will be through the nose.

Yoga teachers like Sam often give people with FMS gentle stretching exercises to help relieve tightness of the fascia, the soft tissue that wraps (and links) muscles and organs in the body. These stretches, particularly when coordinated with the breath, he believes, stretch and loosen the fascia and make movement easier and more pain free. Although the medical profession tends not to pay much attention to fascia, yogis and bodyworkers find it plays a role in many conditions from back pain to carpal tunnel syndrome. It was partly the palpable tightness of her fascia that convinced Sam that Jill had FMS. "The more symptomatic I find people are with fibromyalgia or fibromyalgia-like symptoms, the tighter the skin is to the underlying structures." He says he can often tell where people have pain just by the tactile feel of the fascia.

Sam devises routines that are closely tailored to each patient's needs and abilities. In Jill's case, he noted that she had weakness, numbness, tingling, and some difficulty with coordination. In the aftermath of her neck surgery, her symptoms were more pronounced on the right side of her body. She had poor posture, with shoulders rounded forward and stooped, head protruding forward of the neck.

The asana practice Sam created for Jill was designed to energize her and realign her without causing her to overexert. He wanted to break into the "insidious cycle" that afflicts so many FMS sufferers: a sedentary life, due to the fact that exercise is so painful; the lack of exercise and resulting weight gain can fuel depression, which makes it even harder to overcome the lethargy of FMS. Sam says that almost all the people who come to him in chronic pain are overweight, and Jill was no exception. He describes typical chronic pain sufferers as having "a heaviness about them, a darkness about the eyes, a dullness of the skin."

With all of Sam's exercises, the operative principle is that less is more. He tells every client that on a scale of one to ten, from completely passive with nothing going on to very vigorous and really painful, he wants them to work at a level of two approaching three. This is very subtle work. Though it might seem that such an approach would not yield any results, Sam finds that this is the best way to make steady progress and avoid injuries and other setbacks.

Here is the sequence of the poses and instructions that Sam provided for Jill.

EXERCISE #1. **SUPPORTED RELAXATION POSE (Savasana).** Set up your props to support your body in your most pain-free, neutral, reclining position. Use as many props as you need to completely relax. Once you are comfortable, bring your attention to your breathing, and stay with it for the remainder of Savasana. Don't try to actively control the breath; instead simply tune in to the gentle rhythm of air coming in and going out. If you remain calm and comfortable, you can stay in the pose twenty minutes or longer.

Jill couldn't lie flat on her back because her neck and shoulders were sore, so Sam used various props to create a wedged platform to support her body at a slight angle. He also placed a small pillow under her neck, and supported her arms and legs so they were aligned with her torso (figure 17.1). The net effect is as if she is in a "reclining chair," with the legs elevated and the arms supported.

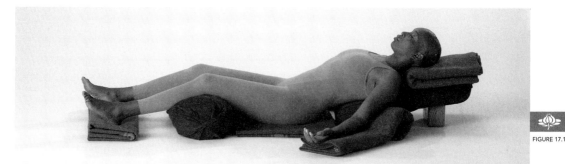

FIGURE 17.1

The length of time that Sam might keep a new student in this supported position depends on what he observes. He says, "I'm like an eagle, watching all the time for their level of agitation or discomfort." With Jill, the timing was twenty minutes or longer because the support allowed her "to be more comfortable than she'd been in ages, even more comfortable than lying in bed."

How much more than Supported Relaxation pose Jill did in a given session depended on how she was doing that particular day. Sam explains that progress in yoga is like the stock market. Some days you're going to feel better and do more, and some days you're going to feel like you've never done yoga before. That's true of Sam's own practice, too. "There are days I walk down the stairs for my morning practice, and I'll be able to do twenty or thirty Sun Salutations like I did the day before. The next day I'll spend my entire session in a supported, relaxed breathing position, because that's all I can do that day—and it doesn't matter." Sam says that it's doing only what you can comfortably do at any moment, even if it's just breathing in a supported position, that's going to take you in the right direction. He knows it may sound far-fetched, because in our culture the emphasis is always on trying hard. "Everybody in gym class from day one is taught to compete and to try." He explains that competing and trying is not going to get FMS sufferers the recovery that they're looking for. To heal, you need to accept the reality of where you are right now and respond appropriately, not try to force something that your body is not ready for.

EXERCISE #2. **ELBOW MOVEMENTS IN RELAXATION POSE** (Savasana). After you have set the basic foundation of body, mind, and breath coordination in Relaxation pose as described above, you can begin to move your arms, one at a time. Keeping your hand cupped and relaxed, inhale and bend your arm at the elbow. Exhale and release your arm back down to the support. Move your arm slowly and mindfully, always coordinating your movement with your breath. Practice this movement three times on one side, then repeat with the other arm.

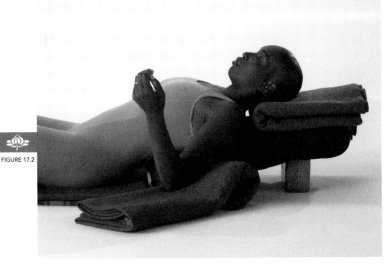

FIGURE 17.2

Key to Sam's philosophy is beginning by moving only one arm at a time. He says that when your sensory system is already overloaded by chronic pain, moving both arms means "two times the sensory input going into a brain that's already compromised."

EXERCISE #3. **HAND AND ELBOW MOVEMENTS IN RELAXATION POSE** (**Savasana**). Repeat the arm movements from exercise #2 while straightening your fingers and thumbs to stretch your palms. Sam believes that when the palm of the hand is active, it helps the elbow and shoulder to open more, and creates a sense of lightness. As in the prior pose, do the arm movement three times on each side, coordinating with breath, adjusting to your capacity, as always.

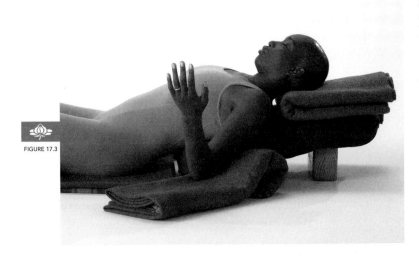

FIGURE 17.3

EXERCISE #4. **SHOULDER MOVEMENT IN RELAXATION POSE (Savasana).** While you are still in Supported Relaxation pose, straighten the fingers and thumb of one hand as in exercise #3, with the palm facing upward to the degree that is comfortable. Keeping the elbow straight, on an exhalation, raise your arm from your shoulder and move it up and over toward your head. As you extend the arm, the thumb will move toward pointing at the ceiling (figure 17.4). How high you lift the arm depends on the mobility in your shoulder at any given time. If you experience any pain at all, you've gone too far. Inhale as you come down. Repeat two more times on that side and then switch sides.

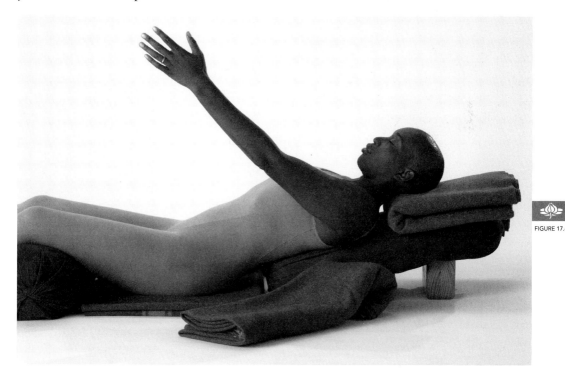

FIGURE 17.4

Because Jill's shoulder mobility was limited, Sam placed props on the floor behind her head to support her arms, so there would be no tension or strain. Because she had less mobility in her right arm, he propped that side about 10 or 15 degrees higher.

The main purpose of the following exercise is to stretch the fascia in the arms, shoulders, trunk, hips, and legs. For example, you gently move the hand away from the shoulder to stretch the arm. To explain the concept of moving two body parts away from each other without strain, Sam picks up an old rubber band and holds it loosely between the index fingers of his two hands. First he demonstrates pulling the rubber band rapidly with one hand and shows how the stretch is uneven and very often the rubber band will snap.

Then he demonstrates pulling the rubber band slowly and evenly with both hands. "You can see how the fibers of the rubber band seem to stretch more evenly along its entire core," he says. "Stretching your arm in this fashion allows the skin of your arm and then the underlying fascia to gently start to stretch."

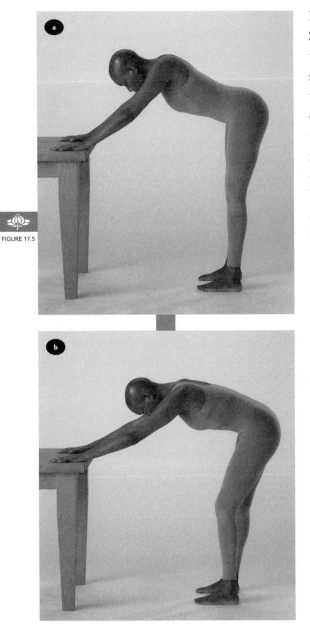

FIGURE 17.5

EXERCISE #5. **WIGGLE AND WAGGLE.** Start by facing a kitchen counter or table-top and placing your palms flat on the surface. Position your feet so they are six to eight inches apart and slightly turned out. As you step backward, fold forward at the hips until your arms are extended fully and you have reached an angle that does not create pain anywhere in your body. Bend your knees as much as is necessary to keep the spine from rounding. From there, subtly "lift your tail feathers" to gently stretch your hamstrings (thigh muscles) and the fascia (connective tissue) at the back of the thighs (figure 17.5a).

To do the pose correctly, make sure you are keeping your shoulders moving downward away from the ears, allowing the neck to remain relaxed. Also, keep your head a little higher than your spine, but not tilted back. When you turn your head from side to side, you should always be able to look above your arms and shoulders.

To begin the wiggle and waggle, bend your left knee without moving your arms. Then, on an exhalation, begin to stretch the right side of your body (figure 17.5b). "Pull your rubber band evenly from both ends, from the hands to the hips," Sam says. On your inhalation, return to neutral. Repeat two more times on the right side only, moving with your breath. Then return to center, making sure your neck is still relaxed, and do the exercise on the other side three times.

Sam calls the wiggle and waggle "the fundamentally most important exercise in yoga for chronically ill and injured people." In fact, he gives it to every single client, from those who are chronically ill and in pain to those who are young and physically agile and very athletic. For people who are significantly out of alignment, and Jill was slightly, he explains that over time the tightness of the soft tissue that's taking them off plumb will resolve itself. Sam says, "Athletes and nonathletes alike get significant release with this exercise, promoting flexibility."

EXERCISE # 6. **THE WINDMILL, thirty to sixty seconds.** Start by standing with your feet hips' width apart and your arms at your sides. Turning your torso, swing your arms from side to side, bending at the knees and pivoting on your back foot like a golfer hitting a drive (figure 17.6). Let your breath flow smoothly. Alternate between the left and right sides, always pivoting on your back foot and allowing your back heel to come off the floor to make sure there's no torque on your knees.

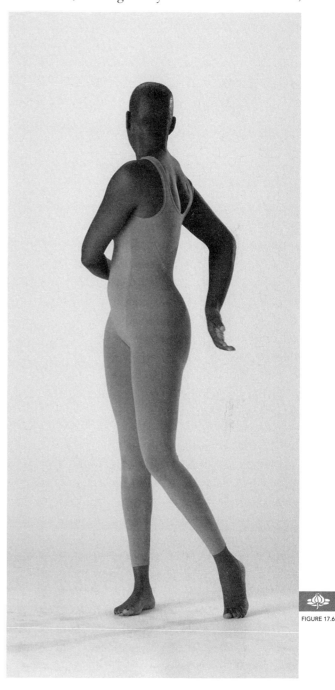

FIGURE 17.6

EXERCISE #7. **SUPPORTED RELAXATION POSE (Savasana).** For the final Relaxation pose, use props to support your head, arms, and legs in a pain-free, neutral, reclining position. You may find that you need considerably fewer props at this point than in the Relaxation pose at the beginning of the practice due to the fascial release (softening of connective tissue) created by preceding poses.

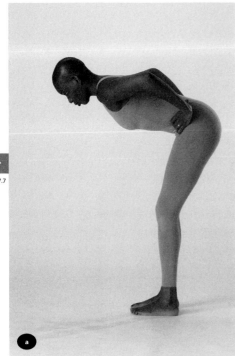

FIGURE 17.7

These seven exercises were the extent of Jill's initial practice sessions with Sam. Later on, as Jill improved, he added gentle Sun Salutations. To make the Sun Salutations less likely to cause problems, he made the following three modifications:

1. Keep your hands on your waist when bending forward and when coming up (figure 17.7a). Sam has found that when students go into or come out of forward bends with their hands over their heads, it can worsen their FMS symptoms.

2. Rather than doing Cobra pose or Upward-Facing Dog, do Sphinx pose, with your forearms on the ground (figure 17.7b).

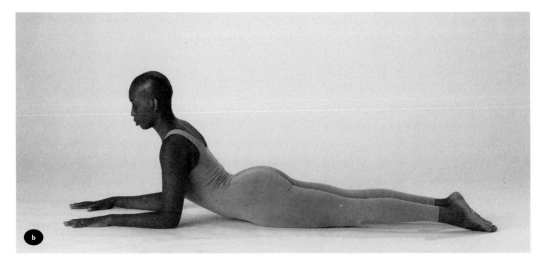

3. Keep your knees bent in Downward-Facing Dog pose (figure 17.7c).

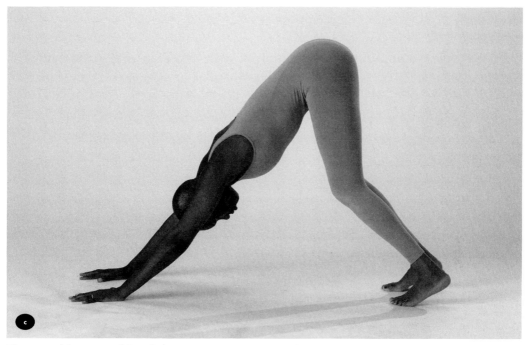

Three modifications of Sun Salutations Sam recommends.

OTHER YOGIC IDEAS

In her long career as a yoga teacher, Ana Forrest has only met one man who said he had fibromyalgia. All the others have been women and, all of them, bar none, breathe poorly, she says. For many of them, she has observed, there is an emotional component to the condition. They seem unable or unwilling to express what they're feeling, so there's a huge emotional backlog that remains lodged in the tissue where it causes pain. She finds deep-breathing practices to be extremely useful. She might tell a student with FMS, "Let's go into where in your body you feel that despair and that sadness, and let's breathe into that, and release as much of it as we can." Says Ana, "If we did our work well, there'd frequently be a whole outpouring of tears," in addition to a lessening of pain.

OTHER YOGIC IDEAS

Roger Cole has heard from several students with FMS that Iyengar restorative poses (see chapter 3) "are what saved them." He thinks it makes perfect sense that restorative poses would be helpful, because they stretch muscles passively, while providing much-needed deep relaxation. He recommends in particular supported forward bends such as Paschimottanasana with the forehead supported by a folded blanket or your arms placed on a chair (as long as you don't have lower back problems) (top) and supine twists such as Jathara Parivartanasana with bent knees, which can be supported by folded blankets (bottom).

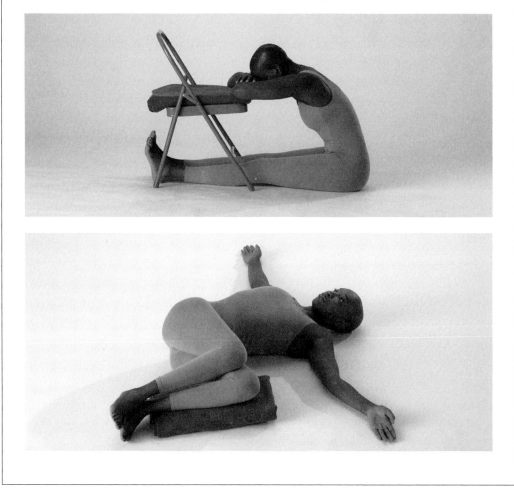

Contraindications, Special Considerations, and Modifications

Some people with FMS get light-headed when they change position quickly. Moving slowly from pose to pose and taking particular care when coming out of standing forward bends, inversions, or other poses when the position of the head moves from low to high can prevent this symptom or lessen its impact.

Many vigorous yoga classes—as well as activities like aerobics, jogging, and basketball—involve jumping. Most experts consider such high-impact activities contraindicated in FMS. On the other hand, perhaps the worst thing you can do is nothing. Being inactive leads to deconditioning of muscles, which over the long run may result in even greater pain.

Normally in yoga, you should always let pain be your guide: If a pose hurts you at all, you should modify it so it doesn't hurt or you shouldn't do it. This rule of thumb may be even more important for people with FMS to follow. If you push yourself to do a yoga pose or any other exercise when you are experiencing discomfort, you may regret it the next day. To prevent overdoing, it can be helpful to take breaks between asana, resting in Child's pose or Savasana before resuming your more active practice.

Kristin Thorson says, "More often than not, people with fibromyalgia do not know that they have overdone it until the next day or a few hours later, once they are home and wondering, 'What did I do?'" To sort out whether a practice is safe, don't just notice how you feel when you are doing it but try to tune in to longer-term trends. Do you have less pain than usual the day after asana practice? Are you more relaxed and energetic? If you practice regularly does your mood improve? How about your sleep? These may ultimately be more reliable indicators of whether the practice is benefiting you than how you feel while doing the poses, though that should feel good, too. If you tune in to yourself carefully, Kristin believes yoga will help you build strength and stamina. It may take you longer than it would the average healthy person, but you can achieve long-lasting results.

One final consideration with FMS is when to do your yoga practice. Most patients experience less pain and stiffness from the late morning through the midafternoon. If this is true for you, and your schedule allows, try to time your asana practice accordingly. Practices such as pranayama, meditation, and deep relaxation can be done whenever it is most convenient. As your internal awareness evolves, you will increasingly be able to tell what times are best to do yoga and you may discover that what works best for you doesn't fit the rules of thumb listed here.

A Holistic Approach to Fibromyalgia

❋ Poor sleep can increase pain and fatigue during the day. Steps to improve sleep include getting up at the same time every day, winding down before bedtime, and if necessary, taking medication such as a low dose of a tricyclic antidepressant (see chapter 23).

❋ Since a significant minority of people with fibromyalgia also have sleep apnea, your doctor may want to investigate this possibility.

❋ Cognitive-behavioral therapy appears to improve coping and mood.

❋ For people with depression, antidepressant medication (at higher doses than that used for sleep) can help. Note: some of the newer drugs like Paxil (paroxetine) and Zoloft (sertraline) can contribute to sleep problems.

❋ Two supplements that may be helpful in depression, S-adenosyl-l-methionine (SAM-e) and 5-hydroxytryptophan (5-HTP), may also improve tender point soreness.

❋ Nonsteroidal anti-inflammatory drugs like ibuprofen and naproxen, as well as the pain reliever acetaminophen, aren't generally effective for FMS pain.

❋ Oral narcotics can be a good option for pain control. Few people with chronic, painful conditions like FMS get addicted to these drugs, though side effects like sedation and constipation are common.

❋ Doctors who have been trained to do it (for example, some rheumatologists and primary care doctors) can treat pain by injecting a local anesthetic directly into tender points. The treatments usually need to be repeated for maximal effect. Note: the skill of the doctor doing the injections is key.

❋ Another potentially helpful technique, which some physicians do, involves spraying tender areas with an anesthetic spray and then stretching the underlying tissue.

❋ Topical pain relievers such as capsaicin rubbed into sore muscles can lessen discomfort.

❋ Acupuncture can be beneficial and is very safe.

❋ A recent survey on nondrug therapies conducted by the Fibromyalgia Network found that massage, which can lessen pain and relieve stress, was the treatment recommended by the highest percentage of patients. Note, however, that vigorous, deep-tissue massage may make pain worse.

❋ Other modalities favored in the survey included the application of heat, either via heat wraps or hot tubs, and chiropractic care, particularly when the treatment was complemented by acupressure techniques.

❋ Some doctors surveyed by the Fibromyalgia Network believed that osteopathic manipulation may be even more effective than chiropractic.

❋ The survey also found that learning all they could about the disease and following developments in research allowed people with FMS to cope better.

Jill found the yoga she was doing with Sam so subtle that for a while she wasn't even sure it was helping. "At first I felt like I wasn't getting anything out of it, but I stuck with it. There were many times when I didn't even want to get up and go." However, if nothing else, she was motivated by the relaxation, which was deeper than anything she'd experienced. As she told a friend in the early days of her sessions with Sam, "I really don't know yet how it's going, but the hour and a half of complete relaxation is worth it all." After several months, she says, "I couldn't wait to get up and go there. And I don't know when that transition was made. It slowly crept up on me."

Now Jill says, "I feel like I've come a long way. As I progressed, I saw changes in my body. My clothes were fitting differently. I've lost some weight. My strength and energy level is better." She adds, "For the longest time, whenever I went somewhere, to a cocktail party or some other kind of gathering, halfway through I'd have to sit down, because I just didn't have the energy level, or I felt my back wasn't going to hold me up. Sam has taught me a lot about the union and balance of my body, and I've gotten better. All of a sudden I notice, my God, I never sat down this evening. I didn't feel the fatigue, and didn't feel a twinge of pain."

Jill says, "Am I 100 percent? No. But, I'm stronger, and I'm doing things with Sam—being able to balance my body, and having the strength to do yogic positions—that I'd never even thought I could do when I was eighteen, much less forty-eight. The pain, when I first came to him, was like having a fifty-pound weight on the upper part of my spine. That's completely gone." Even with the yoga, Jill confesses that her mind still goes nonstop. "I'm someone who's thinking of ten things that have to be done at all times." But yoga, she says, took "the sharp edges and rounded them."

Although her condition is vastly improved, how much Jill can do still varies day to day. Says Sam, "Today Jill might come in, do a couple of windmills, the wiggle and waggle, up to ten Sun Salutations, and start to sweat, with no discomfort at all. Sometimes, though, she only does four Sun Salutations, and we have to modify them so she doesn't exacerbate her pain." Jill has started to practice regularly at home between lessons and, as Sam has taught, has learned to modify her practice as needed.

Perhaps the most satisfying result of Jill's yoga practice is the change in her ability to ride horseback. When she began yoga, she'd get pain after riding for ten or twenty minutes. Now she can ride for an hour or longer and walk away without pain. Not only that, but yoga even seems to be having an effect on the horses. "The reason," Sam explains, is that "in nature, all the horse wants to do is find its balance. Then we take an imbalanced human being and put her on a perfectly balanced horse and we screw the horse up." People who practice yoga have a better sense of both physical and emotional balance. A number of equestrians who have become Sam's students are discovering that "the more yoga they're practicing, the easier it is to get the horses to respond to their commands. It's amazing."

HEADACHES

Before becoming a yogi, RODNEY YEE danced professionally with the Oakland Ballet Company and the Matsuyama Ballet Company of Tokyo. One day in 1980, Rodney and a fellow dancer decided to try a class at the Yoga Room, an Iyengar yoga studio upstairs from the Berkeley Ballet Theatre where they were rehearsing, to see if it might help with their flexibility. Rodney remembers telling his friend afterward, "I can't believe how good I feel." Not only did his body feel fabulous, but he was touched in an emotional and spiritual way as well. A short time later, Rodney began to phase out his dance career in order to pursue yoga full-time. At the time, his family thought he was crazy and would never amount to anything because his earnings from teaching yoga were so meager that he needed to work as a waiter to pay the bills. Today Rodney is featured in over twenty yoga videos and has cowritten two books (with Nina Zolotow), *Yoga: The Poetry of the Body* and *Moving Toward Balance*. He teaches at the Piedmont Yoga Studio in Oakland, California, and internationally.

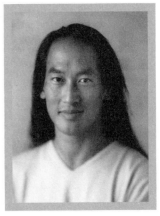

Margaret MacIntyre (not her real name) developed migraines while working as a magazine editor in a fast-paced, deadline-driven environment. To make matters worse, she is, as she herself says, "the type of person who can make anything stressful." She knows there is a strong connection between her stress levels and headaches. Putting it in Ayurvedic terms (see chapter 4), she says, "I have a real pitta-vata constitution. I'll get really caught up in thinking, stress myself out doing it, and end up with a migraine." There is also a history of migraines in her family; both of her grandmothers had them.

"My migraines occur in the right frontal area. Once I get a migraine, without fail it will last for three days. There's no variation in that, though I've found that there is a range of intensity. When it starts, it causes me to feel very drawn. I get a little sensitive to light, I get hypersensitive to smell. Sometimes I get a visual disturbance, too," she says. "Things will become blurry. If I'm having a really bad one, I've got to go lie down. I can't focus on things. It's a complete audio-visual shutdown."

Margaret has been a yoga practitioner for many years, gravitating primarily to active styles like vinyasa flow and Ashtanga yoga. Even so, her migraines persisted, tending to vary with her stress levels. One reason for her continued problems, she admits, was that she tended to push the edge in her yoga practice more than she should, doing advanced poses, intense pranayama exercises, and "high-energy" Sun Salutations. Before meeting Rodney and asking for his recommendations regarding her migraines, she had always avoided doing restorative poses in her home practice.

> **CAUTION** More than occasional headaches that occur at night or first thing in the morning may be related to depression, severe high blood pressure, or to a sleep disorder such as sleep apnea, and should be professionally evaluated. In rare cases, headaches are caused by life-threatening conditions. Ruptured aneurysms and strokes caused by hemorrhages can cause severe head pain, which may come on fairly suddenly. Contrary to what many people believe, brain tumors are rarely the cause of headaches. With tumors, other symptoms like balance problems, seizures, or muscle weakness will usually appear long before headaches. In general, doctors recommend that if you are having "the worst headache of your life" or one that is unlike any you've ever had before, you should seek prompt medical attention This is especially true if you are over the age of fifty.

Overview of Headaches

There are dozens of possible causes of headaches. By far the most common are stress- or tension-related headaches, often associated with tightness in the muscles of the head and neck. People with tension headaches sometimes describe a feeling of pressure or dull pain encircling their head, like an overly tight bandana. In migraines, in contrast, pain is often on only one side of the head and described as pounding or throbbing in nature (which corresponds to the increase in pressure with each heartbeat). Migraines, despite their reputation, range in intensity from mild to incapacitating. Unlike tension headaches, they are often accompanied by nausea, vomiting, and a profound aversion to light and sound. Some people's migraines are preceded by a brief period of visual disturbances (the aura), such as lights dancing in front of the eyes, or, much less commonly, changes to the sense of smell like Margaret sometimes experiences. Pressure in the sinuses, associated with a cold or allergies, or infection in the sinuses if they stay blocked too long, is another relatively common cause of headaches. Sinus headaches can also lead to migraines in people who are susceptible.

> **TIP** Specific yogic tools may be useful for sinus headaches. If you use a neti pot (see chapter 4) to lavage your nasal passages with warm salt water early in a cold or at the first sign of nasal allergies, you remove excess mucus, allowing you to breathe more easily, and you may also be able to wash out viruses before they have a chance to colonize your nasal passages. Inflammatory cells may similarly be removed before they cause congestion. The neti pot may also help prevent blockages of the small openings to the sinuses, known as ostia, potentially heading off a full-fledged sinus infection. A study from Sweden's Karolinska Institute suggests that the humming sounds like those made while chanting can improve ventilation of the sinuses. It appears that the resultant vibrations in nasal cavities help open up the ostia. Try chanting "Om," holding the "m" a little longer than usual and tune in to the vibration in your nose and upper palate. The pranayama technique of Bhramari (see p. 16), where you hum a sound similar to the buzzing of a bee, also causes strong vibrations in the head and may help relieve sinus pressure.

One underrecognized cause of both migraines and tension headaches is the use of pain relievers. The resulting "rebound headaches" can be worse than the ones you originally took the drugs to treat. The problem can result from taking even over-the-counter drugs like aspirin and ibuprofen as infrequently as twice a week. Drugs that combine pain relievers with caffeine and/or the sedative butalbital (e.g., Fiorinal, Esgic) are the ones most likely to cause rebound. The only way to get rid of rebound headaches is to stop taking pain relievers until the headaches go away. Since the withdrawal headaches can be bad, preventive therapy (see p. 332) may be advisable to get you through that phase.

The closer attention you pay to your headaches, the better you can help your doctor do his or her job. Many people with migraines, for example, are not properly diagnosed, but this is sometimes because they do not provide enough details to their doctors to allow for a diagnosis. The better you are able to describe your headaches—including where they are located, how long they last, the quality of the pain, what precipitates them, and what seems to make them better—the more you help the doctor make the correct diagnosis.

This is important since therapies for various kinds of headaches differ. If you are not satisfied with the headache care you get from your primary care doctor, however, probably the best option, if it is available to you, is to consult a doctor specializing in headaches. These physicians can be found in the relatively few headache clinics that exist, in some pain clinics, and at some university hospitals. Even there, be sure to assess whether the doctor takes a comprehensive approach including factors like diet, exercise, and stress levels, or whether the strategy focuses mainly on drugs.

 TIP Yoga teacher and physical therapist Julie Gudmestad suspects that some tension headaches may be *caused* by yoga, specifically by arching the neck too much when doing backbends (top). A solution to this problem is to try to elongate your neck when bending backward, and to prevent the head from moving too far behind the upper spine. In doing Locust

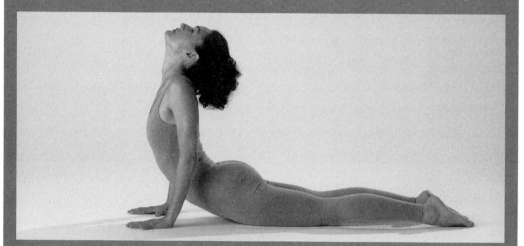

pose, for example, you might keep your gaze toward the ground, rather than lifting your head and trying to look straight ahead. In Cobra, you would keep your gaze straight ahead rather than looking up (bottom). Gary Kraftsow links headaches with the unconscious tendency of many yoga students to arch their necks back as they move into forward bends. If you find yourself doing this, try keeping your neck in a neutral position or let your head drop slightly forward instead.

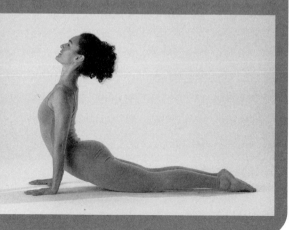

How Yoga Fits In

Since stress is a major factor in both tension headaches and in migraines, yoga can certainly play a role in prevention. Almost any form of yoga, including simple breathing techniques, can be effective in lowering stress levels. But a dedicated practice of yoga—particularly of meditation—may change the entire way you relate to people, situations, and events that are stressful to you, allowing you to respond more calmly, to feel less agitation. Incorporating regular Deep Relaxation (Savasana) into your yoga practice may similarly help you to be more resilient in the face of life's inevitable challenges.

Yoga may also help with muscle tension in the back, neck, and head, which can cause or contribute to headaches. Yoga teaches that releasing the tight muscles improves blood flow to them, and can help relax the mind as well. There are a number of specific yoga postures that can help relieve tightness in these areas. From a yogic perspective, it's not just tightness but muscle weakness and a failure to use muscles properly that can be a factor in headaches. Asana can help strengthen muscles, educate the body in how to use them, and improve bad postural habits like holding the head forward of the spine (see pp. 32–35).

A steady yoga practice causes your ability to observe your internal environment to become more refined. As you become more aware of the way you use your body, you may begin to notice that you scrunch your eyes and forehead when you concentrate on something, or that you crook your neck to hold the phone next to your ear in a way that may be contributing to chronic muscular tightening and headaches (a phone headset is a great solution to this problem). With more subtle awareness, you may start to identify the signs of a headache earlier, sometimes even before the pain starts. You may notice, for example, gripping in your neck or the back of your head. Early detection can be essential for migraines since it's usually much easier to prevent them or treat them in the initial minutes than after the pain is full-blown. By encouraging pratyahara, the ability to turn your senses inward and away from external stimuli, yoga provides respite from the kind of sensory overload of modern life that can trigger headaches (see chapter 3). Because yoga is typically performed in a peaceful setting with dimmed lights, that too can facilitate relaxation. When the nervous system relaxes, muscles are more likely to release tension.

The awareness that yoga encourages also helps you become more sensitive to factors in the external environment that may be responsible for triggering headaches. Many experts suggest that headache sufferers keep a diary listing any headaches, their severity, how long they lasted, and possible precipitating factors. Possible triggers include various foods, bright lights (especially fluorescent), loud noises, skipped meals, sleep deprivation, air pollution, cigarette smoke, menstruation, menopause, estrogen taken either in birth control pills or after menopause, perfumes, changes in barometric pressure, either too much or too little sleep, and of course, stress. Among smokers, the more you smoke, the greater the headache problems tend to be. Looking back over your list may enable you to discern patterns that could help you avoid future attacks. This advice is entirely consistent with the yogic practice of self-study, svadhyaya.

Foods considered most likely to trigger migraines are listed below. If you're unsure if a given food is triggering your headaches, it's best to remove it from your diet for a couple of weeks and see what happens when you reintroduce it. If several foods are suspected, eliminate them all and reintroduce them one at a time. If eliminating all the leading suspects doesn't improve your headaches, you may not have food triggers. But if your headaches do recur when you eat a food again, that's evidence it may be a problem.

FOODS THAT COMMONLY TRIGGER MIGRAINES

Aged cheeses	Bananas, apples
Red wine, beer, and other alcoholic beverages	Citrus fruits
Dried fruits treated with sulfites (organic may be okay)	Eggs
Food made with monosodium glutamate (MSG)	Beans
Food containing artificial sweeteners like aspartame (NutraSweet, etc.)	Chocolate
Freshly baked bread	Wheat
Yogurt, sour cream, and other dairy products	Seeds, nuts, peanuts
Pickled foods	Cured or processed meats (e.g., bologna, pepperoni, ham)

Yogic Tool: **VISUALIZATION.** Just by changing what you are thinking about, you can alter patterns of blood flow in the body. In the case of migraines, the objective is to reduce the amount of blood going to the head. Lie down in Deep Relaxation pose, with a pillow or folded blanket beneath the back of your neck and head. Close your eyes, breathe slowly and deeply through your nose, and imagine that your hands are immersed in warm water and that the blood flow is turning your palms rosy pink. As your fingers and hands heat up, imagine that your head is cooling down at the same time. Stay with these images and follow your breath for five to ten minutes or as long as you feel comfortable. This exercise can also be done in a seated position.

Yoga has been shown to reduce feelings of anger and hostility, and this could be useful for people with headaches. Dr. Robert Nicholson of Saint Louis University did a study which found that anger, particularly bottled-up anger, was a better predictor of headaches than anxiety or depression, two problems frequently linked to headaches. His advice sounds distinctly yogic: take deep breaths to quell your anger, try to figure out why you are angry deep down (self-study), let go of things beyond your control, and forgive. He points out that forgiveness will not change the past but neither will anger. Learning to let go of resentments can change you—and perhaps alter the likelihood of your getting a pounding headache.

The Scientific Evidence

There is scientific evidence that relaxation techniques and biofeedback can be effective for both tension and migraine headaches, lessening the duration as well as the frequency of attacks. Although these techniques are often offered outside of a yoga context, the approaches owe much to yoga. In a biofeedback session, for example, a patient might be taught to relax tight muscles in the face or neck, with instrumentation providing feedback directly from the muscles. After a while, the patient learns to induce the relaxation without the feedback. The process is all about facilitating awareness and conscious control of normally unconscious processes, and there's nothing more yogic than that. Almost all relaxation techniques, including biofeedback, bring the patient's awareness to the breath, another classic yogic tool. Dr. Seymour Diamond conducted two studies, published in the journal *Headache,* on patients with chronic headaches that hadn't responded to conventional treatment. The combination of biofeedback, meditation, and relaxation techniques produced what he describes as "an excellent response." Mindfulness-based stress-reduction programs that include asana and meditation have also been shown in studies led by Dr. Jon Kabat-Zinn to be an effective approach to chronic pain including headaches, improving function and lessening the need for medication (see p. 155–56).

S. Latha and K. V. Kaliappan of the University of Madras studied a yoga program that consisted of gentle asana and pranayama exercises, with twenty patients with either tension or migraine headaches participating. The randomized controlled trial lasted four months, and included two yoga classes a week in addition to home practice. Both the yoga and control groups continued to take their usual headache medications. Only the yoga group showed improvements, all statistically significant, in frequency, duration, and intensity of their headaches. The yoga group was able to decrease the amount of pain medication they took, while usage increased among the controls. In addition, the yoga group reported significant improvements in their levels of stress as well as their ability to cope with it.

In the largest study to date of yoga for chronic tension headaches, Dr. S. Prabhakar and colleagues divided eighty-five people into one group receiving yoga therapy and another on drug therapy. The primary drugs used were antidepressants for those who had depressive features in addition to their headaches, and Valium for those who manifested anxiety. The yoga practice consisted of asana, pranayama, and cleansing techniques (kriyas) done for forty-five to sixty minutes for fifteen to twenty sessions. Results were assessed at six weeks, six months, and one year later. Both the drug and yoga groups showed significant reductions in headache severity, frequency, and duration, though the changes were greater in the yoga group. Both groups showed improvements in anxiety and depression, though the results were again significantly greater in the yoga group. Only the yoga group showed less disruption of their social and work lives by headaches.

Rodney Yee's Approach

Given the role of stress in many headaches, Rodney believes, any kind of yoga can be helpful—including the strenuous practice that Margaret had been doing. "A well-rounded yoga practice is sometimes the best thing." By well-rounded, Rodney means a practice "that has something of everything—some standing poses, some inversions, some backbends, twists, forward bends, and some restoratives. It's a practice that speaks to every part of the body."

But since Margaret's practice didn't seem to be bringing her much relief from her headaches, Rodney reviewed it with her so he could see if there were any characteristics that might explain her lack of response. One problem that stood out to Rodney was that Margaret's practice wasn't well-rounded. She was putting almost all of her time into active, energizing practices, and none on restoratives. Margaret says that in "my personal practice, I almost never did those kinds of poses. I'm basically a prop minimalist. I had a bolster and some blocks and a strap and blankets, but I didn't use them very much." Rodney thought adding gentle restorative poses to her usual practice would help her achieve better balance. For more on restoratives, see chapter 3.

In talking to Margaret and watching her, he noticed that her eyes were very intense and that they didn't blink or move very much. "They had a laser-beam quality. It's like the pupils were fixated." This quality seemed related to Margaret's description of the pressure she felt building in her right eye when a migraine was coming on, as well as the fact that her eyes became dry then. He thought the dryness made sense because of how infrequently she blinks. The fact that she felt the symptoms more sharply in her right eye made sense, too, because she'd had toxoplasmosis ten years before, which had affected the retina in her right eye.

One of Rodney's goals in working with Margaret was to get her "to be able to work intensely in the asanas, or in everyday life, without hardening her eyes so much." Margaret says, "It kind of took me aback a little bit, but then I could see what he was talking about. I do express a lot of mental efforting through my eyes." Rodney asked her to use her fingers, placed gently over her closed eyes, to feel any hardness in her eyes. He wanted her to become aware of the sensations, so that she could consciously work on softening them. The idea was to break down her old habit and replace it with a new one, so that she would associate work not with intensity in the eyes but with relaxation. He viewed the hardening of the eyes as an ingrained habit, what yogis would call a samskara.

As part of the work he did to help Margaret change this habit, Rodney asked her to practice the restorative poses below with her eyes covered with a head wrap. In addition to being deeply calming, he says that the head wrap is particularly good at facilitating awareness of what you are doing with your eyes. He also asked her to try her regular asana practice wearing the head wrap, when feasible, to heighten her awareness.

TIP You can use any wide bandage for a head wrap. Many yogis, including B. K. S. Iyengar, who developed the technique of using head wraps in yoga practice, prefer Indian-made bandages that stretch but don't contain elastic, because they think elastic tends to compress the head. Rodney feels that a plain Ace bandage, properly applied, works fine. To put on a head wrap (also sometimes called an eye bandage), start wrapping clockwise at the forehead, go down by the eyes, and then come back up (left, center). Don't pull tightly; keep the bandage just lightly touching the eyes. Tuck the loose end to secure the bandage in place (right). In order to see when you move from pose to pose, you can roll up the bottom of the wrap, and then flip it back down when you are in the next pose.

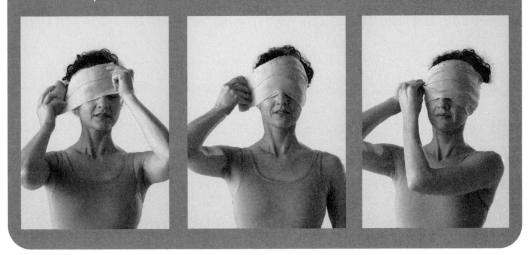

Here is the sequence of practices and instructions that Rodney provided for Margaret.

EXERCISE #1. **LEGS-UP-THE-WALL POSE (Viparita Karani), five minutes or longer.**
Set up for the pose by placing a bolster or stack of blankets folded into long, thin rectangles parallel to the wall and approximately six inches away from it. To come into the pose, sit on one end of the bolster with your side near the wall (figure 18.1a). Then turn toward the wall

FIGURE 18.1

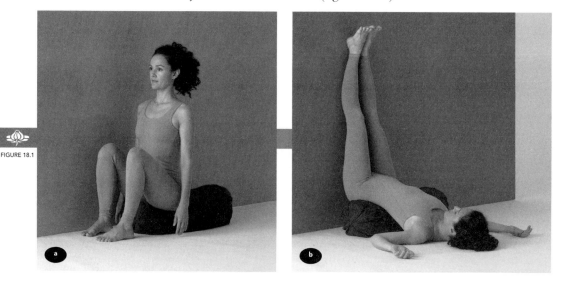

and swing your legs overhead and onto the wall. Keeping your pelvis on the bolster, allow your shoulders and head to come onto the ground. Rest your arms either out to your sides or in cactus position (figure 18.1b). See chapter 3 for more on this and the following pose.

EXERCISE #2. **SUPPORTED COBBLER'S POSE (Supta Baddha Konasana), five minutes or longer.** Set up for the pose by placing a bolster on your mat to support your torso with a folded blanket or pillow at the end of the bolster to support your head. To come into

FIGURE 18.2

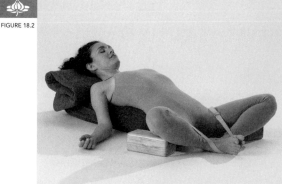

the pose, sit a few inches in front of the bolster (not on it), with the soles of your feet together in Cobbler's pose. Loop a strap around your sacrum and the tops of your feet, running it between your legs (not around your knees). Place blocks, pillows, or folded blankets under your thighs for support so that there is no tension in the groin area. Then slowly lie back over the bolster (see figure 18.2).

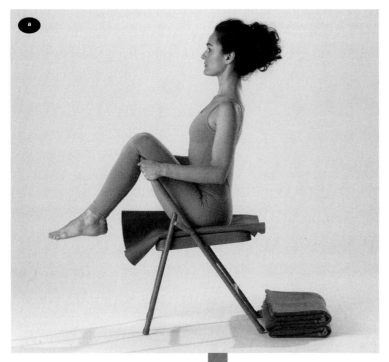

EXERCISE #3. **CHAIR SHOULDERSTAND** (Sarvangasana), **five minutes or longer.** To set up for the pose, place a bolster or two blankets folded into long, thin rectangles in front of a metal office chair. If you are using folded blankets, have the folded edge of the blankets face away from the chair. Place a folded yoga mat or blanket on the seat of the chair. To come into the pose, sit sideways on the chair. Hold on to the sides of the chair and swing your knees over the back (figure 18.3a). Keeping your legs over the back of the chair, slowly lean back until your shoulders reach the folded blankets or a bolster on the floor and the back of your head touches the floor. Then, thread your arms under the chair seat and hold on to the back legs of the chair. When you feel ready, bring one leg at a time to a vertical position (figure 18.3b). Please see pp. 275–76 for more on this pose and precautions to be aware of before attempting it.

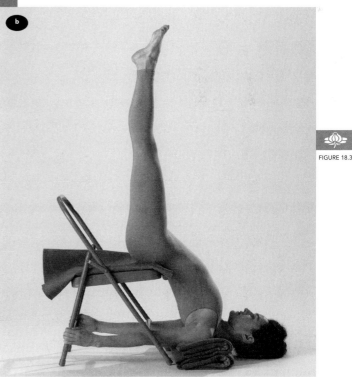

FIGURE 18.3

EXERCISE #4. **HALF PLOW POSE (Ardha Halasana), five minutes or more.** To set up for the pose, fold two or more blankets into wide rectangles (as you would for regular, not chair, Shoulderstand) and stack them in front of the chair, with the folded sides facing the

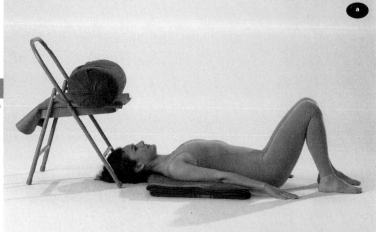

FIGURE 18.4

chair. If you are tall, you may also need to place blankets, a bolster, or other props on the chair seat (the taller you are, the more height you need) so that when you are in the pose, your thighs can be supported. To come into the pose, lie back

on the blankets so your shoulders are supported and your head is on the ground just under the seat of the chair, if you have a chair that doesn't have a bar connecting the legs in the front (or a chair from which the bar has been removed). If there is a support bar between the front legs, position the top of your head just in front of it (figure 18.4a). On an exhalation, roll back and swing your legs up and over so the tops of your thighs rest on the chair seat (or the

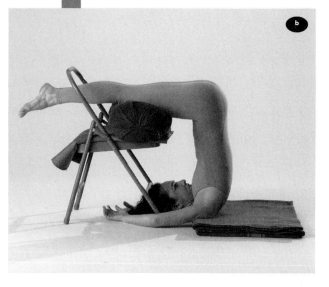

props you have placed on top of it), your feet extend through the back of the chair, and your back is perpendicular to the floor. If your head is under the chair, position it so that the front edge of the seat (or the props on top of the seat) comes to the junction of your hips and thighs (see p. 450). Rest your arms around the chair legs with your elbows bent to 90 degrees, hands up toward the head, palms up (figure 18.4b). If you are tall you may need to turn the chair sideways (if the seat is level) or use a chair with its back removed (available from yoga suppliers, see appendix 2).

EXERCISE #5. **ONE-LEGGED FORWARD BEND (Janu Sirsasana), with head support, two or more minutes on each side.** Start by sitting with your legs extended in front of you. If your lower back rounds when your pelvis is flat on the ground, sit on one or more folded blankets. Bring the sole of your left foot near the inside of your right thigh and place a bolster or stack of folded blankets across your straight leg. On your inhalation, lengthen your spine. On your exhalation, fold forward at your hips so your torso comes over your right leg and your arms and head rest easily on the prop (figure 18.5). If your head does not reach the prop, increase the height of the prop or use the seat of a chair to rest your head. Repeat on the other side.

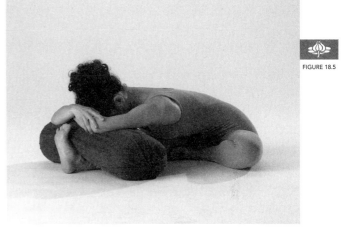

FIGURE 18.5

EXERCISE #6. **SEATED FORWARD BEND (Paschimottanasana), with head support, five or more minutes.** Set up as you did for the previous pose, keeping your legs straight, and placing the props across the tops of both legs. On your inhalation, lengthen your spine. On your exhalation, fold forward at the hips so your torso comes over your straight legs and your arms and head rest easily on the prop (figure 18.6). Again, if your head does not reach the prop, add more props or use a chair seat to rest your head (see p. 312).

(see p. 312).

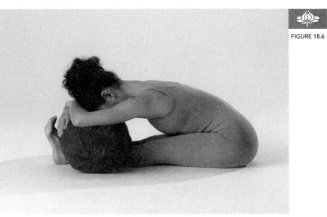

FIGURE 18.6

Note: As an experienced yoga practitioner, Margaret can stay comfortably in this pose for several minutes, but less experienced students should stay only as long as they feel completely comfortable.

Although the primary focus of the plan Rodney devised was relaxation, he says that a secondary effect of many of the postures was to release muscular holding in the neck and shoulders. The supported forward bends and Chair Shoulderstand in particular are useful for this purpose.

EXERCISE #7. **BREATH AWARENESS, with a brief pause after the exhalation, five to ten minutes.** Sit in a comfortable upright position (figure 18.7). When you are settled, slowly inhale and exhale. Then briefly pause after the exhalation. (Rodney says the difference between a pause and a retention is basically a matter of degree. A pause might last only a second.) Continue at your own pace, staying relaxed and never forcing your breath.

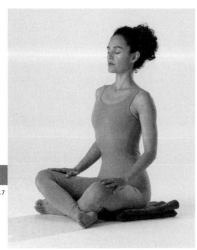

FIGURE 18.7

In addition to prescribing this gentle breathing exercise, Rodney asked Margaret to discontinue her previous pranayama program. She had been doing advanced pranayama exercises with long retentions of the breath, and with fixed ratios of time spent inhaling and exhaling. Rodney believes that in most cases any type of breath retention or ratio breathing, unless you've had first-rate pranayama instruction and are very cautious, could contribute to migraines. He thinks vigorous breathing practices like Bhastrika and Kapalabhati are also potentially problematic. Even though Margaret's personality always pushes her to do more, he says that since she is already stressed out, what she needs to do in her practice is less. "It's obvious that she's driven," Rodney says. So he asked her, "Are you willing to give things up to get rid of these headaches?"

Another modification to Margaret's practice that Rodney suggested was to follow Headstand, which yogis consider a "heating practice" and which she likes to do, with Shoulderstand, which is thought of as "cooling" but which she almost always skips. Shoulderstand can also often relieve tension in the neck muscles that develops from Headstand. Rodney thought it was interesting that just as Margaret had avoided restoratives, she had also avoided "anything that was more cooling."

This understanding of heating and cooling practices comes out of Ayurveda (see chapter 4). Ayurveda teaches that people often prefer foods, yoga practices, and lifestyle choices that increase their constitutional (doshic) tendencies. In other words, their preferences are often precisely those that will put them further out of balance. In Margaret's case, her strong pitta, or fiery constitution, seemed to crave additional heat, when what she actually needed was cooling. Rodney told Margaret there were many signals, including her stress levels and headaches, that indicated she needed to relax more, calm her nervous system and relax her sense organs, especially her eyes.

Rodney also noticed that Margaret held a lot of tension in her groin area and lower abdomen. His sense was that "the energy is going up," which in yogic thinking could contribute to headaches. "It's a visual thing," Rodney says. "Her thighbones were externally rotated and pushing forward." John Friend talks about a similar finding in many women with infertility (see chapter 22). Because Rodney felt there was not much downward release, he surmised Margaret might also have digestive problems, which she confirmed. What Rodney wanted to encourage in Margaret is what yogis call apana, a downward-moving force of prana or life energy in the body. Apana, yoga teaches, helps with bodily functions like digestion, urination, and menstruation. Rodney recommended that Margaret focus on releasing tension in her abdomen and grounding her legs in standing poses.

> **TIP** Focusing on the downward movement in breathing can contribute to headache relief. If asked to take a deep breath, most people lift their chests and actively recruit their neck and facial muscles, which ought to be relaxed. A better way to inhale, Rodney says, is to think of the lungs as being like a sponge which first needs to empty in order to absorb. Exhale as smoothly as you can, using your abdominal muscles to gently squeeze the air out. Then, rather than actively drawing breath in, let your belly relax with the natural downward movement of the diaphragm (see chapter 10), allowing the body to relax and absorb breath.

Contraindications, Special Considerations, and Modifications

While restorative poses can be very helpful in headache prevention, not everyone can simply relax into them right away. Rodney finds that many people "not only have stress, but also sort of a mental looping, where the mind keeps on obsessing over something. That kind of stress can bring on a headache." The problem is that "sometimes the restoratives don't stop the mind from going into this obsessive loop." The solution may be to practice as Margaret now does, first doing an active asana practice to burn off steam, then moving into restoratives and more meditative practices.

If you have a severe migraine or a cluster headache—another type of debilitating headache which typically comes at the same time every day for weeks—you may need to simply lie down in a dark room and not attempt any yoga practices at all. During a less intense headache, it is probably best to avoid an active asana practice in favor of restorative work, or to do only gentle poses to avoid working too close to your "edge," so as not to make matters worse. Inversions may also make symptoms worse, although B. K. S. Iyengar has been known to use them at times as part of the remedy. In general, supported inversions such as Chair Shoulderstand are thought to be preferable to unsupported inversions.

A Holistic Approach to Headaches and Migraines

✳ There have been many changes in the drug treatment of migraines in recent years with the development of new medications (the triptans), such as Imitrex (sumatriptan) to treat, or if caught early enough, to eliminate the headaches entirely. These medications may help control migraines by constricting dilated blood vessels in the head, and they can be effective for severe tension headaches as well.

✳ Some triptans are available as a shot or in a nasal spray. Other medication including the anti-inflammatory indomethacin is available in suppositories. These forms are faster acting than tablets, and are particularly helpful for people too nauseated to keep medication down.

✳ Some migraine sufferers get good relief with over-the-counter medications like ibuprofen and naproxen, or with combination pain relievers that include some caffeine. Liquid forms of ibuprofen are absorbed into the system faster than pills and may therefore be preferable.

✳ Some patients need stronger pain relievers, including narcotics. When used appropriately, these drugs are generally safe and effective, with a low potential for addiction.

✳ Medications to prevent migraines include the tricyclic antidepressants, usually in lower doses than used for depression, beta-blockers like propranolol, which are typically used for high blood pressure, and medications originally targeted at epilepsy.

✳ Headache experts recommend considering preventive treatment if you're getting two or more severe headaches a month that put you out of action for three or more days total, if you don't respond to symptomatic treatments, or if you are using pain relievers so much that you're experiencing rebound headaches.

✳ A study published in the *Journal of the American Medical Association* found that preventive treatment with antidepressants for chronic tension headaches was much more effective if it was combined with stress-reduction techniques. Those who used medication and stress-reduction methods in combination were also more likely to be able to discontinue the drugs later on without a flare in headaches.

* Safe nondrug preventive measures besides yoga include the herb feverfew, vitamin B$_2$, and magnesium.

* Acupuncture appears to be an effective method of preventing migraines and is extremely safe.

* Over-the-counter migraine remedies that contain caffeine can get rid of a headache, but regular consumption of the stimulant may make it more likely to get a migraine at times when the caffeine levels in your system are dropping, and may make headaches worse when you do get them.

* A diet low in fat and high in complex carbohydrates can reduce the frequency, duration, and intensity of migraines.

* Omega-3 fatty acids, found in such deep-sea fish as salmon and mackerel, and in flaxseed oil, have a similar benefit.

* If postural problems are part of the problem, in addition to yoga, instruction in the Alexander Technique may provide relief.

* A number of bodywork modalities can help with tension headaches including Trager work, shiatsu (acupressure), spinal manipulation, physical therapy, and various forms of massage including myofascial release techniques.

* Acupressure can be self-administered: press firmly on the hollow just below the bottom of your skull on both sides of the neck as you tip your head back. Alternatively, pinch the webbed space between the thumb and index finger of your left hand. Try either or both of these techniques, maintaining pressure for two or three minutes.

Contrary to her expectations, Margaret enjoyed the restorative practice that Rodney recommended. "The head wrap is really profound," she says, "very effective in making me feel very deeply drawn inward." Her favorite pose of the sequence is Chair Shoulderstand. "I get this sense of my legs clicking into place, and a sense of relaxation that I've never experienced in any pose before." In retrospect, Margaret sees that she had always avoided the restorative experience, because like a lot of driven people, she felt that she always needed to be accomplishing something. "I had to struggle with myself just to get used to the idea that it's okay to spend this time.

"Rodney has asked me to do some subtle things, like draw the skin of my forehead down, rather than up, when I'm working with the head wrap." (See pp. 11–12 for more on this topic.) She says the difference was palpable. She's also followed his advice about paying attention to her eyes, and to whether or not she's straining, both on and off her yoga mat. Another suggestion she incorporated was to do her yoga practice without wearing her contact lenses, allowing her to relax her eyes even more.

Rodney's program, which she enjoys so much that she does it nearly every day, has reduced her migraines from three or four a month, and twice that many when really stressed, to one or two. Even more impressive, this success came in spite of her moving, just after beginning the program, to another city to take another demanding editing job. Even though she's extremely busy and anxious about the new job—circumstances that are exactly "the kind of environment that breeds my migraines"—she's had many fewer than expected. "I think that's pretty amazing."

HEART DISEASE

 NISCHALA JOY DEVI says, "Before yoga, I realized the American dream." Despite all the material advantages, however, she still wasn't happy. She met her guru, Sri Swami Satchidananda, the founder of Integral yoga, in San Francisco in 1973 and connected with him immediately. She was working as a physician's assistant in a cardiologist's office at the time, but gradually became disillusioned with the narrow approach to healing found in Western medicine. When she moved to the guru's ashram in Connecticut in 1979, she started to teach yoga to a number of seriously ill patients in its holistic health clinic. "It was a natural way for me to combine both parts of my life," she says. A few years later, she met the physician, medical researcher, and author Dean Ornish, another disciple of Satchidananda. When he put together the Lifestyle Heart Trial, a groundbreaking study of a multifaceted program to reverse heart disease, Dean asked her to help design the yoga portion of the program. Nischala taught yoga to the participants as well as training the other yoga teachers, and subsequently served as Director of Stress Management. Nischala was also a cofounder with Dr. Michael Lerner of the Commonweal Cancer Help Program in Bolinas, California, a residential retreat for people with cancer that incorporates yoga, massage, and other healing modalities. She has gone on to write two books, *The Healing Path of Yoga* and *The*

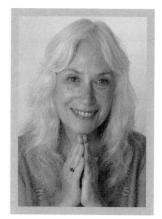

Secret Power of Yoga, and created and directs Yoga of the Heart, a yoga therapy training program for yoga teachers and health professionals working with people with life-threatening diseases. She lives in the San Francisco Bay Area and teaches internationally.

You might have thought that Ron Gross would have been an easy convert to the idea of using a yogic approach to heart disease because he is Nischala's father-in-law. In reality, Ron was as deeply skeptical of yoga's therapeutic potential as he'd been unhappy about his son Bhaskar's decision to renounce the world and become a swami at the Satchidananda ashram years before. Bhaskar's time at the ashram ended when he and Nischala, whom he met there and who had also taken the path of renunciation, came to the realization that they could best be of service by returning to the outside world. They are now married.

A hard-charging businessman, Ron describes himself as "a typical type A. I get up early and work late." During Ron's commute to the office, he says, "I used to get stomach pains because I was so angry that the traffic was moving so slowly going through the tunnel." He'd also get "stomach muscle pains" in real tough business negotiations. "Sometimes," he says, "I'd lose my cool, blow up, start yelling and screaming, pick up and walk out of the negotiations. That might have been good for the negotiations, but it wasn't very good for me."

Ron's other risk factors for heart disease besides his type A personality include a family history. His father died of a heart attack at age fifty-two. Ron's total cholesterol was high, around 230, his HDL or "good" cholesterol was dangerously low, in the mid-20s, while his LDL or "bad" cholesterol was almost 200, much too high. He did have some factors in his favor, however. He wasn't a smoker, didn't have diabetes or high blood pressure, and had exercised regularly his entire adult life. At 5' 8" and 165 pounds, he wasn't more than a few pounds over his ideal weight.

Ron's first indication of heart disease came at the age of sixty-eight. He was swimming to get in shape for an upcoming diving trip when he noticed that he was uncharacteristically out of breath. His doctor ordered an angiogram and discovered his right coronary artery was about 90 percent blocked. Ron had an angioplasty immediately. "The doctor said if I had gone on my scuba-diving trip, they'd have brought me back in a box, because I would never have survived. But I felt pretty good after the angioplasty," good enough to continue being active. Though he gave up diving, he continued his tennis game. He also started to eat a low-fat diet.

"Fast forward to two years later. I was walking across the street, maybe half a block, I have to stop and rest. I was out of breath. Everything was back to where I was before the original angioplasty. It looked like I'd have to go in for another angioplasty." Nischala was teaching the Dean Ornish program at the time, which begins with a week-long residential retreat, in which students walk, attend group meetings, eat a vegetarian diet that derives less than 10 percent of its calories from fat, and are taught yoga postures, breathing techniques, meditation, and imagery. Nischala said, "If you take the week-long program, and you don't feel better, I'll pay for it.

"Of course, I had no money at the time," she says, but based on her experience, it seemed like a pretty safe bet.

Overview of Heart Disease

Heart disease is the number one killer in the modern world, and contrary to popular notions, it is not just men who are affected. While men do tend to come down with symptoms earlier than women, heart disease is the number one cause of death for both sexes, and more women than men suffer heart attacks.

In predicting heart attacks, doctors tend to focus on risk factors like smoking and elevated cholesterol, but science has uncovered strong evidence for other possible contributors. Type A behaviors, which are characterized by anger and hostility, a focus on achievement, and a sense of urgency about time—exactly the behaviors Ron describes—have been strongly linked to heart attacks in a number of studies. Other psychosocial factors include job dissatisfaction, loneliness, and an unhappy marriage. Overweight is not a huge independent risk factor but is problematic in that it contributes to type 2 diabetes, high blood pressure, and elevated levels of a type of blood fat known as triglycerides, all of which are strongly linked to heart problems. There appears to be an unhealthy synergy involving risk factors for heart disease. They don't just add up—they multiply. People with four or five bad ones may be at fifty times the average risk for a heart attack.

 TIP When considering medication to lower your cholesterol, keep in mind that there's generally no rush. Cholesterol wreaks its damage over decades. Whether you start a drug today or six months from now usually won't make much difference. My advice is to give diet, exercise, and nondrug therapies a chance to work before committing to what may be a lifelong regimen of medication.

In recent years, researchers have begun to focus on inflammation as another major factor in heart disease. Supporting this notion is the higher incidence of heart disease among people with inflammatory conditions ranging from rheumatoid arthritis to gingivitis (inflamed gums). Recently, some doctors have been advocating measuring the level of C-reactive protein (CRP), a measure of inflammation, to assess heart attack risk. That inflammation and heart disease are associated isn't news to many yogis and those trained in Ayurveda. What Western doctors call a type A personality has a lot in common with the constitutional type that Ayurvedic medicine calls pitta (see chapter 4). Pittas tend to be intense, fiery, prone-to-anger overachievers. If their fire burns too hot, Ayurveda says, it predisposes them to heart attacks and other inflammatory conditions, and for thousands of years Ayurvedic practitioners have used diet, lifestyle recommendations, herbal remedies, and other treatments to try to cool down the flames.

> **CAUTION** Women often don't have the so-called classic symptoms of heart disease—classic, as it turns out, for males, who until recently were the only ones studied. The classic heart attack symptom in men is crushing chest pain that radiates to the shoulder, jaw, or arm. Women may have milder pain in the chest or abdomen. Often their most prominent symptom is fatigue and a general feeling of weakness. An underrecognized warning sign, which may begin months before a heart attack strikes, is an extreme form of burnout known as vital exhaustion, characterized by excessive fatigue and lack of energy, increased irritability, and feelings of demoralization. Both sexes may have nausea, sweating, or shortness of breath.

How Yoga Fits In

Because the stress response affects the heart in a number of harmful ways, yoga's proven ability to fight stress is a big part of the explanation for how yoga benefits people with heart disease. Stress hormones raise the blood pressure and heart rate, putting added strain on the heart and increasing its need for oxygen. Periods of either physical or mental stress can be particularly dangerous for someone with a heart whose blood supply is compromised by fatty blockages, though evidence suggests that stress can induce a heart attack in the absence of blockages by causing spasm in a coronary artery. Stress hormones also induce changes that cause the blood to clot more easily. Doctors now believe that heart attacks often happen when a clot gets lodged in an artery that is already partially narrowed. The stress hormone cortisol is known to increase both eating and the laying down of fat in the abdomen. Intra-abdominal fat can increase the body's resistance to the effects of insulin, raising blood sugar and further increasing the risk of heart disease.

Yoga's ability to lessen anger may lower the risk of a heart attack. "Anger is a very strong emotion," Nischala says. "It takes at least three hours physiologically for the body to get back in balance, to the place it was before an angry episode—and many heart attacks happen within three hours of an angry episode." She says that anger was very common among the participants in the Ornish program, and most knew and admitted it.

The regular practice of yoga seems to lessen anger by fostering greater psychological equanimity, increasing feelings of compassion for others, and increasing the sense of gratitude. Yoga also helps people achieve a heightened awareness that puts the minor annoyances of life in a larger perspective, so that they are less likely to respond to the traffic jam or the difficult situation at work with the kind of agitation Ron Gross described. And yoga provides specific tools, such as breathing techniques, which can dampen the first sparks of anger and prevent them from being fanned into an inferno.

Yoga as a form of physical exercise, if done vigorously enough, can raise the heart rate into the aerobic range, potentially lowering the risk of a future heart attack (but see below for safety considerations). Even pranayama (yogic breathing) alone has been shown to improve cardiovascular conditioning. The improved efficiency of lung function and better oxygenation that comes with regular yoga practice means that more oxygen reaches the heart muscle even in instances where partial blockages compromise blood flow. Yoga can help people lose weight not just because asana burns calories, but because lower levels of stress hormones lessen appetite, and because practitioners bring conscious attention to what and how they eat (see chapter 27).

Yoga is also a good antidote to depression (see chapter 15), which is a major problem after a heart attack, and greatly increases the likelihood of dying. Doing yoga makes you feel better about yourself and more hopeful about your ability to get better. The resulting increase in optimism can encourage you to keep up your practice and make other lifestyle changes that contribute to better health.

Yogic Tool: **KARMA YOGA.** "My experience is that nothing opens the heart, whether it's a sick heart or a healthy heart, quicker than doing service," Nischala says. "There is always an opportunity to serve." See p. 295 for an example of how karma yoga can help in heart disease.

New breakthroughs in the understanding of heart disease are causing some doctors and scientists to focus not just on large blockages in major arteries—like the 90 percent occlusion that led to Ron Gross's angioplasty—but to smaller blockages as well. Dean Ornish explains why. Those large blockages, he says, "aren't the ones that are likely to kill you," because new blood vessels called collaterals are likely to have grown around the blockage to supply blood to the area at risk, and also because by the time a blockage has gotten that large, "it tends to be stable, calcified." Heart attacks are more likely to be caused "by the 20 to 30 percent lesions," which are "usually fresh . . . not calcified . . . and more likely to become unstable." Given this new understanding, holistic approaches make particular sense. Rather than targeting only the largest blockages, as interventions like angioplasty and bypass surgery do, yoga works in a systemic way and is likely to have effects on blockages large and small.

The Scientific Evidence

In 1948, in what may have been the first reported use of yoga therapy in a Western medical journal, Aaron Friedell, MD, described the use of "attentive breathing" in eleven patients with angina in the journal *Minnesota Medicine*. Attentive, or mindful, breathing consists of inhaling and exhaling slowly, taking brief pauses between each inhalation and exhalation. Dr. Friedell first learned the technique in 1927 from Paramahansa Yogananda, author of the classic *Autobiography of a Yogi*. Friedell later refined the technique, teaching his patients alternate nostril breathing, "closing one nostril while inhaling slowly through the other." The patients, some of whom were debilitated by chest pain and shortness of breath, noted marked improvement of their symptoms. They would begin their mindful breathing as soon as they felt the first signs of an angina attack coming on and could usually make it go away quickly. Some of the patients were able to discontinue all use of nitroglycerin and other medications.

The benefits of yogic breathing were documented again in a Western medical journal fifty years later. A 1998 study, published in *The Lancet,* found that a yoga technique called "complete breathing"—in which you use the abdominal muscles to exhale as fully as possible, allowing a larger inhalation on the subsequent breath—helped patients with congestive heart failure (CHF) to breathe better (see p. 35). After only a month of training, subjects taught this form of yogic breathing were getting more oxygen into their systems and doing it with fewer breaths per minute than controls. They were also able to exercise more.

Dr. Dean Ornish's studies, published in such leading medical journals as *JAMA* and *The Lancet* beginning in 1983, tell us more about the health benefits of a comprehensive program of yoga and lifestyle changes. The yoga portion of the Lifestyle Heart Trial, which was designed by Nischala—a modification of the standard Integral yoga class as taught by her guru Swami Satchidananda—included asana, pranayama, visualization, meditation, and deep relaxation. The rest of the program consisted of a low-fat vegetarian diet, smoking cessation, group support sessions, and aerobic exercise. Following the weeklong intensive training, patients attended regular meetings in their communities and were asked to continue the diet, yoga, and exercise on their own. One year after starting the program, LDL cholesterol levels dropped from an average of 144 to 87 in people who were *not* taking medication to lower their levels. Patients who followed Ornish's program had 91 percent reduction in the frequency of their angina, as well as a significant reduction in severity of attacks.

What was most striking about the Lifestyle Heart Trial is that the patients who did the program showed *reversal* of their heart disease. That is, when they came in for retesting after five years of following the precepts of the program, their blockages had gotten smaller and positron emission (PET) scans showed that the heart muscle was receiving an increased supply of oxygen-carrying blood. When I was in medical school in the 1980s, such a reversal was considered impossible. Everyone "knew" that blockages only got bigger over time, which is precisely what happened to patients in Ornish's control group who followed standard medical care. Subjects in the Ornish program improved quickly, and—even better—their heart disease continued to reverse during the third and fourth years of the program. Though many in the control group were taking medication to lower cholesterol, their disease nonetheless continued to progress. Many in the yoga and lifestyle program were able to get off blood-pressure medication, too, in part because of the average weight loss in the first year of almost twenty-four pounds.

While the Lifestyle Heart Trial involved 48 patients (28 who did the program and 20 controls), the research was later extended to eight medical centers around the country and a total of 440 patients, with similarly impressive improvements in risk factors such as blood pressure, cholesterol levels, and body weight. The authors wrote that the program "may be particularly beneficial for women," given their excellent results and a prognosis generally worse than men's after heart attacks, bypass surgery, and angioplasties. Both men and women were able to avoid bypass surgery for three years without any increase in illness or death due to heart disease. More recently, as part of an effort to gain Medicare coverage for the program, Dean Ornish is compiling data on over 2000 patients like Ron who have taken the week-long training. These data are still being collected and analyzed, but the results so far are very persuasive: Within twelve weeks of beginning the program, patients achieve significant reductions in cholesterol and other blood fats, C-reactive protein, fasting blood sugars, hemoglobin A1c (a measure of long-term control of blood sugar), and systolic and diastolic blood pressure, and these changes are sustained after a year. Patients also enjoy statistically significant improvements in quality of life and measures of depression and hostility.

While it's impossible to say for sure how big a role yoga played in the program's success, those involved in the research view it as crucial. Yoga reduced stress and stress-related behaviors like smoking and dietary excess, Dean says, and made it easier for people to adhere to the program's other elements. In Nischala's opinion, yoga "seemed to be the catalyst for making everything else happen." Whatever the reason, she says that people who practiced yoga at home tended to get quicker relief of angina and other symptoms, as well as greater reversal of the buildup of the plaque in their arteries.

Numerous studies from India have also documented the ability of a comprehensive yoga program to improve heart disease and its risk factors. A controlled trial conducted at the Yoga Institute in Santacruz near Mumbai examined the effects of a comprehensive yogic intervention on 113 patients with angiographically proven coronary artery disease. The yoga program included instruction on yogic techniques, lifestyle recommendations, and a low-fat diet rich in fiber, vitamins, and antioxidants. The controls received standard medical care, and both groups continued prescribed medication. At the end of one year, the yoga group had a 23 percent drop in cholesterol (247 to 185) compared to 4 percent among controls, and a 26 percent reduction in LDL cholesterol (146 to 108) compared to 3 percent in the control group. On repeat angiography after one year, 70 percent of the yoga group had smaller blockages versus 28 percent of controls, while 10 percent of the yoga group had larger blockages versus 36 percent of controls. In addition, the researchers found that even patients who had only a small improvement on their angiograms noted a major reduction in symptoms, likely a reflection of yoga's systemic benefits. A randomized controlled trial of 93 patients conducted by Dr. A. S. Mahajan and colleagues at the All India Institute of Medical Sciences in New Delhi found a yoga program resulted in statistically significant weight loss as well as improvements in total, LDL, and HDL cholesterol, and triglycerides. Two other Indian studies had similar findings.

Nischala Devi's Approach

Nischala is a big believer in the "less is more" philosophy. "Most people I see—and not just the people who have heart disease—push beyond their limit." If you have any questions about your ability to do any of the practices described below, please do less than you think you can (especially if you've got type A traits). Any of the sitting practices can be done in a chair if that's more comfortable.

Nischala incorporates a Deep Relaxation pose at several stages of her therapeutic practice, not just at the end of the practice as is common. She understands that relaxation is not necessarily something that many heart patients like. Indeed, many want to skip it, feeling it's a waste of time. In Nischala's experience, however, it's a critical part of the practice, and the more you do it, the better relaxation feels. She has found it can be useful for lowering heart rate and relieving anginal pain, and cardiologists have told her that when patients engage in deep relaxation during an angiogram, there is a visible release of spasm in the coronary arteries.

> **CAUTION** If you have intermittent angina and the pattern is stable—it comes on with a certain level of exertion, subsides with rest, and does not seem to be getting worse—it's okay to do yoga as tolerated and back off if symptoms appear. However, angina that is new or more pronounced than usual should prompt an immediate medical evaluation as it may herald an impending heart attack.

Here is the sequence of practices and instructions that Nischala provided for Ron, the same one used in the Lifestyle Heart Trial, and found on her audio recording *Relax, Move & Heal,* which Ron used to guide his home practice.

EXERCISE #1. **NECK MOVEMENTS.** Sit in a comfortable position with your back straight but not rigid. Close your eyes. Bring your awareness to the breath, and observe it as it flows in and out, gently and through your nose. Now you are ready to begin the neck movements:

1. Inhale and bend your head forward so that the chin comes toward the chest. As you exhale, allow all the muscles in the back of the neck to relax (figure 19.1a). Inhale and lift your head back up. Exhale and relax.

2. Inhale and bring your right ear toward the right shoulder. Exhale, and feel the stretch on the left side of the neck, making sure you aren't lifting the

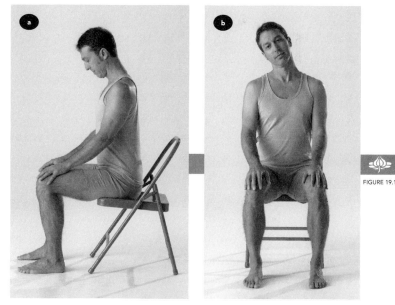

FIGURE 19.1

shoulder to the ear (figure 19.1b). Inhale and bring your head back to center. Exhale and relax. Repeat this stretch on the other side.

EXERCISE #2. **SHOULDER MOVEMENTS.** Sit in a comfortable position with your arms loose at your sides. Practice the following shoulder movements:

1. Inhale and bring your shoulders forward, as if to make them touch in front of your chest, which moves your shoulder blades apart (figure 19.2a). Exhale and relax your shoulders.

2. Inhale and lift your shoulders toward the ears (figure 19.2b). Exhale and release.

3. Inhale and bring your shoulders back, moving your shoulder blades close together, toward your spine (figure 19.2c). Feel your chest expand. Exhale and relax. Gently shake your arms.

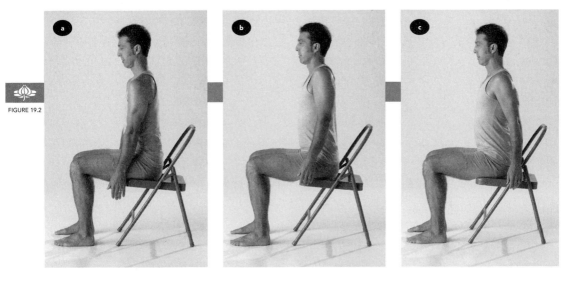

FIGURE 19.2

Now combine all three movements in the following order:

1. Inhale and raise your shoulders up toward the ears.

2. Exhale and move your shoulders forward and toward each other.

3. Inhale and bring your shoulders down.

4. Exhale and bring your shoulders back, moving the shoulder blades together.

Repeat steps 1 through 4 for several cycles, then do several cycles of the same movements, but moving in the opposite direction. When you're done, notice any relaxation that's come in your arms and shoulders, and gently shake out your arms.

EXERCISE #3. **ANKLE MOVEMENTS.** Sit on the floor with your legs stretched out in front of you. Practice the following ankle movements:

1. Exhale and point your toes away from you (figure 19.3a). Inhale and lift your toes toward you (figure 19.3b). Repeat twice more.

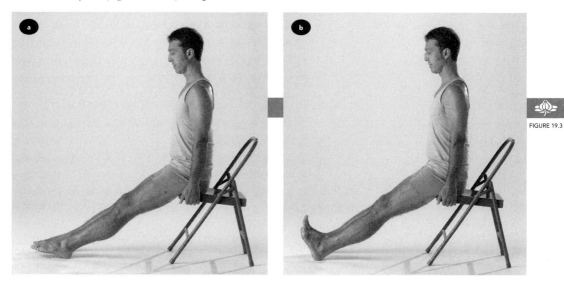

FIGURE 19.3

2. Move your toes in a clockwise direction, keeping your legs still so the movement comes from your ankles, not your legs (figures 19.4a & b). Begin slowly at first, then increase the size of the circle and the speed. Do three repetitions. Repeat in the opposite direction.

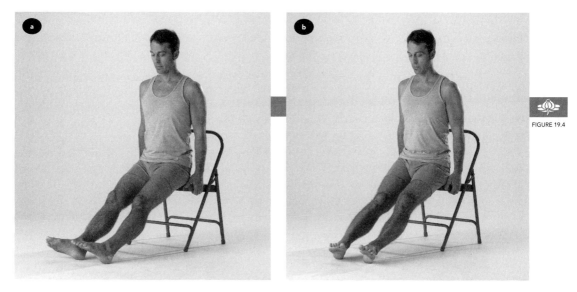

FIGURE 19.4

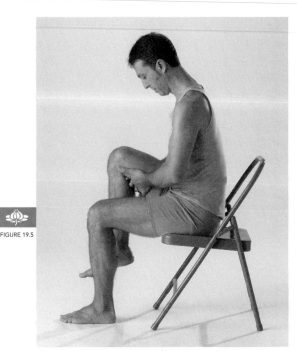

FIGURE 19.5

EXERCISE #4. **KNEE TO CHEST POSE.** Sit with your legs stretched out in front of you. Bend your right knee, leaving the sole of the left foot on the floor. Inhale, and use your hands to bring your right thigh up toward your chest. Exhale, lower your head slightly, and give the leg a good hug (figure 19.5). Inhale, and raise the head. Exhale, and release your arms, allowing the leg to return to the floor. Give your legs a gentle shake. Relax. Repeat on the other side.

EXERCISE #5. **RELAXATION POSE (Savasana)/Body Scan, one minute.** Start by lying on your back with a pillow under your head and another behind your knees. Allow your arms and legs to relax by your sides. Turn your palms up, if that's comfortable. Close your eyes, and breathe slowly and deeply (figure 19.6). When you are settled, begin to mentally observe and release any tension in your body. Start with your feet, lower legs, thighs, and hips. Relax. Next move to your hands, arms, shoulders, abdomen, chest, and throat. Relax. Then move to your back and spine, neck, head, and face. Relax. If you detect any strain or tiredness, use the breath to help release it. On the inhalation, imagine a fresh supply of energy entering each part of your body. On the exhalation, imagine any tiredness or tension being released. Allow your body to relax completely.

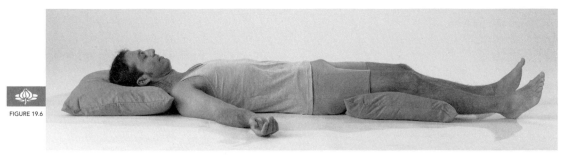

FIGURE 19.6

EXERCISE #6. **COBRA POSE (Bhujangasana).** Start by lying on your belly with your feet parallel and your heels together. Place your palms flat on the floor beneath your shoulders, with your elbows close to your body and your fingers pointing forward. Extend your chin. Inhale, and slowly lift up your head and neck. Lift the upper chest slightly off the floor (figure 19.7). (Do not push the hands into the floor, as this can raise your blood pressure.) Stay for a few relaxed breaths, and then lower back down, touching your chin down before the forehead. Rest for a moment, with your cheek turned to one side and your arms at your sides. Stretch only as far as is comfortable. Each time you may have a different capacity.

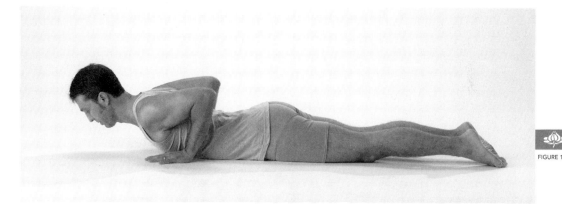

FIGURE 19.7

EXERCISE #7. **HALF LOCUST POSE (Salabhasana), ten seconds.** Start by lying on your belly, facedown with your chin on the floor. Place your arms alongside your body or tuck your arms under your body, if it's comfortable. Keeping your right leg straight, inhale and raise the leg a few inches off the floor (figure 19.8). Holding steady, breathe normally. Then slowly lower your leg and allow it to relax. Repeat with the left leg.

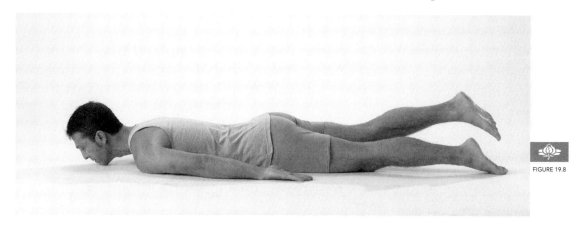

FIGURE 19.8

EXERCISE #8. **RELAXATION POSE (Savasana), one minute.** Return to the relaxation position described above. Tune in to your body. Notice any discomfort, trembling, muscle aches, or disturbed breathing that might have resulted from the backbends (Cobra and Half Locust). Nischala says, "Be aware of the internal signals. Learn the difference between a good stretch and something that is doing harm."

EXERCISE #9. **SEATED FORWARD BEND (Paschimottanasana).** Start by sitting on the floor with your legs stretched out in front of you, and the knees slightly bent. Place one pillow under your hips and a second behind your knees. Lock your thumbs together and raise your arms up toward the ceiling. Inhale and stretch your arms and torso as you look

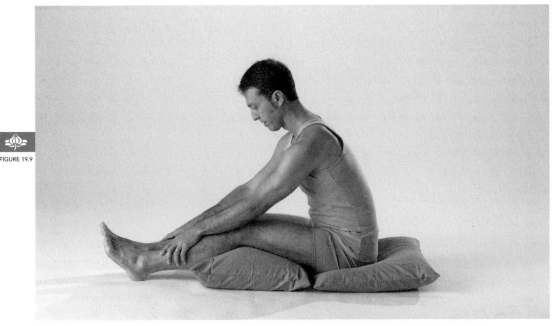

FIGURE 19.9

up. Then exhale and bend forward over your legs. Stopping halfway, inhale and stretch toward the wall in front of you. Then exhale and release forward over your outstretched legs. Hold on to your legs wherever it's comfortable, and relax (figure 19.9). If there is any pain in your legs or back, do not come so far forward. After several breaths, lock your thumbs again, inhale, and stretch your arms as you come up.

EXERCISE #10. **RELAXATION POSE (Savasana), one minute.** Return to the relaxation position described above.

EXERCISE #11. **SUPPORTED SHOULDERSTAND (Salamba Sarvangasana), modified.** Lie on your back near a wall, with your knees bent and your buttocks as close to the wall as possible. Turn your palms down and press them into the floor. Bring the soles of your feet to the wall, and begin to walk up the wall (figure 19.10a). As you do this, bring your hands to your lower back for support. Breathe normally and go up only as high as is comfortable, without any strain. If you're comfortable doing so, straighten your legs, allowing them to lean against the wall (figure 19.10b). If you develop dizziness or feel pressure in your head or neck, come out of the pose right away. Otherwise, stay up for one minute or less, and gradually build up your time in this pose to three minutes. Come out of the pose slowly by walking your feet down the wall and lowering your buttocks to the floor.

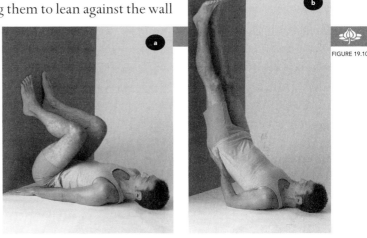

FIGURE 19.10

EXERCISE #12. **RELAXATION POSE (Savasana), thirty seconds.** Lie down in the relaxation position described above.

EXERCISE #13. **FISH POSE (Matsyasana), modified, thirty to sixty seconds.** Start by lying on your back. Bring your legs together and use your hands to grasp the sides of each thigh. Using your elbows for support, come to a half-seated position. Lean back and slowly tilt your head backward as far as you comfortably can and place your head on the floor. Balance your weight between the head, elbows, buttocks, and legs. If this is not comfortable for you, place a pillow under your shoulders and allow your head to tilt over the edge of the pillow (figure 19.11). The chest and heart center are fully expanded, so breathe through your nose, deeply and easily. Relax your shoulders. To come out of the pose, reverse the tilt of your head, and slowly lower your back, neck, and head down to the floor.

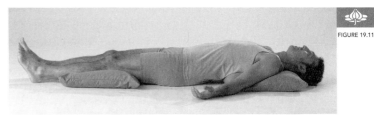

FIGURE 19.11

EXERCISE #14. **DEEP RELAXATION POSE (Savasana), one minute or longer.** Return to the relaxation position described above.

EXERCISE #15. **HALF SPINAL TWIST (Ardha Matsyendrasana), thirty seconds.** Sit on a pillow on the floor with your legs stretched out in front of you, with a slight bend in the knees. Place your left foot outside of your right leg, between the knee and ankle, and place your left arm on the floor behind you. Press your right arm against your left leg, and reach toward and grasp your right knee. If you can't reach your knee, place your right hand on your left hip. Inhale and twist around to the left (figure 19.12). Exhale and relax into the pose, keeping your breath normal and easy. To come out of the pose, inhale and return to your starting position. Gently shake out your legs and repeat the pose on the other side.

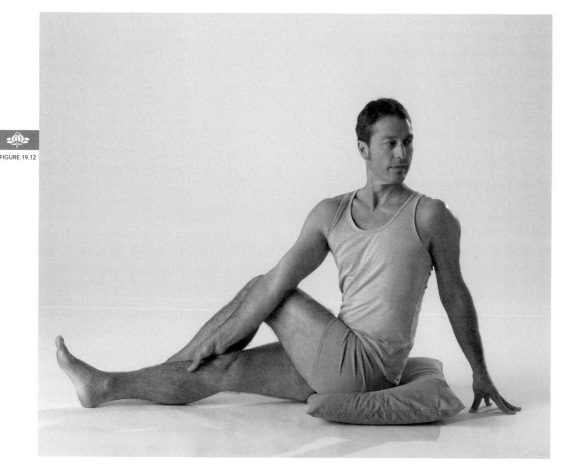

FIGURE 19.12

EXERCISE #16. **YOGIC SEAL POSE (Yoga Mudra), thirty to sixty seconds.** Sit in a comfortable cross-legged position with your eyes closed. Bring your arms behind your back and take hold of your right wrist. Inhale and stretch your arms up. Exhale, extend your chin, and fold your body forward over your legs. When you have come forward as much as you comfortably can, allow your body and head to relax (figure 19.13a). To come out of the pose, inhale, extend your chin, and slowly raise your head and body back to a seated position. As you exhale, bring your palms together at the chest (figure 19.13b), and feel the effects of the yogic seal.

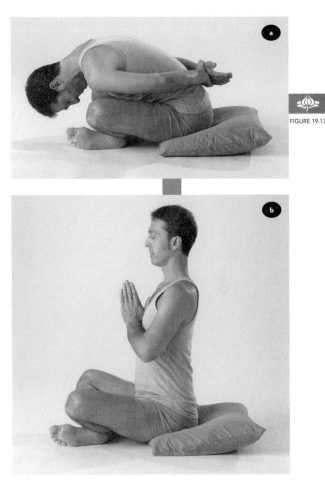

FIGURE 19.13

EXERCISE #17. **RELAXATION POSE (Savasana)/Guided Imagery.** Return to the supine relaxation position described above. When you are settled, observe your body from bottom to top, part by part. Anywhere you notice tension, imagine your breath going there and inducing relaxation. Slowly bring your awareness to the gentle breath as it enters and leaves the body. As it enters, it brings with it oxygen and healing energy. As it leaves, feel yourself letting go of that which you no longer need. Imagine that your entire body is beginning to fill with healing energy, and slowly allow that energy to grow. Gradually begin to deepen the inhalation, and as you do, feel fresh vital energy enter through the top of your head, coming down your face and neck, into the spine and back to the abdomen, into the heart, and down the arms to the hands, the legs to the feet. The whole body fills with fresh, vital, healing energy.

EXERCISE #18. **THREE-PART BREATHING (Dheerga Svasam), three minutes.** Sit on a chair in a comfortable upright position with your eyes closed. Place your right hand on your abdomen, with your thumb resting on your navel and your fingers embracing your belly (figure 19.14).

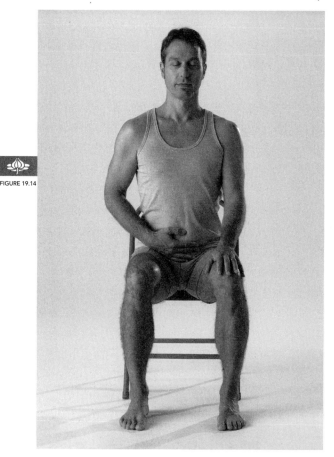

FIGURE 19.14

1. First part: When you are settled, exhale completely through your nose. At the end of the exhalation, gently pull in your abdomen. Begin the inhalation by releasing your abdomen and allowing the lower lungs to fill. Then pull in your abdomen as you exhale. Inhale, expand the abdomen. Exhale, contract the abdomen. Practice this first part of the three-part breath until you feel comfortable with it.

2. Second part: Inhale, expanding the abdomen and then fill the lower ribs. On the exhalation, reverse the order, exhaling from the lower ribs and then the abdomen. Practice the two-part breath until you feel comfortable with it.

3. Third part: After filling the abdomen and lower ribs, inhale into the upper chest, and feel your collarbones rise slightly. On the exhalation, contract the upper chest, the lower chest, and the abdomen, one section following the other. Continue breathing in this manner slowly and deeply.

EXERCISE #19. **ALTERNATE NOSTRIL BREATHING (Nadi Shuddhi), five rounds.** (In many other styles of yoga, this practice is called Nadi Shodhana.) Take the same seated position as in exercise #16. Make a gentle fist with your right hand and then release the

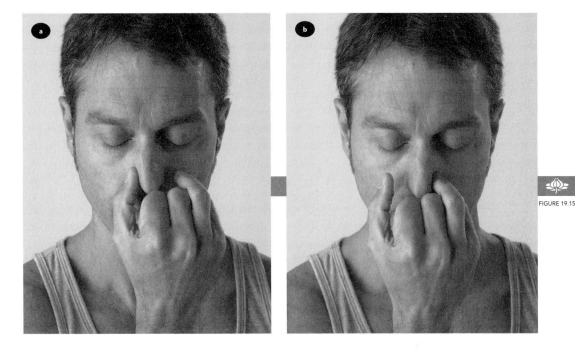

FIGURE 19.15

thumb and the last two fingers. Inhale and then gently close off the right nostril with the thumb (figure 19.15a). Exhale slowly through the left nostril. Inhale deeply through the left nostril, and then gently close off the left nostril with the last two fingers (figure 19.15b). Exhale through the right, inhale through the right and close the right nostril with the thumb. (If holding your hands in this fashion is awkward or uncomfortable, Nischala recommends using any hand position you like to close off the nostrils.) This constitutes one cycle. Repeat one or more times, breathing slowly and deeply. Notice how calm and still the breath and the mind have become, and observe the connection between the two.

EXERCISE #20. **MEDITATION, one or more minutes.** Sitting in your chair or on a pillow, take a comfortable seated position and close your eyes. During the silence, focus the mind on one thing. You may use the breath as you did in Deep Relaxation or just focus on the peace and stillness within. Please check your posture and keep your body still during this entire time. As your body becomes still and quiet, the mind follows. Stay for a minute or longer, building up gradually over time.

Contraindications, Special Considerations, and Modifications

Nischala's program is gentle enough that the risk to heart patients is low. She thinks that more vigorous practices can sometimes be appropriate as long as you build up slowly over time, ideally under the supervision of a skilled teacher. If you have been sedentary, suddenly doing ten Sun Salutations in a row may not be any better an idea than going for a five-mile run. A cardiac-stress test or other tests to evaluate your risk may be appropriate for anyone over fifty (or even younger if you have a number of cardiac risk factors) who plans to begin a vigorous yoga practice.

Other practices that could be too much for heart patients include arm balances, full backbends, and even some of the standing poses, particularly if they are held for a long time or, Nischala says, if done with locked knees (for more on locking the knee, see appendix 1, "Avoiding Common Yoga Injuries"). She says that people with heart disease should "never, ever hold their breath." Vigorous breathing practices like Kapalabhati and Bhastrika are also contraindicated. B. K. S. Iyengar advises against unsupported inversions in

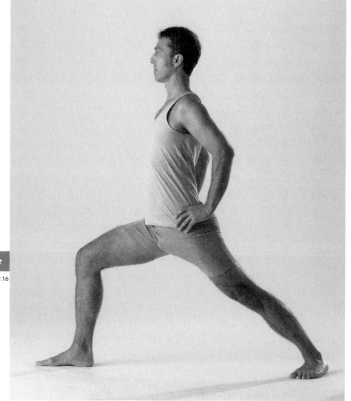

FIGURE 19.16

people with heart disease because he believes that the weight of the abdominal organs puts a strain on the heart. (The modified Shoulderstand Nischala teaches is fine.) He also suggests foregoing long holds of Downward-Facing Dog. Iyengar recommends that heart patients do standing poses like Warrior I with the hands on the hips rather than overhead, to lessen the burden on the heart (figure 19.16). As always, it's not just the poses that are potentially a problem but *how* you do them. Straining or pushing yourself, even in easier poses, invites problems.

For heart patients who have shortness of breath—due to congestive heart failure, for example—Nischala suggests that Deep Relaxation be done with pillows under the upper back and head, aligned in a T shape, and under the knees (figure 19.17a). If you are unable to lie on your back, she suggests the pose be done lying on your right side, with pillows placed under the head, between the arms, and between the knees, which are bent (figure 19.17b). For more marked shortness of breath, she will either prop students up on a number of pillows leaning against a wall or, in even more severe cases, in a chair against a wall.

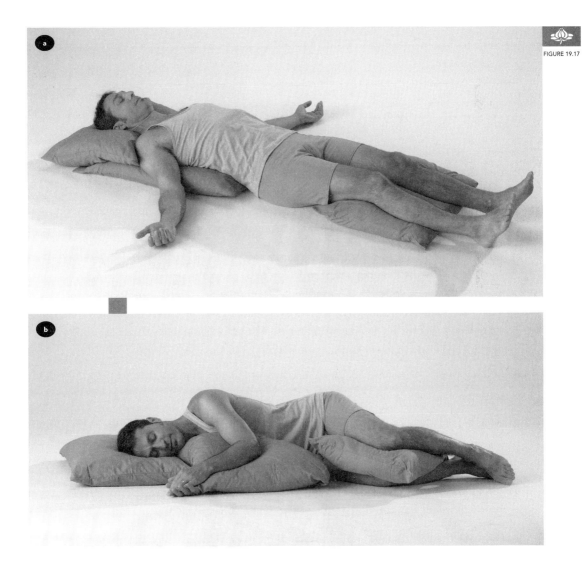

FIGURE 19.17

OTHER YOGIC IDEAS

Restorative chest openers like Bridge pose (Setu Bandha), Reclined Cobbler's pose (Supta Baddha Konasana), and Supported Relaxation pose (Savasana) (see chapter 3) are commonly recommended in Iyengar yoga for the treatment of heart disease. These poses are relaxing, expand the chest, and allow deep breaths to bring oxygen into the system. Although their claims have not been evaluated scientifically, Iyengar yogis believe these poses help the development of collateral blood vessels.

A Holistic Approach to Heart Disease

* Fruits and vegetables are a rich source of healthy phytochemicals, such as bioflavonoids and other antioxidants, which fight heart disease. Bioflavonoids in grapes, grape juice, and wine, especially red wine, as well as in plums, cherries, and blueberries, can help prevent LDL (bad) cholesterol from oxidizing and becoming more dangerous. Antioxidant supplements do not appear to work as well (see chapter 4).

* While low-fat diets can lower cholesterol readings, there is growing evidence that some fats—like the monounsaturated fats in olive oil and the omega-3 fatty acids found in flaxseeds and such fish as salmon, herring, and sardines—are good for the heart. Omega-3 fatty acids fight inflammation and appear to lower the risk for arrhythmias, potentially fatal abnormal rhythms that underlie many cases of sudden death. They also can lower triglyceride levels.

* Nuts and avocados contain heart-healthy fats (though you shouldn't overindulge since they are calorie-rich). Healthy nuts include almonds, pecans, and walnuts.

* While the saturated fats in full-fat dairy products and meats can up your risk, it seems that the "trans" fats—found in some margarines, fried foods, and anything that lists "partially hydrogenated" fat on the label—are even worse.

* Taking low-dose or children's aspirin to thin the blood may lower the risk of a heart attack. Since it's not appropriate for everyone, be sure to talk to your doctor first.

* People with heart disease appear to benefit from getting a flu shot each fall.

* B vitamins, usually included in a multivitamin, may lower the risk for heart disease by dropping the level of a protein called homocysteine, which in recent years has been recognized as an independent risk factor for heart attack.

* The B vitamin niacin, in higher doses, can effectively (and inexpensively) lower LDL (bad) cholesterol and triglyceride levels and boost levels of the HDL (good) cholesterol. Facial flushing, a common side effect, can be diminished by increasing the dose slowly, taking it before bed, and using time-released preparations. Be sure to discuss with your doctor, who will want to check liver function regularly.

* Coenzyme Q10, an antioxidant and natural constituent of human cells, may improve endothelial function (the endothelium is the lining of blood vessels and is crucial in preventing plaque buildup and blood clots). Since some evidence suggests that statins like Lipitor (atorvastatin), Zocor (simvastatin), and Mevacor (lovastatin) lower CoQ10 levels, it may be a particularly good idea for anyone taking these cholesterol-lowering drugs to take CoQ10 as a supplement.

* Not sleeping enough increases the risk of a heart attack (see chapter 23).

* Drinking plenty of fluids throughout the course of the day appears to lower the risk of heart attack, presumably by preventing the increase in clotting that happens with dehydration.

* Fight inflammation of your gums not just by flossing, brushing, and getting regular dental cleanings, but by scraping your tongue daily with a plastic or metal tongue scraper that is available in pharmacies and health food stores.

When Ron began the week-long Ornish program six years ago he was having a lot of angina. He might go through five or six nitroglycerin tablets just warming up to play tennis. After he completed the week-long program, "I didn't feel any big difference physically," he says, "but I did feel a lot more relaxed psychologically. When the program was over, I got one of Nischala's tapes [*Relax, Move & Heal*], and continued the low-fat vegetarian diet." He also began to attend monthly group meetings, which program participants are encouraged to attend.

Once he established a home practice to Nischala's tape every morning, Ron started to notice a huge difference. Nischala says, "Within a few days he couldn't believe how good he felt." Two months after doing the week-long program, his anginal episodes had become so infrequent that he put off having the second angioplasty that had been suggested by his doctors, and he still hasn't needed it.

Although he followed the program's dietary guidelines strictly at first, Ron came to believe that the 10 percent limit on dietary fat was too low in fat for him. "My skin started to dry out; it was peeling all over my face. I needed a little more oil than that." On a trip to rural Japan where food choices were limited, he ended up adding fish, which turned out to be better not only for his skin but for his cholesterol. "My total cholesterol dropped down to 150, which is a very good number." His triglyceride level dropped, too. On the modified diet, however, Ron has gained back most of the fifteen pounds he lost when he started the program.

When he began his home practice, Ron listened to only the first thirty minutes of Nischala's recording (through exercise #16, Yogic Seal pose). Only after three years of doing that was he able to make it through the imagery, meditation, and breathing exercises on the second side of the tape, too. He now does the entire practice every day. Being a typical type A, Ron cautions that most people would find it easier to start with the physical work and only gradually move into the relaxation and breathing work—though he has concluded that the relaxation and breathing have actually been more important to him from a psychological standpoint.

Beyond just improving his heart condition, Ron seems to have developed some of the equanimity that yogis claim is a benefit of the practice. If traffic is tied up on his way to work, it doesn't bother him the way it used to. Now, he says, "If I start to get a little anxious, sitting there in traffic and not moving, I take a couple of real deep breaths and I can reach the point where I can literally relax the muscles in my body." The effects have spilled over into his business as well. "I don't get tight stomach muscle pains because things aren't going my way" in tough negotiations. "If the guy is really hard-nosed, so what? Good luck."

Yoga, he says, "definitely changed my whole personality, my whole character. I stepped off the treadmill." Nonetheless, the essence of the old Ron remains. "I still go to work, and I haven't gotten rid of my type A personality completely. I'm seventy-six and I decided to go back to college." He's studying oceanography and can't keep himself from cramming for the exams to make sure he gets a good grade. Ron has also taken up tap dancing in the last few years, and now gives regular performances. He's still a pitta but he's become a much more sattvic (balanced) one.

HIGH BLOOD PRESSURE

 AADIL PALKHIVALA was seven years old when he began his formal studies with B. K. S. Iyengar in Pune, India. You could say, though, that his first exposure to the master's work was actually in the womb. His mother could not conceive even after seven years of trying, so after exhausting all the medical options, she worked with Iyengar, who developed a special set of practices designed to enable her to conceive and then carry her pregnancy to term. Since Aadil was the result, something seems to have worked! Aadil worked closely with Iyengar throughout his teens, and was certified as a senior teacher of the Iyengar method in his early twenties. Since then he has gone on to study law, naturopathy, Ayurveda, and natural cooking, among a wealth of other interests. His work has been deeply influenced by the Indian spiritual master Sri Aurobindo. Aadil is the founder and director of Yoga Centers as well as the College of Purna Yoga, both in suburban Seattle, and teaches there and internationally.

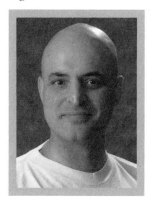

Very early one morning, Dick Hackborn woke up to go to a Microsoft board meeting. When he realized he felt very dizzy and unsteady on his feet, he went back to bed. At 7:00 A.M., he dressed and headed down to the lobby of his hotel, where the staff noticed he wasn't well and called an ambulance. Once he got to the hospital, an emergency CAT scan revealed a small stroke.

At the time of his stroke, Dick was officially retired from a long career at Hewlett-Packard, though that term needs to be qualified. In response to a request from Dave Packard, one of the company's founders, he was serving as chairman of the board of directors, and shortly after he retired, Bill Gates asked him to join the Microsoft board, too. Although he says his board work doesn't involve the same pressure as day-to-day management, it does require long-range strategic thinking—and a lot of hours.

After his stroke, his doctors told him his blood pressure was too high, and he had to get it down. "So I used diet, which was not drastic," he says. "It was just eating healthy food with a good amount of fiber, a lot of vegetables, fruit." As a corporate executive, he'd regularly had business meetings over rich meals at fancy restaurants. In addition, "I started to go to exercise classes three times a week, and would bike and jog in between." With these measures plus a calcium channel blocker, a common type of medication for high blood pressure, he got his upper number, the systolic pressure, down to around 140 (less than 120 is considered normal).

Within a year, he had lost 40 pounds on his new diet and exercise program, and his doctors were able to switch him from the calcium channel blocker to "a diuretic, a water pill, a very small one—it was twelve and a half milligrams of hydrochlorothiazide." Dick was amazed that he had lost the weight so easily. "I wasn't even planning to do it but I got down to my high school weight, which was 180. I'm 6' 1"." Still, his systolic blood pressure wouldn't budge beneath 140.

Next he tried meditation, but that didn't work for him, he says, because he was never able to still his thoughts. He admits that he only gave it a month, which was probably not a fair trial, but he was ready to try the next thing, which turned out to be yoga. His wife had been studying for a couple of years with Camille Thom, who was a student of Aadil Palkhivala. Dick started taking classes with her, and three years later met Aadil when he came to Boise, where Dick lives, to teach a weekend workshop. Afterward, Dick continued to take classes with Camille and practice at home.

Overview of High Blood Pressure

High blood pressure, or hypertension as it's known medically, affects something like one in six people in the Western world, though as many as a third of them are unaware of the problem. When the blood pressure is sky high it can cause symptoms like headaches, but most people have no symptoms whatsoever. The danger of hypertension—and the reason doctors treat it—is the damage it can cause to the body over the long haul. If you think of the heart as a pump and the arteries as something like inner tubes, the higher the pressure, the greater the strain on the pump and the greater the likelihood of getting a blowout.

Among the risks of poorly controlled hypertension are heart attacks, strokes, kidney failure, and even dementia. Much can be done to lower the risk of these problems, but unfortunately, what can be done often isn't. Not only are at least a third of those who have hypertension unaware they have it, only about one-quarter of those who do know keep their blood pressure under good control.

Blood pressure (BP) is typically recorded as two numbers. The top number, the systolic BP, reflects the pressure at the moment when the heart contracts. The diastolic BP, the lower number, is the pressure between beats when the large chambers of the heart relax. This is also the amount of pressure the heart has to overcome to propel blood through the major blood vessels. During my medical education and early years of practice, the focus in treating hypertension was almost entirely on the diastolic pressure. In recent years, however, doctors have come to believe that elevations of the systolic pressure are also worrisome, perhaps even more so than high diastolic BP.

Doctors are continually refining the classification system for hypertension. Recently a panel convened by the US government concluded that optimal BP is under 120/80. From a health standpoint, so long as your pressure is high enough that you don't get light-headed when you stand up, the lower it is the better, because it's easier on your heart and blood vessels.

Keep in mind that blood pressure goes up and down all day long. If you are anxious—as many people are when they go into the doctor's office—that could easily bump your reading by 10 or 20 points. Indeed this phenomenon, known as "white-coat hypertension," leads doctors to prescribe blood pressure medications to some people who don't need them. Similarly, if you are in pain, as people often are when they go to an emergency room or clinic, your BP may be much higher than usual. The more readings you can have done, ideally by taking some measurements yourself at home, the more likely you are to have an accurate representation of your BP.

A number of factors can raise BP, including diet, body weight, and genetic predisposition. Most high blood pressure is what doctors refer to as "essential hypertension," which basically means that your pressure is high but they don't know why. This is distinct from blood pressure that is elevated due to specific conditions like tumors in the brain or adrenal glands, or constriction in the arteries to the kidneys. When there is an underlying cause that can be found—which happens in only a tiny minority of cases—the medical approach is to treat the underlying problem. One sometimes-unrecognized cause of high blood pressure is medication. Pain relievers like ibuprofen and other nonsteroidal anti-inflammatory agents (NSAIDs) can cause a bump in pressure. Thus, using nondrug strategies instead of an NSAID for arthritis and everyday aches and pains may decrease your odds of needing a drug to lower your blood pressure. Birth control pills, steroids like Prednisone, and nasal decongestants can also raise blood pressure.

Repeated readings above 140/90 constitute the typical threshold for the diagnosis of hypertension. Once readings are consistently higher than normal, the rate of complications rises. Some doctors reach for the prescription pad as soon as high BP is discovered, but most experts recommend giving nondrug measures like diet, salt restriction, exercise, and weight loss a chance before resorting to drugs. A major exception to this is when the readings are very high, say 180/110 or over, or when there is already evidence of hypertensive damage to the heart, kidneys, or eyes. If six months to a year of various nondrug approaches doesn't bring your pressure down sufficiently—sooner if your pressure is very high or you have other risk factors for heart attacks and strokes—you may be best off taking medication.

How Yoga Fits In

There are a number of ways in which the practice of yoga can benefit people with hypertension. It is well-known that cardiovascular exercise and the weight loss that often accompanies it can help lower blood pressure. Since a vigorous asana practice, for example a number of repetitions of Sun Salutations, can be intense enough to become aerobic exercise, it therefore has the potential to lower pressure.

Regular yoga practice, whether it's asana, pranayama, chanting, or meditation, can help lower stress levels. Stress can definitely lead to short-term elevations in BP, but what's more controversial is whether sustained stress leads to hypertension. Although most conventional physicians believe there is no clear connection between hypertension and stress, some evidence suggests the link is real. One study, for example, found that people whose bosses were perceived as unfair or unsupportive had higher BP readings. Other studies have found that people with financial worries, long working hours, or high-stress jobs in which they have little autonomy, are more likely to develop high blood pressure. Because of the word *hypertension,* however, some people falsely assume the condition is only about psychological tension. There are plenty of people who are stressed whose BP is fine, and others who seem laid-back but whose BP is dangerously elevated.

There is no controversy about the notion that stress can be a factor in many of the lifestyle choices that raise blood pressure. People under stress are more likely to skip exercise, indulge in unhealthy foods, drink alcohol, or smoke cigarettes, all of which can contribute to increasing blood pressure. Yoga's well-known stress-lowering attributes can help reverse these tendencies and promote healthier lifestyle choices. It also seems that once people experience the natural ease of the body and the peace of mind that a yoga practice promotes, they want to take better care of themselves. Whatever the mechanism, it seems clear that stress reduction through yoga can result in significant improvements in pressure readings—and theoretically in the risk of complications like heart attacks and strokes.

Another aspect of yoga, the emphasis on self-study, svadhyaya, can play a role in controlling hypertension. Checking your BP regularly with a home kit, and attempting to correlate the readings to what else is going on in your life, can help you respond most appropriately. If you keep a log of your readings, make note of the time you took them, your mood, when and what you've eaten, how much sleep you've had, any alcohol or caffeine, and how stressed you feel. Try to figure out if anything in particular seems to raise or lower your readings. Also write down how much yoga or cardiovascular exercise you've done. Looking back over your notebook, you may notice trends that will help you make more informed decisions. You should bring the notebook with you to doctors' visits, and it's a good idea to bring the monitor itself to make sure the readings correlate with the ones taken on the clinic's equipment.

The Scientific Evidence

Two studies examining the effectiveness of yoga as a treatment for high blood pressure were published in the mid-1970s by Dr. Chandra Patel in the British medical journal *The Lancet*. Dr. Patel randomized forty subjects to either three months of yoga relaxation for half an hour three times per week, or to what she called "general relaxation," which consisted of resting on a couch for the same amount of time. The yoga intervention involved lying in Savasana with biofeedback to reinforce relaxation. The intervention was associated with an average 26-point drop in systolic blood pressure and a 15-point drop in diastolic blood pressure after three months of practice, versus a drop of 9 points in the systolic pressure and 2 points in the diastolic pressure for the control group. Follow-up one year later found that in the yoga group, who had been encouraged to maintain the practice, the systolic pressure was still 20 points lower than before the study and the diastolic was 14 points lower. Twelve of the twenty patients in the yoga group were able to reduce their medication requirement by an average of 41 percent, while in the controls there was a slight increase in the need for drugs. Of note, the higher the initial blood pressure, the bigger the drop with yoga. An interesting corollary was that the subjects trained in yogic relaxation sustained less-pronounced bumps in blood pressure in response to emotional or physical stimulation—their nervous systems had become less easily agitated. This is evidence for one of the claimed benefits of yoga: equanimity. Other studies have also documented the blood pressure–lowering effects of Savasana.

A small randomized controlled study, published in the year 2000 in the *Indian Journal of Physiology and Pharmacology*, compared the effects of yoga, drug therapy, and no treatment among thirty-three patients with hypertension. The yoga intervention consisted of Savasana, more active poses, pranayama, and meditation done one hour per day. After eleven weeks the BP among the eleven patients in the yoga group dropped from an average of 156/109 to 123/82. The eleven patients treated with drugs saw their pressure drop from 159/106 to 135/97 on average. The control group went from 155/109 to 151/107 on average, a statistically insignificant change. The yoga group also lost almost seven and a half kilos (over sixteen pounds).

In an attempt to qualify his program for Medicare reimbursement, Dr. Dean Ornish is conducting a demonstration project to show his lifestyle program's cost-effectiveness. Prospective data are being collected on approximately two thousand people with heart disease who have been enrolled in the program, which includes asana, pranayama, meditation, walking, group meetings, and a low-fat vegetarian diet (see chapter 19). Participants experienced statistically significant reductions in both systolic and diastolic BP. After twelve weeks on the program, the systolic pressure dropped from an average of 150 to about 136, while diastolic dropped from an average of about 86 to 78. Still larger drops were evident after one year, though at the time of this writing, not all of the patients being studied had completed a full year in the program.

Transcendental Meditation (TM), a type of mantra meditation, was shown in a 1996 randomized controlled study, published in the journal *Hypertension*, to significantly lower blood pressure in older African-Americans. At the end of the three-month trial, compared with those in the control group, the women practicing TM had a 10-point drop in systolic BP and 6 points in diastolic, and the men dropped almost 13 points in systolic BP and 8 in diastolic. Another randomized controlled study of TM on African-American teenagers at risk of developing hypertension, published in 2004, found reductions in both systolic and diastolic BP.

Devices that slow down breathing, mimicking pranayama techniques, have been shown to lower blood pressure even in those with "resistant" hypertension (BP greater than 140/90 despite taking three or more drugs at maximal dosage). One study of seventeen patients found that simply using one such device for fifteen minutes a day reduced blood pressure measurements by almost 13 points systolic and almost 7 diastolic. More than half of the poorly controlled hypertensives came under an acceptable degree of BP control by doing this breathing practice fifteen minutes per day for eight weeks, making no other changes in their lives. None of the patients suffered any negative side effects. Of note, the higher the blood pressure at the start, the greater the response to the simulated pranayama.

Aadil Palkhivala's Approach

From his perspective as a yoga teacher and a naturopath, Aadil believes that high blood pressure can be divided into two major categories (see table 20.1). "One is when the nervous system is exhausted and therefore jittery," he says. The person with this kind of high blood pressure is the type "who is overworked, who is rushing around all the time, who is brushing his teeth while driving his car." The second category includes those who are, metaphorically speaking, stuck; for example, somebody who is working in a small office with nowhere to go, or someone mired "in a frustrating relationship," who sees no other options. In these people, according to Aadil, "the nervous system is building up energy," and the blood pressure rises as a result. "There are of course multitudes of other reasons" for hypertension, he says, but he finds it useful to make this distinction in his therapeutic work.

Aadil notices physical differences in the two major types of high blood pressure. In the person who is rushing around, he says, "the eyes bulge out slightly. The body trembles almost imperceptibly. It is like somebody who has had too much coffee. Their actions are jittery." In contrast, "the person who is pent up internally" holds "a lot of tension in the jaw and in the neck," especially the muscles that extend from the neck to the shoulder blades, "which become hard and rocklike." In addition to these muscles, which are readily visible, Aadil finds that "internal muscles start to tighten up, trying to protect the body, as it were, from inside." Among these are the psoas deep in the abdomen and the erector muscles that run along either side of the spine in the back. "Those muscles," he says, "start to become very tight very early."

TABLE 20.1 TWO MAJOR CATEGORIES OF HYPERTENSION AS CONCEPTUALIZED BY AADIL PALKHIVALA

"JITTERY" HIGH BLOOD PRESSURE	"PENT-UP" HIGH BLOOD PRESSURE
Overworked, under pressure	Metaphorically "stuck," frustrated
Constant motion, multitasking	Less motion, appearance of calmness
Slight trembling	Muscle tightness
Eyes bulge out slightly, and muscles around eyes are tense	Eyes appear droopy, sunken
Nervous system "exhausted"	Nervous system "pressurized"

When it comes to yoga, Aadil believes that the two categories of high blood pressure should be treated differently. "The person who is exhausted from running around has to be given the slower, restorative postures, including some restorative inversions." The person who has pent-up pressure from inside has to do a more dynamic practice, which might include a number of standing poses and Sun Salutations. Aadil considers jumping from pose to pose contraindicated in people with high blood pressure.

In Aadil's treatment of hypertension, breath plays a critical role, because putting emphasis on the exhalation tends to lower stress levels by shifting the balance of the autonomic (involuntary) nervous system toward the restorative parasympathetic side, and away from the "fight or flight" sympathetic side (see chapter 3). Aadil spends a lot of time teaching students how to release tension from the body by using the exhalation, specifically asking them to extend the exhalation relative to the inhalation throughout their asana practice.

Although Aadil does not recommend formal pranayama to students with hypertension who, like Dick, are beginners, one natural way to extend the exhalation is chanting mantras, a yogic tool that Aadil has found particularly useful for people with high blood pressure. He says that "repeated chanting in a low pitch, in a soft melody, goes deep into the nerves and soothes them as the vibrations of the sound penetrate the body." In particular, he recommends mantras like "Om" and the Gayatri, one of the most ancient and famous of yogic chants. While chanting Om, Aadil suggests extending the "mmm" sound to facilitate relaxation of the nervous system and the mind.

"When I first saw Dick in class," Aadil says, "I noticed that he was extremely tight everywhere." This pattern of muscular tension and a lack of trembling, jitteriness, or bulging in his eyes put Dick into the category of "pent-up" high blood pressure. Aadil says Dick was very bright in the eyes, and paid close attention, but though he tried very hard, he simply had difficulty moving his body. Aadil suspects that the tightness could be a reflection of the high-stress environment Dick worked in for so many years, while striving to remain calm and dignified, and always in control of himself.

Aadil believes that there may be a connection between tightness in the muscles and ligaments like Dick had and hypertension. Aadil says, "It's very rare for me to find a very supple body with high blood pressure." The reason, he suspects, is purely anatomical— tight muscles exert pressure on arteries, creating more resistance to blood flow. If this speculation turns out to be true, asanas as well as massage and other forms of bodywork might have a direct effect on lowering blood pressure.

TIP When doing the exercises below, Aadil recommends using gentle Ujjayi style breathing (see pp. 16–17). He describes this as "full, deep breaths with a soft Ujjayi breathing, with a soft, sibilant 's' sound on the inhalation and an 'h' sound on the exhalation." He does not, however, recommend that anyone with hypertension do the more exaggerated style of Ujjayi found in some styles of yoga. He suggests that students eventually learn to make their exhalations twice as long as their inhalations, which makes the practice more relaxing and meditative, as long as they are never straining for breath. If a person typically inhales for four seconds, for example, Aadil suggests making the exhalation five seconds, and then six seconds, and so on, over the next few months.

Aadil recommends that all his students begin their practices with three brief sequences of poses to warm up.

1. Opening Series—seven seated poses for releasing the stress in the spine. For the first six poses you sit in Virasana, placing your arms in various positions including Prayer pose, stretched overhead with the fingers interlaced, intertwined with the palms facing each other in Eagle pose (Garudasana), and catching the hands behind your back—one coming from above, the other from below—in Cow Face pose (Gomukhasana). The series also includes a seated twist (Parsva Virasana), Staff pose (Dandasana), and Cobbler's pose (Baddha Konasana).

2. Morning Series—nine reclining poses to open and release tension in the back side of the body, from the feet to the head. The series begins and ends with a full body stretch, lying on your back with your arms alongside your ears and your palms facing upward. Also included are ankle stretches and rotations, twists to both sides, Knee to Chest pose, done first one leg at a time, and then with both knees simultaneously, and Supine Hand to Foot pose (Supta Padangusthasana), holding a strap around the ball of the foot of the raised leg when necessary (see p. 163).

3. Hip Opening Series—six reclining poses to open up the hips that begins with Supine Hand to Foot pose as above, next brings the raised leg across the midline, and then out to the side. Next come supine poses that internally and then externally rotate the thigh bones in the hip sockets. Finally, the front of the thigh is stretched by lying back with one leg in the Virasana position and the other knee bent with the foot flat on the floor.

After doing these three series, Aadil suggests moving into standing poses. The sequence of poses and instructions that Aadil suggested for Dick is below. As you'll see in the directions, Aadil uses props liberally, especially with a student like Dick, who is limited in flexibility. The props allow the body to be better aligned in the pose, for maximum benefit.

EXERCISE #1. **TRIANGLE POSE (Trikonasana), with a block, three to nine breaths.**
Stand with your legs three and a half to four feet apart, with your feet facing forward. Raise your arms to your sides at shoulder height, with your palms down. Turn your left foot in about 15 degrees. Moving from the hip joint, rotate your right leg out 90 degrees. Press

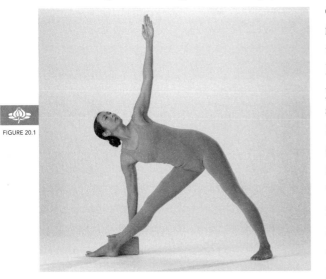

FIGURE 20.1

evenly into the four corners of your feet and use your quadriceps muscles in the front of your thigh to lift your kneecaps up. On an exhalation, tilt your pelvis to the right to bring your spine over your right leg and your right hand onto a block and lift your left arm (figure 20.1). Feel your feet root into the floor with each exhalation, releasing tension into the earth. Stay for three to nine breaths, and then as you inhale, reverse your movements to come out of the pose as you came in. Repeat the pose on the other side.

EXERCISE #2. **SIDE ANGLE POSE (Utthita Parsvakonasana), modified, three to nine breaths.** Stand with your feet five to five and a half feet apart, with your feet facing forward. Raise your arms to your sides, and turn your left foot in and right leg out, as de-

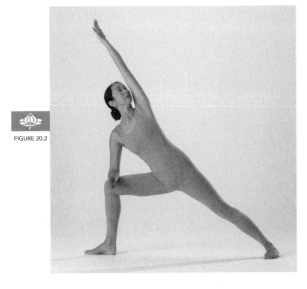

FIGURE 20.2

scribed for Triangle pose. On an exhalation, bend your right leg to a 90-degree angle, and then tilt your pelvis to the right. Rather than bringing your hand down to the floor, do the pose with your right elbow bent, resting on your thigh. With the top of the forearm on your thigh, let the thumb side of your wrist face the ceiling (figure 20.2). Stretch the left side of the body from the waist to the fingertips and from the waist to the outer edge of the left foot. Stay for three to nine breaths, and then inhale as you reverse the steps to come out of the pose. Repeat on the other side.

EXERCISE #3. **HALF STANDING FORWARD BEND (Ardha Uttanasana), against the wall, three to nine breaths.** Stand with your feet hips' distance apart and three to four feet from a wall. On an exhalation, fold forward from your hips and place your hands, with the fingers facing up, on the wall (figure 20.3). The stiffer you are, the closer to the wall you need to stand and the higher up the wall you'll need to place your hands. Grounding your feet and pressing your hands into the wall, try to lengthen the sides of the body. Relax your neck and breathe deeply, grounding the feet into the floor during the exhalations. Stay for three to nine breaths, and then walk in toward the wall to come out of the pose.

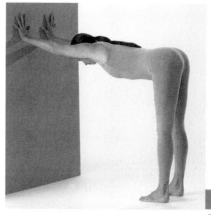

FIGURE 20.3

For students with hypertension, Aadil always substitutes Half Standing Forward Bend for Downward-Facing Dog pose because, he explains, "With hypertension, I don't want to bring the head below the diaphragm." One exception he often uses in students with high blood pressure is Downward-Facing Dog with the head supported and a wrap around the head. He suggests wrapping the head while still standing erect, and removing the wrap after coming out of the pose (see below).

EXERCISE #4. **SIDE STRETCH POSE (Parsvottanasana), against the wall, three to nine breaths.** Stand in Mountain pose a few feet from a wall (the stiffer you are, the closer to the wall you will need to stand). Step your right leg forward toward the wall and your left leg back so your feet are about four feet apart. Angle your back foot in deeply but keep

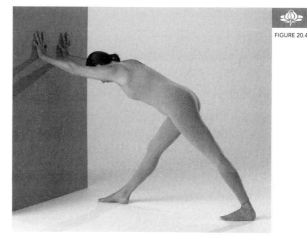

FIGURE 20.4

your hips parallel to the wall. On an exhalation, fold forward from the hips and place your hands on the wall as in the previous pose (figure 20.4). If your hamstrings are tight, move your front foot closer to the wall, with your trunk angling upward, hands higher than your pelvis. Stay for three to nine breaths, breathing deeply, grounding the feet into the floor during the exhalations, then step forward with the back foot and come out of the pose. Repeat on the other side.

EXERCISE #5. **WARRIOR II POSE (Virabhadrasana II), three to nine breaths.** Stand with your feet facing forward, five to five and a half feet apart. Raise your arms to your

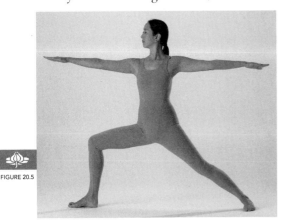

FIGURE 20.5

sides and turn your left foot in and right leg out, as in Triangle pose. Exhale and bend your right knee to a 90-degree angle. Keep pressing into your left heel and reach the left arm strongly back to help keep the spine upright. Drop your shoulder blades down and relax your neck and face. Direct your gaze beyond the middle finger of your right hand (figure 20.5). Stay for three to nine breaths and inhale to come out. Repeat on the other side.

EXERCISE #6. **SEATED TWIST (Bharadvajasana I), three to nine breaths.** Start by sitting on the floor on a folded blanket or other support so the top of your sacrum (the triangular bone at the base of the spine that fits into the back of the pelvis) does not tip backward. The more inflexible you are, the more height you'll need. Extend both legs straight in front of you. Now, bend your knees and bring both feet alongside your right hip, and rest the front of your right ankle in the arch of your left foot. Place both hands behind you (on props the same height as the props you are sitting on) and press them into the floor to help elevate your spine. Reach your left arm behind your back and catch your right biceps muscle near the elbow (figure 20.6a), and on an exhalation, twist to the left. If you are not able to do this, place a strap around the bottom of the biceps and use your right hand to catch the strap from the back (figure 20.6b). Then bring your right hand to the

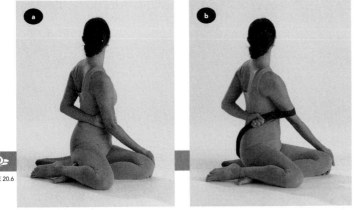

FIGURE 20.6

outside of your left knee. If it is not possible for the right hand to hold the left knee, place a second strap around that knee and hold the end with your right hand. Stay three to nine breaths, and then release your hands and return to center. Swing your legs to the other side and repeat the pose.

EXERCISE #7. **SEATED TWIST (Marichyasana I), three to nine breaths.** Start by sitting on the floor on a folded blanket or other support so the top of your sacrum does not tip backward. Extend both legs straight in front of you. Now, bend your right leg and place the sole of your right foot in front of your right buttock, with the knee straight up. Place the left fingertips on the floor near your left buttock, and pushing down, lengthen the spine. Reach forward with your right hand toward your left foot, and then internally rotate the arm starting at the shoulder blade so that the palm ends up facing the ceiling and your inner elbow faces the floor. Slowly bend the right elbow, wrapping it around the

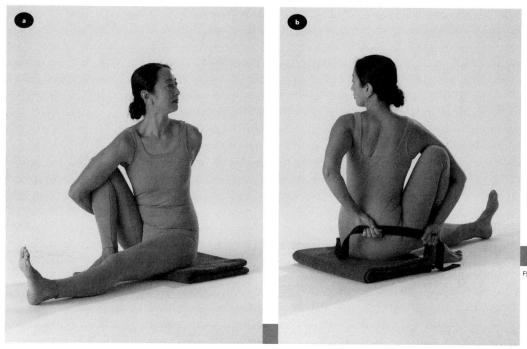

FIGURE 20.7

right leg. Inhaling, lift the sides of the waist as you wrap the left arm behind you, holding the left wrist with the right hand (figure 20.7a). If you cannot reach the wrist, interlock your fingers behind your back, and if that's also not possible, hold a strap with both hands (figure 20.7b). Stay three to nine breaths. Repeat on the opposite side.

TIP "Without Savasana," Aadil says, "the practice of asana is not meaningful. Savasana pulls it all together." For the same reason, he also likes to pause between the poses, not just jump from one to the other, so students can breathe and feel the effect of the pose they have just done.

EXERCISE #8. RELAXATION POSE (Savasana), thirty-six breaths. Lie on your back with your legs stretched out in front of you and your arms at your sides. Place support under your head so that your forehead is not sloping backward (figure 20.8). Allow your legs to fall open and turn your palms up, with your arms a comfortable distance from your body. When you are settled, begin to focus on your breath. For eighteen breaths, make your exhalations slightly longer than your inhalations. For another eighteen breaths, simply observe your breath without trying to change it in any way. Throughout this posture, visualize your body relaxing and melt all your tension into the earth. Let each exhalation be a cue for the body to surrender its hidden clenchings, to unwind, to let go.

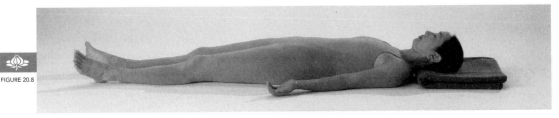

FIGURE 20.8

OTHER YOGIC IDEAS

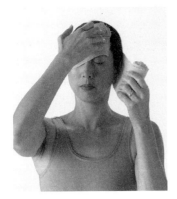

The head wrap is a tool that Aadil often uses with students with high blood pressure, particularly those of the "jittery type," since their focus is too much on the external world. (See chapter 18 for more on the head wrap, also known as an eye bandage.) Aadil suggests wrapping it clockwise in a crisscross pattern (see left), over the bridge of the nose, so as to not put pres-

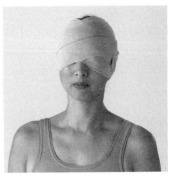

sure on the septum (the cartilage that separates the two sides of the nose). Wearing the head wrap tends to keep the attention inward, an exercise in pratyahara (see chapter 3). Aadil also believes that "it prevents the pressure from building up inside the head" in various poses (see figure at right).

Contraindications, Special Considerations, and Modifications

If you begin a yoga practice after learning that your blood pressure is elevated, in general you want to err on the side of caution. Any form of exercise tends to lower BP over the long run, but blood pressure can rise while actually doing the exercise. Asana such as backbends, inversions, and arm balances are particularly likely to increase BP, as are difficult postures, such as the Warrior poses, especially when held for a long period of time. In fact, any yoga practice, even something as theoretically relaxing as a seated forward bend, can raise your blood pressure if you are uncomfortable or struggling with the pose. Carefully monitoring yourself as you practice is the best way to detect problems. If your breath is smooth and even, and you feel at ease, your blood pressure is likely to be stable.

> **CAUTION** In any posture, avoid what's known as the Valsalva maneuver—holding your breath and bearing down as you would to pass a bowel movement—as doing so can cause a major spike in BP.

A BP under 170/110 with no evidence of what doctors call "end-organ damage," such as thickening of the heart or changes in the retina, is not considered a contraindication to exercise. If the blood pressure is controlled with medication, doctors generally place no restrictions on physical activity, but yogis like Aadil are more conservative. Aadil has often observed that students whose hypertension is controlled with drugs have an exaggerated response to poses like arm balances and backbends, developing trembling or mental agitation much more readily than those with normal BP. Some of his more experienced students have developed the sensitivity to pick up such symptoms early on and regulate their practices accordingly, by coming out of the pose or avoiding it entirely.

Some BP medications can cause brief periods of light-headedness when rising to a standing or sitting position after lying down. Slowing down the transitions to allow time to adjust is often all that is needed to avoid any mishaps.

The higher your BP, the riskier it is to go upside down into inverted postures like Handstand, Headstand, and Shoulderstand. Blood tends to pool in the head and the pressure can build up, possibly increasing the risk of a stroke. In general, the closer the inversion is to straight upside-down, the greater the effect on blood pressure. Thus, because the legs are directly over the head in Headstand, it is likely to cause more buildup of pressure than Legs-Up-the-Wall (Viparita Karani), in which the legs and torso extend upward at an angle.

For someone with hypertension, says Aadil, it is best not to do inversions in a yoga class. One exception he makes is Downward-Facing Dog done with the thighs supported by wall ropes, and the head resting on a bolster or other props. It's even more relaxing, Aadil finds, if you do it while wearing a head wrap. For students who don't have access to a ropes setup, you can improvise at home using a strap and a door (see p. 448 for more details).

Though inversions tend to raise blood pressure while you are doing them, a regular practice of inversions may actually lower it over time. Pressure sensors in the aorta and carotid arteries are stimulated when you are upside down, and a number of hormonal changes result that tend to reduce BP in the long term. However, if your blood pressure is not well controlled (or if you show any signs of jitteriness or agitation), you should avoid inversions, even mild ones like simple standing forward bends and Downward-Facing Dog. Once your pressure is under reasonable control, it's probably safe to slowly introduce inversions, building up to longer holds and more complete inversions like Handstand and Headstand slowly over a period of months. If at any point you find yourself straining or your breath becomes uneven or forced, come right out of the pose and rest in Child's pose, Savasana, or another relaxing position. If your face turns red during inversions, this may be a sign that you should come out of the pose. However, while facial flushing can be a sign of elevated BP, some people always have this response, even when they can do the pose comfortably and safely. If you're in doubt, ask an experienced teacher to check you out while you do the pose.

Aadil believes that gentle Ujjayi (done during asana as discussed above or as pranayama) and Bhramari, the "Bee Breath," in which you make a buzzing sound on the exhalation (see p. 16) are very beneficial and soothing for hypertension and can help reduce blood pressure. He recommends against "heating practices" like Bhastrika or Kapalabhati, or any pranayama that involves breath-holding.

A Holistic Approach to High Blood Pressure

✳ Blood pressure often starts to rise in middle age when people start putting on weight. Losing even a few pounds can make a significant difference in BP.

✳ Regular exercise lowers BP by itself and combined with reducing calories can help with weight loss.

✳ Eating lots of fruits and vegetables, low-fat dairy products, whole grains, and other high-fiber foods like beans not only helps keep weight off, but it provides a number of vitamins and minerals that studies show reduce blood pressure. These include potassium, magnesium, calcium, and vitamin C (supplements may help, too, though evidence for them is weaker).

* Food high in phytoestrogens, such as soy products, also seem beneficial.

* Other factors that can improve blood pressure include not smoking, limiting alcohol consumption, and cutting back on caffeine.

* About 40 percent of people with high blood pressure are "salt-sensitive," meaning that eating too much of it can raise their blood pressure. African-Americans, people with diabetes, and the elderly are most likely to be affected by dietary salt.

* The choice of medication for people with high blood pressure that has not responded fully to such lifestyle changes as diet and exercise is controversial. One major study found that the old standby water pills, which cost pennies a pill, may be more effective in preventing long-term complications than the newer, more highly promoted alternatives like calcium channel blockers.

From the first time he tried yoga, Dick enjoyed it. He even found he could completely let go during Savasana. And that first class had immediate results. When he went home and took his blood pressure, he found it was 120/60, the lowest reading he'd had since he started keeping track of it after his mini-stroke the preceding January, about three months earlier.

Dick was so pleased with the results that he continued with yoga, and over time the benefits appear to have increased. At his most recent checkup, his BP was 108/60 and his physician is now contemplating discontinuing his medication entirely. Dick says he now practices yoga at home three times per week. He does a number of standing poses and regularly does the supported Downward-Facing Dog that Aadil recommends, which he particularly enjoys.

A couple of years after Dick started yoga, he and his wife made a radical decision. Rather than keep all their money for themselves or pass it on to their children, they started a family foundation. (The kids not only approved, by the way; they're involved in the work.) The foundation funds projects in four categories: the arts, special education, local environmental protection, and what they call "people in need," supporting among other causes the Idaho Food Bank. "It's a small foundation but it does good work, and it's really enjoyable being involved." Dick says you just feel better about yourself when you know you're making a difference in people's lives. Without using the words, what he's talking about is service, also known as karma yoga. Whether or not it had anything to do with his and his wife's yoga practice, yogis will tell you that feeling greater compassion for others and wanting to help them is one of the fruits of a steady yoga practice.

In the meantime, Dick is still on Hewlett-Packard's board, and even there he finds that the benefits of yoga are creeping in. When he's at board meetings, "which tend to last the better part of a day and get pretty intense," he'll quietly get up, "go to the back of the room, and do one of the yoga positions where you put your palms together behind your back, and move them up your back." Nobody pays any attention, Dick says, though, "a couple of the women on the board do yoga, so they know what I'm doing." He's found doing it helps him stay calm. "I can relax, feel good, come back, and therefore get involved in the discussion and tone things down for other people as well. It's a fantastic experience. It really is."

HIV/AIDS

 SHANTI SHANTI KAUR KHALSA describes her decision to work with people with AIDS in the mid-1980s as "a calling within a calling," one her guru, Yogi Bhajan, encouraged at every step. "I knew that I needed to be a yoga teacher when I had my first yoga class, and later realized that I needed to do this," she says, although "it was difficult to find places to teach, because people didn't want people with HIV in their building. They didn't want them using their toilets. It was a challenging time." She felt compelled to teach this vilified population after experiencing a "strong, palpable sense" that this was to be her work while attending a celebration for Guru Ram Das, a sixteenth-century Sikh (whom she describes as the "patron saint" of Kundalini yoga). "We all get messages from inside," she says. "Sometimes we listen to them and sometimes we ignore them. But I said yes to this one, and I'm grateful because it brought me into a much deeper sense of my practice and who I am and what I'm on the planet for." Shanti Shanti Kaur holds a PhD in health psychology, and is the founder and director of the Guru Ram Das Center for Medicine and Humanology in Espanola, New Mexico, a nonprofit organization dedicated to serving those with chronic or life-threatening illnesses, conducting research on the medical effects of Kundalini yoga, and training health care professionals to use it in their practice. Her PhD thesis was on using meditation

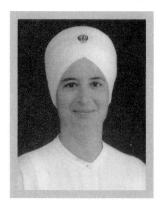

to facilitate healthy behavioral changes in people who are HIV positive. She teaches yoga to people with HIV, a class for people with diabetes, and one for women with breast cancer at the Guru Ram Das Center, and conducts teacher-training workshops internationally.

Jeremy Clark (not his real name) was in his mid-thirties when he first met Shanti Shanti Kaur Khalsa at an event in Los Angeles that author Louise Hay had organized for people with HIV and AIDS. Shanti Shanti Kaur gave a presentation on how Kundalini yoga can help the immune system. She then led the participants through a twenty-minute experience that included breathing, chanting, and physical movements designed to increase lymphatic circulation, as well as meditation and relaxation, all done while sitting in their chairs. Afterward Jeremy felt so good that he decided to ask her to work with him.

Jeremy, who was HIV positive at the time he attended that event in 1987, had been one of the first members of the gay community to get tested for HIV, almost as soon as the test became available. Since there was no effective treatment at the time, many gay men had agonized over whether to be tested, but Jeremy didn't hesitate. He was part of a community that was organized and that fought for early clinical trials of medications.

When Jeremy and Shanti Shanti Kaur began working together, his T-cell count was in the teens (normal is 450 to 1,150), a very low number of these vital immune cells, and for much of the time they worked together it was 0. He must have had some T cells, Shanti Shanti Kaur says, but they were not measurable. "It taught me that T-cell counts alone are not an adequate measure of how someone's doing." She assumes he also had a high viral load, but doctors didn't have a way to measure that then. (Today, monitoring the viral load—the number of copies of the HIV virus circulating in the blood—is one of the principal ways doctors make decisions about treatment.) Although Jeremy looked very healthy when he started working with Shanti Shanti Kaur, he had unexplained fevers and recurring thrush, a fungal infection of the throat. He did not, however, have what was called "an AIDS-defining diagnosis," an opportunistic infection or AIDS-related cancer that signifies the transition from being HIV positive to having AIDS.

Overview of HIV/AIDS

From its discovery in the early 1980s when gay men in Los Angeles and a few other major cities started coming down with unusual infections and cancers, acquired immune deficiency syndrome (AIDS) elicited near panic on the part of the general public. Scientists' suspicion that AIDS was caused by a virus was eventually confirmed when researchers isolated and identified the human immunodeficiency virus (HIV) in 1983.

HIV weakens the body's immune system by destroying T cells, specifically CD_4 lymphocytes, a type of white blood cell that normally helps protect against bacteria, viruses, and some cancers. When the T-cell count is low, the body becomes vulnerable to a wide range of assaults that a normal immune system can effectively withstand. Without treatment, over time the CD_4 count tends to drop lower and lower, putting people with HIV at ever greater risk. Unchecked, HIV can cause neurological damage as well as drastic weight loss, and can ultimately lead to death.

> **CAUTION** An estimated 25 percent of the people infected with HIV in the United States have not been tested (and the numbers may be much higher in other areas of the world). Those at greatest risk of not knowing their HIV status include minorities and people who are infected via heterosexual sex. Since it may be highly beneficial to begin drug treatment before your immune system has been severely compromised, waiting for your first overwhelming infection to get tested is a very bad idea.

For many years, doctors struggled to find effective medications. In 1995 the first of a variety of "highly active" antiretroviral drug combinations that worked on HIV (which is a retrovirus) finally became available. These multidrug regimens radically changed the prognosis for millions of people with the disease. Many who would likely have already died without the drugs have returned to good health. For these people, dealing with the side effects of the medications, which can be significant, has become a bigger day-to-day issue than staying alive. However, for those who cannot afford drug treatment, which typically costs tens of thousands of dollars a year, the situation is still dire. Into this less fortunate group fall most of the infected people in the developing world.

> **TIP** Because the use of drugs is constantly evolving, HIV is one disease where it's important to choose a physician who keeps up-to-date. One study found that patients treated by doctors with fewer than five HIV patients had twice the mortality rate of those treated by doctors with a larger number of HIV patients. The right doctor isn't necessarily a specialist in infectious diseases. What's important is that the doctor puts in the effort to track advances in this constantly changing field.

How Yoga Fits In

Since anything that can increase the effectiveness of the immune system has the potential to limit the damage the AIDS virus will cause, yoga can help people with HIV in several ways. The practice of yoga appears to improve immune function in part by lowering levels of the stress hormone cortisol (see chapter 3), and yoga asana may boost immunity by improving the circulation of lymph, a fluid rich in disease-fighting white blood cells like lymphocytes. Yoga also encourages healthy behavioral change, which can counteract the tendency of people under stress to eat poorly, get too little sleep, and be less than meticulous in following the kind of complicated drug regimens often necessary to protect the health of those who are HIV positive—all behaviors that can further compromise immunity and put them at risk of progressing to AIDS.

Yoga is an excellent remedy for depression (see chapter 15), which is a huge problem for people with HIV. Not only can depression lower your quality of life, but like stress it can adversely affect immunity, lead to unhealthy lifestyle choices, and result in failure to take needed medication as directed, undermining effectiveness and potentially contributing to the development of drug-resistant viruses. The community, or sangha, found in yoga centers and classes can diminish the sense of isolation some people with HIV feel, and help boost mood.

Since highly active antiretroviral medications have greatly diminished the death rate from HIV but can cause a variety of side effects, people who carry the infection need to think of long-term health in a way people early in the epidemic didn't need to. Yoga is perhaps the best overall system of preventive medicine there is. One particular area of concern is that drugs used to treat HIV can adversely affect blood fats, increase abdominal fat deposits, and make the body more resistant to the effects of insulin, all of which increase the risk of heart disease. Yoga can help reduce that heightened risk (see chapter 19).

The increased internal awareness that comes from yoga practice can help with the detection of a variety of infections, allowing your doctors to prescribe medications when they are most likely to be effective. This same awareness can help detect possible side effects from medications, as we saw in chapter 4, when Dolores was able to notice early signs of a fat maldistribution problem, a common side effect of HIV medication, before any serious damage had been done.

The Scientific Evidence

There is preliminary scientific evidence that suggests that mindfulness-based stress reduction (MBSR), which includes meditation practice as well as yoga asana and relaxation, may improve immune function in people infected with HIV. A study of subjects on HIV medications found that twenty-four who were on an eight-week mindfulness program more than doubled the number of natural killer (NK) cells, compared with a control group of ten who showed no change. NK cells help fight viral opportunistic infections in people with HIV, and their numbers tend to decrease as HIV disease progresses. In people who are otherwise healthy, MBSR appears to improve the ability to make antibodies in response to a vaccine (see p. 32). Preliminary evidence also suggests that a long-term practice of MBSR confers greater benefits than a short-term one.

Cognitive-behavioral stress management (CBSM), consisting of relaxation, group support, and instruction in coping strategies, has been shown to lower levels of stress hormones and positively affect mood, anxiety, anger, and levels of some types of immune cells in people with HIV/AIDS. The types of relaxation used in CBSM are varied, including such techniques from the yoga toolbox as guided imagery, deep breathing, and mindfulness meditation. One small study suggested that the yogic tool of imagery could affect the functioning of the immune system. Recently a small randomized controlled trial, led by Dr. Michael Antoni of the University of Miami, found that a ten-week program of CBSM was associated with a greater than threefold decrease in HIV viral load in gay men whose HIV levels were detectable at the beginning of the study, as well as improvements in mood.

A randomized controlled study on using yoga for stress and depression for people with HIV was presented at the 2006 North American Research Conference on Complementary and Integrative Medicine. The study, conducted by Dr. Frederick Hecht of the Osher Center for Integrative Medicine at the University of California, San Francisco, in conjunction with researchers at the Swami Vivekananda Yoga Research Foundation near Bangalore, compared an integrated yoga program that included asana, pranayama, and meditation to a wait-list control. The twenty-three people in the yoga group had hour-long classes three days per week, and were encouraged to practice at home. After three months, as compared to the twenty-five controls, the yoga group had a slightly lower HIV viral load, a higher CD_4 T-cell count, less stress, less anxiety, and improvements in mood, though only the last reached the level of statistical significance. The researchers noted, however, that if the observed differences in the CD_4 count between the yoga group and controls were sustained, it could slow the progression of the disease.

Shanti Shanti Kaur Khalsa's Approach

When Jeremy came for his first lesson, Shanti Shanti Kaur says, he was not visibly ill. "He looked great. He was athletic, and he took really good care of himself." Although Jeremy could have attended Shanti Shanti Kaur's group classes, as did his partner, Mark (also a pseudonym), he preferred to work with her privately.

In both her group and private classes, Shanti Shanti Kaur has her students begin by chanting the mantra "Ong Namo Guru Dev Namo." To do this, you sit in a comfortable cross-legged position with your hands in Prayer position, thumbs pressing into the breast bone. Close your eyes and focus your attention on the area between your eyebrows. You can either chant the entire mantra on a single exhalation or, if that's not possible, take a half breath in after the "Ong Namo." The "Dev" is chanted a minor third higher than the other sounds. Teachers instruct students to chant the entire mantra three or more times, noticing the vibration of the sounds in the skull, throat, and chest.

After Jeremy chanted the mantra, he did a warm-up, consisting of breathing and movement practices which varied, depending on whether Shanti Shanti Kaur felt he needed help with detoxification, building vitality, or becoming calmer (if he was in an anxious state). Following the warm-up there would be a brief Savasana, typically for three minutes.

In Kundalini yoga as taught by Yogi Bhajan's students, each practice centers around a "kriya," a word that has numerous meanings in the yoga world, but is used in this system of yoga to mean a "completed action," or, as Shanti Shanti Kaur puts it, "a sequence that leads to a certain result." Each kriya is taught exactly the way that Yogi Bhajan taught it to his students, and every element of the kriya has a specified duration. If necessary, the teacher may cut the time of each element of the kriya by a certain set fraction, for example, by a third or half, as you would reduce all the ingredients in a recipe if you wanted to make a smaller amount than the recipe called for.

The kriya Shanti Shanti Kaur chose for Jeremy is what they call "Massage for the Lymphatic System." She describes this as an intermediate to advanced program, difficult enough to cause most people to break into a sweat. Due to Jeremy's generally good health, it was appropriate for him. However, during Jeremy's first session, she cut the duration of each element of the practice in half, in order to assess his abilities. Since he did well, for subsequent sessions she increased his times to the standard durations specified in the practice described below.

Not all students and not all people with HIV, including Jeremy later in his illness, would want to do this practice. For anyone debilitated by disease, or anyone with lymphatic congestion or swollen glands, it would not be the kriya of choice.

The first eight practices that Shanti Shanti Kaur provided for Jeremy are all part of the Massage for the Lymphatic System kriya, and, in typical Kundalini yoga style, they have numbers, not names. Although Jeremy did the first three exercises of this kriya, as well as the meditation, sitting on the floor, they can be done in a chair if that is more comfortable. If you practice in a chair, keep your spine aligned, your hips level, and equal weight on both feet on the floor.

EXERCISE #1. **Ten minutes.** Sit in a comfortable cross-legged position with your elbows at your sides. Bend your arms, so that your forearms extend upward and your palms face each other. Then, strongly push one arm out and up at a 60-degree angle, initiating the movement from the armpit, while the other arm stays put (figure 21.1). Then push the other arm out as the first returns to its original position. Continue alternating arms for ten minutes, gradually building up the pace. In this exercise, you can close your eyes or you can choose a focus to promote steadiness of mind. Shanti Shanti Kaur says that the tip of the nose and the third eye are the two most common areas on which to focus.

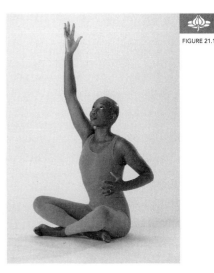

FIGURE 21.1

EXERCISE #2. **Ninety seconds.** Start by sitting in Half Lotus (Ardha Padmasana) or Thunderbolt pose (Vajrasana), ensuring that you have a stable base. Now extend your arms out and up at a 60-degree angle, with your elbows straight, creating a V shape with your arms (figure 21.2a). Inhale. Initiating the movement from your armpits and keeping your elbows straight, exhale and cross your arms over your head, in front of your face (figure 21.2b). Inhale and separate your arms into a V, then exhale and cross your arms again, alternating which arm is on the outside. Keep repeating the arm movements, inhaling as your arms spread apart and exhaling when they cross. The breathing style during this exercise is similar to what is called Kapalabhati in other traditions, with a sharp exhalation moving up and in from the navel, and a brief passive inhalation (see pp. 286–87). Do this exercise for ninety seconds. Says Shanti Shanti Kaur, "If you didn't sweat from the first one, you will with this one."

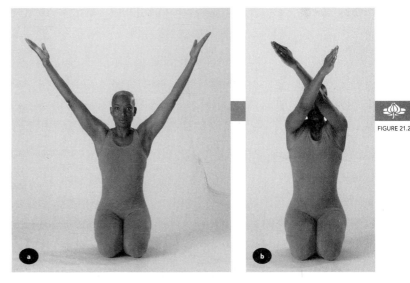

FIGURE 21.2

Shanti Shanti Kaur recommends first working on coordinating the movement with the breath. Once that's established, you can increase your pace. Unless otherwise specified, all breathing in Kundalini yoga is through the nose and is done rhythmically. If the movement becomes vigorous and fast, then the breath speeds up accordingly. When you inhale, think the word *sat* and when you exhale, think *nam*. (Sat nam is a traditional Kundalini yoga salutation and mantra that literally means "truth is my identity.") This coordination of mind, movement, and breath is one of the distinguishing features of Kundalini yoga.

EXERCISE #3. **Two and a half minutes.** Sit in Half Lotus (Ardha Padmasana) or Thunderbolt pose (Vajrasana) as in the previous exercise. Bring your arms out in front of you to around shoulder height, with your palms facing up and your fingers slightly cupped (figure 21.3a). Moving your arms together, lift them up and over your head as if you had water in your hands and were going to release it behind you (figure 21.3b). Or imagine you're holding a bundle with all of your troubles, worries, sorrows, and regrets, which you are going to throw away. Breathe through your mouth and coordinate your breath with your arm movements, inhaling as your arms move up and over and exhaling as you release your arms back down. Keep your inhalations and exhalations of equal length; otherwise, you may become dizzy. Repeat the arm movements for two and a half minutes. If you get light-headed or dizzy for any reason, take a breath through your nose and stop the movement. Breathe at a comfortable rate through your nose until you are feeling stable. Rest if you need to before going on to the next exercise.

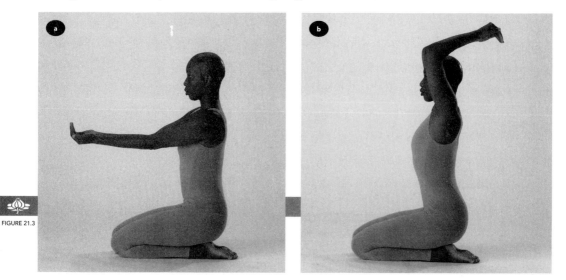

FIGURE 21.3

EXERCISE #4. **Two minutes.** Lie on your back with your arms by your sides, palms facing down (figure 21.4a). Engaging your navel point and pressing your lower spine against the floor so your movement begins with your breath, inhale and simultaneously swing both legs into Plow pose (figure 21.4b). Use your abdominal muscles to initiate the movements. Continue to move back and forth between the reclining position and Plow pose, for two minutes, coordinating your movement with your breath. How you move and breathe in this pose depends on your abilities. If you have strong abdominal muscles and good flexibility, you may be able to do the cycle in one breath, inhaling as you come up and over and exhaling as you come down. But if you are just starting to practice, you will probably need to inhale as you raise your legs, exhale as you bring your feet to the floor behind you, inhale up again, and exhale your feet to the floor in front of you.

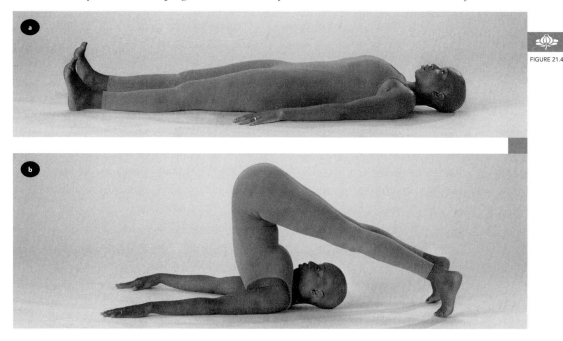

FIGURE 21.4

 TIP Shanti Shanti Kaur says that because doing Plow pose this way challenges both the lower back and abdominal muscles, she sometimes suggests that students put their hands under their hips or at their lower back, or place a blanket roll at their lower backs, to give themselves support and make the exercise easier and less likely to strain the back. Although it's meant to be done with legs straight, many students bend their knees by their ears when in Plow pose, in order to do it comfortably, which is fine. It's also okay to do the exercise in stages as described above. Pace yourself in both breath and movement so that you can do the exercise correctly.

EXERCISE #5. **Three and a half minutes.** Lie on your back, and place your hands under your neck with your elbows pointing toward the ceiling. Do not interlace your fingers, but allow them either to meet in the middle of your neck or overlap. Spread your heels one foot apart. Inhale and press your heels firmly into the floor and lift from the navel point up toward the ceiling, as if you were trying to kiss the ceiling with your belly button, elevating only the area from the thighs to the rib cage (figure 21.5). Exhale and lower back down. Repeat this exercise for three and a half minutes.

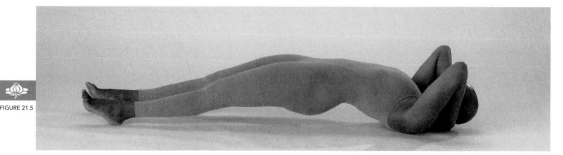

FIGURE 21.5

Although the official Kundalini manual says the knees should stay straight in this exercise, Shanti Shanti Kaur says she has seen few people who can do this exercise and make it look like the pictures in the manual. In real life, many people need to bend their knees for support or they risk hurting their backs. "Yogi Bhajan was a very pragmatic person," she explains. "He didn't want anyone doing anything that wasn't going to be good for them." So just give this your best effort, and don't worry about achieving perfect form.

EXERCISE #6. **One minute.** Remain on your back. Keeping your knees straight, lift both legs up and grasp your toes with your hands (figure 21.6). Breathe through your mouth and

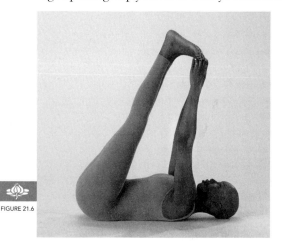

FIGURE 21.6

keep your breath in the back of your throat, and your inhalations and exhalations of equal length. Breathe as slowly and deeply as possible, although it is challenging to do so when your mouth is open. Stay for one minute.

Once again the Kundalini manual specifies straight legs, but Shanti Shanti Kaur says many students need to bend them slightly. Another alternative is to keep your legs straight and hold on to your ankles or calves instead of your feet.

EXERCISE #7. **Eleven minutes.** Start by kneeling with the knees slightly separated and the tops of your feet on the floor. Now release your forehead to the floor as you allow your buttocks to sink to the back of your ankles. Bring your arms back alongside your body with the palms turned up (figure 21.7). You may place a pillow under the forehead or rolled blanket at the heels for support and comfort. Stay in the pose for eleven minutes, breathing slowly and deeply, relaxing fully.

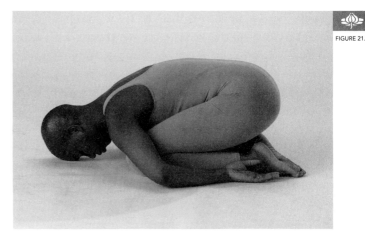

FIGURE 21.7

According to Shanti Shanti Kaur, the intention of this pose, commonly known as Child's pose, "is to lengthen the spine, to have the energy move through the flow of the chakras along the spine, relax deeply, and feel very safe." She has students do Child's pose while listening to a recording called "Naad" by Sangeet Kaur. If you don't have the CD, listen to any music you find relaxing, or focus on your breath.

EXERCISE #8. **Five minutes.** Sit in any comfortable seated position and cross your palms over your heart center, with the left palm on your chest and the right palm on the back of the left hand (figure 21.8). If you have been playing "Naad," sing along with it for five minutes. Otherwise continue to listen to relaxing music of your choice, or just continue to take long, deep breaths. End the exercise with a deep inhalation and a complete exhalation.

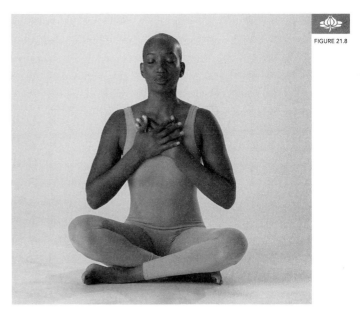

FIGURE 21.8

EXERCISE #9. DEEP RELAXATION (Savasana), eleven to twenty-two minutes.
After completing the kriya, lie on your back with your arms and legs a comfortable distance from the body. Close your eyes and relax (figure 21.9).

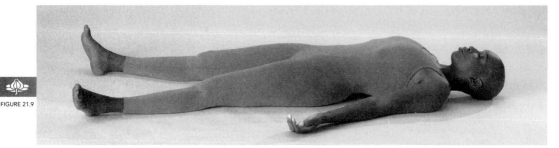

FIGURE 21.9

After the final relaxation, Shanti Shanti Kaur had Jeremy do a meditation practice called "The Inner Sun," which is said to boost the immune system's ability to fight viruses.

EXERCISE #10. INNER SUN MEDITATION, three to fifteen minutes. To retain the heat generated through the practice of this breath meditation, Shanti Shanti Kaur recommends that you cover your head with a scarf, cap, or hat made of natural fabric while practicing. Sit in a comfortable cross-legged position. Bend your left arm and raise the hand to shoulder height, palm facing forward. Place the tips of your ring finger and thumb

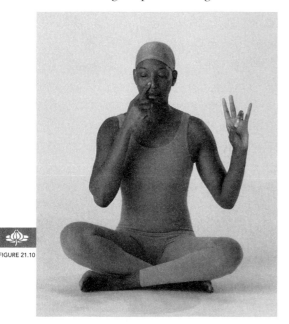

FIGURE 21.10

together. Make a fist with your right hand, extend the index finger, and use it to block your right nostril (figure 21.10). Begin a steady rhythmic breathing through your left nostril similar to that in exercise #2, at what Shanti Shanti Kaur calls "a heartbeat rhythm," approximately one breath per second. You should feel the navel pulsing inward and slightly up with each exhalation. To establish the proper rhythm, you can do this breath with a mantra tape such as "Sat Nam Wahe Guru" by Singh Kaur or "Angel's Waltz" by Sada Sat Kaur, or you can do it without accompaniment. Continue for three minutes, gradually building up to a maximum of fifteen minutes.

To end the exercise, inhale deeply. Retain your breath, being careful not to strain. Now bring your hands together and interlace your fingers, with the right thumb on top, and place the palms in front of your upper chest, at the level of the thymus gland, between the throat and the heart center about six to eight inches from your body (figure 21.11). Pull the fingers apart strongly while simultaneously resisting to create tension. After fifteen to twenty seconds, exhale, and release the tension. Repeat three more times. As Shanti Shanti Kaur explains, "Yogi Bhajan said that this seals the effects of the meditation."

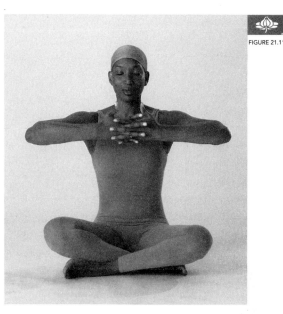

FIGURE 21.11

OTHER YOGIC IDEAS

In Iyengar yoga, teachers commonly prescribe a series of supported inversions and other restorative poses for people with HIV, particularly for those who are weak or tired (see chapter 3). A typical sequence might include: Supported Downward-Facing Dog pose (Adho Mukha Svanasana), Supported Headstand (Sirsasana), which can be done against a wall, hanging from a rope, or between two chairs, Chair Shoulderstand (Salamba Sarvangasana), Supported Half Plow pose (Ardha Halasana), Supported Bridge pose (Setu Bandha Sarvangasa) over two bolsters, and Legs-Up-the-Wall pose (Viparita Karani). See chapters 3, 15, 18, and 25 for more information on these supported inversions. Iyengar teachers believe it essential that the student with HIV never strain in any pose. If doing even a gentle restorative regimen causes fatigue, the student should rest in Child's pose or Deep Relaxation pose before resuming the practice. Those with HIV who are feeling fine are encouraged to do a normal energetic practice balanced with plenty of restorative work.

A Holistic Approach to HIV/AIDS

❋ Dietary changes can improve the workings of the immune system. A diet rich in natural antioxidants and other healthy phytochemicals found in vegetables, fruits, whole grains, legumes, and other whole foods is ideal. Highly processed foods may actually undermine immune function.

❋ Drinking tea, especially green tea, appears to be good for immunity.

❋ Getting adequate amounts of sleep and regular aerobic exercise like brisk walking can boost immune function. Too much exercise, however—for example running marathons or doing intense gym workouts—can actually undermine immunity.

❋ While vitamins are unlikely to confer the same benefits as a balanced diet, one study found that taking a multivitamin supplement was associated with significantly higher T-cell counts and significantly lower viral loads.

❋ Treatment with the supplement coenzyme Q10 appears to benefit asymptomatic people with HIV, as well as those with the drug side effect of fat maldistribution (lipodystrophy).

❋ Marijuana appears to help with peripheral neuropathy, a painful nerve disorder marked by abnormal sensations in the feet and sometimes the hands. (It is illegal to use pot medicinally in most places.) The herb also appears to be useful for the "wasting syndrome," which is marked by severe weight loss, because it stimulates appetite.

❋ Ancient healing systems like Ayurveda and traditional Chinese medicine (TCM) appear to have utility in treating people with HIV/AIDS. Acupuncture may help spur T-cell production. Herbal remedies from Ayurveda and TCM may reduce side effects from conventional drugs, but it's better to consult an expert rather than to self-prescribe.

❋ Massage and other forms of bodywork are relaxing and may have other health benefits.

❋ Reiki, involving light touch designed to change the "energy fields" of the body, may reduce levels of pain and anxiety.

❋ Writing in a journal about emotionally charged events in your life was found in one study to increase the CD_4 count. See p. 174 for more on this practice.

✳ Cognitive-behavioral therapy teaches coping skills and counters dysfunctional attitudes that can contribute to suffering. Studies also suggest it can have beneficial effects on immune function.

CAUTION Many people like Dolores, the woman with HIV whose story appeared earlier in this book, may not feel comfortable revealing their HIV status to their teachers out of concerns about confidentiality. This is not an ideal situation since without that knowledge the teacher won't be able to adjust the practice in light of your condition. If you choose not to reveal your HIV status or other medical information to your teacher, you must assume greater responsibility for not doing things that could adversely affect your health. Pay particular attention to any indications, such as strained breathing, that might signal that a particular practice is not right for you.

Contraindications, Special Considerations, and Modifications

People with HIV run a wide spectrum, from completely asymptomatic to severely debilitated, and the yoga practice that is appropriate will vary accordingly. Since the advent of effective drug therapy, the majority are like Jeremy when he first started working with Shanti Shanti Kaur—strong and energetic, able to do a vigorous practice without problems. But the practice can be adjusted as necessary.

Contraindicated practices are mostly determined by the student's general level of fitness, strength, and energy, or with regard to specific opportunistic infections or disease complications. People who have had a recent bout of pneumonia, for example, may need to avoid intense backbends or vigorous pranayama that may irritate the lung tissue. Since HIV can lead to infections in the retina (cytomegalovirus [CMV] retinitis), it is advisable that people whose immune system is significantly weakened be screened by an ophthalmologist before doing inversions or other postures that can raise pressure in the eyes.

Many people with HIV are dealing with side effects of medication, which may require adjustments in practice. Among the side effects Shanti Shanti Kaur sees frequently are fatigue, headaches, and nausea, all of which she ties to the liver toxicity of many of the drugs. In these situations, she will often substitute gentler kriyas, or cut down the time the student does each exercise. She finds that practices designed to build energy (prana) without taxing the student too much—the idea behind the practices she prescribed for Jeremy—are particularly useful for these complaints.

Another common drug-related side effect Shanti Shanti Kaur sees are joint pains, often in the knees, shoulders, or elbows. She will make whatever adjustments to the practice are necessary to keep the student comfortable. She'll also adjust the practice to deal with the kind of fat maldistribution problem from which Dolores suffered as a result of her HIV medications, often using blankets or other padding to cushion the bones and joints. But in her experience, symptoms can best be reduced (or stabilized) by adjustments in the drug regimen, so she suggests that her students talk to their physicians about possible changes in their medications.

Because people with lowered immunity may be at higher than average risk of catching something from a classmate, I suggest that students with HIV bring their own mat to class. But no such precautions need to be taken to protect other students from those with HIV. Casual contact does not spread HIV—in fact, HIV is much less contagious than influenza, hepatitis B, and other common viruses.

OTHER YOGIC IDEAS

To stimulate the thymus, an important organ in immune function, Pandit Rajmani Tigunait, PhD, the spiritual head of the Himalayan Institute, recommends two breathing practices, Ujjayi and Bhramari (see chapter 1 for instructions). He also suggests meditation with the focus on "the hollow of the throat," a practice described by Patanjali in the *Yoga Sutras.* Each of these practices is very safe and can be done by virtually anyone, including those who are not strong enough for asana practice or more vigorous pranayama.

Jeremy called Shanti Shanti Kaur about a week after he first saw her speak. That was the beginning of a long student-teacher relationship. Shanti Shanti Kaur says of Jeremy, "He was terrific as a student. He was a quick learner. He was very connected to his physicality. He felt things. He was also very subtle. He could feel a shift in his body, he could feel a shift in his energy, he could feel a shift in his mood quickly. That was very satisfying and rewarding for him, and it was motivating for him as well." It only took a couple of classes to cover the basics and "from there we just got deeper and deeper." Jeremy proved to be not only a talented student but also, Shanti Shanti Kaur says, incredibly disciplined. "He was very consistent and thorough with his own practice, and he wouldn't let anything get in the way of it."

Jeremy's dedication to his yoga practice appears to have paid off with major benefits for his health and well-being. As they continued to work together, Shanti Shanti Kaur reports, he had less anxiety, as well as "less depression, more energy, and more endurance." The yoga did not raise his T-cell count, but it almost certainly had reduced Jeremy's opportunistic infections. For example, after he began practicing yoga, his oral thrush disappeared. He also had fewer fevers. It took about three months of practice for them to all but disappear, and they did not return until the last year of his life. From 1987 to 1994 he was more or less asymptomatic. Using a kriya or a breathing technique, "he would nip things in the bud," Shanti Shanti Kaur says. If he had a fever or a minor infection, they would typically do less ambitious and shorter practices. "That was a challenge for him, because he just wanted to do everything. But he also learned how to pace himself."

It seems likely that Jeremy's yoga practice, in addition to minimizing his symptoms and greatly improving the quality of life, increased its length. According to an article in *Patient Care,* prior to the use of highly active drug regimens, people with very low CD_4 counts like Jeremy were likely to survive for an average of only two or three years. But Jeremy survived and even thrived for at least seven years before his health took a turn for the worse.

When Jeremy became ill and symptomatic during the last year of his life, Shanti Shanti Kaur altered his yoga practice. "We did different things, because he needed more support, more comfort. It was very difficult, as you can imagine, for him to see his body not respond the way he was used to." She saw him often in his final days. "We'd do breathing, other things he could do in bed. Sometimes we would just talk and meditate." Shanti Shanti Kaur often led Jeremy through a guided deep relaxation, along the lines of Yoga Nidra (see pp. 67–68), while he lay in bed in Savasana. The goal, she says, was to reduce stress and anxiety, to increase his vitality, and to foster "a deep connection with himself" so that he could face what was happening, and whatever was ahead.

In her work with people with life-threatening diseases, Shanti Shanti Kaur talks very explicitly about death. "We use yogic techniques which are traditionally used to break the fear, and the key one is the breathing. We want people to go more inward and to be more connected to what their experience is, and to learn to face it fearlessly. We want people to be aware, clear, calm. And then, if they get well, they live differently than they did before they got their diagnosis. Or they face death, and they face death beautifully."

Shanti Shanti Kaur visited Jeremy while he was hospitalized several times in his final months. "We regularly chanted, which he loved. It helped regulate his breath, calmed him, and created internal movements at a stage when he otherwise couldn't move much." On a few occasions, she was present at the bedside when he had painful and anxiety-provoking medical procedures done. "We would breathe and do imagery, and he got so relaxed that he just talked through the procedures, which amazed his doctors."

Jeremy eventually died of complications from lymphoma (a kind of cancer). Less than two hours before he died, at home, he called Shanti Shanti Kaur and left a message on her voice mail. "I just called to say I set aside some things for you. I'm getting ready to go." He ended the message with "Sat nam." Shanti Shanti Kaur says, "Like everything else he did, he prepared meticulously for his passing." He made decisions about who was going to get his various belongings, including a rosebush that had been a gift from his beloved mother. When Shanti Shanti Kaur arrived at their home only a few hours after Jeremy had died, his partner, Mark, had already repotted the plant so she could take it with her. Mark also gave her a piece of art Jeremy had made for her, a framed necklace that still hangs in her office. "Jeremy was very, very thorough. He knew he was going to die and he prepared himself for it materially and within himself."

During Jeremy's final hours, Mark and a friend of theirs sat with him, held his hands, and sang some of his favorite yoga chants. Shanti Shanti Kaur describes his death as conscious and peaceful. "He didn't flinch," she says. Looking at Jeremy's path from a mythological perspective, she sees it as a hero's choice. "Some people fight and kick and scream. They do whatever they can to prolong things. I'm not saying that's not an appropriate choice, but that wasn't the route Jeremy took. He did fight for his life and his health, but at a certain point he said he realized that the choices he had available weren't ones he was willing to take. So he very peacefully came to terms with that and he organized himself so he could pass."

With the advent of highly active antiretroviral therapy, a much smaller percentage of HIV patients in the West are dying of the disease than formerly. Today many more people are living with HIV much as they might with any other chronic disease. But the work Shanti Shanti Kaur currently does with her students with HIV is very similar to what she did with Jeremy, including the same kriya and meditation described here. Then as now, she focuses on living, not dying. No matter what their state of health, Shanti Shanti Kaur tells her patients that their lives are "special and sacred and purposeful," and that they should live them that way.

"We work with people to build their sense of the future. People enroll in school and clean up their relationships. They get off of alcohol and drugs. I believe this attitude has a lot to do with how well they do, and why so many of them have lived way beyond what anyone expected." Indeed, some of the early patients Shanti Shanti Kaur worked with are continuing to thrive today.

Even though Jeremy's death occurred before the availability of effective drug therapy for AIDs, and in many ways is no longer typical, Shanti Shanti Kaur and I chose to include it in this chapter because we thought it illustrated a number of important areas, including the yogic approach to life as well as death and dying, which Jeremy exemplified.

INFERTILITY

 JOHN FRIEND's mother introduced him to yoga as a child, reading to him from a book that described yogis and their supernatural powers. "My mother was my main mentor and main guide in my life," John says. "She believed that when you aligned with nature, good things would happen." She also encouraged John at every step. "As I started to practice asana at the age of thirteen, she would say, 'You can do the Handstand.' We'd do it on the driveways and she would be cheering me on. 'I told you so,' she would say. It afforded me a really positive outlook on life so that now when people come to me with problems like infertility, I think, 'Let's just do the best we can and see what happens.' Even if the doctors say a woman can't get pregnant, I try to be open-minded about her chances. My mother was a great example of that kind of thinking." John has studied a variety of styles of yoga over the years, and prior to founding Anusara yoga in 1997 was a certified teacher of Iyengar yoga. Anusara combines the alignment-oriented focus of Iyengar yoga with a life-affirming philosophy shaped by Tantra (see chapter 6). He has been teaching yoga since 1980. He is based in the Houston, Texas, area and teaches internationally.

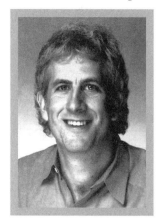

When Ilana Boss Markowitz met John Friend at a yoga workshop he taught near her home in Tucson in 1996, she had been trying to get pregnant for two years. She was thirty-four.

She (and her husband) had already undergone numerous tests, none of which could identify a reason for her difficulties. "Unexplained infertility" was the "diagnosis."

She tried the fertility drugs Clomed and Perganol for a few cycles without success. The entire process was taking its toll. "Anyone who's experienced infertility will tell you, it is the most perpetual and exhausting roller coaster, because every cycle you go through hope, excitement, belief that you might be pregnant, and then it's like the total ultimate crash," she says. "I was definitely less joyful. I was less available in my intimacy with my husband. I was obsessed. Every breath I took was about that. It was horrible."

Yet from outward appearances her life was going well. "I had a really amazing job," she says. "I was the director of a residential program that I created for women and their children. The women were recovering from drug and alcohol abuse. I had a million-dollar federal budget, and twenty-one people on my staff." She was working sixty hours per week at the program and traveling to give presentations about it.

During the weekend workshop Ilana attended, John taught a lot about the bandhas, the yogic locks, and she felt lost. Mula bandha, the root lock, which involves a subtle lifting up from the floor of the pelvis, was particularly mystifying. During the weekend, notably when John taught the Cobbler's pose, Ilana sensed that "the energy was stuck" in her pelvis. She approached John after the last class and told him that she'd been trying to conceive, and sensed that her difficulty accessing mula bandha might be related to her problem. He told her he was doing some work with women having fertility problems and could work with her. "All of a sudden," she says, "I just felt like my whole body relaxed. It was like when you're ill and you go and find a doctor who finally says, 'I can treat you.'" She understood that John was offering no guarantees, but his willingness to try gave her great hope. As John would be leaving town at the conclusion of the workshop, they set up an appointment to speak by phone soon thereafter. They ended up having two phone sessions approximately a week apart.

Overview of Infertility

Four out of five women of childbearing age get pregnant within one year of trying to conceive, though fertility lessens as the woman gets older. If after a year or two no pregnancy results, both the male and female partner may want to be evaluated for infertility since either or both could be contributing to the problem. Because both quantity and quality of a woman's eggs decline as she ages, the longer a woman waits to get pregnant, the less likely she will. For this reason, women over thirty-five who are having trouble getting pregnant may want to consult a fertility specialist sooner than younger women. Besides the decrease in fertility that occurs with age, other reasons for female infertility include congenital abnormalities, scarring from prior pelvic infections, immune system problems (which may result in making antibodies against sperm), endometriosis (the growth of uterine tissue in the abdominal cavity and other locations), and irregular ovulation or failure to ovulate.

Male infertility has been linked to a number of factors. Some men make too few sperm or sperm that don't swim well, or both, lowering the chances of pregnancy. Smoking and drinking as well as pesticide exposure have all been implicated in low sperm counts, and men living in rural areas with high use of agricultural pesticides are known to have higher infertility rates. Even the pressure of a bicycle seat in regular riders can reduce fertility. Sperm are exquisitely sensitive to high temperatures, which is why the scrotum hangs below the abdominal cavity (where the environment is too warm for sperm production). A varicocele, a collection of enlarged (varicose) veins in the scrotum, may reduce fertility because the blood that is backed up in the veins raises the temperature in the testes, where the sperm are produced. There is also some evidence that men over forty become less fertile.

Conventional medical approaches to infertility include drugs to induce ovulation; surgery to correct anatomical problems in the man, the woman, or both; artificial insemination; and in vitro fertilization.

CAUTION There is evidence of a higher rate of major birth defects in babies conceived using high-tech interventions, including in vitro fertilization—about 9 percent versus 4.2 percent when conceived naturally, according to a *New England Journal of Medicine* study. The authors write, "Infants conceived with use of assisted reproductive technology were more likely than naturally conceived infants to have multiple major defects and to have chromosomal and musculoskeletal defects." A recent systematic review of twenty-five similar studies found that such procedures as in vitro fertilization (IVF) and intracytoplasmic sperm injection (ICSI) was associated with a statistically significant 30 to 40 percent increased risk of birth defects. Considering not just the risk of birth defects but the cost, the discomfort and hassle of the fertilization procedures, the risk of undesired multiple births, and questions about the long-term safety of women using powerful hormonal therapies, there are advantages to going a more natural route whenever possible.

How Yoga Fits In

Stress reduction is one of the central ways that yoga can help boost fertility. It makes sense from an evolutionary standpoint that a woman under a lot of stress would not be so fertile. If she is struggling for her very survival, it's probably better not to have to eat for two. One way the body responds to stress is by decreasing blood flow to pelvic organs, so that blood can to be shunted to areas critical for fighting or fleeing, as part of the fight-or-flight response. Yoga can reverse some of the effects of stress by ratcheting down the activity of the sympathetic nervous system and turning up the activity of the parasympathetic nervous system, which controls internal functions, including the reproductive organs (see chapter 3).

Prolonged stress can also have a direct effect on the menstrual cycle. Elevated levels of the stress hormone cortisol can cause menstruation to stop and can also interfere with the release of eggs from the ovaries. Stress can also result in a higher risk of miscarriage. One study found the miscarriage rate was 50 percent higher among women who were stressed during pregnancy. Using stress reduction measures, including yoga, throughout your pregnancy is advisable. Because not all yoga practices are appropriate during pregnancy (see chapter 5), be sure to work with an experienced teacher.

Since stress can play such a huge role in infertility—both in contributing to the problem and in reaction to it—stress-reduction measures can potentially help no matter what the cause (see chapter 3). While yoga and other approaches to stress can provide an alternative to high-tech conception methods, they also may increase the success rate of these procedures by improving blood supply, lowering miscarriage rate, etc. Regardless of the outcome, yoga can improve your quality of life while going through infertility treatments.

Yogis believe that it is possible to learn to relax your pelvic organs and let go of muscular tension, and that doing so can increase blood flow. Various yoga practices help teach you to bring awareness to this area, to notice patterns of muscular holding, and to work systematically to create space in the region. Indeed, these ideas are central to John's approach to infertility.

Yoga teaches that some parts of life are out of your control, and that can help women who are struggling with infertility to acknowledge and accept that reality. This doesn't mean that you should stop making an effort. What's appropriate is to do what you can to change the situation, but let go of the idea that you can control the outcome. Letting go can help reduce stress levels which, of course, paradoxically, increases your odds of becoming pregnant. Yoga also encourages you to look at your attitudes. Many people believe that if they just had something that they lack, in this case a baby, they would then be happy. But yoga teaches that sustained happiness can only be found within yourself. If you don't need a baby to feel okay, you are probably not only more likely to be able to have one, but also better able to give that child what it will need to thrive.

The Scientific Evidence

The best evidence of the role of stress reduction in boosting fertility comes from Dr. Herbert Benson's Mind/Body Medical Institute. Benson is the Harvard physician best known for coining the term "the relaxation response." The MBMI offers a ten-week program which includes gentle yoga, guided imagery, cognitive-behavioral therapy, and instruction in the relaxation response, a demystified form of meditation modeled after yogic mantra meditation. Women who enroll in the program have on average three years of infertility. Their results have included a statistically significant reduction in physical as well as psychological symptoms, and a 44 percent pregnancy rate.

Dr. Alice Domar, who at the time was affiliated with the MBMI, led a randomized controlled study of 184 women who had been trying to get pregnant for one to two years. The women in the experimental group who followed the program described above had a 55 percent chance of a viable pregnancy (a pregnancy that results in a live birth), within the first year, compared to only 20 percent in the control group. Of note, a third group of women who participated in a support group got pregnant at almost the same rate, 54 percent, suggesting that emotional support is another factor that can cut stress and boost fertility. Of note, 11 of the 26 pregnancies (42 percent) in the yoga and cognitive-therapy group occurred naturally without reproductive technologies like in vitro fertilization, compared to only 3 out of 26 pregnancies (11 percent) in the support group. In the control group, 1 of the 5 pregnancies was natural.

Alice Domar has also done research focusing on the high levels of depression among women with infertility. In one study, she found that the degree of psychological distress in these women was similar to people with a terminal illness. Of note, it appears that women with the greatest level of psychological distress were the most likely to get pregnant as the result of the stress-reduction training. Women who entered the ten-week training program with severe depression had a 60 percent chance of a viable pregnancy within six months, compared to 24 percent in the women who entered the program with low levels of depressive symptoms.

John Friend's Approach

During their first phone conversation, John stressed to Ilana that all they were trying to do was set up an environment where pregnancy could happen. They couldn't make it happen. "It's up to Nature, to Destiny," John told her. He felt it was important for Ilana to accept that the outcome was not within her control, which would have the effect of helping her step back and relax. "All we can do," John said, "is do the best we can do and put the results in God's hands. If it's not meant to be, it's not meant to be." John sensed that this message was comforting to her.

Like Ilana, many of the women who suffer from infertility are successful in other aspects of their lives. John says, "If you look at these women's résumés, you'll see they are high achievers. They strive for excellence." They are used to working hard and being rewarded for it, so it is perhaps natural to take this paradigm and apply it to conceiving a child, on the assumption that if they only try harder, they will succeed. Their sympathetic nervous systems are firing, John says, "and it's almost as if they are in attack mode to change the situation." Ilana says, "I think that was part of why I was so frustrated. I was used to basically making happen anything I put my mind to. Anything." Unfortunately, that model doesn't work well with fertility. John goes so far as to say, "It's almost totally contraindicated." They try to go to sleep at night, he says, and their heart is beating fast, their blood pressure is up, and they are not sleeping that well. Of course, poor sleep is itself a stressor and may interfere with fertility.

Beyond this kind of psychological tension, John links fertility problems to a chronic pattern of muscular contraction in the pelvis. In his experience, women with infertility have little awareness of the pattern. While they talked on the phone, John did a diagnostic test to see if the problem she had with the root lock, mula bandha, during the weekend workshop was an indicator of tightness in her pelvic muscles. He asked her to sit in a chair and touch the front of her legs where her thighs met her pelvis, and tell him what she felt. She said that the whole groin area seemed really tight. "All the connective tissue and muscles feel so bound up and my hips and my butt are tight," John recalls her saying.

Here is the sequence of poses and instructions that John provided for Ilana.

EXERCISE #1. **PELVIC AWARENESS EXERCISE, one to three minutes**. Start by coming onto all fours. Bend forward and place the side of your cheek on the floor (figure 22.1). If you prefer, you can bend your arms and use them to create a pillow for your cheek. The position is a version of Child's pose, but with the thighs vertical and the buttocks in the air.

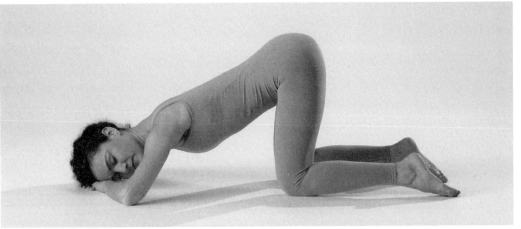

FIGURE 22.1

Relax. Now start to notice the breath in your belly and all the way down into the floor of your pelvis so that you can literally feel the floor of your pelvis, the perineum, the genitalia, and the anus dilating when you inhale and relaxing when you exhale.

When he first put Ilana in this pose, John says, she couldn't feel anything in her pelvic floor. The whole area seemed restricted and without sensation. He says this is pretty common in his female students who are suffering from infertility. He prompted her to try it again. "The second time she did start to feel an expansion in the pelvic floor," he says. "When she exhaled she felt a natural relaxation and shrinking of that area. It was starting to pulsate with her breath."

After she did this exercise for a few minutes John had Ilana sit back up and palpate her thighs again. Wow, she told him, her legs felt so much heavier sitting in the chair. "That's just what I wanted to hear," John says. (His intention was to facilitate body awareness through contrast, a method he frequently employs in his teaching: Feel this, now do this, now go back to the original exercise, now what do you feel?) As a result of letting her pelvic floor pulsate with the breath, her upper thighbones were moving more toward the backs of the legs and that was creating the sense of weight. When you are able to ground your thighbones, the hip creases at the tops of the thighs also start to feel soft.

EXERCISE #2. **CAT/COW, five to ten rounds.** Starting on all fours, inhale, lengthen your spine, and gently arch your back, as you move your face and your sitting bones up (figure 22.2a). Then exhale, round, and tuck under (figure 22.2b). Notice again how your pelvis tends to gently contract with the exhalation and widen on inhalation. Go back and

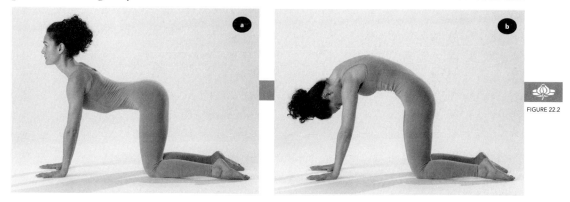

FIGURE 22.2

forth five to ten times, moving with your breath and tuning in to the contrast in the pelvic floor muscles between the Cat and Cow positions. You may not feel much initially, but with practice, John says, you will.

John has noticed that many infertile women feel inhibited in their hip movements. He suggests you can make the Cat/Cow exercise looser and more playful by making the movement more fluid, perhaps bringing in a little side-to-side movement. Sometimes he'll even suggest putting on Latin music to facilitate letting go.

Besides muscular contraction of the pelvis, John has noticed a similar pattern of muscular holding in the abdominal area, which restricts the breathing of many women with infertility. "Their lower abdomen is usually so contracted," he says, "that there isn't a lot of movement in the belly." Part of the problem may have to do with the fact that so many women were taught as teenagers to suck in their gut to appear thinner. When the abdomen is tight, the major muscle of respiration, the diaphragm, can't fully descend on inhalation (see chapter 3). Thus women with infertility tend to be chest breathers. A tight abdomen restricts the flow of blood as well as the breath, which may contribute to infertility. As a remedy, John gave Ilana the following exercise.

EXERCISE #3. **ABDOMINAL BREATHING, five to ten minutes.** Set up for the pose by placing a bolster and/or folded blankets on your mat to support your spine, with a folded blanket on top to support your head. Then sit in front of the bolster (not on it) and lie back. Release your arms and legs to the sides as in Relaxation pose (Savasana). If you are positioned properly, your pelvis will be slightly tipped downward, and the tops of your thighbones will be heavy, that is, pushing toward the floor (figure 22.3). Every time you inhale, let your belly relax and expand. You don't have to push it out, simply allow it to expand naturally, as your lungs fill with breath. You may not have much movement of your belly at first but with awareness and the regular practice of this exercise that will change.

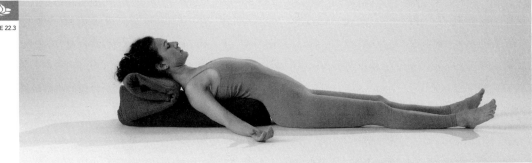

FIGURE 22.3

John asks women working with infertility to focus in particular on their exhalations, which heightens the activity of the parasympathetic nervous system, encouraging relaxation. When teaching these students, he'll often say "slow, deep exhalation," his voice slowing and deepening, taking on a soporific quality. "Let the exhalation take you down. Feel the weight of the feet and the legs as you slowly exhale. With every exhalation feel the breath take you deeper inside." John also sometimes recommends breathing with a 1:2 ratio of inhalation to exhalation. For example, if you normally inhale for three seconds, he suggests you try a three-second inhalation and six-second exhalation. Only do this if you feel completely at ease when breathing.

EXERCISE#4. **PELVIC TIPPING EXERCISE, ten rounds.** Start by lying on your back, with your legs extended. Keeping your right leg flat, bend your left leg and place the left foot on the floor. Now focus on internally rotating your right thigh and grounding it to

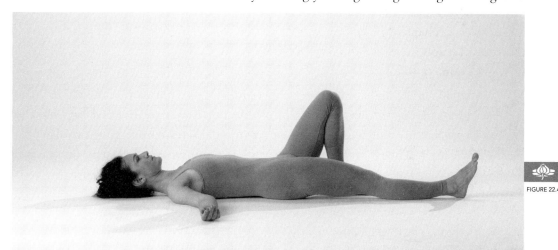

FIGURE 22.4

the floor while you maintain the normal arch in your lower back. This is a principle that John refers to as "Inner Spiral." When you internally rotate the right thigh, you subtly move the thighbone and the muscles surrounding it in a counterclockwise direction but your foot continues to point up. This internal rotation allows you to strongly ground your leg by moving the top of your thighbone closer to the floor. Once you have established that position, start to bring in pelvic tipping. As you inhale, move your sitting bones down toward the floor and arch your lower back. As you exhale, tuck under and let your back flatten, trying to keep your thighbone down (figure 22.4). "Work with the breath," John says, "trying to make it very fluid, even sensual, feeling the pleasure in movement in that area." Repeat the pose on the other side.

Once Ilana understood the principles John was trying to teach her in the exercises above, he asked her to continue her normal yoga practice but to try to bring the same awareness to the other yoga poses she did. For example, he asked her in Downward-Facing Dog pose (Adho Mukha Svanasana) to tune in to the natural pulsations in her pelvic muscles with the breath, and try to re-create the Inner Spiral and the backward movement of the thighs, in the full pose on the floor or with hands on the wall.

Other poses John stresses for his students dealing with infertility include:

- Standing Forward Bend (Uttanasana)

- Extended Side Angle (Utthita Parsvakonasana)

- Pigeon (Eka Pada Rajakapotasana)

- Cobbler's pose (Baddha Konasana)

- Wide-Legged Seated Forward Bend (Upavistha Konasana)

- Head to Knee (Janu Sirsasana)

He believes twisting poses such as Cross-Legged (Sukhasana) twist, the seated twists Marichyasana I and III, and Lord of the Fishes (Ardha Matsyendrasana) can help to create a pelvic floor opening. Inversions like Shoulderstand (Sarvangasana) and Legs-Up-the-Wall (Viparita Karani), which is known to be a particularly restorative pose, can also open up the pelvic floor. While John often recommends the exercises prescribed for Ilana as well as those mentioned above for infertility, he advises that they should be part of a well-rounded yoga practice.

Yogic Tool: **CHANTING.** John finds that chanting is a useful tool to reduce anxiety and stress and increase feelings of gratitude, all of which may be useful in those suffering from infertility. Since the chants John teaches are in Sanskrit, he says most students have only a loose association with the words. The result, he finds, is that students say them in a more emotional than analytical way. Making sounds with feeling creates a release, John says, and afterward students often find that their breathing is more balanced. The literal vibrations of the sound waves may also influence pelvic tissues and perhaps coax opening there. If you experiment, you may notice that chanting lower-pitched sounds, such as those with an "ahh" sound, resonate more in the lower abdomen than higher-pitched sounds.

One thing that differentiates John's style of yoga therapy from many others is the amount of hands-on work he does. With infertility, the goal is not just to detect areas of tightness and create exercise sequences to work on them, but to directly manipulate the fascia, other connective tissue, and even the skeleton, both in order to effect change, he says, and to increase awareness. For example, with the student supine, John will internally rotate her thigh with one hand while simultaneously using his other hand to widen her hip bones in the back. This adjustment reinforces the inner rotation of the thigh and the widening of the pelvis, and helps the student experience what being well-grounded feels like. When they feel this directly, John says, they really get it. While not absolutely essential (and not something he could do with Ilana, since they worked over the phone), John believes the hands-on work can speed up the learning process.

OTHER YOGIC IDEAS

Like John, Jolyon Cowan, a yoga instructor at the Domar Center for Complementary Healthcare at Boston IVF, run by Alice Domar, finds that the majority of women he sees for fertility issues are very driven. His primary focus with these students, influenced by the teachings of the late Italian yoga master Vanda Scaravelli, is to get them to slow down, to bring greater awareness to their bodies and breath. It's more about undoing than doing, he says. "The yoga we do is so gentle the people who have done power yoga or Bikram come in as real beginners. Part of it has to do with our society. People like to be physically active, to keep busy, to be distracted. We teach subtle, internal movements of the sacrum coordinated with the breath. There is so *little* going on, that you can't help but bring your awareness back in." One practice that Jolyon has found particularly effective is the partner yoga the couples in the program do. "Part of the fertility process is reconnecting with yourself and with your partner on a deeper level. There's very little that's more profound than getting in touch with your partner's breath and the movement of their spine as they breathe, and even the temperature of their body. When we do these exercises the students get these huge Cheshire cat grins on their faces." Some students tell him they've been under so much pressure from the infertility that they haven't related to their partners in such a relaxed way for years.

TIP Modern humans spend most of their waking hours sitting. Due to the importance of grounding the thighbones (that is, sinking the femur bones toward the chair) to promote pelvic relaxation, a yogic perspective suggests that if you are concerned about fertility, you need to carefully consider what you sit on (see p. 195). Soft chairs can cause a reflex tightening in the lower abdomen. To ground the femurs, it's best to sit on something firm. Most car seats are badly designed from this perspective—they're meant to feel comfortable on a brief test drive, not for prolonged or repeated use. If your car seat is cushy, consider putting something between you and the upholstery to increase the firmness, giving your sitting bones and your femurs a place to ground.

OTHER YOGIC IDEAS

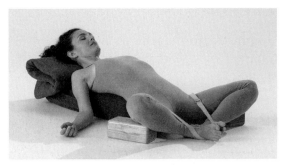

In Iyengar yoga, restorative poses, such as Supported Reclining Cobbler's pose (left) and Supported Bridge pose (below), are often recommended as part of the treatment for infertility (see chapter 3). The idea is to obtain maximal relaxation of the lower abdominal muscles. Even though these muscles are weak in most people, they can also hold a lot of tension. These poses allow the abdomen to widen and relax, and are among the best restorative poses when you are feeling tired or stressed out. In both poses try to let go of all holding in the abdominal and pelvic region, to let the breath flow freely. If there is any tension whatsoever in the groin in Reclining Cobbler's pose, support the thighs with blankets or blocks to allow for complete relaxation there.

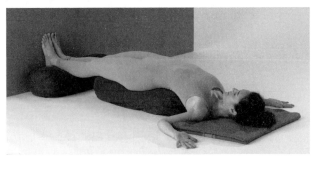

Contraindications, Special Considerations, and Modifications

Almost any style of yoga can be an effective way to reduce stress. Too much exercise of any kind, however, including extremely vigorous styles of hatha yoga, can potentially contribute to female infertility by reducing body fat and suppressing ovulation. Part of the yogic remedy for these women might be giving up their normal practice in favor of a slower, gentler routine. John ties inappropriately strenuous yoga practice to striving and "over-efforting," perennial problems for women with infertility. He believes, however, that if you can learn to do difficult poses with the minimum effort necessary, never losing the balancing ease that Patanjali talked about, it's less likely to be problematic. In other words, it's not just how vigorous your practice is but how you do the vigorous practice.

Headstand tends to narrow the pelvic floor, John finds. People often let their backs sag into a banana shape with their tailbone tucked under and their legs turned out. Doing so can increase tension in the pelvis, potentially exacerbating infertility problems. One potential solution, other than simply avoiding the pose entirely, is to do the pose with your back against the wall (as opposed to in the middle of the room), as it may be easier to relax the groin and internally rotate the thighbones when you don't have to worry about balancing. If you can't find ease and relaxation even with the wall supporting you, it's best to refrain from the pose.

> **TIP** Although it's never been validated in a scientific study, some yogis would tell you that high heels can interfere with a woman's fertility. When you walk on high heels, your weight falls mostly on the balls of your feet and your toes. That translates into a locking of the knee, which John believes causes a chain reaction up the leg that makes it harder to relax the pelvic floor and the surrounding area. You can feel it yourself, John says. If you walk on your tiptoes, the area at the top of the thighs (the same area he had Ilana palpate) gets hard. Hyperextension of the knee can also occur in a number of yoga poses (see appendix 1, "Avoiding Common Yoga Injuries"), which John thinks women with infertility should strive to be aware of and to minimize.

Ilana incorporated John's suggestions into her practice and almost immediately started to notice more awareness of her pelvic muscles, as well as an increased ability to relax them. She practiced the poses John taught her every day for thirty days, and brought the awareness she developed from doing them into the rest of her practice. In addition, Ilana decided to increase the duration of her meditation to fifteen minutes per day. During those meditations, which she describes as "exquisite," she focused on the breath, sometimes imagining that she was breathing in hope and breathing out peace. She says this practice, in particular, "really started changing my thinking."

A Holistic Approach to Infertility

❉ Women who have a very low percentage of body fat may stop ovulating. Gaining as little as five pounds can restore fertility.

❉ Conversely, obesity can also reduce fertility by interfering with ovulation, though being moderately overweight does not lead to fertility problems.

❉ Food and drinking water are potential sources of pesticide exposure, which may affect male fertility. Organic food (see chapter 4) and filtered or bottled water may help reduce the risk.

❉ Beyond pesticides, other toxic exposures, often work related, that can affect male fertility include lead and benzene.

❉ Due to the high temperatures, men with infertility should avoid hot baths, saunas, steam rooms, and even working with a notebook computer in their lap, which may generate enough heat to interfere with sperm production.

❉ It's debatable whether boxer shorts, as opposed to tighter underwear, can really help male fertility, but they can't hurt and are probably worth a try.

❉ Prescription drugs, including blood-pressure medication, can affect male fertility. If this is a possibility, discuss with your doctor whether a change in medication or a switch to nondrug measures could be employed.

❉ As few as five alcoholic drinks per week has been shown to reduce a woman's ability to get pregnant and can interfere with men's fertility as well.

❉ Caffeine can also be deleterious to women's fertility. Try to have no more than two cups of coffee daily, or the equivalent in caffeine from other sources such as tea or soft drinks.

❉ Tobacco can impair fertility in both men and women. Even secondhand smoke should be avoided as much as possible.

❉ Women who hope to become pregnant should avoid douching.

❉ Depression is potentially more harmful to fertility than stress alone. Anyone who is suffering from persistent feelings of sadness, lack of worth, or who has lost pleasure in formerly enjoyable activities should seek professional help (see chapter 15).

* Some herbs such as St. John's Wort, echinacea, and ginkgo biloba may adversely affect both male and female fertility.

* Acupuncture and combinations of traditional Chinese herbs have been shown to effectively treat some types of infertility in both men and women.

As you may have already guessed, Ilana's story has a happy ending. During her very next cycle, she got pregnant. "Two weeks later," she says, "I was puking my guts out—I had such bad morning sickness, it was unbelievable." In retrospect she thinks it was probably a good thing that it took her so long to conceive. The idea that it had taken years before her wish had been granted, she says, "was probably the only thing that gave me any sanity when I was so sick that I felt I just couldn't go on." She found yoga helpful not just in conceiving and during pregnancy, but during labor, too, when she used yogic breathing to help her relax during contractions, and was able to avoid having an epidural or using other forms of pain relief. She felt that what John taught her about feeling the expansion in her pelvic muscles on inhalation was something she was able to use to ease the pain and anxiety of childbirth. By viewing the period of time between contractions as an expansion, she says, she was able to experience labor as a rhythmic flow, "like a breath."

Looking back, she views her experience with infertility as a "blessed journey." She found solace in particular by looking to her Jewish heritage. "In the Old Testament, what we call the Torah, we are introduced to women who enter their spiritual path through infertility. For men, it's about leaving their home. For women, it's about barrenness. It's Sarah, who didn't conceive until she was ninety-nine, Hannah, who is really the model for prayer in our tradition, Leah, Rebecca. It's really a rite of passage."

Ilana believes that some of what she learned by going through this process helped her be a better, more patient mother, too. You can't control whether you'll get pregnant, she says, "you don't have control over what sex your child is, you don't have control over what temperament your child comes into the world with, you don't have control over the chemistry between you and your child. It's such a metaphor for life."

INSOMNIA

ROGER COLE, PhD, is a certified Iyengar yoga teacher who has taught yoga since 1980, and a research scientist who studies the physiology of sleep, relaxation, and biological rhythms. When Roger was a teenager, his sister came home from college with a book that showed a yogic breathing exercise. He recounts that when he first tried that practice, he didn't think it was doing anything, but then he noticed that "in times of stress it made me more calm." This realization "had a profound effect on me." While an undergraduate at Stanford a couple of years later, he began an asana practice, which he also initially learned from a book. Gradually his interest in yoga found expression in his academic work. While in graduate school in health psychology at the University of California, San Francisco, he did studies of brain waves in various yoga poses and also demonstrated how a common blood pressure reflex (the baroreflex) causes reclining and inverted body positions to promote sleep while standing positions inhibit it. Roger teaches yoga in San Diego and gives workshops throughout the United States.

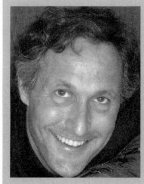

Chris Martin is a physician who takes care of newborns in need of special attention due to difficult deliveries or medical problems. The work schedule of a neonatologist, as his specialty is called, is necessarily erratic. He works several days in a row on call at the hospital, and has an "extremely irregular sleep pattern." Nights on call, he often goes to bed after midnight, regularly gets interrupted in the middle of the night to evaluate and treat newborn babies in distress, and if he's not already up, wakes at around 5:30. Sometimes he gets back to sleep fairly easily after one of those middle-of-the-night interruptions, but if it was a difficult case, he may lie in bed in a state of hyperarousal for a long time, second-guessing medical judgments he's made.

Chris's difficulty sleeping comes and goes, he says. His insomnia was at its worst a few years ago when he went through a divorce. His physician gave him prescription drugs to help him sleep, first Ativan, an antianxiety agent from the Valium family, and then one of a newer class of sleeping pills, Ambien. The drugs, which he used only intermittently, did help him sleep, but he didn't view them as a real solution because he would only take one when he was "at home, off call." Given how frequently he was at the hospital or on call, he was often unable to take the drugs during the worst of his sleep problems.

Chris met Roger when Roger came to teach a workshop at a studio near Chris's home in Tennessee. Chris had been studying Iyengar yoga, the style Roger teaches, for a year. Although he attended classes when he could and took the occasional workshop, he'd never been able to establish a regular home practice. At the time he took Roger's workshop, Chris was stressed enough that he was having wakeful periods several nights in a row, even when he wasn't in the hospital, and he was having trouble breaking the cycle. After the workshop he sent Roger an e-mail asking for his help and they began to correspond. After assessing Chris's problem, Roger suggested several yoga practices he could try to remedy the situation. In addition, Roger recommended a behavioral program that limited the time Chris spent in bed when he wasn't sleeping. Studies have shown that such a program can make it easier to fall asleep.

Overview of Insomnia

The definition of insomnia is the inability to fall asleep or to stay asleep long enough to feel rested. Practically speaking, if you have trouble staying awake during the day, but experience difficulty either falling or staying asleep at night, you have insomnia. Probably the most serious risk from insomnia is its effect on the alertness level of drivers—thousands of accidents every year are believed to be caused by people falling asleep at the wheel.

The first step in addressing sleeplessness is to see a doctor to rule out any underlying problem that might require medical attention. Poor sleep can be the result of a variety of medical conditions ranging from depression to chronic pain, and it can in turn worsen these and other problems. Depression, for example, is often characterized by an inability to get back to sleep after waking in the early morning. Insomnia can be related to hormonal changes, heartburn, and "restless leg syndrome," discomfort combined with an irresistible urge to move the limbs.

The most common type of sleeping problem Roger sees is what's known as sleep maintenance insomnia. This involves falling asleep for a few hours, but then waking and being unable to drop off again. Sleep maintenance insomnia, according to Roger, is a hyperarousal disorder. "Your nervous system is just turned on too high, the sympathetic nervous system is active, the brain circuits that keep you awake are active, and you can't stop thinking."

> **TIP** Ayurveda, the system of traditional medicine in India, views hyperarousal and insomnia as manifestations of an excess of vata, the dosha associated with movement and restlessness (see chapter 4). Key to the Ayurvedic approach to insomnia is establishing a regular routine. Go to bed and get up in the morning at the same time every day. Try to eat warm, nutritious meals at regular times. Creating a bedtime ritual of winding down prepares your nervous system for sleep. Stop all work an hour or two before bed and listen to soothing music or read a relaxing novel (but skip the thrillers if you find them overstimulating). For more information on yoga practices that can help reduce vata, see p. 83.

Less frequently, Roger sees cases of insomnia caused by circadian rhythm disorders, in which the body's internal clock is out of sync with the schedule people are trying to maintain. They have trouble getting to sleep because they go to bed at a time when their body isn't ready to sleep. Circadian rhythm disorders are common among teenagers who may have to get up early in the morning, so they try to go to bed early even though their natural body clock is programmed to stay up later and get up later. People on night shifts or rotating shifts, and people who travel across time zones also frequently experience circadian rhythm disorders. Other factors that may contribute to poor sleep are major life changes—good and bad—such as the death of a loved one, having a new baby in the house, or getting a new job (or losing one).

What you ingest can also affect your sleep, and you may not always know what you've consumed. Caffeine, for example, is found not only in coffee, soft drinks, and chocolate, but also in some nonprescription pain relievers. Cold medicine and over-the-counter diet pills may contain caffeine or other stimulants that can interfere with sleep. Prescription medications, including blood pressure pills such as beta-blockers, asthma drugs, and anti-depressants like Prozac, can all contribute to insomnia, and the same is true for many recreational drugs from cocaine to marijuana. Although alcohol has the reputation of aiding sleep because it may help you drop off, it generally causes more harm than good by contributing to early-morning waking and less-than-refreshing sleep. It is also potentially dangerous when combined with prescription and even nonprescription sleep aids. Nicotine is another common culprit in sleep problems.

How Yoga Fits In

Yoga offers a number of tools that turn down the level of arousal, by shifting the balance from the activating sympathetic nervous system to the relaxing parasympathetic one (see chapter 3). Such tools can offer real hope to insomniacs, since insomnia often afflicts people whose nervous systems are in a near-constant state of arousal. This is not a subjective assessment but something that can be measured in the form of high levels of stress hormones like cortisol and adrenocorticotropic hormone (ACTH) circulating in the bloodstream. Insomniacs show not just higher levels but more frequent bursts of stress hormones, which can occur in response to either stimulation in their environment or to their thoughts. Research indicates that people who sleep poorly don't have more stressful events in their lives than others, but tend to perceive them as more stressful, and react to them more intensely. When your fight-or-flight system is always activated, it doesn't take much to set you off. By relaxing your nervous system, you put yourself in a state of lower responsiveness, so that thoughts or events that might otherwise precipitate a full onset of the fight-or-flight mechanism are met with greater equanimity.

The practice of yoga has been found by numerous studies to lower high levels of cortisol. Since cortisol increases the effects of adrenaline surges that are part of the body's stress response, yoga's ability to lower it helps to explain why the practice could have other benefits, too, leading to the kind of equanimity which makes you less likely to be involved in situations which in turn might interfere with sleep—arguments with your family, conflicts at work, short-temperedness in general. In particular, yogis believe that the regular practice of inversions like Headstand and Shoulderstand, if you're able to do them safely and comfortably (see appendix 1), is calming to the nervous system and mind.

While many forms of exercise can improve sleep, asana is one of the few that works specifically on reducing muscle tension, which can affect both the ability to get to sleep and the quality of sleep. It's possible, says Judith Hanson Lasater, to sleep and be tense. If your muscles haven't let go, she says, you may wake up with a headache or a clenched jaw.

TIP If muscle cramps interfere with your sleep, yoga can help, using the principle known as "reciprocal inhibition." The idea is that when you contract a muscle on one side of a bone, it causes relaxation in a corresponding muscle on the other side. Since many nighttime leg cramps are in the calf muscles, yoga exercises that contract the muscles in the front of the shin can help the calves to relax, relieving the cramps. Next time you have a calf cramp, try this: Lie in bed in Supine Mountain pose and flex your ankles to bring your toes up toward your knees. A regular asana practice also appears to make cramps less likely to occur in the first place, by working out some muscular tension before you get into bed.

Many people with frequent insomnia worry about not sleeping and put pressure on themselves to fall asleep. Unfortunately, sleep does not respond to pressure. Quite the opposite: pressure can contribute to a cycle in which the fear of not being able to sleep becomes the biggest obstacle to sleep. Yoga teaches you to give your best effort and then to let go of any attachment to the results. Letting go—accepting sleeplessness rather than obsessing about it—helps you avoid the kind of repetitive thinking that can directly interfere with sleep. In yogic parlance such a groove is called a samskara. Yoga teaches you how to replace such dysfunctional grooves with ones that serve sleep better (see chapters 1 and 7).

Yoga promotes slow, deep breathing, which can raise levels of carbon dioxide (CO_2), a natural sedative that helps you sleep. (When your breath is quick and shallow, you lose CO_2 from your body and it becomes harder to sleep, which is one reason it can be difficult to sleep at high altitudes if you're not acclimated.) A regular practice of pranayama and meditation may further help sleep by increasing the body's ability to tolerate even higher levels of carbon dioxide, Roger says. Various yogic practices also appear to increase nighttime melatonin levels, which would theoretically improve sleep. (Melatonin is manufactured by the pea-sized pineal gland in the brain, and helps regulate the body's internal clock. Levels of the hormone naturally go up at night and drop during the day because secretion is inhibited by light.) The fact that these practices are so effective in reducing stress is another aspect of their potential impact on insomnia.

Yogic Tool: **DIRECT OBSERVATION.** Yoga teaches that direct observation—particularly if you've developed your sensory abilities through a dedicated practice—is often more reliable than the opinions of experts. Once you've learned to tune in to your body's subtle reactions during yoga practice, you may find yourself becoming more aware in general, which often translates to being able to connect the quality of your sleep with what you eat and drink, what you read, what you watch on TV, or even what you talk about before going to bed. Consider caffeine. It's standard for sleep experts to recommend abstaining from caffeine after noon. This is generic advice, however, which may not apply equally to everyone. There are people who can drink a double espresso an hour before bed and have no problems dropping off. Conversely, if my mother has a small piece of chocolate after dinner, it will keep her up all night. The yogic approach is to look closely at your direct experience to tell you what to do. While not discounting what well-designed scientific studies have to contribute to our knowledge, the experienced yogi learns that the results of careful self-study (svadhyaya) can be trusted and can serve as a valuable complement to those findings. One technique to facilitate the process of self-study is to keep a sleep diary, a notebook that you write in every morning. Jot down when you went to sleep, your subjective impression of how long it took you to fall asleep (don't look at the clock), whether you woke in the night, when you got up, and how rested you felt in the morning. Note any factors that may have affected your sleep— stress or anxiety, whether you took a nap during the day, when you exercised or did yoga, what you ate or drank, etc.

The Scientific Evidence

Several studies have found that meditation can be an effective treatment for insomnia. Research led by Gregg Jacobs, PhD, from Harvard Medical School's Mind/Body Medical Institute found that a multifaceted approach that includes the relaxation response (similar to the mantra meditation used in Transcendental Meditation)—and cognitive-behavioral therapy improved sleep among a group of 102 people with chronic insomnia. While the study did not have a control group whose results could be contrasted with the treatment group, the results suggested that the treatment effects were real and significant. Every single patient noted an improvement in sleep and over 90 percent of those who had been using sleep medication were able to reduce or eliminate entirely their reliance on the drugs. Six months later, 90 percent of respondents said they had maintained or augmented their initial improvement in sleep.

Also at Harvard Medical School, Dr. Sat Bir Khalsa conducted a pilot study of Kundalini yoga techniques on a group of forty patients with chronic insomnia. The intervention consisted of slow, deep breathing exercises. Those who completed the protocol showed an overall improvement in the amount they slept by more than half an hour per night. They also got to sleep on average more than fifteen minutes faster. The National Institutes of Health has funded a larger, controlled study of the same techniques.

A study by Dr. Lorenzo Cohen at the M. D. Anderson Cancer Center, published in the journal *Cancer* in 2004, found that a Tibetan style of yoga involving gentle movements, breathing techniques, guided visualization, and meditation significantly improved the sleep of nineteen people with lymphoma, a form of cancer, compared with a similarly sized control group that was put on a waiting list for the classes. Patients attended seven weekly sessions and were encouraged to practice at home every day. After only a few classes, they reported getting to sleep sooner, sleeping longer, and needing fewer sleeping pills, statistically significant results. In addition to better sleep, there was a trend toward a decrease in depression, fatigue, anxiety, and the number of unwanted thoughts.

A randomized controlled trial of sixty-nine elderly people with insomnia, conducted by Dr. Shirley Telles and N. K. Manjunath of the Swami Vivekananda Yoga Research Foundation, divided them into a control group, a group practicing yoga, and a group given an Ayurvedic sleep aid. The yoga intervention consisted of asana, pranayama, meditation, yoga philosophy, and chanting done for sixty minutes a day, six days per week. The Ayurvedic sleep aid was a combination of herbs recommended in ancient texts, at a dose suggested by an experienced practitioner. After six months, the yoga group averaged an additional hour's sleep per night, got to sleep ten minutes sooner, and felt more rested in the morning, results that were all statistically significant. Controls showed no improvement. The group receiving the Ayurvedic sleep aid improved but the results did not reach the level of statistical significance.

Roger Cole's Approach

Most people, according to Roger, need a calming practice to help them with insomnia, and those who are sedentary will need not just a calming practice but also a more active practice to help them release pent-up tension. In general Roger believes that a well-rounded yoga practice is an excellent prescription for improving sleep. By well-rounded he means a practice that includes in addition to relaxation all the major groups of asana—forward bends, backbends, twists, and inversions.

The trick is to learn how to achieve the right balance between active and calming practices, which is not just a matter of which asanas and other practices to do, but when and how you do them. Roger has observed that many of the people who attend his workshops and classes have an active yoga practice, but still don't sleep well. Often, he feels, these people are trying too hard, taking on too many activities, which can be counterproductive. For example, doing too active a practice too close to bedtime can make it harder to fall asleep, he says. These people need to counterbalance their ambitious approach to yoga with some calming yoga, but they also need to figure out the right time for doing the active yoga and the calming yoga, which is a very individual matter. Conversely, doing restorative poses within a couple of hours of bedtime may cause you to fall asleep during the practice, which could make you more resistant to sleep at bedtime, or more likely to wake up during the night. Roger thinks that most people who would benefit from a calming practice should do the practice "after work, to help them transition between the workday and the evening." In addition to restorative asana, Roger recommends using pranayama to help settle the nervous system, in order both to get to sleep and to get back to sleep if middle-of-the-night wakefulness is a problem.

Although Roger believes yoga can help with sleep, the primary intervention he suggested for Chris was a behavioral program (for nights when Chris was not at the hospital and had control over his sleep choices) based on restricting time in bed to the average amount that you are actually sleeping each night. So-called sleep restriction is one component of a cognitive-behavioral therapy that studies suggest is more effective than sleeping pills, particularly in the long run. At the time Chris began the program, he'd been getting around six hours of sleep a night, even though he often spent a much longer time in bed. Roger told him to limit himself to six hours a night in bed. He might, for example, choose midnight to 6:00 A.M.

The challenge of this program, Roger explains, is that it requires real discipline. When your time comes for sleep, you go to bed. If you're not asleep in fifteen minutes, you have to get up and do something soothing in the dark, but not in bed. If you feel like you might be able to fall asleep you go back to bed, but if you're not asleep in fifteen minutes, you get up again. Same thing if you wake up in the middle of the night. No matter what, you never lie awake in bed for more than fifteen minutes. One of the requirements of the program is that the only activities you're allowed in bed are sleep and sex. "You can't read in bed, balance your checkbook in bed, watch TV, none of that stuff," says Roger. At the time you've chosen for yourself, you get up no matter how much or little you've slept, and no napping is allowed during the day.

If you manage to sleep all the way through the night, you're allowed to add fifteen minutes of sleep the following night; in Chris's case, for example, a total of six hours and fifteen minutes. Each night you sleep well you can add another fifteen minutes, but if you sleep poorly, you either stay at that level or subtract fifteen minutes from the time spent in bed. "After a few days of this," Roger says, "you are pretty sleep deprived, so what happens is that as soon as you get in bed you tend to fall asleep."

Roger believes that the key to the effectiveness of this program is that you begin to change all your associations with being in bed. Instead of bed being the place you associate with not being able to fall asleep and worrying, it becomes your refuge for sleep. Such an approach is entirely consistent with yogic philosophy, in that it works on overcoming an old, dysfunctional samskara, by employing a strategy to lay down a new groove (see p. 21).

PRACTICES TO PROMOTE BETTER SLEEP

As part of a well-rounded yoga practice (and assuming you have no contraindications), Roger suggests the following sequence of inverted poses to promote sleep. Ideally this calming sequence should be done in the early evening, several hours before bed.

EXERCISE #1. **SUPPORTED DOWNWARD-FACING DOG POSE (Adho Muhka Svanasana), with a block or bolster, two minutes.** Kneel on all fours on your mat, your hands slightly in front of your shoulders. On an exhalation, straighten your legs, raise your hips, and lengthen your spine to come into the pose. Take the block or bolster and position

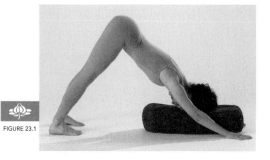

FIGURE 23.1

it so that it just supports your forehead as your head hangs down. As you stay in the pose, the weight of your head will cause it to sink lower and soon it will be resting on the prop and being supported by it, not just touching it (figure 23.1). If you are quite flexible, you will be able to place the crown of your head directly on your mat and won't need support.

EXERCISE #2. **HEADSTAND (Sirsasana), three to five minutes.** Kneel, interlace your fingers, and place your forearms on the floor so your forearms and the space between them form an equilateral triangle. Place the crown of your head on a folded yoga mat and the back of your head into the palms of your hands, which are open. Gradually transfer weight to your arms and head as you straighten your legs (figure 23.2a). When you are ready, bend your knees, exhale, and raise your legs off the ground until your hips come over your spine. Then straighten your legs to come into the pose (figure 23.2b). You can do this pose either at the wall or standing in the middle of the room. The length of time you hold it depends on your experience. Never stay longer in the pose than you feel comfortable (see chapter 4 and appendix 1 for safety considerations for this and the next pose).

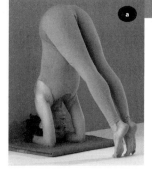
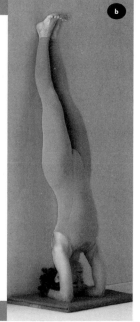

FIGURE 23.2

EXERCISE #3. **SUPPORTED SHOULDERSTAND (Salamba Sarvangasana), five to eight minutes.** Set up for the pose by folding three or four blankets into rectangles and placing them in a stack on a folded mat. Adjust a strap so that the loop will hold your arms shoulders' width apart when placed just above your elbows. Hold on to the strap with one hand for now. Lie back on the blanket with your shoulders a couple of inches from the rounded edge of the stacked blankets so that your head and part of your neck extend past the edge, and the back of your head touches the floor. Bend your knees and place your feet flat on the floor and your arms along the sides of your body, palms down. On an exhalation, push down with your arms, and gently push off with your feet to come briefly into Plow pose (Halasana). In Halasana, slide the strap around your arms just above the elbows, and place your hands on your back, if possible directly on your skin for a better grip (figure 23.3a). On an exhalation, bend your knees and raise your hips over your shoulders. Then inhale and straighten your knees to come into the pose (figure 23.3b). Again, the appropriate length of time depends on your level of experience. Longer holds tend to be more calming to the nervous system.

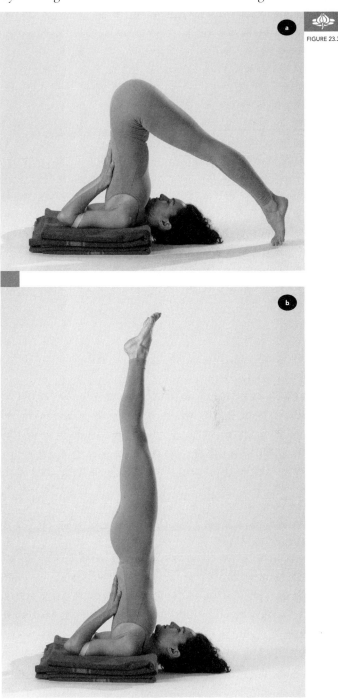

FIGURE 23.3

EXERCISE #4. **SUPPORTED LEGS-UP-THE-WALL POSE (Viparita Karani), ten minutes or longer.** Set up for the pose by placing a bolster or a stack of blankets folded into rectangles approximately six inches from the wall. Sit on one side of the support and move

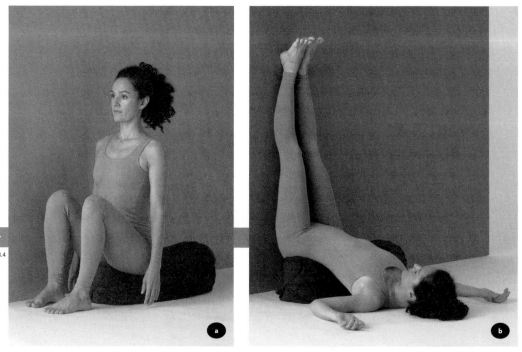

FIGURE 23.4

your buttocks as close to the wall as possible (figure 23.4a). Lower one shoulder toward the floor. From there, swing your legs up so that your heels are on the wall and your thighs are as close to vertical as possible (figure 23.4b). Those with tight hamstring muscles should move the bolster farther from the wall, and not try to get the legs to a 90-degree angle. Place your arms in cactus position, as shown, or alongside your torso as in Savasana. A strap looped around the upper thighs can increase the relaxation. If your feet become uncomfortable due to a lack of circulation, Roger says, bring them down, and cross your legs, as if sitting cross-legged on the wall (see p. 66).

PRACTICES FOR WHEN YOU CAN'T SLEEP

Roger had a number of suggestions for what Chris could do if he couldn't fall asleep or if he woke up in the middle of the night. "If you don't know how to occupy your time while lying in bed for fifteen minutes waiting to see if you fall asleep, try some pranayama." His thinking was based on the observation that many people, including himself, have a hard time staying awake while practicing supine breathing exercises.

EXERCISE #1. **BREATH COUNTING IN UJJAYI PRANAYAMA.** Lie on your back with your head supported. With each inhalation and exhalation, narrow your vocal cords to make a "hhhhhhhh" sound (if you don't know how to do Ujjayi breathing, see pp. 16–17). The key is never to strain at any time. Pause and take normal breaths if your breathing becomes disturbed or difficult. Continue to breathe this way, counting each exhalation. When you reach ten, start counting over again. If you become distracted before you reach ten, calmly pick up where you left off.

"This is a win-win situation," Roger says. "If you successfully follow and count each breath, it is a wonderful meditative practice. If you become distracted and lose count, it probably means you drifted off to sleep for a moment. If you just feel that you are too sleepy to practice, then stop practicing and go to sleep. So you either get a good pranayama practice or fall asleep trying." While doing pranayama, Roger suggests you not think of it as something you are doing in order to fall asleep. Rather you are simply practicing pranayama, and it's possible that sleep will be a result.

EXERCISE #2. **NORMAL INHALATION WITH PROLONGED UJJAYI EXHALA-TION.** Inhale through your nose normally. This time, on the exhalation only, make the sibilant Ujjayi sound. The slight obstruction to the flow of your breath increases the length of the exhalation relative to the inhalation, which slows the heart rate down and calms the sympathetic nervous system. Roger recommends breath retention after the exhalation, which can deepen the relaxation, but only for experienced practitioners of pranayama. You certainly don't want to be trying to learn this some sleepless night.

If you wake up in the middle of the night, the typical advice might be to get up and read or do the dishes, but as Roger points out, "Reading requires light and doing the dishes requires standing up," neither of which is conducive to sleep. Light exposure, whether from reading, watching TV, or surfing the Internet, can reset your internal clock, interfering with sleep in the future. Standing up activates the sympathetic nervous system, which releases the stress hormone norepinephrine into your blood, where it will remain in circulation for an hour or more, stimulating the brain and making it harder to go back to sleep.

A better approach, Roger suggests, is to sit on the floor and do supported forward bends such as those shown below (assuming, he says, you don't have acute back problems or other contraindications). Roger recommends putting blankets under the pelvis, and possibly behind your knees, and then resting your forehead on the seat of a padded chair. If you are quite flexible, you could rest your head on a folded blanket or a bolster, as shown, instead of the seat of a chair.

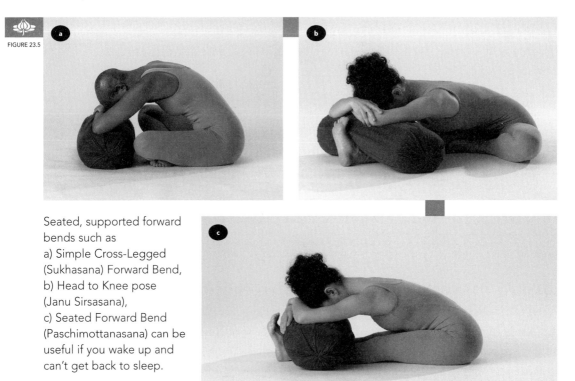

FIGURE 23.5

Seated, supported forward bends such as
a) Simple Cross-Legged (Sukhasana) Forward Bend,
b) Head to Knee pose (Janu Sirsasana),
c) Seated Forward Bend (Paschimottanasana) can be useful if you wake up and can't get back to sleep.

Roger also suggests practicing Legs-Up-the-Wall pose when you can't sleep, though he cautions that if you fall asleep while doing it, that could interfere with being able to fall asleep once you return to bed. He also recommends Child's pose with the trunk and head supported at hip level, head turned to one side then the other for equal amounts of time (figure 23.6).

FIGURE 23.6

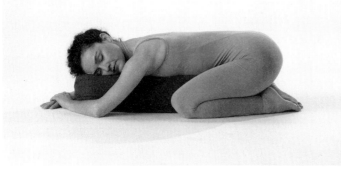

OTHER YOGIC IDEAS

When I visited the Krishnamacharya Yoga Mandiram in India, D. K. Shridar gave me a routine to help with my occasional sleeplessness. A central feature was slow breathing with the emphasis on gradually lengthening the exhalation. This practice can be done lying in bed if you like. Breathing through the nose, inhale for a count of four and exhale for a count of four. Do that twice, then inhale for four and exhale for six. After two times, increase the count of the exhalation to eight and so on, going up to ten and twelve as tolerated. Be sure never to stretch the exhalation any longer than is perfectly comfortable, or you will activate your sympathetic nervous system. If your next inhalation is not perfectly relaxed and smooth, you are probably pushing too hard. Once you reach the maximum exhalation length at which you are comfortable, you can continue at that level as long as you like (though you may find yourself falling asleep).

Because people vary in their responses, Roger says, you may require some trial and error to find out which poses and practices work for you. "If your brain is spinning and the pose helps you settle down and sleep, then it's working. If it seems to relax you but between getting out of it and back to bed, you feel more stimulated, it may not be right." Roger adds that the darker you can keep the room and the less time you spend upright the better. He generally advises people who get up out of bed to do just one posture. Or if you start a sequence and find that one pose seems to be working for you, stay in it.

If what is keeping you awake are work problems or interpersonal conflicts, Roger suggests the following approach. Say to yourself: "I'm going to think about that problem at 9:00 tomorrow morning." Making an appointment with yourself allows you to put that thought off till later and move it out of your mind.

If you prefer to sleep on your side, it may be better to lie on your right side while you're trying to fall asleep. Yogis have realized that the nostril that is higher tends to dominate, that is, air flows preferentially through that side (see chapter 4). Since breathing through the left nostril tends to be calming and contribute to increased activity of the parasympathetic nervous system, lying on your right side may be more conducive to sleep (see p. 62).

If nasal congestion (from allergies, for example) contributes to difficulty sleeping, try using the neti pot right before bed (see pp. 80–81). Be sure to blow your nose gently afterward rather than use forceful Kapalabhati exhalations (as is sometimes recommended) to clear your nasal passages. Such vigorous breathing has been shown to activate the sympathetic nervous system.

A Holistic Approach to Insomnia

❋ Taking a hot bath in the evening may make it easier to fall asleep.

❋ Gentle massage can help promote sleep.

❋ Keep your bedroom as close to totally dark as possible, and reasonably cool and quiet. Run a small fan or other source of white noise to block out extraneous sounds that may interfere with sleep, and wear an eye mask, if necessary.

❋ If your clock is visible in the dark, turn it to face the wall. Watching the clock during wakeful periods may make you more anxious and less likely to sleep.

❋ Avoid napping during the day. The longer the nap and the later in the day you take it, the more likely it will disrupt nighttime sleep.

❋ Studies suggest that guided imagery, biofeedback, hypnosis, and progressive relaxation techniques—in which you sequentially contract and relax various muscles—can aid sleep.

❋ Acupuncture appears to be useful in some cases of chronic insomnia.

❋ Sleeping pills have a role in the temporary treatment of insomnia tied to a stressful life situation, such as after the death of a spouse. Used long-term, however, they lose effectiveness and can cause rebound insomnia. If you do need sleeping pills, use the smallest possible dose for the shortest possible time and try to take them only intermittently.

❋ Melatonin supplements may help with jet lag and can be useful in weaning people off prescription sleeping pills. There is little data, however, on long-term safety of supplemental melatonin. Used occasionally, melatonin may not be dangerous—and may even prove beneficial for sleep—but until more data are available, I recommend against its regular use for insomnia.

❋ Cognitive-behavioral therapy is more effective than sleeping pills in the long term, particularly if you are unable to break the habit of worrying about getting to sleep.

* Over-the-counter sleeping aids containing antihistamines aren't very effective and cause unpleasant side effects such as a dry mouth or a "spaced-out" feeling. I recommend avoiding them.

* Valerian root, an herbal remedy, appears to be safe for short-term use, though some users note daytime grogginess or lethargy. Other safe herbal sleep aids include passion flower, lemon balm, and hops.

* A small 1995 study published as a letter in *The Lancet* found that aromatherapy using diffused essential lavender oil helped elderly patients sleep longer with fewer periods of restlessness.

* For older people, in particular, who tend to fall asleep in the early evening and who wake earlier than they like, light exposure in the early evening can delay their bedtimes. A light box, an electric light that provides very bright full-spectrum light, can be effective, but natural outdoor light is an easy and cheap alternative. A half-hour walk is sufficient (and brings the added benefit of exercise). Even on a cloudy day, outdoor light is much brighter than standard indoor lighting.

* To keep your internal clock set correctly, get up as close to the same time as possible every day, even on weekends.

Contraindications, Special Considerations, and Modifications

Because yoga tends to reduce stress levels and relax muscles, doing an asana practice can be very beneficial for people who have trouble falling or staying asleep. A number of poses can activate the nervous system, however, and care must be taken not to do them too close to bedtime. In general, active backbending poses stimulate the sympathetic nervous system, and the effects can last for hours. In contrast, a sattvic backbend practice, backbends done in a relaxed way, particularly if they are followed by more restorative postures and a long Savasana, may be okay. Other practices that can be stimulating and potentially interfere with sleep include Agni Sara (abdominal churning), vigorous Sun Salutations, and rapid breathing techniques, including Bhastrika and Kapalabhati. People vary in their sensitivities, so let your experience guide you. Although many people like to do yoga with music in the background, Roger believes that it could interfere with inner reflection and the processing of emotions that can often be conducive to sleep.

TIP If your feet are cold it can have an activating effect on the sympathetic nervous system. Keeping the feet warm by wearing socks to bed can facilitate sleep. Best to put them on half an hour before you go to bed, which can help dilate the blood vessels in the feet and encourage relaxation. Keeping your extremities warm during restorative poses is also a good idea. Says Roger, "I always have people cover their hands and feet during restoratives, and it seems to help the relaxation a lot." A simple way to cover your hands is to place each one into the folds of blankets that have been put on either side of you on the floor.

Chris seems to have benefited greatly from his consultation with Roger. He followed the sleep restriction plan Roger outlined for several weeks, until his sleeping improved so much that he found he didn't need it anymore. He's also found it particularly useful to do Legs-Up-the-Wall (Viparita Karani) in the call room at the hospital. Using hospital pillows to support his hips, he'll often do the practice to wind down from the hectic pace of call nights.

Since he and Roger last talked, Chris has also broadened his approach to yoga. After attending an introductory Ashtanga workshop last month, he started going to classes, and when he can't get to class, he does thirty- and forty-five-minute subsets of the longer Ashtanga primary series (see chapter 27) that he learned from a David Swenson video. So now he is making use of one of the most important yogic tools for fighting insomnia—establishing a regular home practice.

Despite the ongoing—even escalating—pressures of his medical practice, his unavoidably irregular work schedule, and his share of parenting responsibilities for his fourteen-year-old son, Chris has experienced a major improvement in his sleep. Referring to the prohibition against staying in bed if sleepless, he says, "There have been very few times that I have had to get out of bed. When I do wake, if I am unable to go right back to sleep, counting breaths seems to work most of the time."

IRRITABLE BOWEL SYNDROME

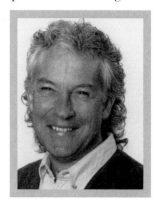

Thirty years ago, MICHAEL LEE was working for the South Australian Public Service Board, studying how people behaved in the workplace and running workshops on how to effect change. He gradually came to realize that the behavioral principles that were the basis of his workshops were insufficient. "I felt the piece that was missing was the body," an insight he thinks had been awakened by starting a yoga practice. "When I first began to practice yoga, I realized that there was a real connection between what was going on in my body and in my life." One day his young daughter said to him, "Daddy, I like when you do your yoga. When you do your yoga you don't get so mad at me." That was a powerful confirmation. In 1984, he took a sabbatical from the work he was doing for the government of Australia and went to the Kripalu Center for Yoga and Health in Lenox, Massachusetts, for the express purpose of developing new programs. Michael admits that the Australian government never got their money back on that investment. "I got so into yoga that I went back and resigned." He developed Phoenix Rising Yoga Therapy in 1986 and ran their center and teaching programs until 2006, when he stepped down to pursue writing and other interests. Michael has written two books: *Turn Stress Into Bliss* and *Phoenix Rising Yoga Therapy.* He has two master's degrees, one in behavioral psychology, the other in holistic health education.

Michael Faber started to develop digestive problems after returning from a trip to South America. His major symptoms early on were constipation and gas. In search of a diagnosis, he went to several doctors, none of whom were able to figure out what the problem was. Finally, after three or four years, he was given the diagnosis of intestinal parasites and treated with antibiotics that got rid of the infection. Even so, some digestive symptoms persisted.

During a stint as a volunteer in the kitchen at the Kripalu Center for Yoga and Health, at a time when he was still having digestive problems (mainly diarrhea and some abdominal discomfort, as well as gas and bloating), he began to be aware that he was living with a lot of anxiety.

As he gained more awareness of his mental state, he was able to correlate it with his symptoms—or lack thereof. For example, on backpacking and camping trips when he was able to relax, "I realized that some of these symptoms that I experienced almost disappeared." When he could see that there was a psychological component to his digestive issues, he saw a therapist, who suggested he try meditation. Around that time, he saw a flyer for Michael Lee's eight-week program using Phoenix Rising yoga and mindfulness meditation to help irritable bowel syndrome. He decided to give it a try.

Overview of Irritable Bowel Syndrome

Irritable bowel syndrome (IBS), formerly known as spastic colon (among other names), is an intestinal problem of unknown cause, though stress appears to be a prominent factor. Its symptoms often include diarrhea, constipation, or both, as well as bloating and cramping. Uncoordinated intestinal contractions, in which one area contracts, attempting to push the food being digested forward, before the area below it is ready, help account for the crampy abdominal pain reported by IBS sufferers. Typically the pain will be relieved by a bowel movement—a pattern that is one of the markers of IBS. Symptoms range from mild to severe and can be intermittent—manifesting, for example, only at times of heightened stress—or nearly constant.

CAUTION In IBS there is no blood in the stool, no fever, chills, or weight loss. The presence of any of these should prompt a trip to the doctor to look for another cause.

While bothersome and at times painful, IBS does not cause permanent damage to the body and does not increase the risk of developing cancer later on. Some people believe that a prior intestinal infection, such as Michael had with parasites, may predispose you to developing IBS, but scientists have come to no definite conclusions on this score. Those with IBS appear to be more sensitive to sensations in their bowels. The same degree of bowel distention or bloating, for example, causes more discomfort in someone with the syndrome than someone who doesn't have it.

TIP Such problems as lactose intolerance (sensitivity to the natural sugar found in milk) or gluten sensitivity can cause diarrhea and bloating. If you notice such digestive symptoms after eating dairy products or high-gluten foods like bread and pasta, be sure to consult your doctor. Another source of unexplained gastrointestinal symptoms, sometimes leading to a mistaken diagnosis of IBS, is fructose intolerance. Like lactose, fructose is a naturally occurring sugar (found in fruit and in high-fructose corn syrup, a low-cost sweetener used in soft drinks and a wide variety of processed foods) that can cause digestive problems in people who don't absorb it normally. A study, published in the *American Journal of Gastroenterology*, found that 134 out of 183 patients with unexplained intestinal symptoms had a positive breath test for fructose intolerance. Commonly reported symptoms included flatulence (83 percent), pain (80 percent), bloating (78 percent), belching (70 percent), and altered bowel habits including diarrhea (65 percent). If you suspect you might have fructose intolerance, ask your doctor about scheduling a breath test.

How Yoga Fits In

The smooth functioning of digestion depends on the action of the autonomic (involuntary) nervous system, especially the parasympathetic branch, associated with relaxation and restoration (see chapter 3). Stress activates the sympathetic side, the fight-or-flight system, which can interfere with the bowels.

Exercise is known to lower stress levels. Beyond this general effect of physical activity, specific yoga postures can offer help with a wide variety of IBS symptoms. For example, people with constipation often benefit from gentle yoga stretches and twists, and, if they are able, more vigorous poses like Sun Salutations and inversions. Since stress can lead to both constipation and diarrhea (as well as cramps, bloating, and other symptoms commonly seen in IBS), a variety of practices, from asana to breathing exercises designed to calm down the sympathetic nervous system and shift the balance more toward the restorative parasympathetic side of the equation, can facilitate better bowel function.

Meditation can help, too. Even in situations where "you can't change the stress," Michael Lee says, "you can change your relationship with it. That's fundamentally where the shift needs to take place." Yogis believe that meditation may be particularly valuable in this regard because it teaches you to separate your symptoms from your thoughts and worries about them. For someone like Michael Faber, letting go of the worry that so often attaches to symptoms can be transformative.

Self-study (svadhyaya) is also part of the yogic prescription for IBS. Self-study can help you figure out what your stressors are and whether there is a connection between them and your symptoms. Self-study also entails looking at the link between the foods you eat and how they make you feel. If you know that certain foods don't agree with you but you choose to eat them anyway, yoga would suggest you look further to ascertain why that might be. Keeping a journal in which you write down your symptoms and any possible connection between them and stress, diet, or other factors can facilitate this process of self-discovery.

Another area to study is *how* you eat. Eating rapidly can lead to swallowing air, which worsens gas and bloating. Taking the time to chew your food thoroughly aids digestion by allowing enzymes in your saliva to mix with food before it gets to your stomach. Bringing more yogic awareness to the entire process of eating can facilitate relaxation by making it more of a meditation (see chapter 27). Be advised, however, that eating quickly may be a deep samskara (behavioral groove), and you may need to repeatedly bring your attention to it before it changes (see chapters 1 and 7).

Yoga also looks at possible psychological contributors to conditions like IBS. Michael Lee says that you need to ask yourself "What are the life issues involved? We can give you all sorts of yoga postures, breathing techniques, and herbs to take but if you don't fundamentally change what's causing the stress, you can't effect healing in a complete sense." He believes that if you walk the path of yoga, you almost inevitably choose to make changes that are life-enhancing. Once you start to experience the calm and peacefulness that lies at your center, it becomes so much easier to treat yourself better by eating healthier, making time for relaxation, and honoring the messages that come from within about what's good for you and what isn't.

The Scientific Evidence

A small randomized controlled study conducted at the All India Institute of Medical Sciences in Delhi compared yoga asana and pranayama to treatment with the antidiarrheal drug loperamide in twenty-two males with diarrhea-predominant IBS. Both yoga and the drug proved effective in reducing bowel symptoms as well as anxiety levels at the end of the two-month study. The yoga, however, showed additional beneficial effects, shifting the balance of the autonomic nervous system toward the parasympathetic branch and, for this reason, was judged to be more effective than the drug.

The relaxation response, a technique developed by Dr. Herbert Benson based on yogic mantra meditation, was shown to effectively reduce symptoms in a small randomized controlled experiment conducted at the State University of New York at Albany. Thirteen patients completed a six-week training in the relaxation response and were then asked to practice it for fifteen minutes twice a day. At the end of six weeks, the meditation group experienced better relief than the controls, who had been placed on a waiting list for treatment, noting improvement in flatulence and belching. In a follow-up at three months, the meditation group also noted improvements in bloating and diarrhea. When ten of the original thirteen patients were surveyed one year after beginning the program, they noted significant additional reductions in pain and bloating, which the authors found tended to be the most distressing symptoms of IBS.

Another randomized controlled study of one hundred patients with IBS was conducted at Banaras Hindu University. The patients were divided into three groups. One group was given drug treatment, one a yoga program, and one a combination of drugs and yoga. The yoga intervention consisted of asana, pranayama, kriyas (yogic cleansing techniques), and meditation. The drug therapy included antianxiety drugs, medication to reduce intestinal cramps (antispasmodics), and fiber supplements. After an initial two-week training, the thirty-six members of the yoga group and twenty-eight members of the combined group were asked to practice half an hour per day for the next two months. Both drugs and yoga used alone proved effective in significantly reducing abdominal pain, constipation, diarrhea, anxiety, and other symptoms, with yoga generally more effective than medication. The combination of yoga and modern drug therapy was consistently more effective than either modality alone, eliminating essentially all symptoms within six weeks, with the benefits persisting at the conclusion of the study.

There are also studies suggesting that biofeedback, which shares many features with yoga, especially in the area of heightening bodily awareness and increasing control over normally involuntary processes, can be effective in IBS. Other studies have found utility in hypnosis that involves guided imagery, another technique that is used in yoga. Mixed programs that include meditation and cognitive-behavioral therapy also appear to reduce symptoms.

Michael Lee's Approach

Normally Phoenix Rising Yoga Therapy (PRYT) is done in a one-on-one setting. But when the idea of forming a group for IBS patients came up, Michael felt he could adapt the principles and guide the students through experiences that would give them close to 90 percent of what they would get in one-on-one sessions. He also thought the group might benefit people through camaraderie. So he and Michael Taylor, a medical doctor trained in Jon Kabat-Zinn's mindfulness-based stress reduction, formed a group with Taylor teaching basic mindfulness meditation techniques and Lee teaching yoga.

Mindfulness meditation, Michael Lee says, involves watching your mind and noticing: "'There I am worrying again' or 'There I am obsessing about my food again.'" As he explains, you watch your thoughts but try not to get caught up in the drama of them. The yoga he taught was about "entering a deeper level of awareness through the body. The body is used as the focus in stretches that are held at the edge: not too much, not too little. The physical sensation is the initial focus, but then you expand your awareness to "being present to the experience in all its aspects." What yogis call their "edge" is a place where a pose is intense but not painful, what Michael calls "a tolerable degree of discomfort." He encourages people to find their own edge, not to compare themselves to someone else (see p. 93 for more on this topic).

"There's a learning curve around doing this kind of body-mind work," Michael says, "first getting comfortable just being present in the physical. Once that's achieved you can go to other levels. It might be thoughts, it might be feelings, images, sensations." People almost always end up hitting on "a recurring theme, and it usually has some deep connection to what's going on in their life at the present time." As the students go through the exercises, Michael encourages them to explore whatever is arising in their bodies and minds.

Another part of the Phoenix Rising experience is what Michael calls a "facilitated group process." This is not the same as group therapy. Rather, he says, "It's an opportunity for people to talk about their experience in the group, where it can be received without judgment and without criticism. It's part of the process that we use in the one-on-one Phoenix Rising sessions, where at the end of the session people talk about what happened for them. The goal, he says, is acceptance of what is, so the process does not involve the kind of skilled intervention that a psychotherapist offers.

The practice Michael Lee gave to the students varied from week to week. The following practice is what the group did in the second week, and as homework later on, when they were given a CD recorded during the class to practice along with.

All of the exercises should be done with conscious breathing. As Michael explains, "We teach breathing a little differently than a lot of other people. We begin with a long slow inhale followed by an exhalation that's basically a letting go. We sometimes call it the 'surrender breath,' the 'what-the-heck breath.' If you hear people who've had a sudden fright and it's all over, they give a sigh of relief. It's an inner message to the body: 'Oh I can relax now, it's okay.'"

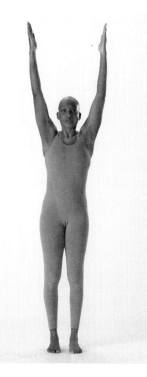

FIGURE 24-1

EXERCISE #1. **BREATHING WITH ARM MOVEMENT, four to six breaths.** Start by standing with your feet together or close together and your arms at your sides, breathing comfortably. Inhale and draw your arms up above your head and hold them there (figure 24.1). Then exhale, encouraging a surrender breath, and lower your arms back down. Repeat twice. Then take stock of the experience you've just had. Close your eyes, and feel your whole body and the breath coming and going, in and out.

EXERCISE #2. **SIDE BENDS, three to four breaths.** Start by standing with your hands by your sides. Make a loose fist with your left hand. Slowly inhale and draw your left hand

under your left armpit (figure 24.2a), lean to your right side and let your right hand drop toward the knee. From that position, reach up with your left arm and turn your head to look up at it. Then lengthen your left arm alongside your left ear (figure 24.2b). To come out of the pose, lift your torso and lower your arms. Repeat on the other side.

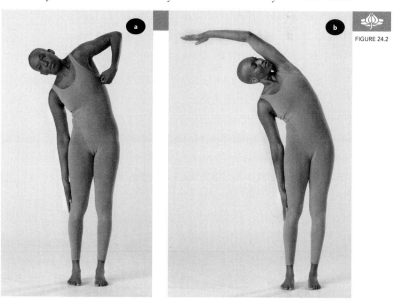

FIGURE 24.2

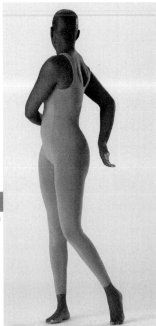

EXERCISE #3. **SWINGING TWIST, sixteen times on each side.** Start by standing with your feet hips' width apart. Swing your arms, and with them your torso, first to one side then the other, pivoting on the foot opposite to the direction in which you are turning, and allowing the heel to lift as you twist (figure 24.3). Keep your whole body long, and let your arms hang loose by your sides like empty coat sleeves. Take deep breaths in and out. Speed up the motion a few times, then slow it down. Inhale, exhale, swing to the left, inhale, exhale, and swing to the right, using the long focused inhalation and the surrender exhalation.

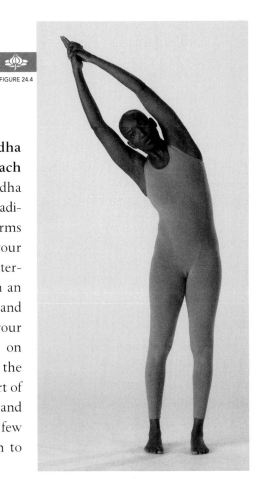

EXERCISE #4. **HALF MOON POSE (Ardha Chandrasana), three to four breaths on each side.** (Note: this pose differs from the Ardha Chandrasana taught in some other yoga traditions.) From a standing position, raise your arms over your head and make a "steeple" with your fingers by extending your index fingers and interlacing the others. Slowly inhale, and then on an exhalation extend your arms to the side, up and over to the right, lengthening the left side of your body (figure 24.4), slowly finding your edge on that side. Notice whether you try to push the edge, and if you do, just notice that. This is part of a three-part process: awareness, acceptance, and making an adjustment if necessary. Stay for a few more breaths. Then on an inhalation, return to center. Repeat on the other side.

EXERCISE #5. **STANDING FORWARD BEND (Uttanasana), with hands in prayer (Namaste) position, three to four breaths.** Start by standing with your feet hips' width apart. Take your hands around behind your back and join your palms together, with your fingers facing up toward your head. Squeeze your shoulder blades together. As you exhale, bend forward from the hips, and as you do, slide your hands up your back. You can separate the palms if you like, and just lace the fingertips together. Allow your head to release downward and bend your knees if you need to. Find the edge in terms of how far your hands go up behind you, so they're not too far up and not too far down, but just right. Take full, deep breaths. Then as you inhale, slowly roll up out of the pose and then exhale with a sigh.

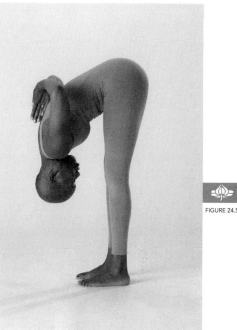

FIGURE 24.5

EXERCISE #6. **STANDING BACKBEND, three to four breaths.** Start by standing with your feet hips' width apart. Place your fists on either side of your lower back. Then look up at the ceiling, press your pelvis forward, and lean back. See if you can open up your throat and let your head go back to where it feels extended but comfortable. Find an edge there, which might be in either your neck or in your back. If you can't take a full, deep breath, it's probably too much, so come up a little and take that full, deep breath. Feel the expansion into your chest and notice the quality of the posture. What's happening now? Sigh with your exhalation, then inhale as you slowly come back up.

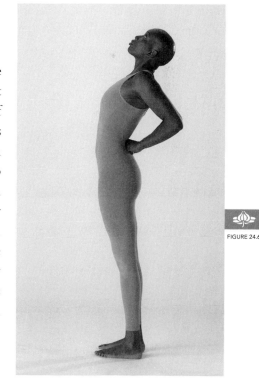

FIGURE 24.6

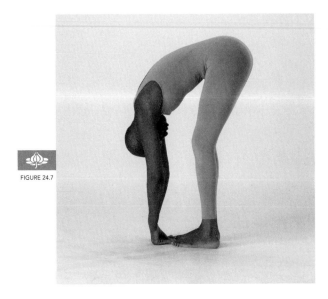

FIGURE 24.7

EXERCISE #7. **STANDING FORWARD BEND (Uttanasana), three to four breaths.** From a standing position, release your arms and your entire body, and bend forward into a rag doll position as you exhale (figure 24.7). Just hang—let your arms and your whole upper body release. You might want to open and close your mouth a few times and roll your jaw around. Let your head be heavy. Bend your legs at the knees a little if you need to. Take slow, deep breaths in and out. To come out of the pose, slowly roll back up to standing as you inhale.

EXERCISE #8. **LOCUST POSE (Salabhasana), three to four breaths.** Lie flat on your belly with your arms stretched straight in front of your head. Lengthen your body, and then inhale and lift your arms and legs simultaneously off the ground (figure 24.8). Breathe deeply. Staying elevated, lengthen from your left arm to your left leg, then do the

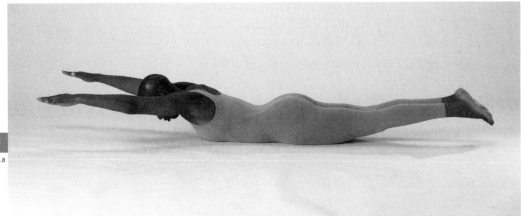

FIGURE 24.8

same on the right side. Notice whether any struggle is present. If there is, see if you can come to the place of just being with the posture, holding it at the edge but letting go of the struggle. Let the breath hold the posture for you, as you breathe from the belly. Slowly come back down, allowing your body to melt into the floor and turning your head to one side.

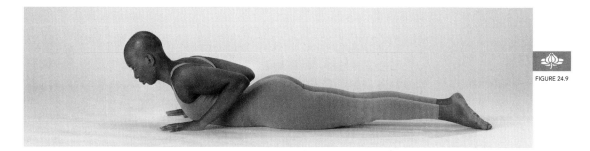

FIGURE 24.9

EXERCISE #9. **COBRA POSE (Bhujangasana), three to four breaths.** Lie on your belly with your head facing downward. Place your hands under your shoulders, keeping your elbows tucked into your sides. Press your pelvis toward the floor and slowly lift your head, looking forward. Slowly, take a deep breath in and come up a little bit farther, lifting your chest off the floor. Stay a few breaths, coming up a little higher if you can, but never taking your navel off the floor (see figure 24.9). To come out of the pose, push into your hands as you slowly lower yourself down. Turn your head to one side and relax.

EXERCISE #10. **ROCKING AND ROLLING, sixteen repetitions.** Start by lying on your back. Bring your knees in toward your chest on an exhalation, and wrap your arms around your legs, drawing them farther toward your chest. Start by gently rocking from side to

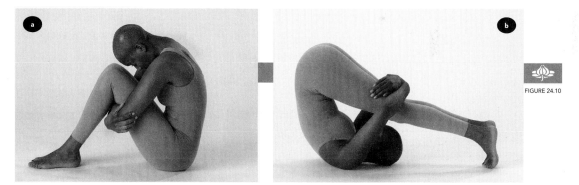

FIGURE 24.10

side, just to give your low back area a little massage on the floor. Let yourself be a little playful. Then begin rocking forward and back, exhaling as you come forward, inhaling as you move back (figures 24.10a & b). Try putting your hands underneath your knees and rocking up to a seated position and back down again. If you can't get up to sitting, that's okay.

Michael says that this is traditionally a pose of self-nurturing, like giving yourself a hug.

OTHER YOGIC IDEAS

Reclined Cobbler's pose (Supta Baddha Konasana) is a restorative pose that allows the abdominal muscles to relax almost completely and is considered soothing for intestinal conditions. It can also be a profoundly relaxing and calming pose to the nervous system, particularly if you hold it for ten minutes or longer. Supporting the thighs increases the ability of the muscles around the groin to let go, further facilitating abdominal relaxation (see p. 326). Inversions, supported (restorative) like Chair Shoulderstand (see pp. 275–76) or regular versions, may also be particularly helpful for constipation, both by reversing the effects of gravity on the body and because they can be deeply relaxing.

EXERCISE #11. **SEATED FORWARD BEND, three to four breaths.** Start by sitting with your legs stretched in front of you. Bend your left leg and place your left foot on the mat outside of your right knee (not inside as shown). Cradle your bent leg in your arms, as you

FIGURE 24.11

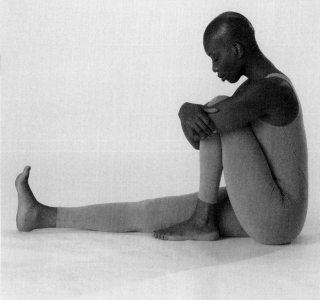

sit up tall, lengthening your back. On your next exhalation, bend forward from your hips just an inch or two, reaching with your chin toward your foot. Breathe and then come farther forward still cradling your leg (figure 24.11) until you find your edge. Stay a few breaths. To come out of the pose, inhale and roll back up. Take your arms behind you and lean back, releasing your head if you like. Shake out your legs and notice how you feel. Repeat on the other side.

EXERCISE #12. **MINDFULNESS MEDITATION, five to ten minutes.** Sit in a comfortable, upright position, either on the floor or on a chair. For the first minute, simply become a witness to your thoughts. Michael says one way to do this is to imagine your thoughts as little boats sailing across a lake, coming in from one side and disappearing out the other. As a thought comes in, simply watch it. Put it in the little boat, and let it sail by and out the other side. In doing that, you're watching the thought, acknowledging it, and letting go of it. If you prefer to use a different image, that's fine. Just do whatever works for you. If it helps, you can focus on your breath, just noticing the breath move in and out, and as you do so, watching the mind's eye.

In addition to taking the weekly class, Michael asked the students to practice for one hour at least six days a week. In each practice session, they were asked to do both some asana as well as meditation.

OTHER YOGIC IDEAS

The Viniyoga pose Apanasana can be soothing for the abdominal region and may be helpful for both diarrhea and constipation. To do the pose, lie on your back, bend your knees, and place each hand on its respective knee. As you exhale, gently bring your knees in toward the chest (left). As you inhale, let the knees drop back to their original position (right). Make the movements slow and deliberate so that they last the entire length of the breath. This exercise can be repeated several times.

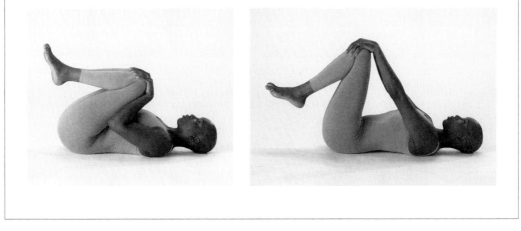

Contraindications, Special Considerations, and Modifications

For people with diarrhea, certain yoga practices, such as strong abdominal twists, should be avoided, as they can increase intestinal activity, potentially worsening symptoms. These poses may also be problematic for people with constipation, although gentle twisting may be beneficial. As always with yoga, you need to adjust your practice to how you're feeling. If you're more symptomatic than usual, you may need to back off in favor of gentler and more meditative practices.

A Holistic Approach to Irritable Bowel Syndrome

* Several types of food can exacerbate IBS symptoms, including fatty and fried foods, foods containing wheat, carbonated beverages, chocolate, caffeine, and some vegetables including cabbage, broccoli, and beans. Let your experience guide you.

* A study found that when IBS patients changed their diet and excluded beef and all cereals except rice-based ones, cut back on citrus fruits, caffeine, and yeast, and used soy products instead of dairy, they had less abdominal pain, fatigue, diarrhea, and constipation.

* Food additives such as monosodium glutamate (MSG) and the artificial sweetener Aspartame can trigger IBS symptoms.

* To reduce gas, avoid carbonated beverages, don't chew gum, and watch your consumption of beans, grapes, and raisins.

* Avoid sugarless gum if it contains sorbitol, a sweetener that can cause diarrhea.

* Soluble fiber can be very helpful for people with IBS whose predominant symptoms include constipation, and for some people with diarrhea. Fruits, vegetables, and whole grains are rich in fiber, particularly soluble fiber. If you start adding fiber to your diet, do so slowly over several weeks and be sure to drink plenty of additional water.

* If you don't get enough fiber from dietary sources, try psyllium, a natural source of soluble fiber.

* Avoid insoluble fiber, which is found in bran, eggplant skins, and bell peppers. It can make IBS symptoms worse.

* Digestive enzymes are safe and appear to effectively reduce gas. For those who are vegetarians, health food stores sell enzymes derived entirely from plant sources, such as papaya.

* Probiotics, essentially natural healthy bacteria like acidophilus in supplement form, appear to be very safe and possibly helpful for IBS.

* Tricyclic antidepressant drugs like desipramine, typically prescribed at one-half to one-third the typical dose used for depression, may help in IBS by modulating pain sensations in the central nervous system. Since tricyclics are often constipating, this treatment may be particularly useful for individuals whose IBS is marked by frequent diarrhea.

* People with diarrhea can get symptomatic relief with the antidiarrheal medication loperamide (Imodium).

* Peppermint is an herb that relaxes the smooth muscle of the bowel wall and can help ease symptoms such as cramping, abdominal distention, and the frequency of bowel movements. Enteric-coated capsules containing peppermint oil are very safe, don't cause the heartburn of non-coated peppermint oil or peppermint teas, and have been found to be effective.

* Acupuncture is safe and there is some evidence that it can help with IBS.

* A randomized controlled study published in *JAMA* found that treatment with a combination of Chinese herbs significantly improved IBS symptoms. While both standardized and individualized herbal combinations proved effective in the short term, fourteen weeks after the end of treatment, those who took the personalized prescription maintained greater improvement.

When Michael Faber began the eight-week program, he found it very difficult, partly because of how much anxiety he had about his health, and about how the foods he ate were affecting it. He realized at one point during his meditation practice that he was worrying about how much he was worrying. Then, he says, "I realized that me noticing that I was worrying about worrying was actually part of the practice. As I was able to see that more and more, a lot of the anxiety and fears started to dissolve." Seeing his worries as just thoughts that he could observe and let go of "was very freeing."

Through the program, Michael came to realize that the tension he felt in his mind was also present in his breathing. "It's often very shallow and rushed, which parallels my mind, which wants to do, do, do, and go, go, go." When he slowed his breath during sitting meditation, he noticed his heart was also slowing down. Through the yoga postures, he discovered that he held a lot of tension in his body, including in his throat and abdomen. "I started noticing that, through the practice, that was changing."

Michael Lee observed the changes in Michael Faber. "He experienced an incredible degree of relaxation. What he reported to the group was that he had never before been able to let himself go that much." During his time at the workshop, his symptoms, which had been very bad before he started, almost disappeared.

However, he found it challenging to stick with the practice, even though its benefits were so significant. "I guess I've struggled with having the discipline about sitting every day, doing yoga every day." Part of the problem is that he's always found satisfaction in achievement but when he's doing yoga or meditating, he always feels he should be doing something else—which, he concedes, "is on some level precisely why I need to practice."

The program, he says, helped him see the value in taking time for himself, "just doing nothing, just relaxing next to a river—that downtime that I didn't necessarily give myself before. In the past I really pushed myself beyond what was really healthy."

Summing it all up, he says that his symptoms recur, though in a milder form, when he doesn't do his practice, and they abate when he does. So he's trying to make the practice a regular part of his life. "It's kind of a work in progress, I guess."

MENOPAUSE

 ELISE BROWNING MILLER was a Peace Corps volunteer in Brazil more than thirty years ago when her back muscles went into painful spasms. Although she'd known for several years that she had scoliosis, a sideways curvature of the spine, this was the first time she'd had any serious pain related to it. Another Peace Corps volunteer, a handsome blond surfer, offered to teach her some yoga stretches, and it was an offer she couldn't refuse. The poses helped her, and upon returning to the States she became a follower of Integral yoga's Swami Satchidananda. Later, she was drawn to B. K. S. Iyengar's focus on anatomical alignment, which she found particularly helpful for her back. Elise now holds a master's degree in therapeutic recreation from the University of North Carolina; is a senior certified Iyengar yoga teacher; and has been teaching yoga since 1976 in Palo Alto, California, throughout the United States, and internationally. She is featured on the instructional videos *Yoga for Scoliosis* and *Intermediate Yoga in Fiji*.

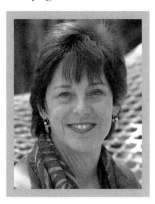

Connie Priddy has been doing yoga for over thirty years, and has studied with Elise since 1990. She originally took up yoga to help her deal with migraine headaches and back pain due to scoliosis, and it was Elise's expertise in that subject that first brought Connie to her. Several years later, she turned to Elise for guidance on dealing with the menopausal symptoms she had begun to develop. Although she had been on hormone therapy for several years, she had to go off the hormones after being diagnosed with breast cancer. Hot flashes soon followed, and they intensified in both duration and frequency when Connie was put on Tamoxifen, a cancer drug that blocks the effects of the female hormone estrogen. During the two years she remained on Tamoxifen she experienced other menopausal symptoms, such as memory problems, "but the hot flashes were the worst—two or three times an hour, and I would just get soaking wet, and weak." It was during this period that she consulted Elise for these symptoms.

Connie had started on hormone replacement therapy (HRT) when she was forty-five. Her doctors had done blood tests and told her that she was perimenopausal, and prescribed estrogen and progestin. She took the hormones right up until she was diagnosed with breast cancer, then had to stop them abruptly. "There was no history of breast cancer in my family, but I suspect that I'm one of those who got it as a result of taking those two medications," she says.

The stress Connie was under because of the breast cancer diagnosis and treatment, and severe menopausal symptoms, were only part of what she was going through. Four months before she learned she had breast cancer, her husband had died of brain tumors after a long period of serious depression that had begun when he was fired from his job, effectively ending his career. With a daughter in college and many bills to pay, she had to sell their house, move, and go back to work for the first time in twenty years, all while still getting radiation treatments.

Overview of Menopause

Menopause refers to the time after the ovaries have stopped releasing eggs, levels of the female hormones estrogen and progesterone drop, menstrual periods cease, and it is no longer possible to conceive a child. Menopause can come on naturally or it can be the result of chemotherapy for cancer or the surgical removal of the ovaries. Natural menopause typically occurs in a woman's late forties or early fifties, but there is a wide age range. Perimenopause is the transitional phase when periods are often irregular. During both perimenopause and menopause it's common to experience mood swings and such symptoms as hot flashes, vaginal dryness, and memory problems. Symptoms vary enormously from woman to woman. Many pass through this stage with few symptoms and minimal disruption to their lives, while others are nearly incapacitated.

For years, doctors prescribed HRT for the treatment of menopausal and perimenopausal symptoms, as well as the prevention of heart disease and osteoporosis. The thinking on HRT has changed radically as recent scientific studies suggest that, if anything, the risk of heart disease as well as of strokes, blood clots, and breast cancer is higher in women who take HRT, specifically those who take a combination of estrogen derived from the urine of mares (Premarin) and synthetic progesterone. This particular combination was found to lower the risk of osteoporosis as well as of colon cancer but most experts now believe that the heightened risk of breast cancer, heart attacks, and other problems makes the long-term use of this drug regimen inappropriate for most women.

> **TIP** It is not yet known whether so-called bioidentical or bioequivalent hormones will prove safer than the conventional versions that Connie had been on. But for women with debilitating night sweats, mood swings, and other menopausal symptoms that haven't responded to more benign measures like soy or herbal remedies (see below), a year or two of hormone therapy might seem worth the risk. Every woman needs to weigh the risks and benefits and make her own decision.

How Yoga Fits In

Women of menopausal age are typically at the stage of life when they are facing a lot of stress from juggling the responsibilities of work, kids, and aging parents. And some, like Connie, may face even worse life stressors, including illness and death in the family. Since many yogis (and a growing number of people in the medical and scientific communities) believe that stress plays a significant role in the severity of menopausal symptoms, reducing stress is thought to be helpful in dealing with hot flashes and mood swings. As discussed in chapter 3, in addition to asana, the yogic tools of pranayama, restorative poses, and meditation are particularly useful for minimizing the effects of stress.

Yoga can help address another big concern for women at menopause and beyond: thinning bones. Although many people don't realize it, stress and osteoporosis are linked. Mental tension raises levels of the stress hormone cortisol, which contributes to the loss of calcium from bones and interferes with new bone growth. In addition to its effectiveness in dealing with stress, yoga offers weight-bearing postures that help build bone strength, and unlike many other forms of exercise, a number of asanas such as Downward-Facing Dog and Handstand involve weight-bearing in the hands and arms, building those bones as well. Since wrist fractures are among the most common breaks related to thinning bones, these poses can be particularly helpful for older women.

While much of the focus in the postmenopausal period is on keeping the bones strong, many women (and men) also lose significant muscle mass as they age. This loss of muscle can contribute to a number of problems, including poor posture, arthritis, and the risk of falling. Since some of the asanas that increase bone strength also build muscle, and since standing poses and balancing postures also improve the sense of balance, potentially lowering the risk of falls—a leading cause of injury, disability, and even death—yoga, independent of its effects on building bone, is likely to help prevent fractures and other injuries.

Heart disease, the other major condition that HRT was supposed to help prevent, remains the number one killer of women in the industrial world, with the incidence of heart attacks climbing substantially after menopause. Here, again, yoga can help. Yoga can lower levels of stress, improve cholesterol readings, lower blood pressure, improve aerobic conditioning, bring additional oxygen to the heart, and reduce levels of frustration and anger (see chapter 19). With this multiplicity of beneficial effects, yoga is likely to significantly lower the risk of heart disease.

Menopause is a time of change, and change, yoga teaches, is inevitable. Coping with unwanted change is above all a spiritual issue. Elise says, "It's hard when we go through the menopause to acknowledge that we're getting older." Denial, anger, and resistance are common, she finds. Yoga's emphasis on meeting challenges with acceptance and gratitude acts as an antidote to these negative, self-defeating attitudes.

The Scientific Evidence

In the large survey done by the Yoga Biomedical Trust mentioned in chapter 1, 83 percent of women reporting "menopausal disorders" found their regular yoga practice helpful.

A randomized controlled trial of thirty-three women with hot flashes done at Harvard's Mind/Body Medical Institute evaluated the effects of stress-reduction training. The women who practiced the relaxation response, a technique based on yogic mantra meditation, had statistically significant reductions in hot flash intensity as well as in measures of anxiety and depression as compared to the control group.

Another randomized controlled study of thirty-three women with hot flashes, published in the *American Journal of Obstetrics and Gynecology,* found that slow, deep, regular breathing led to statistically significant reductions in the frequency of hot flashes. The women taught the breathing technique also developed slower breathing rates and larger lung volumes, which serve to increase the efficiency of breathing.

A pilot study led by Dr. Beth Cohen at the University of California, San Francisco, followed thirteen women with moderate to severe hot flashes for eight weeks who were taught eight restorative yoga postures (see chapter 3). The women attended ninety-minute classes once a week and were encouraged to practice at home on other days, which they did on average for almost half an hour per day. Since there was no control group, the researchers compared each woman's symptoms before and after the program. At the end of eight weeks, the women experienced an average of a 31 percent reduction in the number of hot flashes, and a 34 percent reduction in their severity. In addition, the women lost on average almost three pounds, had a significant increase in HDL (good) cholesterol, and reported improved sleep.

Elise Miller's Approach

Elise pays attention not just to the physical symptoms of women going through the change, but their mental state. "With perimenopause," Elise says, "women are often surprised by not only the irregularity of their periods, but the irregularity of emotions." The emotions are similar to the premenstrual tension that many women experience before their periods, but the timing is completely unpredictable. "So one of the things that I focus on is supported standing poses, which help with getting grounded." These poses use either the wall or a chair for support (see pp. 465–68). Elise encourages her students to get in and out of the poses slowly, and to bring their attention to their breath and to the grounding they get from their feet and their legs.

The sequence of practices that Elise provided for Connie is described below. Note that props are required for a number of the poses. Elise requires all her clients working on menopausal symptoms to have a bolster and one or two blocks.

EXERCISE #1. SUPPORTED DOWNWARD-FACING DOG (Adho Mukha Svanasana), one minute or longer. Place a bolster, block, or folded blanket on your mat to support your head. Come down on all fours, with your arms slightly in front of your shoulders and your feet hips' width apart, with your toes turned under. On an exhalation, straighten your legs and push up through your arms to come into the pose. Allow your head to rest comfortably on the prop (figure 25.1), without compressing the neck or shoulders.

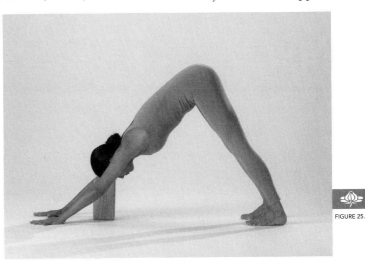

FIGURE 25.1

When Elise taught Connie this pose, she used ropes mounted on the wall of her studio to support Connie's thighs, making this pose even more supported. If you want to support your hips but don't have wall ropes, Elise offers a simple solution. Loop a ten-foot yoga strap around both knobs of an open door and place the prop for your head close by. Then step into the loop and bring the strap to the upper part of your leg bones. Bend your knees and place your hands on the floor, reach out with your arms and walk your feet back to go into the pose, adjusting your hands and feet as necessary. Bring the backs of your legs near the two doorknobs and place the prop under your head so your head can rest comfortably on it. (Some modern doors have knobs that cannot bear much weight. If you're concerned about yours, Aadil Palkhivala suggests looping the strap around the center hinge of the door and then around your hips.)

EXERCISE #2. **WIDE-LEGGED STANDING FORWARD BEND** (Prasarita Padottanasana), one minute. Stand with your feet approximately four feet apart and

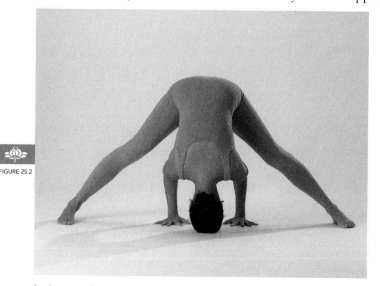

FIGURE 25.2

your toes facing directly forward. With an exhalation, bend forward at the hips and bring your hands to the floor under your shoulders. Inhale and lengthen your spine. Exhale and bring the top of your head down toward the floor, placing your hands parallel to your feet with fingers facing forward. If the top of your head does not comfortably reach the ground, place a block, bolster, or other prop underneath it. When your head is supported by the floor or a prop, the pose is more calming and restorative. To come out of the pose, place your hands on your waist, step your feet slightly closer together, inhale, and come up.

Connie found this pose very helpful for her hot flashes. "It cooled me off, calmed me down, helped me feel centered and rooted."

EXERCISE #3. **STANDING FORWARD BEND (Uttanasana), with head support, one minute.** Set up for the pose by placing a block, bolster, or chair in front of your feet to support your head. Stand with your feet together. As you exhale, bend at the hips and bring your hands to the floor and the crown of your head to the prop. If you are less flexible, you can rest your head on the seat of a chair or even on props that you have placed on top of the chair seat.

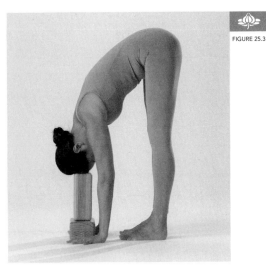

FIGURE 25.3

EXERCISE #4. **UNSUPPORTED SHOULDERSTAND (Niralamba Sarvangasana), two to five minutes.** To set up for the pose, fold three or more blankets into rectangles and stack them with the rounded edges on one side of the stack. Place the stack about eighteen inches from a wall, with the rounded edges facing the wall. Then lie down on the blanket stack so that your shoulders are on the blankets and your head is between the blankets and the wall. Place your hands alongside your body, bend your knees, and put the soles of your feet flat on the floor. As you exhale, push down with your hands and swing your hips over your shoulders. Bring your hands to your back to support yourself. Straighten your legs, placing the toes and balls of your feet on the wall. If you are a more advanced student and secure in your balance, bring your hands to the fronts of your thighs, as Connie does. If not, and you need support, place your hands on your back in the traditional manner (see p. 419). To come down, place your hands on your back to support yourself as you bend your knees and roll out of the pose.

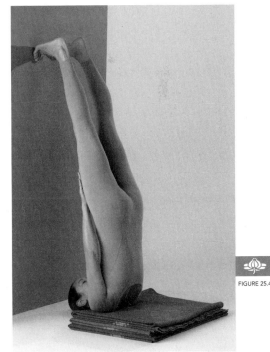

FIGURE 25.4

For Shoulderstand and Plow pose, Elise recommends students support their shoulders on an average of three blankets, which is how many Connie used. For students who are just beginning or are not comfortable with Shoulderstand, she recommends substituting Legs-Up-the-Wall pose (Viparita Karani, see p. 64).

EXERCISE #5. **HALF PLOW POSE (Ardha Halasana), two to five minutes.** To set up for the pose, place your folded blankets in front of a chair, with the rounded edges facing the chair. Then lie back on the blanket stack with your shoulders on the blanket and your

FIGURE 25.5

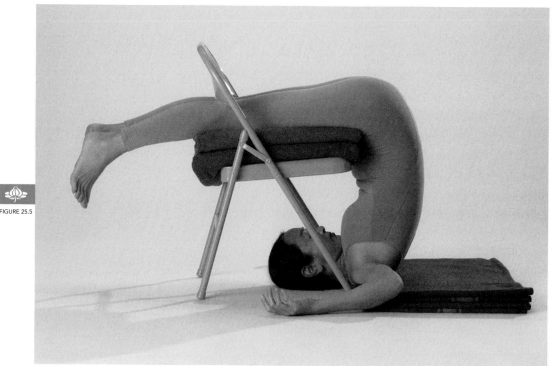

head just over the edge of the blankets, looking up toward the bottom of the seat of the chair. Place your arms alongside your body and push down with them as your elevate your hips and bring your thighs to the top of the chair seat for support. If your thighs do not rest easily on the chair seat, you can place folded blankets or a bolster on the chair seat. Extend your legs through the space at the back of the chair. Your back should be straight, not rounded. Ideally the edge of the chair should come right to your hips. (If your chair has a support bar between the front legs, this may not be possible. See p. 328.) The hips should be directly over the shoulders (see figure 25.5).

Elise recommends this pose for hot flashes and also for headaches, as long as they are not too severe.

EXERCISE #6. **SUPPORTED BRIDGE POSE (Setu Bandha Sarvangasana), two minutes.** To set up for the pose, place one yoga block on its side at the wall and have a second block nearby. Position yourself near the wall so that when your legs are extended, the soles of your feet just come to the wall. Lie on your back with your knees bent and your feet flat on the floor near your buttocks. Place your arms alongside your torso with your palms up.

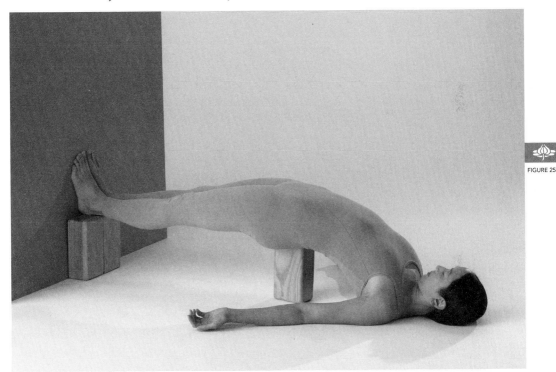

FIGURE 25.6

On an exhalation, push down on your hands and feet and lift your hips. Once your hips are elevated, slip a yoga block on its tall side underneath your sacrum at the back of your pelvis. Then, one at a time, extend your legs and place your feet on the block at the wall (see figure 25.6). Stay two minutes.

If Connie was exhausted or having a lot of menopausal symptoms, Elise had her do a more restorative version of the same pose (which she also recommends for beginning students). Set up for the pose by placing two bolsters in a line, then place a folded blanket near the end of one bolster to support your head and shoulders. Make a loop with a yoga strap and keep it nearby. To enter the pose, sit on the bolster closer to the blanket, and swing your feet onto the second bolster, keeping your knees bent. Loop the strap loosely around your upper thighs. If you want an even more restorative pose, you can loop a strap

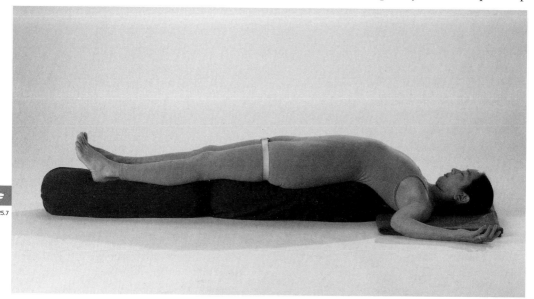

FIGURE 25.7

around your ankles, too. As a trial run, lie back on the bolster so the bottom tips of your shoulder blades touch the edge of the bolster, and the tops of your shoulders and your head rest comfortably on the blanket. Scoot your torso into position if necessary. Come back up and tighten the yoga strap(s). When you are all set up, lie down again and rest the tops of your shoulders and your head on the blanket. Straighten your legs, and bring your arms out to the sides or into cactus position (figure 25.7).

The straps provide additional support and help you feel more grounded. For even more grounding, you can place sandbags on the tops of your thighs. Elise says, "That pose is so powerful. It starts quieting the nervous system almost immediately." If you only have one bolster, you can do the same pose with your feet resting on a block.

EXERCISE #7. **UJJAYI II PRANAYAMA, five minutes.** You can do this exercise either sitting up, if you are experienced with pranayama, or lying down. If you do this exercise upright, sit in a comfortable cross-legged position with your spine tall. Without rounding your lower or upper back, lower your chin toward your breastbone into jalandhara bandha, the chin lock (figure 25.8a). If you do this exercise lying down, use a pranayama pillow or fold your blankets so that they are about eight inches wide and several feet long

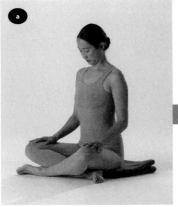

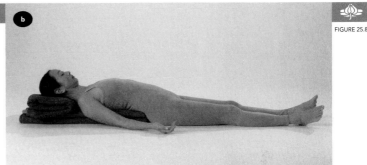

FIGURE 25.8

(figure 25.8b). Sit in front of the prop (not on it) and lie back with your spine on the prop and extra support under your head to ensure your chin is lower than the forehead. Let your arms and legs rest at your sides as in Relaxation pose. Close your eyes.

Breathe in normally through your nose (not using Ujjayi), and then use Ujjayi to slow your exhalation (if you don't already know how to do Ujjayi breathing, see pp. 16–17). Elise says, "The inhalation is an observation of the breath. The exhalation is long and slow, like a balloon slowly deflating, seeping out." It's a subtle breath just loud enough to keep your attention but not so loud that it disturbs your psyche.

EXERCISE #8. **RELAXATION POSE (Savasana), ten minutes.** If you are comfortable doing Relaxation pose with the same support as for reclined pranayama above (a practice that in the Iyengar system is known as Savasana II), Elise recommends doing it that way. Otherwise remove the blankets and lie flat, with support under your head as needed. To facilitate relaxation, you can place a bolster sideways under your knees (figure 25.9).

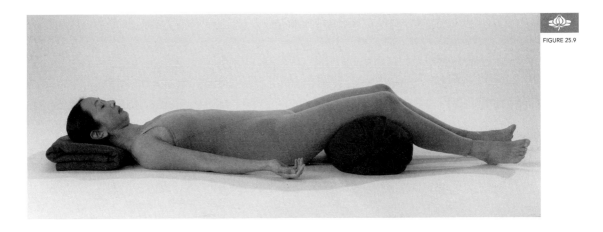

FIGURE 25.9

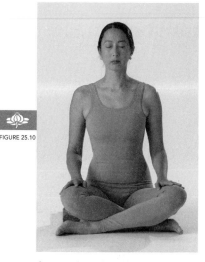

FIGURE 25.10

EXERCISE #9. **MEDITATION, five minutes.** Sit in a comfortable position with your spine tall but relaxed. Close your eyes. Begin to tune in to your breath, noticing the air moving through your nose. Listen to the sound it makes. If you find your focus has wavered, simply return your attention to the breath without judging yourself.

The restorative style of yoga described above is what Elise recommends when a student is having hot flashes and other bothersome symptoms. After symptoms abate, her approach changes to a more vigorous form of asana, focused on keeping your body and mind healthy for the years to come. "Then I work with arm balances, standing poses, Downward- and Upward-Facing Dog, even some weight-bearing backbends." These poses not only strengthen bones but also the spirit. For example, Elise says, "I encourage women in my classes in their fifties and sixties to work with Elbow pose, Pincha Mayurasana, the arm balance." (See figure 25.9.) "It's a way of saying, 'I've still got my vitality.'"

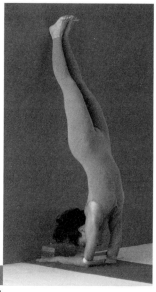

FIGURE 25.11

OTHER YOGIC IDEAS

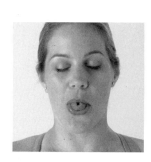

Yogis consider the pranayama technique Sithali, in which you curl your tongue and slowly inhale through your mouth (see left), to be cooling and therefore helpful for hot flashes. (Those unable to curl the tongue can do a related technique where you keep your tongue flat and inhale through your mouth.) The exhalation is through the nose. Try the practice for one to five minutes.

Contraindications, Special Considerations, and Modifications

Women going through menopause may need to avoid certain strenuous yoga practices that can bring on hot flashes. Connie often got hot flashes when she did intense backbends like Upward Bow pose (Urdhva Dhanurasana). But if she did a backbend lying through a chair (figure 25.12), a supported pose that allowed her to focus on her breathing, that usually solved the problem. On the occasional days when even this proved too much, Elise would substitute poses like Supported Bridge pose (see figures 25.6 and 25.7). Intense abdominal work, such as in the Boat pose (Navasana) and twists, vigorous Sun Salutations, and Headstands may also bring on hot flashes. Elise had Connie do a more restorative version of Headstand, hanging from ropes, which she likes. Forward bends can be soothing, but only if done in a relaxed manner.

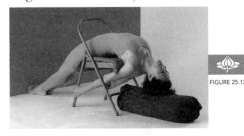

FIGURE 25.12

> **TIP** The recommendations in this chapter to do "cooling" practices and avoid "heating" ones are informed by Ayurveda, the traditional system of medicine in India (see chapter 4). Ayurveda views hot flashes as a pitta problem, that is, too much "fire" in the body. To diminish pitta, it would suggest you drink plenty of water and limit your intake of spicy food, hot drinks, and alcohol in favor of sweet fruits like apples and pears, and watery vegetables like cucumber and zucchini.

Kripalu yoga teacher and physical therapist Sara Meeks warns that in women with significant bone loss due to osteoporosis—particularly those who have already had fractures due to thinning bones—forward bends, especially seated ones, can lead to compression fractures of the vertebrae and should be avoided entirely. Dropping the head in these poses increases the pressure on the spine even more. Other poses that are contraindicated in people with known osteoporosis include Knee-to-Chest pose and straight leg raises. High impact movement, like jumping from pose to pose, is also to be avoided. Even simple Child's pose (figure 25.13), she says, can compress the front of the spine and cause a fracture.

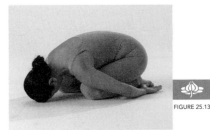

FIGURE 25.13

Also of concern for those at risk of osteoporosis are any postures in which you might lose your balance and fall. These would include inversions like Headstand, balancing poses like Tree pose, and even some standing poses. Doing the poses close to a wall or using a chair for support, however, can allow you to safely do these poses, and there is good reason you ought to. Because these asanas test your balance, practicing them regularly is one of the best ways to improve it. Better balance learned on your yoga mat could help you avoid a disastrous fall at home.

A Holistic Approach to Menopause

✳ Increasingly, doctors are favoring conventional drugs like Fosamax (alendronate) and Evista (raloxifene) over hormone therapy to keep bones strong. These drugs won't help hot flashes and other symptoms, but raloxifene appears to have the advantage of actually lowering the risk of breast cancer.

✳ If you smoke, quitting can keep bones healthier, in addition to lowering the risk of cancer, heart disease, and menopausal symptoms like hot flashes.

✳ Calcium is essential for bone health. You need around 1,500 mg of calcium per day, either through diet or supplements. Foods high in calcium include dairy products, sardines, and green leafy vegetables.

✳ If you take calcium supplements, be sure to space the doses since most people can only absorb about 500 mg at a time. Adding vitamin D aids absorption. Since calcium can lead to magnesium depletion, take supplemental magnesium along with calcium (at about half the dose; for example, 250 mg of magnesium with 500 mg of calcium).

✳ Soft drinks should be avoided since the high phosphorous content can leach calcium from bones.

✳ Symptoms like hot flashes are far less common in countries like Japan and Korea where diets are high in soy products. Foods like tofu, soy milk, miso, and tempeh are rich in natural phytoestrogens (plant estrogens) that may account for this difference. Phytoestrogens are also found in other natural foods including whole grains, nuts, flaxseeds, carrots, and chickpeas.

✳ There is less evidence that supplemental soy-derived isoflavones can fight peri-menopausal symptoms—and more reason to worry about safety (see chapter 4).

✳ Some women find, and there is some scientific evidence, that an herbal remedy, black cohosh—another source of natural phytoestrogens—is useful for hot flashes (though a recent large study found it no better than a placebo). Other evidence suggests that it may help with vaginal dryness and sensitivity, and have some utility in preserving bone and in improving levels of blood fats after menopause.

* Other supplements that may help with menopausal symptoms, though the evidence is not strong, include red clover, dong quai (usually used in combination with other Chinese herbs), evening primrose oil, and vitamin E. Of these products, evening primrose oil may be the safest. Keep in mind that it can take a few months for herbal preparations to take full effect.

* There is evidence that acupuncture can effectively reduce menopausal symptoms, and it has other health benefits.

Connie says, "Yoga saved my life. Yoga helps keep me centered and rooted, and helps keep me physically fit, too." She found so much relief from her yoga practice that after a lumpectomy and the removal of some of her lymph nodes, she could hardly wait to get back to it. Three weeks later she was already testing herself with a few poses to see if she was strong enough to do a practice.

Later, when her hot flashes became really bad, she found that the deep Ujjayi breathing Elise recommended was very helpful. Other poses she found helpful besides those described in the sequence above included Baddha Konasana (Cobbler's pose), both sitting and supine versions, and Upavistha Konasana (Wide-Legged Forward Bend).

Community, what yogis call sangha, has been a major source of healing for Connie. She says she could not have gotten through that period in her life without her friends, half of whom she met through yoga. Her yoga buddies helped her move, brought her meals, and were part of a group that completely surprised her the morning after she'd moved into her new, more modest house not far away. "The doorbell rang and I went to the door, and there were fifteen people out there. It was like an old-fashioned barn raising. A lot of my friends brought their husbands, and by the end of that day my bookshelves were up and the books were on them, everything was unpacked and put away in the kitchen, pictures were hung on the wall, and the boxes were knocked down and taken away."

"You know," Connie says, "you can't help but have an open heart if you seriously practice yoga. And having an open heart brings compassion and love, and you give it, then it's given back to you. I will never give up yoga. I may have to do fewer and fewer of the postures, or do them less and less flexibly, but I will never give up yoga."

CHAPTER 26

MULTIPLE SCLEROSIS (MS)

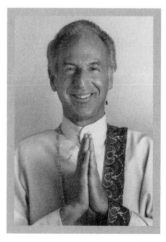

When ERIC SMALL says he comes from a long line of horse traders, he means it literally. From a very early age Eric learned how to look a horse in the mouth. "You never believed what the owner told you; you had to make your own evaluation." It was under his horse-trading father's tutelage that Eric first became a teacher—at the age of six. "My father would put me on a box in the middle of the ring—a little kid, blond hair, big, thick glasses, skinny as a rail—and I could teach people how to ride horses. And I could project my voice. I knew what to look for." When he began practicing yoga more than fifty years ago after developing MS at the age of twenty-two, the transition to teaching was natural. It was what he'd been doing all his life. His commitment to teaching yoga became even stronger when he studied with B. K. S. Iyengar, whose work forms the basis of what he now gives to his students. Eric says Iyengar's approach is so powerful that "you don't want to keep this to yourself." He runs the Beverly Hills Iyengar Yoga Studio, is the coauthor of *Yoga and Multiple Sclerosis,* and is featured in the video *Yoga with Eric Small.* Eric and his wife, Flora Thornton, have funded two major yoga programs, The Eric Small Adaptive Iyengar Yoga Program, available nationally through local chapters of the MS Society, and The Eric Small Living Well with MS program, offered in Southern California.

By the time Jack Cullin (not his real name) was finally diagnosed with multiple sclerosis at the age of thirty-one, he had developed double vision, extreme fatigue, and a balance problem, as well as numbness in his legs and left arm. The diagnosis was made only after he had already had three flare-ups of symptoms. The symptoms abated again after the diagnosis, and the residual symptoms didn't seem serious enough to move him to radically change his lifestyle. He continued to work in a very stressful, upper-level job as an account executive for a large marketing firm, which left him little time to spend with his wife and two young children.

However, eight months later, after yet another flare-up left him with some difficulty balancing while walking, a friend finally convinced him to try Eric's class. He'd been resistant to his friend's earlier suggestions, Eric says, because he thought yoga "was just some kind of mystical chanting or something." In spite of his skepticism, he was curious and also perhaps just desperate enough to give yoga a shot.

Overview of Multiple Sclerosis

Multiple sclerosis is an autoimmune disease of unknown cause in which the immune system attacks the fatty tissue, known as myelin, which acts as insulation for nerve cells in the brain and spinal cord. Lacking myelin, nerve cells are inefficient at passing their messages down the line, and as a result, the functions those nerves serve can be affected. Recent evidence also suggests that the immune system attacks the nerve fibers themselves. For years, researchers have postulated that a viral infection results in an immune response that turns on the body, though the theory remains unproven. There is clearly also a genetic component, as the disease is more common in people who have an affected relative. People of northern European ancestry as well as those who grow up in cold climates are more likely to be affected.

The clinical course of MS is highly variable, from fairly mild to rapidly debilitating. The classic and most common form is what is known as relapsing-remitting MS. In this type, attacks result in discrete losses in nerve function, different from one attack to the next, which fully or partially disappear between attacks. This is the form of the disease that both Jack and Eric have. Less commonly, the disease progresses steadily without remissions. Sometimes, for unknown reasons, MS goes into long-term or permanent remission.

Symptoms from MS are extremely diverse, reflecting the different parts of the nervous system involved. Common symptoms include a clumsiness or loss of feeling in the arms and legs, difficulty with balance, a reduction in bowel or bladder control, and sexual dysfunction. Also common are blindness in one or both eyes due to involvement of the optic nerve, double vision like Jack experienced, painful contractions in muscles, overwhelming fatigue, emotional problems, and difficulty with thinking and memory.

> **CAUTION** There is no definitive test for MS. Making the diagnosis depends on taking a careful history of symptoms and looking at suggestive but not definitive findings on MRI scans and other tests. It is vital—particularly if you are contemplating drugs that have potentially serious side effects, cost thousands of dollars a year, and are meant to be long-term regimens—to be sure you truly have the disease. Experts debate how frequently MS is incorrectly diagnosed, but estimates vary from one-tenth to one-third of cases. If you have any doubt about your diagnosis, don't hesitate to get a second and third opinion.

How Yoga Fits In

There are a number of ways that yoga can help with MS. Though the idea remains controversial among some physicians, studies suggest that stress is an important factor in increasing the likelihood of developing the disease and in flare-ups after the initial onset. Precisely how stress causes these effects isn't known, but it is hypothesized that elevated levels of the stress hormone cortisol increase levels of proinflammatory cytokines, internal messengers of the body's immune system, which fuel inflammation and contribute to the destruction of the myelin lining of nerve fibers.

Beyond stress's possible role in the physiology of MS, stress is certainly an offshoot of living with the disease, which can be very challenging. If only because yoga can be so effective at combating stress and depression, it can be useful medicine for those trying to cope with the illness, helping to improve quality of life both during and between flare-ups.

Yoga can help in other ways, too. Gaining heightened awareness of the body, breathing more deeply and regularly, improving balance and coordination, and learning to let go of holding in muscles—these are all areas where yoga practice, specifically the practice of asana and pranayama, can make a big difference. People with MS can develop contractures, areas where the connective tissue around joints tightens, leading to a loss in movement. Over time, a regular yoga practice and the slower, deeper breathing that comes with it can help reverse these detrimental changes.

Poor posture can contribute to muscle tightness and pain. Asana practice can improve posture as can a regular practice of pranayama and meditation. All of these practices appear to be useful in boosting mood, as well. A regular meditation practice may be particularly useful in helping with pain control (see chapter 3).

The yogic tool of karma yoga, selfless service, may be useful, too. One study found that people with MS who volunteered to work on a telephone support line for other people with the disease noted significant improvements in their self-esteem, confidence, and mood. In that study, in fact, the volunteers showed greater benefits than those they counseled. Your local chapter of the MS Society may have information about volunteer opportunities, which, beyond any health benefits, provide social contacts in what can be an isolating disease.

The course of MS tends to be quite variable, and one of the beauties of yoga is that it can be adapted to meet the student's changing needs. If fatigue is a problem, a more restorative practice can be used. If a particular limb is weak, props can be used to help the person do the poses with more ease. If balance is an issue, postures can be done standing against the wall or holding a chair for support. For people who are unable to stand, even with assistance, asana practice can be modified to accommodate them. Some breathing, guided meditation, and meditation practices can be done in bed if necessary. Sam Dworkis, who has had MS for a number of years, says yoga is about "learning how to accept what your body allows you to do at any given moment, and understanding that's the reality." If you think you're not healthy enough or flexible enough to do yoga, he believes you're focusing too much on what you can't do, and not enough on what you can. "The thing that's so interesting to me is that my yoga practice enables me to pay more attention to the things I do have control over."

Yoga can also help build hope. Even though yoga can't cure the disease, doing it can lessen your symptoms and enhance your sense of well-being, encouraging faith and maybe even optimism. When you realize you are feeling better as a direct result of something you have done, it gives you a sense of empowerment, because of the concrete steps you have taken to improve your own situation.

Yogic Tool: **TAPAS.** Tapas (see pp. 21–23) is the dedication and discipline that fuels your yoga practice. Eric stresses that the key to success with yoga is the work you do. "I'm not interested in somebody coming here and dropping their body in front of me, and letting me do all the work. This is not what yoga is about. Yoga is what you do for yourself. And that's a big step—a *big* step. You can easily say, 'Oh, I can't do this because I have MS. So I'll just sit here and be helpless.' Or, 'If I do it for three weeks, will I be better?' My requirements are that you meet me halfway. As much as I give you, you must also practice to give yourself." The minimum amount of practice that Eric recommends is half an hour daily. "And they have to bring me their homework sheets indicating how much time they spent doing each one of the exercises."

The Scientific Evidence

In a 2002 survey conducted by Oregon Health Sciences University (OHSU), 30 percent of the almost two thousand people with MS interviewed said they had taken yoga. Of that group, 57 percent reported that yoga was "very beneficial," a better result than any MS drug elicited.

To date there is only one controlled study that has examined the effects of yoga on MS. Not surprisingly, Eric Small served as a consultant on the project. Led by Barry Oken, MD, a professor of neurology at OHSU, the study randomized sixty-nine people with different types of MS into three study groups for six months. The first group took part in a weekly Iyengar asana class specifically adapted for people with MS. The second group took a weekly exercise class using stationary bicycles. Members of the exercise group were given a stationary bike for home use, and those doing yoga were encouraged to practice at home every day in addition to the weekly class. Members of the third group continued their usual activities. Both the yoga and exercise interventions resulted in a statistically significant improvement in fatigue, one of the most prevalent and potentially debilitating symptoms of MS. Subjects in the yoga and exercise groups also reported a statistically significant improvement in their overall health. The researchers noted some improvement in mood, too, though the magnitude of the change wasn't statistically significant.

Eric Small's Approach

In the *Yoga Sutras,* Patanjali speaks of the need to balance effort and ease. Trying too hard either on or off your yoga mat can actually interfere with what you hope to achieve, a major problem for people with MS, who Eric says "are all type A personalities." (See chapter 19.) Wanting badly to keep up with those around them and to maintain appearances, "They all push themselves too hard." Doing so, he believes, takes a toll on already taxed nervous systems, increasing stress. Eric says that even students who have tremors or sudden weaknesses often don't want to use the props and supports he recommends. "They're the tough ones," he says. "Those are the people you need to slow down."

Eric likes to put his new students with MS in restorative poses right away, particularly those who tend to try too hard. It slows them down and gives him a chance to evaluate them. One focus of his observations is how well the student follows instructions. "That gives you a fairly good idea of their cognitive function, and their retention of information. It also gives me an idea as to how the body has been affected by the disease—whether there's a general weakness, specific weaknesses, spasms, what is the range of motion."

Based on what he sees in those first restorative poses, Eric adjusts the program. If he notices a loss of range of motion in the hip, for example, he'll use extra props to brace that area. For him it's all about individualizing the therapy to the specific needs of the student. "You modify and modify, with blankets, other props, chairs, pillows, and belts, and blocks. You support, you keep supporting." In addition to taking a case history, including flare-ups and residual symptoms, he finds out what medications they're taking and does a hands-on assessment. He notices their posture and breathing; he even inspects the pattern of wear on their shoes.

On first examination, Eric saw that Jack appeared to be a relatively healthy man of average weight, with muscle tone that was average to above average—perhaps attributable to the fact that Jack had been a runner and hiker. Eric noticed that Jack listed dramatically toward the left, although Jack was not aware of it. This told him that Jack's left side was the weak side. "I also noticed that he had a tendency to go forward and backward, almost imperceptibly," an indication that Jack was struggling with his balance. This suggested to him that Jack had a problem with his inner ear. Because Jack had a suitable chair at home, Eric made liberal use of a chair prop in the routine he designed. He likes the support and the help with balance that chairs provide his MS students.

The sequence of poses and instructions that Eric provided for Jack follows. None of the poses are held longer than ten seconds, because he feels that when you are dealing with people who fatigue easily, have problems with balance, and often have short attention spans, the poses should be comfortable and quick. If fatigue becomes a problem, he allows for relaxation time between poses.

EXERCISE #1. **CHANTING OM.** Sit in a comfortable upright position on the floor or on a chair, and close your eyes. If you sit on a chair, place folded blankets on the seat of the chair (figure 26.1), or on the floor in front of the chair, depending on your height, so that your knees and hips are at the same level and your knees are directly over your ankles, with your feet flat on the floor. Inhale. On your exhalation begin making the sound "O" for several seconds. While continuing to exhale, close your lips and hum the "M" sound for a few more seconds. Repeat twice.

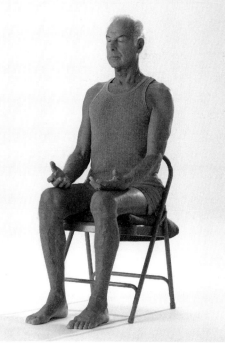

FIGURE 26.1

Eric asks students to make chanting of Om part of their home practice because he believes the vibrational component of the sound waves has therapeutic value, particularly with a neural disorder.

>
> **TIP** In all the asana Eric teaches, breath remains a major focus. "Any expansive movement is done on the inhalation, and any contraction is on the exhalation. Standard operating procedure." For example, you inhale on moving into a backbend or raising the arms above the head, because these movements open the body and are considered expansive. You exhale on going into forward bends, which brings the body in on itself, and is considered a contraction.

EXERCISE #2. **COBBLER'S POSE (Baddha Konasana), in a chair.** Set up for the pose by placing one or two bolsters or a second chair in front of your chair to support your feet. The stiffer you are, the lower the support should be. To come into the pose, sit upright on your chair, bend your knees, and bring the soles of your feet together on the prop. Allow your knees to gently drop to the side.

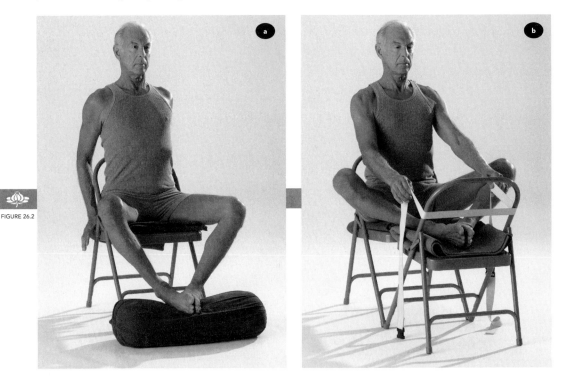

FIGURE 26.2

Due to some stiffness, Jack started with his feet on a bolster placed on the floor in front of the chair (figure 26.2a) and later went up to two bolsters. After three months of regular practice, he was easily able to put his feet up onto the seat of a second chair and to drop his knees to at least 60 degrees (figure 26.2b).

EXERCISE #3. **SUPPORTED WARRIOR II (Virabhadrasana II), holding a strap.** To set up for the pose, place a chair on a yoga mat and have a looped yoga strap nearby. Now step your right foot through the back of the chair, and bend your knee so your thigh is supported by the seat of the chair and your front foot is on the floor. If balance is a problem, turn the chair sideways (figure 26.3), since putting the foot through the back could lead to a fall. Extend your left leg behind you and turn the left foot slightly in. Putting your weight more onto the leg on the chair seat may allow you to bring your legs into better alignment. Next, extend your arms to the sides, holding the strap looped around the right hand between your thumb and your palm, extending around the back of your neck and between the thumb and palm of your left hand. When the belt crosses your neck, it should pass over your seventh cervical vertebra (C7, the prominent bump on the lower part of the back of your neck). Do a little "push-pull" between your two hands. Repeat the pose on the other side.

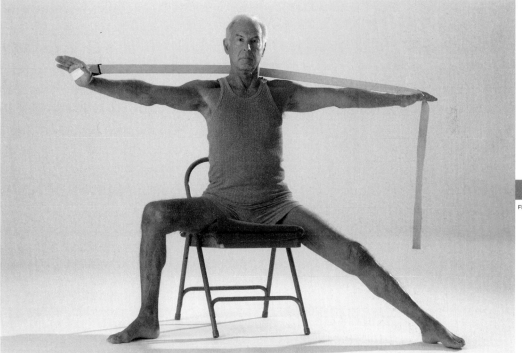

FIGURE 26.3

The strap, says Eric, is "to steady the nerves, where the nerves come out of the spine." You are also supporting C7 and your arms so your arms don't get the shakes.

FIGURE 26.4

EXERCISE #4. SUPPORTED EXTENDED SIDE ANGLE POSE (Utthita Parsvakona-sana), using two chairs.

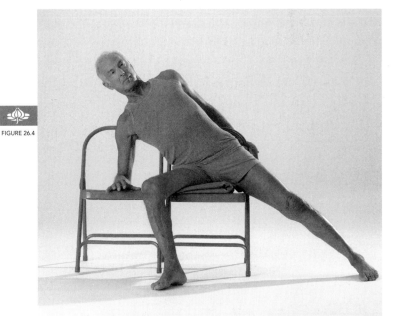

To set up for the pose, place two chairs on your yoga mat, one next to the other.

Sit on the left chair, place your right forearm and palm on the seat of the right chair, and lean into them. Turn your right leg out to the right and bend the right knee. Use your other arm to hold on to the back of the first chair (figure 26.4).

"That opens the chest, gets the kidneys working, releases the pressure of the liver, and stimulates the transverse colon and the descending colon." Repeat the pose on the other side.

EXERCISE #5. **SUPPORTED TRIANGLE POSE** (Trikonasana) at the wall, using chair. Set up for the pose by placing your mat next to a wall, with a chair on your mat, and the back of the chair against the wall. Extend your right leg out to the side as best you can, with your foot turned out 90 degrees. Then step your left leg out to the left side with the foot turned slightly in. Lengthen the right side of your torso, bend from the right hip, and place your right hand on the seat of the chair (figure 26.5). Lengthen your left arm straight up. If this is not possible, place your hand on your hip, as shown. Allow your rib cage to rotate toward the ceiling. To come out of the pose, reverse your steps. Repeat the pose on the other side.

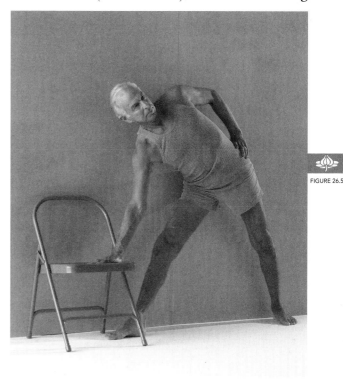

FIGURE 26.5

EXERCISE #6. **WARRIOR I** (Virabhadrasana I), using chair. Set up for the pose by placing a chair sideways on the mat. Stand facing the side of the chair, and bring your right leg over the seat and put your foot on the floor. Bend your knee to 90 degrees. Lift your left heel and turn your left leg so that the front of the thigh is touching the edge of the chair seat. Straighten your left leg as much as possible. Holding your right hand on the back of the chair, raise your left hand overhead. Using your hand on the chair for leverage, lift your chest (figure 26.6). Step out of the pose. Repeat the pose on the other side.

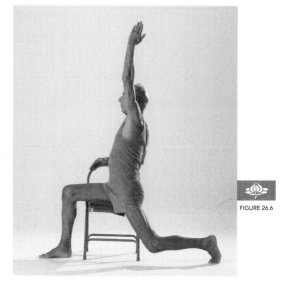

FIGURE 26.6

EXERCISE #7. REVOLVED SIDE ANGLE POSE (Parivrtta Parsvakonasana), using the chair. Sit down on a chair, with your legs straddling the sides and your feet touching the floor. Turn to the right so that your left leg is behind you and the top of your left thigh

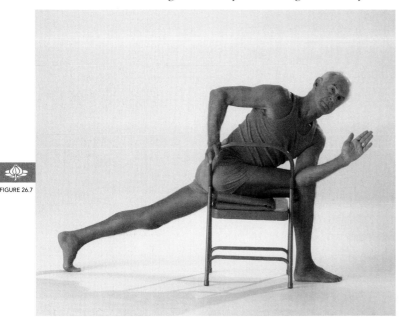

FIGURE 26.7

is touching the chair seat. Bend your right knee to 90 degrees. Place your left elbow on the outside edge of your right knee. Hold the back of the chair with your right hand while keeping your head facing forward. Use the motion of the left elbow to open your chest, continuing to face forward with your head. Repeat the pose on the other side.

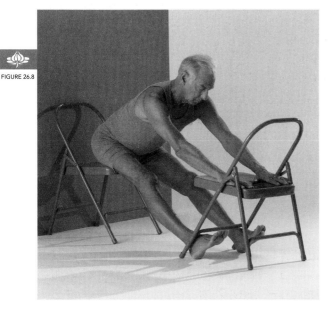

FIGURE 26.8

EXERCISE #8. SEATED FORWARD BEND (Paschimottanasana), using two chairs. Set up for the pose by placing one chair against a wall with a second chair facing it. Sit on the chair that's touching the wall. Extend your legs out toward the second chair and place your hands on the seat of the second chair. Then push the second chair forward until you feel a mild stretch of your hamstrings (back thigh muscles).

EXERCISE #9. **SEATED TWIST (Bharadvajasana I), with a chair.** Sit sideways on the chair facing to the right, with the knees and feet hips' width apart. Turn to your right and use both hands to take hold of the back of the chair, using your arms to help you twist. With each inhalation, lengthen your spine. With each exhalation, turn from your navel and twist a little more deeply into the pose, but keep your head facing the same direction as your chest. Keep your shoulders level. To come out of the pose, swing your legs to the other side of the chair. Repeat the pose on the other side.

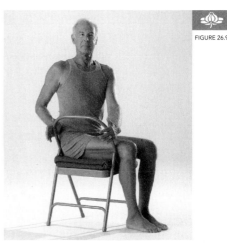

FIGURE 26.9

EXERCISE #10. **SUPPORTED FRONT BODY STRETCH (Purvottanasana), on two chairs.** Set up for the pose by placing one chair with its back about two feet from the wall and a second chair facing the first. Sit backward on the chair farther from the wall and put your legs through the back of the other chair (figure 26.10a), then slide your buttocks onto the other chair, bend your knees, and brace your feet against the wall. From this position, lie back onto the two chairs with your head near the back of the seat of

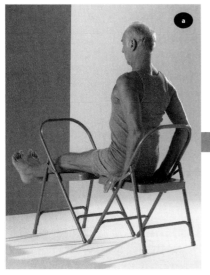

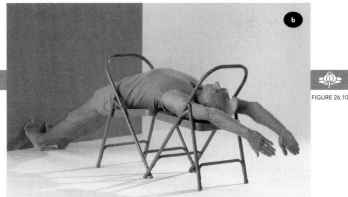

FIGURE 26.10

the second chair. You can lay your head directly on the seat of the second chair, or if your chin is higher than your forehead when your head is flat, place a support under your head. Holding on to the first chair with your hands, use your legs to push away from the wall, until they are straight. From there, thread your arms through the back of the second chair and stretch them toward the center of the room (figure 26.10b).

Normally in this pose Eric does not use padding on the chairs but if a student finds the surface too hard, he will put a sticky mat and a blanket on the chair seat. However, in general, he prefers not to because he wants students to be able to slide their buttocks back and forth, which is hard to do with a blanket or a sticky mat.

"It's a very gentle, easily accomplished backbend," Eric says. He chose this supported backbend for Jack to alleviate the depression he suspected Jack had, and because he believed it would improve Jack's digestion.

EXERCISE #11. **SUPPORTED RELAXATION POSE (Savasana), with legs on a chair.** Set up for the pose by placing a chair sideways on your mat. (If you have long legs, you may need to use two chairs.) Fold a blanket into a long rectangle and place it perpendicular to the chair. Sit on the blanket with your buttocks near the chair and swing your legs up onto the chair, resting your calves on the chair seat or on a folded blanket on top of the seat. Your thighs should be perpendicular to the floor and your calves parallel to it. Now lie

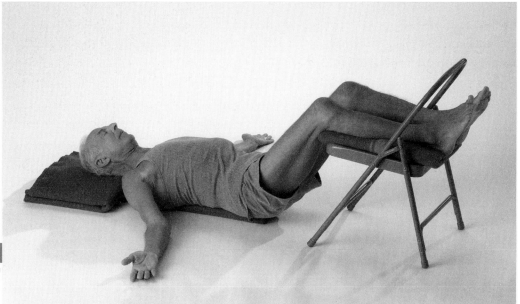

FIGURE 26.11

back on the folded blanket so that it supports your entire spine, from your hips to your head. If you have difficulty reaching the floor with your arms, place blankets under your arms, from the shoulder to the fingertips. If your chin is higher than your forehead when you lie back, place an additional blanket under your head.

Eric says, "With MS, any time the student is lying on the floor, or in an inversion, the spine and the head have to be supported."

EXERCISE #12. **BREATH AWARENESS PRANAYAMA, three minutes.** Place a bolster lengthwise on your mat. Sit in front of it (not on it), and loop a strap around your thighs. If necessary, place a folded blanket under your head, as shown, so that your chin is lower than your forehead when you are in the pose. Lie back. Now tune in to the sensation of the breath in your nose. Encourage your inhalation to come at the base of your nostrils and the exhalation to be through the tip of your nostrils. In this relaxed breath do not puff up your abdomen as is done in belly breathing. Breathe smoothly in and out with no retention of breath whatsoever.

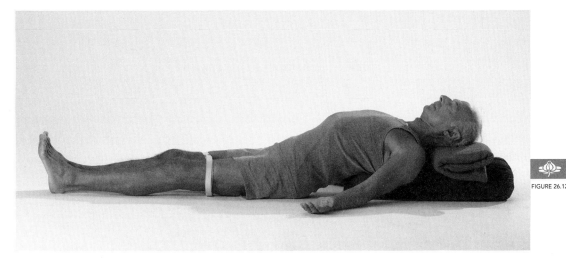

FIGURE 26.12

Eric says that he teaches this pranayama in the very first lesson to MS students because he finds it so beneficial. As with Savasana, all pranayama he teaches to these students is done in a supported reclined position. As his students progress with pranayama over the coming weeks, he moves from the smooth breath described above to Ujjayi, making a gentle sibilant sound on both the inhalation and exhalation (see pp. 16–17). The instructions for the abdomen are the same.

On days when Jack is exhausted Eric recommends he switch to a more restorative practice, including such poses as Legs-Up-the-Wall pose (Viparita Karani, see p. 64) and Reclined Cobbler's pose (Supta Baddha Konasana, see p. 326). In both of these poses, he often suggests placing sandbags on the shoulders to facilitate a deeper level of relaxation. Weighted sandbags strategically placed can also encourage spastically contracted muscles to let go. "I use a lot of weights with MS," Eric says. He might, for example, put sandbags on the hands when a student is on the floor in Reclined Cobbler's pose or in Relaxation pose. At other times he puts weights on students' hands, arms, groin muscles, and even on their heads. Since sandbags placed incorrectly can cause harm, they should be used only under the guidance of a seasoned teacher.

Contraindications, Special Considerations, and Modifications

One of the biggest risks to people with MS is overheating, which can make symptoms worse because it slows nerve conduction. For this reason, yoga in hot rooms and vigorous styles that heat up the body are generally contraindicated for people with the disease. Eric keeps the room temperature at 67 degrees and watches activity levels very carefully. During the summer, he doesn't teach any afternoon classes because it's too hot in Southern California, where he lives. If the weather is very warm, or if a student is having an MS flare-up or is very fatigued (a common experience for Eric's students because with public access transportation it may take them hours to get to the class), he'll lead a primarily restorative practice.

People with MS and other neurological conditions should avoid any poses that require a sudden burst of energy to come into the pose, like the full backbend Upward Bow (Urdhva Dhanurasana) or Handstand. Some people with MS find that exercise can increase problems with muscle spasticity. Gently and slowly warming up and focusing on maintaining smooth, deep, slow breathing throughout the practice can help prevent this problem.

A Holistic Approach to Multiple Sclerosis

❊ Studies suggest that pain is undertreated in people with MS. Since normal pain relievers are not always effective, doctors often suggest tricyclic antidepressants (prescribed at lower doses than typically used for depression) and some medications normally used to treat epilepsy. Often, a combination of different medications proves more effective than any single drug alone.

❊ Nondrug measures like meditation and cognitive-behavior therapy to learn coping skills may lessen the need for pain-relieving drugs or allow you to use smaller doses.

* In MS patients who are depressed, treatment with either medication or psychotherapy has been shown to decrease levels of chemical messengers (proinflammatory cytokines) that fuel inflammation. Thus reducing depression may have a beneficial effect on the disease process itself. Treating depression also appears to reduce fatigue (see chapter 15).

* A diet high in vegetables and fruits and whole grains fights inflammation and has other healing properties (see chapter 4).

* Saturated fats and trans-fatty acids, which are found in many processed foods, appear to promote inflammation and should be avoided. Omega-3 fatty acids damp down inflammation (for more details, see p. 167).

* Ginger and the Indian spice turmeric have anti-inflammatory properties. They can be used in cooking or taken as supplements.

* The combination of dietary fiber and plenty of water can help prevent constipation, especially if combined with regular asana practice, walking, or other forms of exercise.

* The Ayurvedic herb triphala is also useful to improve digestion. Although you can find this in health food stores and it's generally very safe, the best approach is to consult an Ayurvedic practitioner.

* Many patients with MS find some relief using medicinal marijuana for such symptoms as pain, muscle spasticity, and tremors, though using the herb, with certain exceptions, is illegal.

* Many people with MS find traditional Chinese medicine of benefit.

* Massage and other forms of bodywork are relaxing, can help with muscle spasticity, and are a valuable complement to asana practice.

* Since community can be therapeutic with MS and many people with the disease have limited mobility, the Internet can be a useful tool. Online support groups for MS are abundant.

Despite his initial misgivings about yoga, Jack was so moved emotionally by his first exposure to Eric's class that at the end of the hour he told Eric, "I'm yours." He started coming regularly to the weekly class.

Many MS students find Eric, who has had MS for over fifty years, to be an inspiration. When they see how active and productive he is, "they suddenly make the connection that if I'm fifty years down the road from them, and I'm doing what I'm doing, why not get on the bandwagon?"

Beyond asana and pranayama, Eric encourages the kind of yogic self-study that can bring about changes in attitudes and behavior. During class he tells students, "We all have to take responsibility for where we are and what we do. If you are in a very stressful employment situation, why are you wasting your time in here? Because nothing's going to get better unless you make some life changes." Jack appears to have gotten the message. "Jack has been with me for four years now. He's still in the same field, but now he's in business for himself, so he has much less stress, and he can pace his day according to how he functions." Because working for himself has allowed Jack to set his own schedule, he is able to arrange his work so that he and his wife both have enough time to spend with their children and with each other.

Another part of the stress-reduction strategy Eric recommends is honesty, the yama that Patanjali called satya (see chapter 1). "In most cases, people do not tell their employers that they have MS. They try to get through the best way they can. But I tell them, You are protected by the Americans with Disabilities Act. They cannot discriminate against you because you've contracted a disease. You have to go back and tell your employers, or your supervisor, exactly what your situation is, exactly what you think you can do. And once you get rid of this deep dark secret, then you reduce 80 percent of your stress."

Eric says that since Jack started yoga, he has put on around ten pounds of muscle and looks good. Eric describes Jack's mood when they started working together as "sour, strident, worried, and depressed, but he has a wonderful attitude now." Eric adds, "He's gained flexibility through his practice and his sex life improved, which was another issue." He believes the opening of the pelvis that comes through regular practice helps both men and women in this regard.

Jack also seems to have embraced the philosophy of karma yoga. "He is very eager to pass the word around, and he does volunteer work for the MS Society," Eric says. "As soon as you start giving to other people, your problems aren't as serious. So start listening to other people's problems, and yours in perspective are practically nothing."

In essence, Eric asks of his students what his teacher B. K. S. Iyengar asked of him. He summarizes it: "Take responsibility. Develop your own practice, learn where your strengths are, learn where your fears are, face your fears, develop strength in your weaknesses."

OVERWEIGHT AND OBESITY

RICHARD FREEMAN first got interested in yogic philosophy at the age of thirteen when he read Henry David Thoreau's *Walden*. In Richard's soft-spoken presence, you can readily envision him as a shy teenager drawn to the ascetic writer, himself inspired by a copy of the *Bhagavad Gita* he'd brought with him to that cabin in the woods. In 1970 Richard took his first trip to India, studying with many teachers

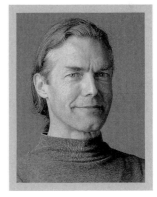

including B. K. S. Iyengar. After spending eight years in Asia learning yoga and meditation, Richard moved back to the United States where he met the man who would become his principal teacher, Pattabhi Jois, the central teacher in the lineage of Ashtanga yoga. Richard continues to teach this system in his own unique way, deeply informed by his study of Sanskrit and yogic philosophy. Richard is the director of the Yoga Workshop in Boulder, Colorado, and teaches there and internationally. He is featured on the instructional videos *Yoga with Richard Freeman* and the audio series *The Yoga Matrix*.

James Vitale has been severely overweight since childhood, and as an adult has weighed as much as 360 pounds (he is 6' 2"). He tried various diet and exercise plans over the years and had some success, but the regimens were never sustainable and the results were never long-lasting.

James has worked hard at understanding what led to his weight problem. Unlike many obese people, he does not feel that he eats for emotional reasons, whether it's sadness, anxiety, or boredom. He sees his overeating as a habit, and says that he recently had an epiphany about its origin. While visiting his mother he came across two baby books, his and his sister's. "I found hers first, and it had events in there, like baby's first step and baby's first solid food—which for my sister was at five or six months. I looked at mine, and my mother had written 'one week' after first solid food. I asked my mom, 'Is this a mistake? How could I possibly have been eating solid food at one week?' She said, 'No, it wasn't a mistake. For some reason, I didn't produce milk and you had a bad reaction to all the formulas we tried you on so I had to start you on strained fruit and vegetables.'" His mother further explained that she had a major problem feeding him because whenever she removed the spoon from his mouth, he screamed and became totally unmanageable. When she consulted a doctor about the problem, he said that since a baby's natural instinct is to suck, which produces a steady stream of milk, the spoon-feeding was frustrating for him. So in order to re-create the experience of a constant food supply, she devised a strategy of using two spoons, one spoonful after the other. The conversation with his mother was a revelation. "I can never explain that moment. It just brought clear so much in my relationship to food."

Not so much out of a desire to improve his body but more to find happiness, James became a Buddhist and began to study yoga, starting with Jivamukti yoga, a vigorous style similar to Ashtanga yoga, and later developing an interest in Kundalini yoga as well. James began to study at Richard's studio after he moved to Boulder, where he lived for two years. During his time there, James's yoga practice consisted mostly of the classes he took several times a week at Richard's studio, working with both Richard and some of his protégées.

Overview of Weight Loss

The epidemic of overweight and obesity is no longer confined to those in the West, as dietary habits have changed and people all over the world have become more sedentary. This is a matter of serious concern because there is little doubt that being overweight can have major health consequences, including type 2 diabetes, sleep apnea, high blood pressure, heart disease, and some forms of cancer. Particularly dangerous is fat around the middle. Extra body weight makes back problems more likely, increases the strain on the joints, and can contribute to or worsen injuries to ankles, knees, hips, and other vulnerable areas of the body. Not surprisingly, being overweight can be both a cause and a consequence of depression and low self-esteem.

Beyond the negative health consequences of being overweight are the consequences of trying to lose weight. Many diets are nutritionally imbalanced and unhealthy, and there is very little evidence that any of them are effective in the long term. Yo-yo dieting, which sometimes causes extreme weight swings, may be riskier than simply being fat. While extreme calorie reduction can result in quick weight loss, if you eat much less than 1200 calories per day, your body breaks down muscle tissue for energy. Losing muscle mass lowers your metabolic rate, minimizing the expenditure of the calories you consume. As soon as you slip off this kind of extreme diet (and everyone eventually does, because these diets are so onerous that they are virtually unsustainable), the weight you put on will likely be predominantly fat.

There can be a vicious cycle regarding weight. Given the societal pressure to be thin, people who are overweight may be highly self-critical. As a result of this chronic dissatisfaction, they may develop elevated levels of the stress hormone cortisol, which in turn encourages stress-related eating ("food-seeking behavior," as scientists who study rats call it), which, of course, results in further weight gain, which may then fuel more stress and stress-related eating. Another unfortunate effect of cortisol is that it makes the conversion of calories into fat, particularly fat in the abdomen, much more efficient. The resulting apple-shaped body type has been linked with diabetes and heart disease, whereas excess weight in the hips and a pear-shaped body has not been.

> **TIP** Contrary to popular belief, when it comes to body weight, it does not matter whether the calories you consume come from carbohydrates, proteins, fat, or alcohol. As far as the body is concerned, a calorie is a calorie. There is, however, truth to the idea that excess carbohydrates, such as white rice and white flour, and particularly in the form of simple sugars, found in such foods as desserts and soft drinks, may cause a spike in insulin levels and a rebound in hunger that may lead you to eat more later on. Alcohol can cause a similar insulin response. The idea that rich desserts and white flour would contribute to being overweight is consistent with the ancient teachings of Ayurveda (see chapter 4). Ayurveda says that these foods increase kapna, the dosha associated with obesity and inactivity. For an Ayurvedic perspective on weight loss, see chapter 16.

How Yoga Fits In

Yoga can be helpful in weight loss in a number of ways. The most obvious perhaps has to do with the number of calories you burn on the yoga mat. Some of yoga's more vigorous varieties, such as those practiced in many gyms, as well as power yoga and Ashtanga, the style Richard teaches, can raise the heart rate into the aerobic range. Yet many people who take to milder yoga practices such as gentle asana and breathing techniques also drop weight, so it's about more than just burning calories. Because of stress's role in overeating and in the formation of fat, yoga's proven ability to fight stress (and lower cortisol levels) is another aspect of its effectiveness as an aid to weight loss.

Yoga may also help with weight loss through its focus on seeing clearly—one of the key tenets of yogic philosophy (see chapter 7). Before you can change something, yoga teaches, you must acknowledge it for what it is, which can be a problem for people with weight issues. A 1992 *New England Journal of Medicine* study looked at obese people who considered themselves resistant to diets. They told their doctors that they exercised and restricted their calories but didn't lose weight. These people tended to view their weight problems as genetic, their metabolisms as slow, and their dietary habits as normal. When researchers carefully measured what these people were actually eating and the number of calories they were burning, they discovered that the patients had on average underestimated their food intake by 47 percent and overestimated their exercise by 51 percent. When compared to a control group there was no significant difference in metabolic rates. Thus their primary problem was not a slow metabolism, it was a failure to see clearly, or as Richard puts it, "being tricked by their own minds."

Keeping a food and exercise diary, a form of self-study, or svadhyaya, is one way to improve your ability to see clearly. If you write down everything you eat, that very process brings awareness to what may be unconscious habits. You might also jot down what your emotional state was when you were eating. Don't judge it, just notice. If you find that you are judging yourself, notice that, too. Use the diary as a tool to facilitate the process of tuning in. Reviewing your diary regularly can be an effective way to spot patterns that you might not otherwise identify.

Another concept from yoga that is relevant to weight issues is that of samskaras (see chapter 1), the behavior grooves we dig through repeated actions. Many people who overeat are on automatic pilot and don't necessarily even notice the taste of their food. James describes an epiphany he had after he first started to practice yoga and meditation. He went out to dinner with a group of friends. Normally he talks a lot but that evening he was feeling more reflective than usual. "All of a sudden I noticed how awesome the food tasted. I realized I am never really conscious when I'm eating. I'm not there to experience it." Yoga, of course, encourages being mindful of the moment, which helps you notice and savor your food instead of gulping it automatically.

Introspective practices and meditation in particular may hold the greatest opportunity to study yourself and your relationship to food and body weight. As you refine your ability to tune in to bodily sensations, you may notice when you are not hungry but simply eating out of habit or emotional neediness. Meditation can also help you respond differently to hunger pangs by teaching you to observe the sensation before reacting to it. The space between observation and reaction makes it obvious how much your response is a matter of habit, of conditioning. And that, Richard says, is "the method that breaks the conditioning."

Yoga philosophy is opposed to the setting of specific weight-loss goals, such as "I want to lose ten pounds in the next month." Doing so makes you too attached to particular outcomes, which may or may not happen. Being focused on the end also distracts you from paying attention to what's going on right now, in favor of fantasizing about some imagined future—which is the antithesis of yoga. It is, however, desirable to set an intention for what you plan to do for the next day, month, or year. This is the yogic tool of sankalpa (see chapter 7). You might decide, for example, that you are going to practice asana for fifteen minutes, six days a week, or that you are going to eliminate bread or white rice from your evening meals, or allow yourself only half a cup of ice cream after dinner. You can exert control over your actions but not over how your weight responds to them. Simply do your work, yoga says, and the future will take care of itself.

Although it can be very effective, the yogic process of weight loss is slow and requires patience. When I worked as a primary care doctor, patients often asked me to give them a plan that would enable them to lose a lot of weight quickly—for example, fifty pounds in two months. While possible, that kind of rapid weight loss can only occur as a result of extreme deprivation diets, which aren't good for the body and are impossible to sustain. From a yogic perspective, there is something wrong with the whole concept of diets— artificial regimens that require you to ignore hunger pangs and eat food that is often nutritionally inadequate and aesthetically unappealing; to torture yourself, if necessary, to achieve an external result. None of this involves cultivating the skills you will need to maintain a healthy weight when the diet is over—hence relapse rates on most diets that approach 100 percent. My response to my patients was to suggest that if they could just lose one ounce per day, that would be almost half a pound a week, which adds up to twenty-three pounds in a year. To lose an ounce per day, you've only got to burn about 250 calories more than you take in. A minimal change in diet or exercise (or both) is all you need, and it doesn't have to feel like torture.

It's all about taking one small step in the right direction, and then taking the next one. Yoganand Michael Carroll, a Kripalu yoga teacher, tells a story of his now deceased guru Swami Kripalu. Years ago, the swami thought he had been eating too much, so at his next dinner he counted the number of bites he ate. For the next six weeks, he ate one bite less than that at each meal and noted the effect. For six weeks after that he ate two bites less, and so on, until he'd reached an intake of food that seemed right to him. Using his subtle awareness, he had determined precisely the correct amount to eat. What the swami knew was one of the fundamental principles of yoga: a small action done repeatedly can make an enormous difference.

The Scientific Evidence

Evidence from scientific studies conducted in both India and the United States suggests that a multifaceted yoga program that includes dietary modifications, as well as asana, breathing exercises, and meditation can facilitate weight loss. In the Yoga Biomedical Trust survey of yoga practitioners mentioned in chapter 1, 74 percent of those who were obese found yoga helpful, though specific weight-loss results were not quantified.

A study led by Dr. Alan Kristal of the Fred Hutchinson Cancer Research Center in Seattle linked yoga to weight control and weight loss. The researchers studied more than 15,000 healthy men and women between the ages of 53 and 57, 132 of whom had been regular yoga practitioners for at least four years (though no effort was made to determine which styles of yoga individuals practiced). During the previous ten years, overweight people in the yoga group lost an average of 5 pounds, compared to a 13.5 pound gain among overweight nonpractitioners.

A study by Dr. Anand Shetty of Hampton University, presented at the annual meeting of the American Heart Association in 2006, found that yoga helped overweight high school students lose weight. Sixty overweight teens were randomly divided into a group that did yoga and a control group that pursued their usual activities. There were no dietary restrictions in either group. The yoga group did asana and pranayama for forty minutes four days per week. After twelve weeks, the yoga practitioners had lost an average of six pounds while the control group showed a slight weight gain.

In the Lifestyle Heart Trial, led by Dr. Dean Ornish (see chapter 19), patients following a comprehensive program that included asana, pranayama, and meditation, along with a low-fat vegetarian diet, walking, and support group meetings, averaged almost twenty-four pounds of weight loss over the first year. Five years later, they had maintained more than half of that original weight loss. The control group, prescribed a low-fat diet as part of their medical care, gained three pounds on average in the first year, and maintained the weight at five years. One advantage of the program's diet is that you do not need to count calories or control portion sizes: As long as you choose the right foods, you can eat as much as you like.

Aside from its ability to aid weight loss, yoga also appears to improve self-image in general, and body image in particular. Dr. Suzanne Engelman and colleagues from Georgia State University compared group therapy to yoga classes. After ten weeks, the 45 people in the therapy group had a statistically significant improvement in self-image but not in body image, compared to a control group of 42 undergraduate psychology students. The 33 yoga students, all of whom were new to yoga, took a generic hatha yoga class, but did not do any therapy. After ten weeks, compared to controls, the yoga group had significant improvements in both their feelings about themselves and their bodies.

Richard Freeman's Approach

Many overweight people view food as the enemy. This is very different from yogic thinking on food, which, as Richard explains, views it as a manifestation of the divine, a gift from God. Richard cites the *Taittiriya Upanishad,* an ancient Hindu text, which equates food with Brahman, the divine force in the universe. Yoga would say go to your direct experience: food is one of life's great pleasures.

> **TIP** Especially for people who struggle with their weight and their relationship to food, Richard suggests bringing yogic awareness to mealtimes. One way to do this, he says, is through ritual, which might be prayer or chanting before you eat. He also suggests eating in silence. On meditation retreats, Richard says, people eat mindfully and it's a powerful practice. "They're not engaged in conversation, they're simply watching and tasting, looking at the food, noticing the texture of food." Chewing each bite thoroughly is another way of getting yourself to savor your food and slow down the eating process. Richard believes fine food eaten mindfully can be both an aesthetic and spiritual experience.

The asana practice that Richard teaches in his studio is based on the six progressive series of Ashtanga yoga. When James studied with Richard, his practice was based on what is known as the primary series, which consists of dozens of poses, done in a specific sequence, beginning with a number of Sun Salutations, and including standing poses, a number of forward bends, and a few backbends, twists, and inversions. (To see the complete primary series, go to http://ashtangayoga.info/asana-vinyasa/primary-series/index.html.) Later, as James's practice advanced, he added portions of the intermediate series, including a number of backbends such as Bow pose (Dhanurasana) and Camel pose (Ustrasana). One universal aspect of Ashtanga yoga is smooth, audible Ujjayi breathing (see pp. 16–17) done throughout the practice. The only exception is Deep Relaxation pose (Savasana), when the breath is free with no constriction in the throat.

Richard's approach with James was to encourage James to do whatever he was comfortable with in the regular classes, and to modify certain postures as necessary. Rather than go through the entire primary series, this chapter will simply describe some of the modifications that Richard and James made to the standard asana practice in order to accommodate James's weight.

EXERCISE #1. **JUMPING.** In Ashtanga as in some other styles of yoga, students often jump from pose to pose. But James says that when he began he wasn't able to jump, primarily because his weight made it hard for him. So if jumping is difficult for you, you can simply step from one pose to another.

For example, when you move from Standing Forward Bend (Uttanasana) to Downward-Facing Dog pose (Adho Mukha Svanasana), bend both knees and then step with the right foot back into a Lunge pose with your left knee in front. Then step with the left foot back to meet the right. At this point, you can move into Downward-Facing Dog pose.

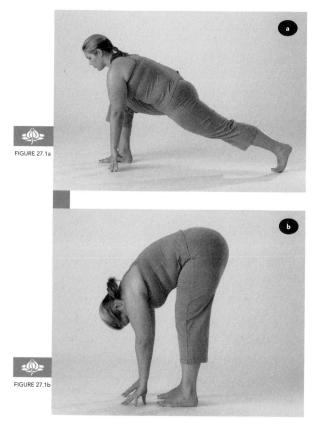

FIGURE 27.1a

FIGURE 27.1b

To reverse this move, shift your hips forward and step with your right foot, placing it between your hands into a Lunge pose (figure 27.1a). From Lunge, step with the left foot forward to meet the right, moving into Standing Forward Bend (figure 27.1b).

Now that he had lost some of his excess weight and is more familiar with the practice, James does the jumps. Watching him jump between poses in his Sun Salutations brings to mind old films of Jackie Gleason dancing; he demonstrates a grace and ease that people weighing half as much would have trouble emulating. However, for most people who weigh as much as James does, jumping from pose to pose is generally not a good idea: one false move could result in a significant injury. The fact that James is still young and very well coordinated lets him get away with it.

EXERCISE #2. **STEPPING INTO LUNGE.** Richard also had James move his front foot out to the side (figure 27.2) when stepping back into Lunge pose from Standing Forward Bend. Otherwise he could barely get onto his fingertips, because his large belly and thighs got in the way. If he left his foot in the normal position, his knee tended to splay out to the side into a potentially injurious misalignment, and since he was unable to put part of his weight on his hands, that knee was also bearing additional weight. Moving his foot to the side gives him a little more space. Similarly, keeping the feet a little farther apart than usual in some forward bends (figure 27.1b) gives him enough room to keep his belly out of the way.

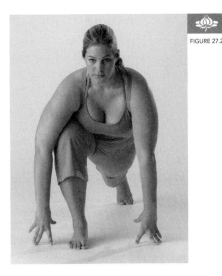

FIGURE 27.2

If Lunge pose with the back leg straight is too demanding, you can drop your back knee to the mat. If you use a thin yoga mat and no other padding, however, this and poses such as Camel pose may be hard on the knees because of all the weight brought to bear on them. James always keeps a blanket nearby, so that anytime he gets onto his knees he can pad them; otherwise his knees always hurt by the end of the practice.

EXERCISE #3. **DOWNWARD-FACING DOG POSE (Adho Mukha Svanasana).** Richard had James reduce the time he stayed in some poses like Downward-Facing Dog pose to make the practice safer and more comfortable. "Anytime I have to bear a lot of weight on my upper body, I have to rest frequently because my muscles get exhausted quickly." If he stayed too long in Downward-Facing Dog pose, his wrists began to hurt,

though he's learned to remedy that aspect of the problem by pressing down hard onto his knuckles and the pads of his fingers and using the strength of his forearms to lift up and away from the wrists. To reduce the strain on the wrists in Dog pose, it's also possible to substitute Dolphin pose (figure 27.3). Similar modifications can be made for other problematic poses. You can either find substitute poses, or reduce the time you hold

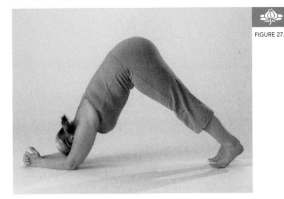

FIGURE 27.3

them. Standing poses like Triangle pose (Trikonasana) and the Warrior poses (Virabhadrasana I and II) as well as inversions can all be challenging if held for long.

EXERCISE #4. **PUSH-UP POSE (Chaturanga Dandasana) AND UPWARD-FACING DOG (Urdhva Mukha Svanasana).** The yoga push-up, an element of the Sun Salutation,

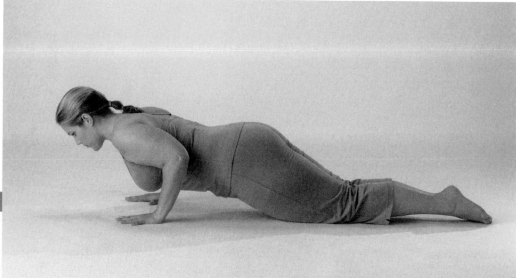

can be hard on the wrists as well as the shoulders. James learned to just skip it entirely and instead rest on the floor until the next pose. Another possibility is to do the push-up with your knees on the ground (figure 27.4). Similarly, rather than doing Upward-Facing Dog pose, another pose that is hard on the wrists, James substituted Cobra pose (figure 27.5).

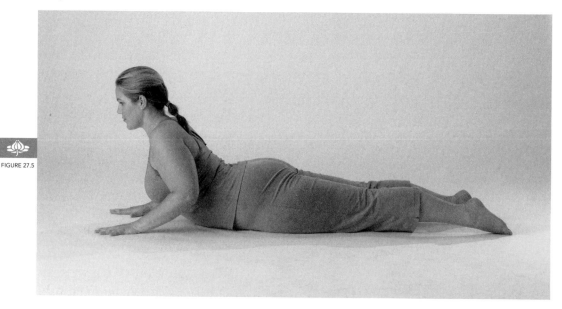

OTHER YOGIC IDEAS

People who are successful at weight loss tend not to undermine their success with negative self-talk. If you catch yourself saying things like "This is never going to work. I might as well give up," do as the sage Patanjali suggested in the *Yoga Sutras*, and counter that defeatism with the opposite kind of self-talk. Tell yourself that you intend to take small steps in the right direction and that you have faith in yourself and your yoga practice. Self-defeating thoughts can also take the form of excuses. "I had a stressful day. I deserve to eat whatever I feel like." You might counter that by telling yourself that when you are stressed, you want to give your body food that is fresh and light, to do something that is good for it, not something that will end up leaving you feeling worse.

EXERCISE #5. **EXTENDED SIDE ANGLE POSE (Utthita Parsvakonasana).** When James does Extended Side Angle pose, rather than dropping his hand to the floor and trying to rotate his chest, he's found taking an intermediate position first works better (figure 27.6a). "I am flexible enough to turn my chest and look up at my

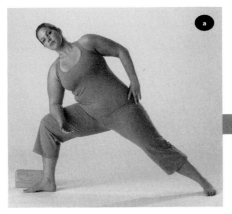

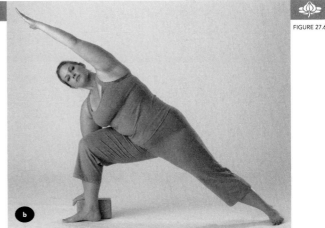

FIGURE 27.6

hand," he says, "but my flesh will get in the way. So I have to start out with my elbow on my knee, turn my chest, and then go down" (figure 27.6b).

OTHER YOGIC IDEAS

Yoga teacher Ana Forrest, who has had her own struggles with an eating disorder, finds that the urge to eat when she shouldn't usually lasts about twenty minutes, then passes. She suggests that, rather than indulging yourself, if you are fit enough, immediately start doing Sun Salutations and continue for twenty minutes, going as fast as you can and breathing as deeply as you can. When you're done, bring your attention inward. Ask yourself, "What is it I'm really needing and wanting right now? It's not the cheesecake, but what is it I think I'll get from the cheesecake, and is there some other way I can get that?"

EXERCISE #6. **TWISTS.** There are a lot of twists that are hard for James because his belly and thighs get in the way. If he's in class and the teacher calls for a twist he can't do and doesn't present him with an alternative pose, he'll do a simple cross-legged twist (figure 27.7) or perhaps a twist sitting in a chair (see p. 469).

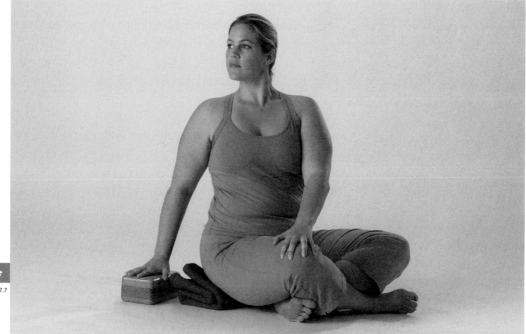

FIGURE 27.7

> **TIP** James has found that twists are easier if he uses his hands to move his flesh out of the way. Doing this may add 20 degrees to the amount he is able to rotate his spine in some poses. He realizes that some people might find moving their belly in a class embarrassing, but his first teacher, Kirin Mishra, then a Jivamukti yoga instructor in New Jersey, was matter-of-fact about it. "She really trained me—don't be embarrassed , just grab it and move it out of the way."

EXERCISE #7. **TAKING BREAKS.** Another consideration if you are overweight and/or out of shape is to not overdo it. Taking breaks, as James did when he just rested while the class did yoga push-ups, can allow you to have more energy for the next pose. Such breaks also provide a necessary cool-down period before moving into any of the more introspective practices. If you are sweaty and out of breath it's hard to settle into Relaxation pose, pranayama, and meditation (all of which are regularly taught in the Ashtanga tradition).

Contraindications, Special Considerations, and Modifications

Some yoga positions may be extremely difficult for those who are heavy. Excess weight can put a strain on the low back, knees, ankles, and other joints. The heavier you are, the more work it is to move the body and the greater the weight borne by whatever part of the body is holding you up. That could be the hands and wrists in a pose like Downward-Facing Dog, or the feet, knees, and ankles in standing poses.

Overweight also makes yoga more challenging aerobically, and Richard therefore tries to be careful not to overwork heavy students. For those who have been largely sedentary, for safety it is essential to build your practice slowly over a period of months. This is doubly true if you do yoga in hot and humid conditions, as is common in some styles. Focus on keeping your breath smooth and regular, as any strain in the breath is often the first indicator of overdoing. It's much better to simply rest in Child's pose (see p. 201), for example, while the rest of the class moves on, than to push yourself to do something that might result in an injury. Yoga teacher Sandra Summerfield Kozak suggests coming in and out of a pose, holding it briefly each time, rather than doing one long hold.

Good alignment is even more important in people who are heavy because excess weight contributes to potentially injurious joint compression when the bones aren't situated properly in relationship to one another. Thus if your knee drifts to the side instead of staying directly over the ankle in the unmodified version of Lunge pose, as James's did, the result could be compression in the hips, knee, or ankle joints. If you are significantly overweight, please pay particular attention to appendix 1, "Avoiding Common Yoga Injuries," as you are at greater risk for almost all of them.

Yoga teacher and physical therapist Julie Gudmestad cautions that any poses in which you stand on one leg may be risky if you're overweight. Many people who are heavy already have knee, foot, ankle, and/or hip problems, or arthritis from carrying around so much weight. Asana like Tree pose, she says, put enormous pressure on the knee of the standing leg. One solution she's found is to practice the same poses lying on the mat instead of standing. Instead of Utthita Hasta Padangusthasana (figure 27.8a), one element of the Ashtanga primary series that James didn't modify, you could do Supta Padangusthasana (figure 27.8b), which is essentially the same pose with a different orientation. Julie says many standing postures can be modified in this fashion.

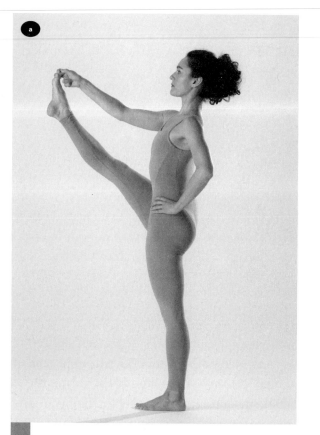

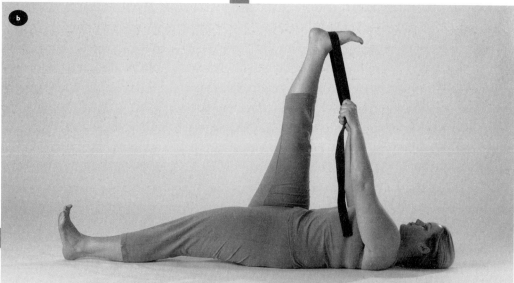

FIGURE 27.8

Richard says that inversions can be particularly challenging for people who are heavy. There may simply be too much weight on your head and neck in Headstand for the pose to be safe, for example, and with rare exceptions he advises that obese students skip it. Inversions and balancing poses also bring the risk of falling; if you are significantly overweight a fall is more likely to injure you, or if you are in a class, someone next to you. Shoulderstand and Plow pose (see p. 90) are especially difficult for women with large breasts. Often, the solution can be to either modify the pose or use blankets and other props. For example, instead of doing a vertical Shoulderstand, substitute the version where the body is in a piked position (figure 27.9). Ideally, modifications and substitutions, as well as the proper arrangement of props, should be discussed with an experienced yoga teacher.

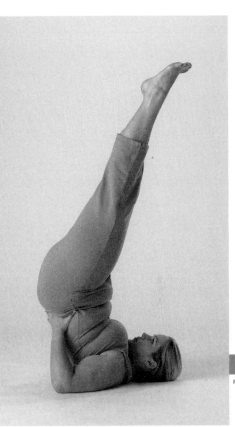

FIGURE 27.9

TIP James recently had a breakthrough with Shoulderstand. He was taking a workshop with Roger Cole who suggested that he put much more support under his shoulders than he'd ever tried before—five blankets. Roger also taught James to wrap a mat around the folded blankets to prevent slippage. According to James this made a huge difference in his ability to do the pose securely, without the blankets shifting beneath him.

James credits his yoga practice with everything from muscle building to inner peace. Eventually the yoga practice led to weight loss, too—about 60 pounds over the course of two years of study with Richard, from 340 down to 280 pounds. But even before he lost any weight, he experienced more ease in his everyday life—better balance, more energy, fewer injuries. "The yoga practice," James says, "allowed me to do a lot more." He gained enough confidence in the abilities of his body to start skiing and hiking in the mountains near

A Holistic Approach to Weight Loss

❋ Strength-training exercise (which could include asana) to maintain and even build muscles can help with a weight-loss plan because muscle tissue burns calories and will help keep your metabolic rate from dropping in response to weight loss.

❋ To increase your awareness of how active you really are, consider buying a pedometer. These small devices, which can be attached to your clothing, measure the number of steps you take each day. Fewer than 5,000 steps per day is considered a sedentary lifestyle; more than 10,000 steps is considered active.

❋ High-protein diets like the Atkins plan can help people drop weight quickly, but any diet that favors fatty meats and fatty dairy products, and doesn't include generous portions of vegetables, fruit, and fiber, is unhealthy in the long term (see chapter 4).

❋ Avoid diet drugs and dietary supplements to lose weight. Any drug powerful enough to suppress appetite or raise your metabolic rate is bound to have other unhealthy side effects, and the withdrawal of popular weight-loss drugs from the market supports this notion. Since pills don't get at the root causes of overeating and inactivity, you may need to take them for the rest of your life, and that's not a good idea.

❋ Drastic weight-loss surgeries such as stomach stapling are appropriate in extreme cases, but my recommendation is use them only as a last resort. Even surgery may not be enough by itself, as it's estimated that 30 percent of people who have the operations will start gaining weight back if they don't take a comprehensive approach to weight loss.

Boulder. At first, he often developed sore ankles and knees after exercising, but after a few months of yoga practice that disappeared.

Yoga has changed not just his body but his attitude about his body weight. "When you're overweight, you just hate your body," he explains. "You feel excluded from doing things that other people do automatically. It's like, I'm too heavy for that, or I don't want to look stupid, or I don't want people to see how out of shape I am." But the way Richard treated him helped him move toward self-acceptance. "I experience Richard as one of the most compassionate and loving presences I've ever been in." James first got this sense when he showed up for a class that was too advanced for him. At one point, James says, Richard approached his mat. "I felt like I was a school kid about to get into trouble. I looked up into his face, and he was just smiling at me." Richard's demeanor said to James that he was thinking, "You're in this situation, and maybe it's a little more than you can handle, but there's a way you can get through it." James says, "He didn't have to say anything. Whatever he did, however he adjusted me, I can't explain it. It was like grace. I felt like I fit in the class again, even though I still couldn't do the exact posture he was teaching."

James's growing yogic awareness is also changing his attitudes about eating. "For any person who's more than fifty pounds overweight, I'd say they have no clue when they're physically hungry." At one point he read a book about fasting and decided to try a five-day fast. "That was the first time I experienced a physical sensation that I realized was hunger. I was like, 'Whoa, this is hunger!'" Until then, eating was just something he did by habit and by opportunity. Now, he says, physical cues from his body much more than the availability of food guide what and when he eats. One benefit he found in fasting was that it gave him much more awareness of his samskaras. When you're finished with a fast and "you go back to the old habits," he says, "the consequences of those behaviors stand out in much sharper relief."

James has found Richard's suggestion to turn his mealtimes into a meditation particularly useful, though challenging. He recognizes that his worst periods of being overweight always coincided with the bad habit of eating while doing something else: reading, watching TV, conversing. Now he tries to make a ritual of his meals by cooking his own food, eating alone in silence, focusing on the taste and textures of the different parts of the meal, and chewing slowly and deliberately. "When I do that, I inevitably feel better. I end up eating a lot less, and digesting better. There are innumerable benefits to it." Although it's not easy to get himself to do this on a regular basis, the results are so positive he always wonders why he doesn't eat this way all the time.

Like many of Richard's students, James has made a definite connection between his diet and the quality of his yoga practice. "I know that how I eat directly affects how motivated I'll be to practice asana. If I'm eating light, I have lots of energy, my body feels really free, I enjoy practicing. If I'm eating heavy foods, or I'm not being very conscious about it, I don't want to practice at all." Sometimes when he sits down to eat, he'll ask himself, "Will I want to practice yoga a couple hours after eating this meal? And that," he says, "may decide something for me."

In addition to his asana and pranayama practice, James meditates regularly and has developed a strong interest in chanting, all practices that Richard encourages his committed students to pursue. Despite the enormous physical benefits of these practices, it's even more the feeling of spiritual well-being that keeps James interested in yoga and Buddhism. All the suffering he endured as a teenager trying to fit in, he says, "pushed me into a search for what was meaningful about living. In terms of bringing about happiness, these are the most effective methods I've encountered."

James eventually moved from Boulder to the East Coast to take a lucrative job in a high-technology start-up firm. The demands of the job have meant less time to exercise and practice yoga, more eating on the run, with the result that over the last few years he's gained back almost a third of the weight he lost while studying with Richard. He's beginning to question, though, whether it's worth it, and is planning to scale back his responsibilities in the coming months. "Earlier in my life," he says, "I chose to sell out for career and financial advancement. I'm not willing to do that that anymore."

Lately James has been thinking about the link between his yoga and meditation practice and what happens in the rest of his life. "When I'm consistent in my pracice, it's as if the things I want just start coming to me, versus my having to go out and aggressively try to get them. If I practice consistently, I have a lot more health and energy, my mind is more calm, my body feels better, I want to play. I'm like a kid at the sandbox. If I'm not practicing, I'm all stiff, and I'm eating bad food, and I'm not sleeping right. Forget it."

THE FUTURE OF YOGA AS MEDICINE

DEPENDING ON WHICH ESTIMATES YOU BELIEVE, between 15 and 20 million people practice yoga in the United States. As with the overall movement toward alternative medicine, the growing interest in yoga and its applications to health has come from the general public, not from the medical profession—in part because people weren't getting the answers and the help they needed from their doctors or other health care providers.

The ascent of yoga therapy may be coming in the nick of time. As the baby boomers move into the decades when they are increasingly likely to suffer from chronic conditions like high blood pressure, arthritis, diabetes, and heart disease, many will find yoga's ability to help prevent, relieve, and heal these ailments a welcome complement to the offerings of the medical profession. They will also appreciate the money that yoga may enable them to save, thanks to the fact that a regular practice can decrease the amount of medical care needed. Yoga can also make essential medical interventions more effective. Better still, there's no pre-approval from an insurance company required to proceed.

Considering how effective yoga therapy appears to be, it's a real bargain. After an initial, quite modest investment in equipment and instruction, you can pursue it on your own at home for free. If you decide that ongoing instruction is worth your while, you can get it. For now, of course, with rare exceptions, any cost connected with yoga instruction or yoga therapy comes from your own pocket, but someday perhaps the government and insurance companies will see the wisdom of covering these expenses. It would certainly be in their interest to do so.

Yoga makes economic sense not just for individuals, but for the insurance industry, and the entire country. Health care costs continue to rise each year, growing faster than overall inflation, a pace that is unsustainable. The likely result will be further cost-cutting, denial of benefits, larger numbers of people without medical insurance, and people who do have coverage having to jump through higher hoops to get it. If therapeutic yoga were to come into much greater use in the United States, the result could be billions of dollars in savings, not to mention a major reduction in suffering. Many cardiac procedures like angioplasty and bypass surgery could be prevented. The number of back pain operations could be cut to a small fraction of what it currently is. Among people practicing yoga as medicine, expenditures for drugs to treat diabetes, heart disease, hypertension, asthma, and arthritis would likely decline. Reduced use of prescription drugs and lower doses of those used would mean substantial reductions in serious drug side effects and dangerous drug interactions, themselves among the leading causes of hospitalization and of death.

Right now, however, the yoga world isn't sufficiently prepared for the likely boom in the demand for therapy. While more teachers are being trained all the time, if yoga as medicine grows the way I suspect it will, the need for qualified therapists could far outstrip availability. I really hope that yoga teachers and others reading these words will think about yoga therapy as a career option. This is likely to be a growth industry for years to come.

To health care professionals like nurses and physical therapists, I say consider adding therapeutic yoga to what you do, or even making it your main focus. Your training gives you the background in anatomy, physiology, and clinical care that most yoga teachers lack, and makes you ideally suited for this field. For any health care professional who has chafed under the restrictions of managed care, shrunken hospital budgets, and penny-wise-pound-foolish cost-cutting efforts, bringing yoga to people who are suffering is a way to reconnect with why you likely got involved in patient care in the first place.

I recommend yoga to physicians, too. Even if you don't decide to get professionally involved in yoga therapy, practicing yoga could bring you great personal benefits. It's excellent preventive medicine in general, and particularly good for anyone living under stress—which certainly applies to the medical profession these days. In the process of learning yoga you would gain valuable understanding of tools that could benefit the majority of your patients—especially those with the chronic diseases and psychosomatic complaints that take up so much of your time and emotional energy and for which conventional medicine doesn't have fully satisfactory solutions. You can read all you want about yoga—including every study ever published—but to truly understand it, you must do it.

To medical researchers, I say please consider putting your efforts into investigating this healing system. While the evidence so far strongly suggests yoga's healing potential, more research is needed. Well-done yoga studies could boost yoga's scientific legitimacy in the minds of doctors, policy makers, and the general public. This could prove vital in the years to come if yoga therapy is to help meet the needs of our aging population. Be advised, however, that you may need to tackle yoga research in creative ways. Yoga is not a perfect fit with Western science, which is best at detecting the effects of single variables. Yoga, however, is a holistic system that affects multiple variables simultaneously. There are hundreds of different tools in the yoga toolbox that can be combined in an almost infinite number of ways. While this complexity makes yoga harder to study, it is also probably the key to its effectiveness. Moreover, some of yoga's purported benefits, like greater psychological equanimity and heightened feelings of compassion and connection to others, are difficult if not impossible to quantify, yet may have very real effects on health and healing.

Even though it's a lot easier to study standardized protocols, the best yoga therapy I've observed is tailored to each patient. Thus, when researchers insist on standardizing the approach for the purposes of science, what they are studying may well be second-rate yoga therapy. I believe it's a testament to the power of yoga how many of these studies have found positive results anyway. What I suggest as an alternative is a type of research known as "outcomes studies." In such experiments, no effort need be made to standardize the approach or to isolate single interventions. In outcomes studies, you simply compare how well people with a condition do when treated with one approach versus another. Dr. Dean Ornish's landmark studies on reversing heart disease used this technique to investigate a comprehensive lifestyle program that included yoga, a low-fat vegetarian diet, walking, and other elements. Outcomes studies allow the kind of improvisation and changes in protocol (to reflect the students' needs on any particular day) that the best yoga therapists routinely employ.

To help bring yoga as medicine to people in need, I have what may seem like an outlandish proposal. What if we as a society said that we'd seen enough of yoga's potential to consider a leap of faith? What if we decided to spend one billion dollars on yoga for one year and see what happens? We could teach yoga in nursing homes and community centers and schools. We could buy bolsters, mats, and straps for YMCAs, retirement communities, and for chronically ill people who want to do yoga at home but can't afford the equipment. We could train doctors, nurses, and other health care professionals to work with patients interested in yoga therapy. And we could simultaneously do scientific studies of the results. We could also survey people about their experience and assess whether they thought that yoga improved their health and well-being. Then as a society, we could look at the data and decide whether that was a good way to spend our money and whether, as I suspect, the result would be a net savings of health care dollars. A billion dollars is a lot of money, of course, but there are many things on which we spend much more that give us very little return on our investment.

Finally, I would like to mention the future of *Yoga as Medicine*, the book. This project is in many ways a work in progress. The field it covers is enormous and, although I've done my best to get things right, in some instances I undoubtedly have not. I therefore welcome your feedback and constructive criticism. For the material on doing yoga safely and the sections in part 3 on contraindications to specific practices, in particular, I've assembled whatever information I could find and extrapolated from what is known, but these efforts are really only a first attempt. I hope readers will write me and describe their experiences, good and bad, so that future editions of this book can fill in some of the gaps and correct any errors. You can send letters to me in care of the publisher, contact me via my website, www.DrMcCall.com, or email me at YogaDoctor@gmail.com. While I cannot respond to individual requests, I'll look at everything and what you write will shape my future work. Thanks very much.

Namaste,

Timothy McCall
Berkeley, California
April 2007

AVOIDING

COMMON YOGA INJURIES

While yoga can help prevent and treat many health conditions, it can also lead to injuries, especially if it isn't done appropriately and mindfully. Please see chapter 5 for an overview of how to do yoga safely. Below I'll cover eight major categories of common yoga injuries, and how to prevent them. If you don't know anatomy well, some of what follows may be hard to follow. If so, you may find it useful to consult a book such as *Anatomy of Hatha Yoga* by H. David Coulter or *Anatomy of Movement* by Blandine Calais-Germain. Photos of some poses mentioned, but not shown in this book, can be found at www.yogajournal.com by clicking on Pose Finder.

Back and Spinal Problems

Forward bends, especially seated forward bends such as Paschimottanasana and Head to Knee pose (Janu Sirsasana), are riskier than they look if your tendency is to bend from the waist rather than from the hip joints. To bend at the hips, you need to tip your pelvis forward, which is difficult to do when you are sitting, and which requires flexibility in the hamstring muscles in the backs of the thighs. People who have tight hamstrings tend to hump their backs so that they can get their upper body farther forward, but this is really only giving the appearance of going deeper into the pose since the hips aren't moving. When the lower back rounds, the front portions of the lumbar vertebrae get compressed. The disks between the vertebrae get pushed backward and, if they are weak, may even bulge or rupture, compressing nearby spinal nerves. This kind of nerve compression is a common cause of sciatica, pain that can radiate all the way down the leg to the toes. If you already have sciatica, forward bends could make it worse. Even riskier, forward bends can cause compression fractures of vertebrae already thinned by osteoporosis.

Many people when they first begin yoga are so stiff that if they try to do seated forward bends, their lower back is already humped before they attempt to go forward. A potential solution is to sit on a folded blanket (or a stack of blankets if necessary) or other prop to raise your hips until you are able to get a natural inward curve in the lumbar spine. Another possibility is to slightly bend your knees. That takes the pressure off the hamstrings and allows you to tip your pelvis farther forward. Another remedy for a rounded lower back is to hold a strap over the balls of your feet and stay more upright (see p. 100).

A forward bend done from a standing position—like Uttanasana—is less risky to the back than a seated forward bend but still can put a lot of pressure on the spinal disks, the shock absorbers between the vertebrae. The lumbar spine can still get compressed, but with the change in orientation of the body, gravity now tends to create an opening between the vertebrae, making the standing pose somewhat safer from this aspect than the seated version. Still, if your tendency is to round the back, placing your hands on blocks or even the edge of a chair can relieve the strain. In anyone with an acute back injury, the safest forward bends are done lying on your back, as when you bring your knees to your chest. Pressure in the spinal disks in this position is much less than in either seated or standing forward bends.

Backbends such as Camel pose (Ustrasana), Upward-Facing Dog (Urdhva Mukha Svanasana), and Cobra pose (Bhujangasana) can cause back problems, too. Many people have a lot of flexibility in the lower back but not so much in the upper back. In doing backbends, they tend to overly arch the lumbar spine to make up for the lack of movement up higher. Although it's not as risky to the nerve roots as rounding the lower back in forward bends, too much arching can compress the lumbar vertebrae and cause pain.

The neck can similarly be overarched in some poses. When doing backbends, rather than opening the upper chest—a stubborn area for many people—some students compensate by arching the neck way back (see p. 320). Some students have an unconscious habit of overarching their necks as they fold into both standing and seated forward bends.

Once again, the result can be compression of the vertebrae and pain. Taken to extremes, arching the head back can cut off blood flow to the brain and may cause such symptoms as dizziness or even a stroke.

Neck Injuries

Upside-down poses in which the head rests on the ground including Shoulderstand (Sarvangasana), Plow pose (Halasana), and Headstand (Sirsasana) can lead to neck injuries (all three poses are shown on p. 90). The standard versions of Shoulderstand and Plow cannot be safely done by most people without placing folded blankets or other support under the shoulders. The blankets help maintain the natural inward curve of the cervical spine (the neck vertebrae), and prevent it from flattening out in a way that would make injury far more likely. Rupturing of the cervical disks, the shock absorbers between the vertebrae in the neck, can lead to a painful compression of nerves in the neck if these poses are done incorrectly. A more insidious process is a gradual overstretching of the ligaments that help the neck keep its natural inward curve. A flattened neck is structurally less efficient at bearing weight than an arch, potentially setting the stage for arthritis. If you have no props, or are not sure how to use them, you can substitute what is sometimes called Half-Shoulderstand, in which the hands support the lower back and the legs angle up from the hips (see p. 489). Yoga teacher and physical therapist Julie Gudmestad suggests that students with any kind of neck pain or injury such as whiplash or a history of disk problems do this modified version.

In Shoulderstand, be sure to never turn your head to the side. A student of Aadil Palkhivala's did this in her home practice and immediately herniated two disks in her neck. This seemingly innocuous movement can also strain the muscles and ligaments and, even more worrisome, could tear vertebral arteries in the back of the neck, potentially causing a stroke. The older you are and the more fragile your arteries, the greater the risk. While tearing an artery in this fashion isn't likely, even a small risk of a very bad side effect is worth taking seriously.

If your body is ready for it, Headstand can be a wonderful pose to calm the mind and build strength. Many students, however, lack the openness in their shoulders and chest that is required to avoid compressing their spines in the pose. That's what my problem was, and the result was thoracic outlet syndrome, as I described in chapter 5. Among those who may want to skip Headstand are anyone with carpal tunnel syndrome, thoracic outlet syndrome, or degenerative arthritis of the neck. For students with scoliosis, an abnormal curvature of the spine, any compression of the chest from Headstand could increase pain, muscle stiffness, and other symptoms. Leslie Kaminoff points out that due to anatomical differences some students can't do the pose safely without using props such as blankets to adjust for the length of their head and neck relative to their upper arms—something only an experienced teacher is going to be able to discern.

Unfortunately, the negative effects of Headstand can be insidious. It may take years, for example, for degenerative arthritis of the cervical spine to become apparent. Thus people could be practicing the pose every day and even noting benefits, not realizing that they were setting themselves up for later problems. For safety reasons, I have come to believe that Headstand should not be taught in general yoga classes unless the teacher has the ability to sort out which students shouldn't be doing it. The problem, Roger Cole believes, is that "it's way too easy to get up there and balance before you're ready." If you can't get and maintain good alignment, skip this pose and focus on preparatory poses like Wide-Legged Standing Forward Bend (Prasarita Padottanasana). If your head doesn't reach the floor, place a block or other prop under the crown of your head for support (see p. 271).

N.B. Going upside down raises the pressure in the eyes and can be risky for those with glaucoma and diabetes, and even people who are extremely nearsighted may be at risk for a retinal tear. It's advisable if you have any of these conditions to get clearance from an ophthalmologist in addition to your regular doctor. Having a cataract doesn't make inversions riskier, although having had cataract surgery, particularly if you had it recently, increases the risk of a retinal tear or detachment. Upside-down poses are also potentially risky for people with poorly controlled blood pressure (see chapter 20).

Hamstring Tears

The hamstrings are the three muscles at the back of each thigh that run from the pelvis to the back of the lower leg. These muscles are often injured in yoga practice, particularly from an overly aggressive practice of forward bends—the riskiest being standing forward bends. It's important to listen to the feedback from your body and never push to get a certain result, such as being able to place your hands on the floor, even if you were able to do it the day before. While it is possible to tear the belly of the muscle, the more common site of injury is right near where the tendons attach to the sitting bones in the pelvis. Hamstring injuries are more likely to occur with sudden movements, particularly when the room is cold or you haven't warmed up sufficiently, but they may also occur when you are warm and tired, such as near the end of a long practice session when your attention may be flagging. This can happen to people who are stiff and who push too hard, but is more common among students who are flexible but who lack muscle strength. Julie Gudmestad says she hasn't seen hamstring tears near the sitting bones in anybody but yoga practitioners. The reason, she suspects, is that a lot of classes and most people's home practice include a lot of hamstring stretching but relatively little hamstring *strengthening*. Poses like Bridge pose (Setu Bandha) and other backbends build hamstring strength. When doing Bridge, think about moving your sitting bones, the ischial tuberosities, toward your knees, and using this action to lift the pelvis higher. The longer you hold the pose, and the more often you do it, the more you'll strengthen the hamstrings.

Any pose where the hamstrings are stretched is especially risky once a tear has occurred, even if it's a small one, so forward bends must be avoided, often for many months, and then only slowly reintroduced after the muscles have been strengthened with other postures. Any attempt to do forward bends before the injury has healed can put you back to square one and can even exacerbate the initial injury. Even poses like Triangle pose (Trikonasana, see p. 368) and Downward-Facing Dog (Adho Mukha Svanasana, see p. 275) contain an element of forward bending and are potentially troublesome. Using blocks under the hands in Dog pose reduces the stretch to some degree.

Shoulder Injuries

Shoulder irritation is endemic in the modern world. Unlike the hip, the shoulder socket isn't fully formed. To hold the ball of the humerus, the arm bone, in place, the tendons of four muscles form a kind of "pseudo-socket." These tendons are easily inflamed with activity and the result is what's known as rotator cuff tendinitis. Yoga can cause rotator cuff injuries, or reactivate old ones. Any kind of repetitive movement in which the arms are raised over the head can be problematic. The best way to prevent injuries is to maintain good alignment of the arm and shoulder, being particularly careful not to allow the head of the arm bones (near the shoulder) to jut forward. This is a particular concern in such asanas as Reverse Prayer pose (Namaste), and Cow Face Pose (Gomukhasana). If your shoulder starts to bother you, it's best to lay off and return carefully to practice when you are symptom-free. It's also possible to modify poses, for example, doing Warrior I (Virabhadrasana I) keeping the hands on the hips rather than overhead.

Probably the worst offender for causing rotator cuff problems is the yoga push-up, Chaturanga Dandasana. If you don't keep the head of the arm bones—the humerus bones—firmly lodged in the shoulder socket or if you allow the bones to jut forward in the joint, you make yourself vulnerable to injury. This is most likely to happen in rapid flowing yoga sequences such as in Ashtanga and vinyasa classes where you jump into the pose multiple times and usually only stay a few seconds before moving on to the next one.

It's best to practice Chaturanga more slowly so that you can focus on getting the alignment right before doing quickly flowing sequences. If you can't keep your shoulders back, try practicing the pose with your knees on the mat, which takes some of the weight off your arms (see p. 484).

Sacroiliac Strains

The sacroiliac (SI) joint sits in the irregularly shaped surface between the outside edge of the sacrum, the triangular bone at the base of the spine, and the ilium, one of the bones that comprise the pelvis. Painful misalignments and irritation of the sacroiliac joint, which usually happen on only one side at a time, are among the most common yoga injuries. As with hamstring tears, Roger Cole finds that SI problems usually occur to people who are fairly flexible, often seasoned yoga practitioners or former dancers. There is not a lot of movement in the SI joints, and indeed in some people these joints become fused as they get older (these people don't get SI strains). If the joints still move, however, and you twist the sacrum relative to the pelvis—which can happen in everything from Triangle pose to Marichyasana I (see p. 371)—you end up putting an unhealthy torque on them.

Roger says that it's common for the top part of one side of the sacrum to get out ahead of the ilium and get stuck there. This can happen in seated forward bends, particularly those like Head-to-Knee pose (Janu Sirsasana), in which there is also an element of twisting involved (see p. 329). If you have an SI problem you may need to avoid such poses or do them in a modified fashion, for example by placing support under the thigh of the bent leg. Also potentially aggravating according to Roger are poses like Cobbler's pose (Baddha Konasana) and wide-legged forward bends, either seated or standing. To prevent SI problems in twisting poses, Judith Hanson Lasater recommends releasing your pelvis, that is letting it turn slightly in the direction of the twist, instead of keeping it fixed (as is often taught). This helps the pelvis and sacrum to twist in unison, reducing the potential for unhealthy torsion between them.

Knee Injuries

Lotus pose (Padmasana) is perhaps the most famous of all asanas, dating back thousands of years, but it can be a killer for the knees. While it may not be initially obvious, the area of the body that needs to be flexible to get into Lotus is the hips. If the ball of the femur (leg) bones can't externally rotate sufficiently in the hip socket, there is simply no way to get your feet into the proper position—unless you use your hands to pull your ankles over the opposite thigh—which puts tremendous torque on the knee joint. Roger Cole says,

"When the thigh stops rotating, the only way to get the foot up higher is to bend the knee sideways. Knees are not made to do this." Many eager yoga students have ruptured the ligaments in the knee trying to get into this pose—and unlike some of the potential dangers from asanas described in this appendix, the damage is immediate.

Another potential safety issue for the knees is the tendency to hyperextend, that is overstraighten or lock the joint, in some poses. Even many people who are otherwise quite stiff have excessive mobility in the knee which can show up in asanas like Triangle (Trikonasana), Tree pose (Vrksasana), and even Mountain pose (Tadasana). Locking the knee joint compresses it and puts too much strain on the medial meniscus, the shock-absorbing cartilage in the knee. Worse, Tom Alden says, is that "the medial meniscus is pinned in a way that it can be torn when you move." If you find yourself locking your knee, it's safer to think of keeping a "micro-bend" in the joint. Actually what you are doing is keeping the knee straight, not allowing it to hyperextend, but if you're used to locking the knee, it will probably feel as if you are bending it slightly. In fact, doing standing postures like Triangle pose and Mountain pose without hyperextending the knee and strongly engaging the quadriceps muscles in the front of the thigh is good preventive medicine. Most people with hypermobile knees are weak in these muscles. Yoga teacher Donald Moyer finds that most people who lock the knee put the majority of their weight on their heels. Shifting the weight more to the ball of the foot tends to remedy the problem.

The medial meniscus can also be damaged in Hero's pose (Virasana) a kneeling pose similar to Thunderbolt pose (Vajrasana), but with the feet farther apart. In order to prevent this injury, Tom says, it's vital to keep neutral alignment in the leg bones so that there is no torsion in the knee. If you slowly lower yourself in the pose, at some point you may notice that you are developing a feeling of twisting or compression in the joint. The remedy, Tom says, is to put a block or folded blanket under your buttocks, high enough that you can maintain good alignment.

The knees are at risk in standing poses like Warrior II (Virabhadrasana II, see p. 370) if the front knee isn't well aligned over the ankle. Many students have a tendency to allow the knee to drift toward the big-toe side, so that it is no longer in line with the ankle. Since the knee functions as a hinge joint, when the knee drifts, the result can be compression of the joint. It's also potentially risky to allow the front knee to extend past the front ankle. This position can create a shearing force in the joint and can damage the cartilage. If you find this happening in Warrior pose, you need to widen your stance.

Even sitting in a simple cross-legged pose for meditation can damage the knees. Similarly, Lotus and Virasana, two traditional postures for sitting practice, can strain the knee because to sit safely in these positions for long periods of time requires flexibility in the hips. This is one reason why meditators should consider doing a regular asana practice.

Leslie Kaminoff says the incidence of arthritis among serious Buddhist meditators, who usually don't do asanas, is very high. They look really nice when they're sitting, he says, but when they get up, they walk like they just got off a horse. Some Buddhist traditions ask students not to change their position no matter how much pain they are in. While such discipline may help train the mind, from a medical standpoint it's ill-advised. You are much better off meditating comfortably in a chair than torturing yourself on the floor. T. K. V. Desikachar told me that any position, even lying down, is fine for meditation so long as you don't fall asleep.

Ankle Injuries

Hero's pose (Virasana) and Supta Virasana, the reclining version of the same pose, can be very challenging to people who have tightness over the tops of the feet. If that area hurts, you are probably compressing bones in your ankles and may be stretching ligaments on the top of your foot, neither of which is desirable. One possible solution is to roll a small towel up and place it under the ankles. Roger Cole has had good results using a shelf of blankets placed under the shins to protect the ankle joints. What you do not want to do, he says, is take the pressure off the ankles by allowing the feet to turn out to the side in this pose, which twists the knees, compresses the cartilage, and stresses the ligaments. It's safest if the feet don't splay to the sides, but point straight back, and if they are positioned immediately adjacent to the pelvis on either side.

Another potentially risky pose for the ankles is Lotus, and, as with the knee problems mentioned earlier, it's related to limited mobility in the hips and forcing yourself into the posture. In order to get into the pose, many students overstretch the tops of their feet, using their hands to force the feet into position. The result is an unhealthy sickling of the ankle joint. This stretches the joint's ligaments in the same way that an ankle sprain can. Doing this repeatedly can lengthen the ligaments, leading to instability and the possibility of future ankle sprains. Sickling of the ankles also puts added pressure on ligaments, in the knee. Although it requires greater flexibility in the hips, keeping your ankles in a more neutral alignment is safer.

Wrist Injuries

Certain asanas, including Downward-Facing Dog pose, the yoga push-up Chaturanga Dandasana, and Handstand can put a lot of pressure on the wrist joints, specifically the carpal tunnel. Many students tend to collapse their wrists, letting the weight fall almost entirely on the heel of the hands. Pressure there can directly compress the carpal tunnel, the small passageway through which tendons and the median nerve pass from the arm to the hand (see chapter 13). The more you weigh and the smaller your wrists, the greater the compression tends to be.

If your weight falls predominantly on your hands in Downward-Facing Dog instead of the feet, bend your knees slightly to relax the hamstring muscles and lessen the burden on the wrists. Ideally, the pressure on each hand should be evenly distributed between the heel of your hand and the knuckle side and between the thumb side of the hand and the pinky side. Pressing the index finger and thumb more firmly into the mat can help achieve this. If you feel compression in your wrists in Downward-Facing Dog pose, try placing a rolled-up mat, a slant board, or a book underneath your wrists and see if it allows you to redistribute some of the weight to your knuckles. See chapter 13 for more suggestions on avoiding wrist compression.

Learning to change where the weight falls on your hands could help prevent injuries in poses like Handstand, Upward Bow (Urdhva Dhanurasana), and many arm balances like Crane pose (Bakasana, also sometimes called Crow pose). These asanas put even more strain on the wrist than Downward-Facing Dog because you are bearing weight with the wrist bent to almost 90 degrees. As in Dog pose, see if you can bring more weight to the knuckles and the thumb-and-index-finger side of the hands.

SOURCES OF

FURTHER INFORMATION

Books

The Heart of Yoga: Developing a Personal Practice by
T. K. V. Desikachar

The Tree of Yoga by B. K. S. Iyengar

Yoga and the Quest for the True Self by Stephen Cope

The Yoga Sutras of Patanjali: Commentary on the Raja Yoga Sutras by Sri Swami Satchidananda

Yoga: The Iyengar Way by Silva Mehta, Mira Mehta, and Shyam Mehta

Video

The Wisdom of Yoga by Carlos Pomeda

Yoga Unveiled on the history and essence of yoga by Gita and Mukesh Desai

Audio

Meditations for Life by Rod Stryker

Moving into the Garden of Your Heart: Yoga Nidra by Betsey Downing, PhD (available at www.betseydowning.com)

Information on Yoga and Yoga Therapy

International Association of Yoga Therapists
www.iayt.org

Yoga Alliance
www.yogaalliance.org

Yoga Journal
www.yogajournal.com

Yoga Research and Education Foundation
www.yref.org

Traditional Yoga Studies
www.traditionalyogastudies.com

Complementary, Alternative, and Mind-Body Medicine

Mind/Body Medical Institute
Harvard Medical School
www.mbmi.org

National Center for Complementary and
Alternative Medicine
www.nccam.nih.gov

Dr. Andrew Weil
www.drweil.com

Yoga Props and Clothing

Gaiam
www.gaiam.com

Green Yoga (information on environmentally
sensitive yoga props)
www.greenyoga.org

Hugger Mugger
www.huggermugger.com

Tools for Yoga
www.toolsforyoga.net

Yoga.com
http://yoga.com/

Contact Information for Featured Teachers

Chapter 8: Anxiety and Panic Attacks
Rolf Sovik, PsyD
Himalayan Institute of Buffalo, New York
www.himalayaninstitute.org

Chapter 9: Arthritis
Marian Garfinkel, EdD
B. K. S. Iyengar Yoga Studio of Philadelphia
www.philayoga.com

Chapter 10: Asthma
Barbara Benagh
www.yogastudio.org

Chapter 11: Back Pain
Judith Hanson Lasater, PT, PhD
www.judithlasater.com

Chapter 12: Cancer
Jnani Chapman, RN
Osher Center for Integrative Medicine
www.osher.ucsf.edu

Chapter 13: Carpal Tunnel Syndrome
Tom Alden, DC
www.tomalden.com

Chapter 14: Chronic Fatigue Syndrome
Gary Kraftsow
American Viniyoga Institute
www.viniyoga.com

Chapter 15: Depression
Patricia Walden
www.yoganow.net

Chapter 16: Diabetes
Sandra Summerfield Kozak, MS
International Yoga Studies
www.internationalyogastudies.com

Chapter 17: Fibromyalgia
Sam Dworkis
Recovery Yoga & Extension Yoga
www.extensionyoga.com

Chapter 18: Headaches
Rodney Yee
www.yeeyoga.com

Chapter 19: Heart Disease
Nischala Joy Devi
www.abundantwellbeing.com

Chapter 20: High Blood Pressure
Aadil Palkhivala, JD
College of Purna Yoga
www.yogacenters.com

Chapter 21: HIV/AIDS
Shanti Shanti Kaur Khalsa, PhD
Guru Ram Das Center for Medicine
and Humanology
www.grdcenter.org

Chapter 22: Infertility
John Friend
Anusara yoga
www.anusara.com

Chapter 23: Insomnia
Roger Cole, PhD
www.rogercoleyoga.com

Chapter 24: Irritable Bowel Syndrome
Michael Lee
Phoenix Rising Yoga Therapy
www.pryt.com

Chapter 25: Menopause
Elise Browning Miller, MA
www.ebmyoga.com

Chapter 26: Multiple Sclerosis
Eric Small
Beverly Hills Iyengar Yoga Studio
www.yogams.com

Chapter 27: Overweight and Obesity
Richard Freeman
The Yoga Workshop
www.yogaworkshop.com

Other Teachers/Experts Cited in the Book*

Ana Forrest
Forrest Yoga
www.forrestyoga.com

Pandit David Frawley, OMD
American Institute of Vedic Studies
www.vedanet.com

Julie Gudmestad, PT
www.gudmestadyoga.com

Jon Kabat-Zinn, PhD
Center for Mindfulness at the University of
Massachusetts Medical School
www.umassmed.edu/cfm/index.aspx

Leslie Kaminoff
The Breathing Project
www.thebreathingproject.com

Dean Ornish, MD
Preventive Medicine Research Institute
www.pmri.org

Rod Stryker
Para Yoga
www.parayoga.com

Types of Yoga

Ashtanga Yoga
www.ashtanga.com

Bikram Yoga
Bikram's Yoga College of India
www.bikramyoga.com

Himalayan Institute
(Hatha, Raja, and Tantric Yoga)
www.himalayaninstitute.org

* For others not listed here, see www.DrMcCall.com.

Integral Yoga
Satchidananda Ashram Yogaville
www.yogaville.org

Iyengar Yoga
B. K. S. Iyengar Yoga National Association of the
United States
www.iynaus.org

Kripalu Yoga
Kripalu Center for Yoga and Health
www.kripalu.org

Kundalini Yoga (in the style of Yogi Bhajan)
www.kundaliniyoga.org

Transcendental Meditation
www.tm.org

Viniyoga
American Viniyoga Institute
www.viniyoga.org

Yoga Centers in India
Mentioned in *Yoga as Medicine*

Kabir Baug
Sun-Jeevan Yoga Darshan
51, Narayan Peth
Pune 411 030 India
www.kabirbaug.com

Kaivalyadhama Yoga Institute
Lonavla
Pune 410 403 India
www.kdham.com

Krishnamacharya Yoga Mandiram
New No.31 (Old #13) Fourth Cross Street
R. K. Nagar
Chennai 600 028 India
www.kym.org

Ramamani Iyengar Memorial Yoga Institute
1107 B/1 Hare Krishna Mandir Road
Model Colony, Shivaji Nagar
Pune 411 015 India
www.bksiyengar.com

Vivekananda Yoga Research Institute
Swami Vivekananda Yoga Anusandhana
Samasthana (VYASA)
19, Eknath Bhavan, Gavipuram Circle
K. G. Nagar
Bangalore 560 019 India
www.vyasa.org

The Yoga Institute
Shri Yogendra Marg, Prabhat Colony
Santacruz (East)
Mumbai 400 055 India
www.yogainstitute.org

SANSKRIT GLOSSARY

Agni. The Ayurvedic principle of digestive fire, which is said to not only help digest food but emotional and intellectual experience as well.

Agni Sara. Stomach churning, a yogic practice said to build digestive fire.

Ahimsa. Nonviolence to yourself and others. The first of Patanjali's yamas and the foundation of the practice of yoga.

Apana. The downward flow of prana in the body, hypothesized in yoga and Ayurveda. Apana is said to regulate biological functions such as urination, defecation, and menstruation.

Aparigraha. Nonhoarding. The fifth of Patanjali's yamas.

Asana. Yogic postures. The third limb of Patanjali's eight-limbed system of yoga.

Ashtanga yoga. Patanjali's eight-limbed system of yoga. Also the name of a style of yoga propagated by Pattabhi Jois.

Asteya. Nonstealing. The third of Patanjali's yamas.

Ayurveda. The ancient science of Indian medicine that includes dietary and lifestyle suggestions, bodywork, herbal remedies, and even surgery.

Bandha. Literally locks, bandha involve muscular contractions that subtly alter the position of the spine, and are said to effect the flow of prana during certain yogic practices. See *Mula bandha, Jalandhara bandha,* and *Uddiyana bandha.*

Bhakti yoga. The yoga of devotion. Worshipping a deity or chanting verses from sacred texts like the *Bhagavad Gita* are examples.

Bhastrika. Literally "bellows." A breathing technique in which the breath is forcefully inhaled and exhaled, often at rapid rates. See *Kapalabhati.*

Bhramari. The Bee Breath, a pranayama technique involving humming.

Brahmacharya. Sometimes interpreted as celibacy, but also less strictly understood as having integrity and following the other yamas in sexual relationships. The fourth of Patanjali's yamas.

Chakras. Literally wheels, chakras are energy centers that yoga teaches run along the spine from the base (the root chakra) to the crown of the head. Pronounced CHOCK-rahs, not SHOCK-rahs.

Dharana. Concentration, the sixth limb of Patanjali's eight-limbed system of yoga.

Dharma. One's duty or destiny in life, and by extension one's purpose and path.

Dhyana. Meditation, the seventh limb of Patanjali's eight-limbed system of yoga.

Dosha. Literally, that which goes out of balance. The Ayurvedic doshas are kapha, pitta, and vata. Each person is said to be a specific balance of the three, which predisposes them to certain body types, personality traits, and medical conditions.

Drishti. The focus of the eyes in yoga practice; for example, looking out over the front hand in Warrior II pose.

Duhkha. Suffering. The opposite of sukha. Patanjali taught that future suffering can be avoided.

Gunas. The three qualities of activity (rajas), inertia (tamas), and balance (sattva) that in yogic and Ayurvedic teaching are said to infuse everything.

Guru. One who removes darkness. A teacher.

Hatha yoga. Literally "forceful" yoga. The yogic path that includes the yamas, niyamas, asana, pranayama, mudras, and in some people's definition, meditation as well. In the West, it has come to be used as a generic term for various styles of yoga that include the physical poses.

Ida. Postulated energy pathway, or nadi, running along the spine. Ida extends to the left nostril and is associated with relaxation and activation of the parasympathetic nervous system.

Ishvara. The Lord. Ishvara is the term for God that Patanjali used in the *Yoga Sutras.*

Ishvara pranidhana. Literally "devotion to God," metaphorically "giving up the illusion of being in control of what happens." The fifth of Patanjali's niyamas.

Jalandhara bandha. The chin lock, used, for example, in Shoulderstand.

Japa. Fingering mala beads while reciting mantra.

Jnana yoga. The yoga of knowledge which involves study of yogic texts as well as direct experience of practices including meditation.

Kapalabhati. Literally "skull-shining." A breathing technique in which the breath is forcefully exhaled and passively inhaled, often at rapid rates. Also sometimes referred to as Breath of Fire. See *Bhastrika.*

Kapha. The Ayurvedic dosha associated with water and earth. Characterized by inertia and stability.

Karma. Literally "action," karma refers to the laws of cause and effect. In the yogic view, every thought, word, and deed creates karma and affects what happens later.

Karma yoga. The yoga of work, of selfless service. Karma yoga, as articulated in the *Bhagavad Gita*, is about giving your best effort and letting go of any attachment to what happens as a result.

Kosha. The sheaths or layers of human existence as postulated in yogic lore. The five sheaths include the physical, prana or energy, lower mind (manas), higher mind (buddhi), and bliss (ananda).

Kriya. Cleansing practices. Also used to specify yogic practice designed to have a specific effect. Patanjali defines kriya yoga, the yoga of action, as tapas, svadhyaya, and Ishvara pranidhana, the last three niyamas.

Kumbhaka. Breath retention, usually done during pranayama. Holding can be done either after inhalation (Antara Kumbhaka), after exhalation (Bahya Kumbhaka), or both.

Kundalini. The "serpent energy," said to lie at the base of the spine in yogic lore. When activated, Kundalini rises up the spine to the crown of the head.

Mala beads. Precursor to the Roman Catholic rosary, a string of beads to finger while chanting mantra.

Mantra. A word or phrase, often from a sacred text, chanted or said silently to oneself. "Om" is probably the most famous one.

Moksha. Enlightenment or liberation. The ultimate goal of yoga.

Mudra. Literally a "seal." Various gestures and positions of the hands and body.

Mula bandha. The root lock. A subtle muscular contraction of pelvic muscles said to bring energy up the spine.

Nadis. Postulated energy pathways in the body, analogous to the traditional Chinese medical concept of meridians. See *Ida*, *Pingala*, and *Sushumna*.

Nadi Shodhana. Also sometimes called Nadi Shuddhi. Alternate nostril breathing. The pranayama practice is said to balance the energy between the left and right nostrils and with that the sympathetic and parasympathetic nervous systems. See *Ida* and *Pingala*.

Neti Kriya. Rinsing the nasal passages, usually with warm salt water. A small pot with a thin spout, sometimes called a neti pot, is often used to deliver a stream of liquid into one nostril which then flows out the other.

Nidra. Sleep as in the guided meditation Yoga Nidra.

Niyamas. The "do's" or personal observances. The second limb of Patanjali's eight-limbed system of yoga, which includes tapas, sauca, santosha, svadhyaya, and Ishvara pranidhana.

Patanjali. Compiler of the *Yoga Sutras*, the approximately two-thousand-year-old collection of aphorisms that many consider the most important text on yoga.

Pingala. Postulated energy pathway or nadi running along the spine. Pingala extends to the right nostril and is associated with activation of the sympathetic nervous system, causing physical and psychological stimulation.

Pitta. The Ayurvedic dosha associated with fire. Characterized by intelligence, passion, and anger.

Prakriti. One's inborn Ayurvedic constitution, kapha or vata-pitta, for example.

Prana. The breath or life force. Analogous to the Chinese concept of chi.

Pranayama. Yogic breathing exercises. The fourth limb of Patanjali's eight-limbed system of yoga.

Pratyahara. The turning of the senses inward as when one concentrates on the internal sound of the breath. The fifth limb of Patanjali's eight-limbed system of yoga.

Rajas/rajasic. The quality of activity or restlessness. One of three gunas or qualities described in yoga and Ayurveda. See also *Tamas* and *Sattva.*

Raja yoga. "Royal" yoga is a synonym for the classical yoga of Patanjali.

Samadhi. The state of complete absorption. The eighth limb of Patanjali's eight-limbed system of yoga.

Samskara. Ingrained patterns or "grooves" of thought or behavior. In yoga, old samskaras are overcome by establishing new ones.

Sangha. Community.

Sankalpa. The yogic tool of intention. Intention is what you plan to do, a promise to yourself, not what you hope will happen as a result.

Santosha. Contentment. The second of Patanjali's niyamas.

Sattva. The quality of calm, clearheadedness, and balance. One of three gunas or qualities described in yoga and Ayurveda. See also *Tamas* and *Rajas.*

Satya. Non-lying or truthfulness. The second of Patanjali's yamas.

Sauca. Purity, cleanliness. The first of Patanjali's niyamas.

Seva. Selfless service. The work of karma yoga.

Sitali. Literally "cooling." A pranayama done with the inhalation through a curled tongue. Pronounced SHE-tah-lee.

Sthira. The principle of steadiness and firmness. Asana, Patanjali says, should be a balance of steadiness and ease.

Sukha. Happiness or ease.

Sushumna. The postulated central channel or nadi through which prana or Kundalini energy flows up the spine from the root chakra to the crown of the head. In yogic teaching, sushumna is only opened when ida and pingala are balanced and breathing is equal between the two nostrils, as happens in meditation.

Svadhyaya. The traditional meaning was study and chanting of the scriptures. In more modern usage it means self-study. The fourth of Patanjali's niyamas.

Tamas/tamasic. Characterized by inertia or dullness. One of three gunas or qualities described in yoga and Ayurveda. See also *Rajas* and *Sattva.*

Tantra. An ancient yogic path that stresses that enlightenment can come through the body, and not just by transcending it as is taught in the more ascetic, classical yoga.

Tapas. Fire, discipline, devotion. The third of Patanjali's niyamas.

Uddiyana bandha. The solar plexus lock. Drawing up the abdomen inward and upward. This is best appreciated when done during breath holding after a complete exhalation.

Ujjayi. Victorious breath. A sibilant sound made by narrowing the vocal cords. This is a type of pranayama and can also be performed during asana.

Vata. The Ayurvedic constitutional type or dosha associated with air. Characterized by creativity, movement, and indecision.

Vinyasa. A flowing sequence. A style of hatha yoga in which practitioners flow from pose to pose.

Yamas. The "don'ts" or moral injunctions. The first limb of Patanjali's eight-limbed system of yoga, which includes ahimsa, satya, asteya, brahmacharya, and aparigraha.

Yoga. The state of connection or union. A technology of life transformation. Also often used as shorthand to refer to the practices, particularly asana, that comprise yoga.

Yogi. One committed to the path of yoga. Technically, the term yogin is used for a male practitioner, and yogini for a female, though the term yogi is sometimes used for either.

SANSKRIT WORDS IN ASANA NAMES

Adho. Downward, as in Adho Mukha Svanasana, Downward-Facing Dog pose.

Anga. Limb, as in Sarvangasana, Shoulderstand.

Ardha. Half, as in Ardha Chandrasana, Half Moon pose.

Asana. Pose or posture.

Baddha. Bound, as in Baddha Konasana, Bound-Angle pose, also known as Cobbler's pose.

Baka. Crane, as in Bakasana, Crane pose (sometimes called Crow pose).

Bala. Child as in Balasana, Child's pose.

Bheka. Frog, as in Bhekasana, Frog pose.

Bhuja. Arm, as in Bhujapidasana, an arm-balancing pose.

Bhujanga. Snake or cobra, as in Bhujangasana, Cobra pose.

Chandra. Moon, as in Ardha Chandrasana, Half Moon pose.

Chatur. Four, as in Chaturanga Dandasana, Four-Limbed Staff pose, the yogic push-up.

Danda. Staff or stick, as in Dandasana, Staff pose.

Dhanura. Bow, as in Urdhva Dhanurasana, Upward Bow (full backbend) pose.

Dwi. Two, as in Dwi Pada Viparita Dandasana, Two-Legged Inverted Staff pose.

Eka. One, as in Eka Pada Rajakapotasana, One-Footed Royal Pigeon pose.

Garuda. Eagle, as in Garudasana, Eagle pose.

Go. Cow, as in Gomukhasana, Cow Face pose.

Hala. Plow, as in Halasana, Plow pose.

Hasta. Hand, as in Padahastasana, Hand to Foot pose.

Janu. Knee, as in Janu Sirsasana, Head to Knee pose.

Jathara. Stomach or abdomen, as in Jathara Parivartanasana, a supine twisting pose.

Kapota. Pigeon, as in Kapotasana, Pigeon pose.

Karna. Ear, as in Karnapidasana, Ear Pressure pose.

Kona. Angle, as in Utthita Parsvakonasana, Extended Side Angle pose.

Kurma. Turtle, as in Kurmasana, Turtle pose.

Makra. Crocodile, as in Makrasana, Crocodile pose.

Mala. Garland, as in Malasana, Garland pose.

Marichi. A mythological sage, as in Marichyasana, Sage pose.

Matsya. Fish, as in Matsyasana, Fish pose.

Matsyendra. Literally, Lord of the Fishes, a famous yoga teacher from the tenth century CE, as in Ardha Matsyendrasana, Half Lord of the Fishes pose.

Mayur. Peacock, as in Pincha Mayurasana, Feathered Peacock pose, also known as Forearm Balance pose.

Mukha. Face or mouth, as in Adho Mukha Svanasana, Downward-Facing Dog pose.

Namaste. Refers to the position of the hands in the traditional Indian salutation, with the palms pressed together in front of the chest. Sometimes called Prayer position.

Nava. Boat, as in Navasana, Boat pose.

Nirlamba. Without support, as in Nirlamba Sarvagasana, Unsupported Shoulderstand.

Pada. Foot (or sometimes leg), as in Padahastasana, Hand to Foot pose.

Padangusta. Big toe, as in Padangusthasana, Hand to Big Toe pose.

Padma. Lotus, as in Padmasana or Lotus pose.

Parivrtta. Reverse or revolved, as in Parivrtta Trikonasana, Revolved Triangle pose.

Parsva. Side, as in Utthita Parsvakonasana, Extended Side Angle pose.

Paschima. Westward, as in Paschimottanasana, Seated Forward Bend pose. (Yoga practitioners traditionally faced east, hence a stretch of the back of the body was of the westward portion.) See *Purva*.

Pida. Pressure, as in Karnapidasana, Ear Pressure pose.

Pincha. Feather as in Pincha Mayurasana, Feathered Peacock pose, also known as Forearm Balance pose.

Prasarita. Spread out, as in Prasarita Padottanasana, Wide-Legged Standing Forward Bend.

Purva: Eastward, as in Purvottanasana, a backbending pose that stretches the front or eastward side of the body. See *Paschima*.

Salabha. Locust, as in Salabhasana (pronounced shah-lah-BAH-sah-nah), Locust pose.

Salamba. Supported, as in Salamba Sarvangasana, Supported Shoulderstand.

Sama. Together, and hence harmonious, as in Samasthiti, another name for Tadasana, Mountain pose. The same root is found in the word *samadhi*.

Sarvanga. Literally, "all limbs," as in Sarvangasana, Shoulderstand.

Sava. Corpse, as in Savasana, Corpse pose, also known as Deep Relaxation pose. Pronounced SHAH-vah.

Setu. Bridge, as in Setu Bandha Sarvangasana, Bridge pose. Pronounced SAY-too.

Sirsa. Head, as in Sirsasana (pronounced sheer-SHAH-sah-nah), Headstand.

Sthiti. Standing, as in Samasthiti, another name for Tadasana, Mountain pose.

Supta. Supine, as in Supta Baddha Konasana, Reclining Cobbler's pose.

Surya. Sun, as in Surya Namaskar, Sun Salutations.

Svana. Dog, as in Adho Mukha Svanasana, Downward-Facing Dog pose.

Tada. Mountain, as in Tadasana, Mountain pose.

Tri. Three, as in Trikonasana, Triangle pose.

Upavista. Seated as in Upavista Konasana, a seated, wide-legged forward bend.

Urdhva. Upward, as in Urdhva Mukha Svanasana, Upward-Facing Dog pose.

Ustra. Camel, as in Ustrasana, Camel pose.

Utkata. Fierce, powerful, as in Utkatasana (usually known as Chair pose).

Utthita. Extended, as in Utthita Parsvakonasana, Extended Side Angle pose.

Vajra. Thunderbolt, as in Vajrasana, Thunderbolt pose.

Viparita. Inverted, as in Viparita Karani, Legs-Up-the-Wall pose.

Vira. Hero, as in Virasana, Hero's pose.

Virabhadra. Literally, blessed warrior and the name of a mythic fighter, as in Virabhadrasana I, Warrior I pose.

Vrksa. Tree, as in Vrksasana, Tree pose.

Chapter 2

p. 26
"Recently scientists have described a fifth type, gamma waves…"
Lutz A, Greischar LL, Rawlings NB, Ricard M, Davidson RJ. Long-term meditators self-induce high-amplitude gamma synchrony during mental practice. Proc Natl Acad Sci USA. 2004 Nov 16; 101(46):16369–73.

p. 28
"Alcoholism and Other Drug Abuse"
Shaffer HJ, LaSalvia TA, Stein JP. Comparing hatha yoga with dynamic group psychotherapy for enhancing methadone maintenance treatment: a randomized clinical trial. Altern Ther Health Med. 1997 Jul; 3(4): 57–66.
Gelderloos P, Walton KG, Orme-Johnson DW, Alexander CN. Effectiveness of the Transcendental Meditation program in preventing and treating substance misuse: a review. Int J Addict. 1991 Mar; 26(3):293–325.
Raina N, Chakraborty PK, Basit MA, et al. Evaluation of yoga therapy in alcohol dependence. Indian Journal of Psychiatry. 2001; 43, 171–74.

"Anxiety," see chapter 8.

"Asthma," see chapter 10.

"Attention Deficit Hyperactivity Disorder"
Jensen PS, Kenny DT. The effects of yoga on the attention and behavior of boys with Attention-Deficit/Hyperactivity Disorder (ADHD). J Atten Disord. 2004 May; 7(4):205–16.

"Chronic Obstructive Pulmonary Disease (e.g., Emphysema)"
Tandon MK. Adjunct treatment with yoga in chronic severe airways obstruction. Thorax. 1978 Aug; 33(4):514–7.

Kulpati DD, Kamath RK, Chauhan MR. The influence of physical conditioning by yogasanas and breathing exercises in patients of chronic obstructive lung disease. J Assoc Physicians India. 1982 Dec; 30(12):865–8.
Behera D. Yoga therapy in chronic bronchitis. J Assoc Physicians India. 1998 Feb; 46(2):207–8.

"Congestive Heart Failure"
Bernardi L, Spadacini G, Bellwon J, Hajric R, Roskamm H, Frey AW. Effect of breathing rate on oxygen saturation and exercise performance in chronic heart failure. Lancet. 1998 May 2; 351(9112):1308–11.

"Drug Withdrawal"
Chauhan, SKS. Role of yogic exercises in the Withdrawl [sic] Symptoms of Drug Addicts, Yoga Mimamsa. 1992 Jan; 30(4): 21–23.

"Eating Disorders"
Daubenmier, JJ. The relationship of yoga, body awareness, and body responsiveness to self-objectification and disordered eating. Psychol of Women Q, 2005 June; 29(2): 207–219.

"Epilepsy"
Panjwani U, Selvamurthy W, Singh SH, Gupta HL, Thakur L, Rai UC. Effect of Sahaja yoga practice on seizure control & EEG changes in patients of epilepsy. Indian J Med Res. 1996 Mar; 103:165–72.
Rajesh B, Jayachandran D, Mohandas G, Radhakrishnan K. A pilot study of a yoga meditation protocol for patients with medically refractory epilepsy. J Altern Complement Med. 2006 May; 12(4):367–71.

"Fibromyalgia," see chapter 17.

"Heart Disease," see chapter 19.

"High Blood Pressure," see chapter 20.

"HIV/AIDS," see chapter 21.

"Infertility," see chapter 22.

"Insomnia," see chapter 23.

"Irritable Bowel Syndrome," see chapter 24.

"Menopausal and Perimenopausal Symptoms," see chapter 25.

"Mental Retardation"
Uma K, Nagendra HR, Nagarathna R, Vaidehi S, Seethalakshmi R. The integrated approach of yoga: a therapeutic tool for mentally retarded children: a one-year controlled study. J Ment Defic Res. 1989 Oct; 33 (Pt 5):415–21.

"Migraine and Tension Headaches," see chapter 18.

"Multiple Sclerosis," see chapter 26.

"Neuroses (e.g., Phobias)"
Vahia NS, Doongaji DR, Jeste DV, Kapoor SM, Ardhapurkar I, Ravindranath S. Further experience with the therapy based upon concepts of Patanjali in the treatment of psychiatric disorders. Indian Journal of Psychiatry. 1973; 15:32–37.

"Obsessive Compulsive Disorder"
Shannahoff-Khalsa DS, Beckett LR. Clinical case report: efficacy of yogic techniques in the treatment of obsessive compulsive disorders. Int J Neurosci. 1996 Mar; 85(1–2):1–17.
Shannahoff-Khalsa DS, Ray LE, Levine S, Gallen CC, Schwartz BJ, Sidorowich JJ. Randomized controlled trial of yogic meditation techniques for patients with obsessive compulsive disorders, CNS Spectrums: The Int J of Neuropsychiatric Medicine. 1999; 4(12): 34–46.

"Osteoarthritis (Degenerative Arthritis)," see chapter 9.

"Osteoporosis"
Greendale GA, McDivit A, Carpenter A, Seeger L, Huang MH. Yoga for women with hyperkyphosis: results of a pilot study. Am J Public Health. 2002 Oct; 92(10):1611–4.

"Pain (Chronic)"
Kabat-Zinn J. An outpatient program in behavioral medicine for chronic pain patients based on the practice of mindfulness meditation: theoretical considerations and preliminary results. Gen Hosp Psychiatry. 1982 Apr; 4(1):33–47.

"Pancreatitis (Chronic)"
Sareen S, Kumari V. Yoga for rehabilitation in chronic pancreatitis. Gut. 2006 Jul; 55(7):1051.

"Pleural Effusion (Fluid Collection in the Lining of the Lung)"
Prakasamma M, Bhaduri A. A study of yoga as a nursing intervention in the care of patients with pleural effusion. J Adv Nurs. 1984 Mar; 9(2):127–33.

"Post-Heart Attack Rehabilitation"
Tulpule TH, Tulpule AT. Yoga: a method of relaxation for rehabilitation after myocardial infarction. Indian Heart J. 1980 Jan–Feb; 32(1):1–7.

"Postoperative Recovery"
Tyagi I, Sharma UD, Bajaj P, Husain T, Gupta S, Lamba PS, Khan A. Evaluation of pink city lung exerciser for prevention of pulmonary complications following upper abdominal surgery. Indian J of Anaesthesia. 1991 Dec; 39(6):198–203.

"Post-Polio Syndrome"
DeMayo W, Singh B, Duryea B, Riley D. Hatha yoga and meditation in patients with post-polio syndrome. Altern Ther Health Med. 2004 Mar–Apr; 10(2):24–5.

"Pregnancy (Both Normal and Complicated)"
Narendran S, Nagarathna R, Narendran V, Gunasheela S, Nagendra HR. Efficacy of yoga on pregnancy outcome. J Altern Complement Med. 2005 Apr; 11(2):237–44.
Narendran S, Nagarathna R, Gunasheela S, Nagendra HR. Efficacy of yoga in pregnant women with abnormal Doppler study of umbilical and uterine arteries. J Indian Med Assoc. 2005 Jan; 103(1):12–14, 16–17.

"Rheumatoid Arthritis," see chapter 9.

"Rhinitis (Inflammation of the Nose)"
Sim MK. Treatment of disease without the use of drugs. VI. Treatment of rhinitis by a yogic process of cleaning and rubbing the nasal passage with a rubber catheter. Singapore Med J. 1981 Jun; 22(3):121–3.

"Schizophrenia"
Gangadhar, BN, Ganesan D, Jagadisha, Nagendra HR. Yoga therapy in the treatment of schizophrenia. Presented at the 15th International Conference of Frontiers in Yoga Research and Its Applications, December 16–19, 2005, Bangalore, India.

"Scoliosis (Curvature of the Spine)"
Zaba R. [Effect of intensive movement rehabilitation and breathing exercise on respiratory parameters in children with idiopathic stage-I scoliosis] Przegl Lek. 2003; 60 Suppl 6:73–5 (in Polish).

"Sinusitis"
Rabago D, Zgierska A, Mundt M, Barrett B, Bobula J, Maberry R. Efficacy of daily hypertonic saline nasal irrigation among patients with sinusitis: a randomized controlled trial. J Fam Pract. 2002; 51:1049–55.

"Tuberculosis"
Visweswaraiah NK, Telles S. Randomized trial of yoga as a complementary therapy for pulmonary tuberculosis. Respirology. 2004 Mar; 9(1):96–101.
Prakasamma M, Bhaduri A. A study of yoga as a nursing intervention in the care of patients with pleural effusion. J Adv Nurs. 1984 Mar; 9(2):127–33.

"Urinary Stress Incontinence"
Milani R, Valli G, Bhole MV. Yoga-eutonia in Genuine Stress Incontinence—an exploratory study, Yoga Mimamsa. 1992 Jan; 30(4):10–20.

p. 29
"more and better research being published in both India and the West."
Khalsa SBS. Yoga as a therapeutic intervention: a bibliometric analysis of published research studies. Indian J Physiol Pharmacol. 2004; 48:269–85.

p. 31
"Increases Flexibility"
Ray US, Mukhopadhyaya S, Purkayastha SS, Asnani V, Tomer OS, Prashad R, Thakur L, Selvamurthy W. Effect of yogic exercises on physical and mental health of young fellowship course trainees. Indian J Physiol Pharmacol. 2001 Jan; 45(1):37–53.

Ray US, Hegde KS, Selvamurthy W (1983). Effects of yogic asanas and physical exercises on body flexibility in middle-aged men; Yoga Rev. III 2:75–79.

"yoga appears to build endurance and delay the onset of fatigue"
Ray US, Hegde KS, Selvamurthy W. Improvement in muscular efficiency as related to a standard task after yogic exercises in middle aged men. Indian J Med Res. 1986 Mar; 83:343–8.

"Improves Balance"
Gauchard GC, Jeandel C, Tessier A, Perrin PP. Beneficial effect of proprioceptive physical activities on balance control in elderly human subjects. Neurosci Lett. 1999 Oct 1; 273(2):81–4.

p. 32
"almost four times as likely to have complete clearing of their skin"
Benhard JD, Kristeller J, Kabat-Zinn J. Effectiveness of relaxation and visualization techniques as an adjunct to phototherapy and photochemotherapy of psoriasis. J Am Acad Dermatol. 1988 Sep; 19(3):572–4.
Kabat-Zinn J, Wheeler E, Light T, Skillings A, Scharf MJ, Cropley TG, Hosmer D, Bernhard JD. Influence of a mindfulness meditation-based stress reduction intervention on rates of skin clearing in patients with moderate to severe psoriasis undergoing phototherapy (UVB) and photochemotherapy (PUVA). Psychosom Med. 1998 Sep–Oct; 60(5):625–32.

"The group developed a higher level of influenza antibodies in their blood"
Davidson RJ, Kabat-Zinn J, Schumacher J, Rosenkranz M, Muller D, Santorelli SF, Urbanowski F, Harrington A, Bonus K, Sheridan JF. Alterations in brain and immune function produced by mindfulness meditation. Psychosom Med. 2003 Jul–Aug; 65(4):564–70.

"As part of a larger study looking at osteoporosis ..."
Kado DM, Huang MH, Karlamangla AS, Barrett-Connor E, Greendale GA. Hyperkyphotic posture predicts mortality in older community-dwelling men and women: a prospective study. J Am Geriatr Soc. 2004 Oct; 52(10):1662–7.

"This notion is backed by an experiment done in Italy ..."
Di Bari M, Chiarlone M, Matteuzzi D, Zacchei S, Pozzi C, Bellia V, Tarantini F, Pini R, Masotti G, Marchionni N. Thoracic kyphosis and ventilatory dysfunction in unselected older persons: an epidemiological study in Dicomano, Italy. J Am Geriatr Soc. 2004 Jun; 52(6):909–15.

p. 33
"New research suggests that excessive kyphosis is not only ..."
Huang MH, Barrett-Connor E, Greendale GA, Kado DM. Hyperkyphotic posture and risk of future osteoporotic fractures: the Rancho Bernardo study. J Bone Miner Res. 2006 Mar; 21(3):419–23.

"A pilot study, published in the *American Journal of Public Health* ..."
Greendale GA, McDivit A, Carpenter A, Seeger L, Huang MH. Yoga for women with hyperkyphosis: results of a pilot study. Am J Public Health. 2002 Oct; 92(10):1611–4.

p. 35
"Yoga practice has been shown to improve vital capacity..."
Telles S, Nagarathna R, Nagendra HR, Desiraju T. Physiological changes in sports teachers following 3 months of training in yoga. Indian J Med Sci. 1993 Oct; 47(10):235–8.

"Leads to Slower and Deeper Breathing"
Bernardi L, Spadacini G, Bellwon J, Hajric R, Roskamm H, Frey AW. Effect of breathing rate on oxygen saturation and exercise performance in chronic heart failure. Lancet. 1998 May 2; 351(9112):1308–11.

p. 36
"Yoga has also been shown to increase levels of hemoglobin and red blood cells..."
Chohan IS, Nayar HS, Thomas P, Geetha NS. Influence of yoga on blood coagulation. Thromb Haemost. 1984 Apr 30; 51(2):196–7.

p. 38
"An unpublished study done at California State University..."
Professor Steven A. Hawkins, PhD, and former faculty yoga teacher Bee Beckman of the Department of Kinesiology and Physical Education at California State University, Los Angeles, personal communication.

p. 39
"One study of forty young men in the Indian army..."
Ray US, Sinha B, Tomer OS, Pathak A, Dasgupta T, Selvamurthy W. Aerobic capacity & perceived exertion after practice of hatha yogic exercises. Indian J Med Res. 2001 Dec; 114:215–21.

"In people with heart disease, a comprehensive lifestyle program..."
Ornish D, Scherwitz LW, Doody RS, Kesten D, McLanahan SM, Brown SE, DePuey E, Sonnemaker R, Haynes C, Lester J, McAllister GK, Hall RJ, Burdine JA, Gotto AM Jr. Effects of stress management training and dietary changes in treating ischemic heart disease. JAMA. 1983 Jan 7; 249(1):54–9.

"subjects who practiced just pranayama could work harder..."
Raju PS, Madhavi S, Prasad KV, Reddy MV, Reddy ME, Sahay BK, Murthy KJ. Comparison of effects of yoga & physical exercise in athletes. Indian J Med Res. 1994 Aug; 100:81–6.

"one study found significant reductions in fat folds..."
Bera TK, Rajapurkar MV. Body composition, cardiovascular endurance and anaerobic power of yogic practitioner. Indian J Physiol Pharmacol. 1993 Jul; 37(3):225–8.

p. 40
"Yoga appears to improve both of these measures."
Bowman AJ, Clayton RH, Murray A, Reed JW, Subhan MM, Ford GA. Effects of aerobic exercise training and yoga on the baroreflex in healthy elderly persons. Eur J Clin Invest. 1997 May; 27(5):443–9.

"A study by Italian researcher Luciano Bernardi..."
Bernardi L, Sleight P, Bandinelli G, Cencetti S, Fattorini L, Wdowczyc-Szulc J, Lagi A. Effect of rosary prayer and yoga mantras on autonomic cardiovascular rhythms: comparative study. BMJ. 2001 Dec 22–29; 323(7327):1446–9.

"the vibrations generated in the head from humming sounds...",
Maniscalco M, Weitzberg E, Sundberg J, Sofia M, Lundberg JO. Assessment of nasal and sinus nitric oxide output using single-breath humming exhalations. Eur Respir J. 2003 Aug; 22(2):323–9.

"Improves Brain Function"
Manjunath NK, Telles S. Spatial and verbal memory test scores following yoga and fine arts camps for school children. Indian J Physiol Pharmacol. 2004 Jul; 48(3):353–6.
Naveen KV, Nagarathna R, Nagendra HR, Telles S. Yoga breathing through a particular nostril increases spatial memory scores without lateralized effects. Psychol Rep. 1997 Oct; 81(2):555–61.
Jedrczak A, Toomey M, Clements G. The TM-Sidhi programme, age, and brief tests of perceptual-motor speed and nonverbal intelligence. J Clin Psychol. 1986 Jan; 42(1):161–4.
Dash M, Telles S. Yoga training and motor speed based on a finger tapping task. Indian J Physiol Pharmacol. 1999 Oct; 43(4):458–62.

p. 41
"Activates the Left Prefrontal Cortex"
Davidson RJ. Anterior electrophysiological asymmetries, emotion and depression: Conceptual and methodological conundrums. Psychophysiology. 1998; 35:607–614.

"Changes Neurotransmitter Levels"
Devi SK, Chansauria JPN, Udupa KN. Mental depression and Kundalini yoga, Ancient Science of Life. 1986; 6 (2): 112–8.

"Yoga has been found to lower fasting blood sugar..."
See chapter 16.

"improve sensitivity to the effects of insulin."
Mukherjee A, Banerjee S, Bandyopadhyay SK, Mukherjee PK. Studies on the interrelationship between insulin tolerance and yoga. Indian Journal of Physiology and Allied Sciences. 1992; 46:110–115.

p. 42
"Improves Levels of Cholesterol and Triglycerides"
Mahajan AS, Reddy KS, Sachdeva U. Lipid profile of coronary risk subjects following yogic lifestyle intervention. Indian Heart J. 1999 Jan–Feb; 51(1):37–40.
Damodaran A, Malathi A, Patil N, Shah N, Suryavansihi, Marathe S. Therapeutic potential of yoga practices in modifying cardiovascular risk profile in middle aged men and women. J Assoc Physicians India. 2002 May; 50(5):633–40.

"Thins the Blood"
Chohan IS, Nayar HS, Thomas P, Geetha NS. Influence of yoga on blood coagulation. Thromb Haemost. 1984 Apr 30; 51(2):196–7.
Schmidt T, Wijga A, Von Zur Muhlen A, Brabant G, Wagner TO. Changes in cardiovascular risk factors and hormones during a comprehensive residential three month kriya yoga training and vegetarian nutritions. Acta Physiol Scand Suppl. 1997; 640:158–62.

p. 43
"people who imagined the exercises ..."
Ranganathan VK, Siemionowa V, et al. From mental power to muscle power—gaining strength by using the mind. Neuropsychologia. 2004; 42:944–956.

"reduces pain in people with arthritis, back pain, fibromyalgia, carpal tunnel syndrome ..."
See chapters in part 3 on these individual conditions for more details on scientific studies.

"Jon Kabat-Zinn finds that mindfulness meditation ..."
Kabat-Zinn J. An outpatient program in behavioral medicine for chronic pain patients based on the practice of mindfulness meditation: theoretical considerations and preliminary results. Gen Hosp Psychiatry. 1982 Apr; 4(1):33–47.

"obsessive-compulsive disorder to lower their dosage of medications ..."
Shannahoff-Khalsa DS, Beckett LR. Clinical case report: efficacy of yogic techniques in the treatment of obsessive compulsive disorders. Int J Neurosci. 1996 Mar; 85(1–2):1–17.
For information of studies on asthma, heart disease, high blood pressure, and type 2 diabetes, please see the relevant chapters in part 3 of this book.

p. 44
"Improves Psychological Health"
Arpita. Physiological and psychological effects of Hatha yoga: a review of the literature. The Journal of The International Association of Yoga Therapists. 1990, 1(I&II):1–28. A review of more than 100 studies.
Steptoe A, Patel C, Marmot M, Hunt B. Frequency of relaxation practice, blood pressure reduction and the general effects of relaxation following a controlled trial of behavior modification for reducing coronary risk. Stress Medicine. 1987; 3(2):101–107.

"a finding documented for students of TM ..."
Monahan RJ. Secondary prevention of drug dependence through the transcendental meditation program in metropolitan Philadelphia. Int J Addict. 1977 Sep; 12(6):729–54. (This is one of many studies of TM finding healthier habits, such as decreased smoking and use of alcohol. See descriptions of others at www.tm.org/research/508_studies.html.)

Chapter 3

p. 49
"A study published in the journal *Health Psychology* ..."
Cartwright M. Stress and dietary practices in adolescents. Health Psychology. 2003; 22(4):362–369.

p. 50
"Some studies link the tendency toward stress ..."
Wilson RS, Evans DA, Bienias JL, Mendes de Leon CF, Schneider JA, Bennett DA. Proneness to psychological distress is associated with risk of Alzheimer's disease. Neurology. 2003 Dec 9; 61(11):1479–85.
Wilson RS, Barnes LL, Bennett DA, Li Y, Bienias JL, Mendes de Leon CF, Evans DA. Proneness to psychological distress and risk of Alzheimer disease in a biracial community. Neurology. 2005 Jan 25; 64(2):380–2.

p. 62
"Effects of left-nostril breathing ..."
Shannahoff-Khalsa DS, Kennedy B. The effects of unilateral forced nostril breathing on the heart. Int J Neurosci. 1993 Nov; 73(1–2):47–60.
Jella SA, Shannahoff-Khalsa DS. The effects of unilateral forced nostril breathing on cognitive performance. Int J Neurosci. 1993 Nov; 73(1–2):61–8.
Kennedy B, Ziegler MG, Shannahoff-Khalsa DS. Alternating lateralization of plasma catecholamines and nasal patency in humans. Life Sci. 1986 Mar 31; 38(13):1203–14.

Chapter 4

p. 77
"Less powerful treatments are often the best place to start ..."
For an in-depth discussion of this topic, see my first book, *Examining Your Doctor,* or excepts of it on my Web page, www.DrMcCall.com

p. 79
"Organic fruits, vegetables, and grains may also have higher vitamin ..."
Worthington V. Nutritional quality of organic versus conventional fruits, vegetables, and grains. J Altern Complement Med. 2001 Apr; 7(2):161–73.

p. 80
"David Rabago, MD, and colleagues ..."
Rabago D, Barrett B, Marchand L, Maberry R, Mundt M. Qualitative aspects of nasal irrigation use by patients with chronic sinus disease in a multimethod study. Ann Fam Med. 2006 Jul–Aug; 4(4):295–301.

Chapter 8

p. 134
"people suffering from the autoimmune skin condition psoriasis ..."

Fortune DG, Richards HL, Kirby B, McElhone K, Markham T, Rogers S, Main CJ, Griffiths CE. Psychological distress impairs clearance of psoriasis in patients treated with photochemotherapy. Arch Dermatol. June 2003; 139:752–56.

p. 134
"when psoriasis patients listened to guided meditation tapes…"
Bernhard J, Kristeller J, Kabat-Zinn J. Effectiveness of relaxation and visualization techniques as an adjunct to phototherapy and photochemotherapy of psoriasis. J Am Acad Dermatol. (1988) 19: 572–73.

p. 137
"Voluntarily slowing the breathing…"
McCaul KD, Solomon S, Holmes DS. Effects of paced respiration and expectation on the physiological and psychological responses to threat. J Pers Soc Psychol. 1979; 37:564–571.

"Increasing the length of exhalation…"
Cappo BM, Holmes DS. The utility of prolonged respiratory exhalation for reducing physiological and psychological arousal in non-threatening and threatening situations. J Psychosomat Res. 1984; 28:265–273.

"Training in relaxed, diaphragmatic breathing…"
Clark DM, Salkovskis PM, Chalkley AJ. Respiratory control as a treatment for panic attacks. J Behavo Ther Exper Psychiat. 1985; 16:22–30.

p. 138
"A 1973 double-blind controlled study…"
Vahia NS, Doongaji DR, Jeste DV, et al. Further experience with the therapy based upon concepts of Patanjali in the treatment of psychiatric disorders. Indian J Psychiatry. 1973; 15:32–7.

"Another small study by the same authors…"
Vahia NS, Doongaji DR, Jeste DV, Ravindranath S, Kapoor SN, Ardhapurkar I. Psychophysiologic therapy based on the concepts of Patanjali. A new approach to the treatment of neurotic and psychosomatic disorders. Am J Psychother. 1973 Oct; 27(4):557–65

"In a 1991 study done as part of a doctoral dissertation…"
Harrigan JM. A component analysis of yoga: the effects of diaphragmatic breathing and stretching postures on anxiety, personality and somatic/behavioral complaints. Dissertation Abstracts International. 1981; 42(4-A):1489.

"In a study of forty children and adolescents…"
Platania-Solazzo A, Field TM, Blank J, Seligman F, Kuhn C, Schanberg S, Saab P. Relaxation therapy reduces anxiety in child and adolescent psychiatric patients. Acta Paedopsychiatr. 1992; 55(2):115–20.

"Dr. Andreas Michalsen…"
Michalsen A, Grossman P, Acil A, Langhorst J, Ludtke R, Esch T, Stefano GB, Dobos GJ. Rapid stress reduction and anxiolysis among distressed women as a consequence of a three-month intensive yoga program. Med Sci Monit. 2005 Dec; 11(12):CR555–561.

"A study by Jon Kabat-Zinn..."
Kabat-Zinn J, Massion AO, Kristeller J, Peterson LG, Fletcher K, Pbert L, Linderking W, Santorelli SF. Effectiveness of a meditation-based stress reduction program in the treatment of anxiety disorders. Am J Psychiatry. 1992; 149:936–943.

p. 139
"These results were maintained..."
Miller J, Fletcher K, Kabat-Zinn J. Three-year follow-up and clinical implications of a mindfulness-based stress reduction intervention in the treatment of anxiety disorders. Gen Hosp Psychiatry. 1995; 17:192–200.

"It's worth noting that another study..."
Kabat-Zinn J, Chapman A, Salmon P. The relationship of cognitive and somatic components of anxiety to patient preference for alternative relaxation techniques. Mind/Body Medicine. 1997; 2:101–109.

Chapter 9

p. 155
"Marian Garfinkel's doctoral dissertation..."
Garfinkel MS, Schumacher HR Jr, Husain A, Levy M, Reshetar RA. Evaluation of a yoga based regimen for treatment of osteoarthritis of the hands. J Rheumatol. 1994 Dec; 21(12):2341–3.

"More recently, Marian and several colleagues..."
Kolasinski SL, Garfinkel M, Tsai AG, Matz W, Dyke AV, Schumacher HR. Iyengar yoga for treating symptoms of osteoarthritis of the knees: a pilot study. J Altern Complement Med. 2005 Aug; 11(4):689–93.

"A small controlled trial, published in the *British Journal of Rheumatology* ..."
Haslock I, Monro R, Nagarathna R, Nagendra HR, Raghuram NV. Measuring the effects of yoga in rheumatoid arthritis. Br J Rheumatol. 1994 Aug; 33(8):787–8.

"Another study at Vivekananda..."
Dash M, Telles S. Improvement in hand grip strength in normal volunteers and rheumatoid arthritis patients following yoga training. Indian J Physiol Pharmacol. 2001 Jul; 45(3):355–60.

"Dr. Jon Kabat-Zinn..."
Kabat-Zinn J. An outpatient program in behavioral medicine for chronic pain patients based on the practice of mindfulness meditation: theoretical considerations and preliminary results. Gen Hosp Psychiatry. 1982 Apr; 4(1):33–47.

p. 156
"The majority of patients in mindfulness-based..."
Kabat-Zinn J, Lipworth L, Burney R. The clinical use of mindfulness meditation for the self-regulation of chronic pain. J Behav Med. 1985 Jun; 8(2):163–90.

p. 174
"monitoring symptoms may be just as valuable..."
Powell H, Gibson PG. Options for self-management education for adults with asthma. The Cochrane Database of Systematic Reviews. 2002 March.

"A study published in the *Journal of the American Medical Association...*"
Smyth JM, Stone AA, Hurewitz A, Kaell A. Effects of writing about stressful experiences on symptom reduction in patients with asthma or rheumatoid arthritis. A randomized trial. JAMA 1999; 281:1304–1309

p. 175
"In 1967, the first clinical trial..."
Bhole MV. Treatment of bronchial asthma by yogic methods: a report. Yoga-Mimamsa, 1967; Jan; 9(3):33–41.

"In a later study there, Bhole..."
Bhagwat JM, Soman AM, Bhole MV. Yogic treatment of bronchial asthma: a medical report. Yoga-Mimamsa. Oct 1981; 20(3):1–12.

"Dr. Virendra Singh and colleagues..."
Singh V, Wisniewski A, Britton J, Tattersfield A. Effect of yoga breathing exercises (pranayama) on airway reactivity in subjects with asthma. Lancet. 1990 Jun 9; 335(8702):1381–3.

"S. C. Jain and B. Talukdar..."
Jain SC, Talukdar B. Evaluation of yoga therapy programme for patients of bronchial asthma. Singapore Med J. 1993 Aug; 34(4):306–8.

"A randomized controlled study, published in the *British Medical Journal...*"
Nagarathna R, Nagendra HR. Yoga for bronchial asthma: a controlled study. Br Med J. 1985 Oct 19; 291(6502):1077–9.

p. 176
"The same authors tracked 570 asthma patients..."
Nagendra HR, Nagarathna R. An integrated approach of yoga therapy for bronchial asthma: a 3–54-month prospective study. J Asthma. 1986; 23(3):123–37.

"Another found that a yoga group and a control group..."
Sabina AB, Williams AL, Wall HK, Bansal S, Chupp G, Katz DL. Yoga intervention for adults with mild-to-moderate asthma: a pilot study. Ann Allergy Asthma Immunol. 2005 May; 94(5):543–8.

"A third study found no improvement in lung function..."
Vedanthan PK, Kesavalu LN, Murthy KC, Duvall K, Hall MJ, Baker S, Nagarathna S. Clinical study of yoga techniques in university students with asthma: a controlled study. Allergy Asthma Proc. 1998 Jan–Feb;19(1):3–9.

Chapter 11

p. 193
"A program of mindfulness-based stress reduction . . ."
Kabat-Zinn J, Lipworth L, Burney R. The clinical use of mindfulness meditation for the self-regulation of chronic pain. J Behav Med. 1985 Jun; 8(2):163–90.

"Another survey supporting yoga's effectiveness . . ."
Klein AC, Sobel D. Backache relief: the ultimate second opinion from back-pain sufferers nationwide who share their successful healing experiences. Times Books, New York, 1985, p. 43.

"A recent randomized controlled study of twenty-two people . . ."
Galantino ML, Bzdewka TM, Eissler-Russo J, et al. The impact of modified Hatha yoga on chronic low back pain: a pilot study. Altern Ther Health Med. 2004; 10:56–58.

p. 194
"A randomized controlled trial led by Kimberly Williams . . ."
Williams K, Steinberg L, Petronis J. Therapeutic application of Iyengar yoga for healing chronic low back pain. International Journal of Yoga Therapy. 2003; 13:55–67.
Williams KA, Petronis J, Smith D, Goodrich D, Wu J, Ravi N, Doyle EJ Jr, Gregory Juckett R, Munoz Kolar M, Gross R, Steinberg L. Effect of Iyengar yoga therapy for chronic low back pain. Pain. 2005 May; 115(1–2):107–17.

"A randomized controlled trial, published in the *Annals of Internal Medicine* . . ."
Sherman KJ, Cherkin DC, Erro J, Miglioretti DL, Deyo RA. Comparing yoga, exercise, and a self-care book for chronic low back pain: a randomized, controlled trial. Ann Intern Med. 2005 Dec 20; 143(12):849–56.

Chapter 12

p. 208
"Recent research published in *The Lancet* . . ."
Brenner H. Long-term survival rates of cancer patients achieved by the end of the 20th century: a period analysis, Lancet. 2002 Oct 12; 360(9340):1131–5.

p. 210
"suggestive evidence comes from Dr. Dean Ornish . . ."
Dean Ornish, MD, presentation at American Urological Association 98th Annual Meeting: Abstract 105681. Presented April 27, 2003.

p. 211
"Researchers from the University of Calgary . . ."
Culos-Reed S, Carlson LE, et al. Discovering the physical and psychological benefits of yoga for cancer survivors. International Journal of Yoga Therapy. 2004; (14): 45–52.

"Preliminary findings are encouraging from a pilot study of Iyengar yoga..."
Deborah Garet, MPH, personal communication.

"A randomized controlled study conducted at the M. D. Anderson..."
Cohen L, Warneke C, et al. Psychological adjustment and sleep quality in a randomized trial of the effects of a Tibetan yoga intervention in patients with lymphoma. Cancer. 2004 May 15; 100(10):2253–60.

p. 212
"Studies of mindfulness-based stress reduction . . ."
Speca M, Carlson LE, Goodey E, Angen M. A randomized, wait-list controlled clinical trial: the effect of a mindfulness meditation-based stress reduction program on mood and symptoms of stress in cancer outpatients. Psychosom Med. 2000 Sep–Oct; 62(5):613–22.

"Guided imagery and relaxation . . ."
Walker LG, Walker MB, et al. Guided imagery and relaxation therapy can modify host defences in women receiving treatment for locally advanced breast cancer. Br J Surg. 1997; 84(1S):31.

"A program of cognitive-behavioral therapy . . ."
Fawzy FI, Cousins N, Fawzy NW, Kemeny ME, Elashoff RE, Morton D. A structured psychiatric intervention for cancer patients. I. Changes over time in methods of coping and affective disturbances. Arch Gen Psychiatry. 1990; 47:720–5.
Fawzy FI, Kemeny ME, Fawzy NW, Elashoff R, Morton D, Cousins N, Fahey JL. A structured psychiatric intervention for cancer patients. II. Changes over time in immunological measures. Arch Gen Psychiatry. 1990; 47:729–35.

"When the researchers followed up on the melanoma patients ..."
Fawzy FI, Fawzy NW, Hyun CS, Elashoff R, Guthrie D, Fahey JL, Morton DL. Malignant melanoma: effects of an early structured psychiatric intervention, coping, and affective state on recurrence and survival 6 years later. Arch Gen Psychiatry. 1993; 50:681–9.

"A recent randomized controlled study done by Dr. Raghavendra Rao..."
Dr. Raghavendra Rao. Personal communication.

p. 222
"acupuncture can diminish pain after surgery for breast cancer."
He JP, Friedrich M, Ertan AK, et al. Pain-relief and movement improvement by acupuncture after ablation and axillary lymphadenectomy in patients with mammary cancer. Clin Exp Obstet Gynecol. 1999; 26:81–84.

Chapter 13

p. 230
"the first scientific evidence of its effectiveness..."
Garfinkel MS, Singhal A, Katz WA, Allan DA, Reshetar R, Schumacher HR Jr. Yoga-based intervention for carpal tunnel syndrome: a randomized trial. JAMA. 1998 Nov 11; 280(18):1601–3.

Chapter 14

p. 246
"The best evidence to date . . ."
Bentler SE, Hartz AJ, Kuhn EM. Prospective observational study of treatments for unexplained chronic fatigue. J Clin Psychiatry. 2005, May; 66(5):625–632.

Chapter 15

p. 265
"A study conducted at Benares Hindu University . . ."
Devi SK, Chansauria JPN, Udupa KN. Mental depression and Kundalini yoga. Ancient Science of Life. 1986; 6(2): 112–8.

p. 266
"a controlled study from Punjabi University . . ."
Khumar SS, Kaur P, Kaur S. Effectiveness of shavasana on depression among university students. Indian J Clin Psychol. 1993; 20:82–87.

"In a randomized controlled trial, Alison Woolery . . ."
Woolery A, Myers H, Sternlieb B, Zeltzer L. A yoga intervention for young adults with elevated symptoms of depression. Altern Ther Health Med. 2004 Mar–Apr; 10(2):60–63

"Long-term follow-up shows these results persist . . ."
Miller JJ, Fletcher K, Kabat-Zinn J. Three-year follow-up and clinical implications of a mindfulness meditation-based stress reduction intervention in the treatment of anxiety disorders. Gen Hosp Psychiatry. 1995 May; 17(3):192–200.

"A randomized controlled trial of a program that combined MBSR . . ."
Teasdale JD, Segal ZV, Williams JMG, et al. Prevention of relapse/recurrence in major depression by mindfulness-based cognitive therapy. Journal of Consulting and Clinical Psychology. 2000; 68:615–623.

"Recent evidence from Dr. Richard Davidson's lab . . ."
Davidson RJ, Kabat-Zinn J, Schumacher J, Rosenkranz M, Muller D, Santorelli SF, Urbanowski F, Harrington A, Bonus K, Sheridan JF. Alterations in brain and immune function produced by mindfulness meditation. Psychosom Med. 2003 Jul–Aug; 65(4):564–70.

p. 284

"A small, early study on yoga for diabetes…"
Shembekar AG, Kate SK. Yoga exercises in the management of diabetes mellitus. Journal of the Diabetes Association of India. 1980; 20:167–171.

"As published in *Diabetes Research and Clinical Practice*…"
Jain SC, Uppal A, Bhatnagar SO, Talukdar B. A study of response pattern of non-insulin dependent diabetics to yoga therapy. Diabetes Res Clin Pract. 1993 Jan; 19(1):69–74.

p. 285

"A small randomized controlled trial of yoga asana…"
Monro RE, Power J, Coumar A, Nagarathna R, Dandona P. Yoga therapy for NIDDM. Complementary Medical Research. 1992; 6:66–88.

"As part of a Medicare Demonstration Project…"
Dean Ornish, personal communication.

"statistically significant decreases in fasting blood sugars…"
Singh S, Malhotra V, Singh KP, Madhu SV, Tandon OP. Role of yoga in modifying certain cardiovascular functions in type 2 diabetic patients. Assoc Physicians India. 2004 Mar; 52:203–6.

"increases in measures of lung function."
Malhotra V, Singh S, Singh KP, Gupta P, Sharma SB, Madhu SV, Tandon OP. Study of yoga asanas in assessment of pulmonary function in NIDDM patients. Indian J Physiol Pharmacol. 2002 Jul; 46(3):313–20.

"the hemoglobin A1c dropped from 8.8 . . ."
Singh S, Malhotra V, Singh KP, Sharma SB, Madhu SV, Tandon OP. A preliminary report on the role of Yoga Asanas on oxidative stress in non-insulin dependent diabetes mellitus. Indian Journal of Clinical Biochemistry. 2001 Jul; 16(2):216–20.

"In a third, the yoga group…"
Malhotra V, Singh S, Tandon OP, Sharma SB. The beneficial effect of yoga in diabetes. Nepal Med Coll J. 2005 Dec; 7(2):145–7.

"an increase in measures of nerve conduction…"
Malhotra V, Singh S, Tandon OP, Madhu SV, Prasad A, Sharma SB. Effect of Yoga asanas on nerve conduction in type 2 diabetes. Indian J Physiol Pharmacol. 2002 Jul; 46(3):298–306.

p. 296

"people with diabetes who walked…"
Gregg EW, Gerzoff RB, Caspersen CJ, Williamson DF, Narayan KM. Relationship of walking to mortality among US adults with diabetes. Arch Intern Med. 2003 Jun 23; 163(12):1440–7.

Chapter 17

p. 303
"A 1999 study led by Dr. Patrick Randolph..."
Randolph, PD, Caldera YM, Tacone AM, et al. The long-term combined effects of medical treatment and a mindfulness-based behavorial program for the multidisciplinary management of chronic pain in West Texas. Pain Digest. 1999; 9:103–112.

"A study by Kenneth Kaplan..."
Kaplan KH, Goldenberg DL, Galvin-Nadeau, M. The Impact of a meditation-based stress reduction program on fibromyalgia. General Hospital Psychiatry. 1993; 15:284–289.

"Other studies of MBSR..."
Kabat-Zinn J. An outpatient program in behavioral medicine for chronic pain patients based on the practice of mindfulness meditation: theoretical considerations and preliminary results. Gen Hosp Psychiatry. 1982 Apr; 4(1):33–47.

Chapter 18

p. 319
"A study from Sweden's Karolinska Institute..."
Weitzberg E, Lundberg JO. Humming greatly increases nasal nitric oxide. Am J Respir Crit Care Med. 2002 Jul 15; 166(2):144–5.

p. 323
"Dr. Robert Nicholson of Saint Louis University..."
Nicholson RA, Gramling SE, Ong JC, Buenaver L. Differences in anger expression between individuals with and without headache after controlling for depression and anxiety. Headache. 2003 Jun; 43(6):651–63.

"Dr. Seymour Diamond conducted two studies..."
Diamond S, Montrose D. The value of biofeedback in the treatment of chronic headache: a four-year retrospective study. Headache: The Journal of Head and Face Pain. 1984; 24(1):5–18.
Diamond S. Biofeedback and headache. Headache: The Journal of Head and Face Pain. 1979; 19(3), 180–184.

"Mindfulness-based stress-reduction programs..."
Kabat-Zinn J. An outpatient program in behavioral medicine for chronic pain patients based on the practice of mindfulness meditation: theoretical considerations and preliminary results. Gen Hosp Psychiatry. 1982 Apr; 4(1):33–47.

"S. Latha and K. V. Kaliappan..."
Latha S and Kaliappan KV. Efficacy of yoga therapy in the management of headaches. Journal of Indian Psychology. 1992; 10(1&2): 41–47.

p. 324
"In the largest study to date of yoga for chronic tension headaches..."
Prabhakar S, Verma SK, Grover P, Chopra JS. Role of yoga in the treatment of psychogenic headache. Neurology India. 1991 Jan; 39(1):11–18.

p. 332
"A study published in the *Journal of the American Medical Association*..."
Holroyd KA, O'Donnell FJ, Stensland M, Lipchik GL, Cordingley GE, Carlson BW. Management of chronic tension-type headache with tricyclic antidepressant medication, stress management therapy, and their combination: a randomized controlled trial. JAMA. 2001 May 2; 285(17):2208–15.

Chapter 19

p. 339
"Even pranayama (yogic breathing) alone..."
Raju PS, Madhavi S, Prasad KV, Reddy MV, Reddy ME, Sahay BK, Murthy KJ. Comparison of effects of yoga & physical exercise in athletes. Indian J Med Res. 1994 Aug; 100:81–6.

p. 340
"In 1948, in what may have been..."
Friedell A. Automatic attentive breathing in angina pectoris. Minnesota Medicine. 1948; 31, 875–881.

"The benefits of yogic breathing..."
Bernardi L, Spadacini G, et al. Effect of breathing rate on oxygen saturation and exercise performance in chronic heart failure. Lancet. 1998 May 2; 351(9112):1308–11.

"Dr. Dean Ornish's studies..."
Ornish DM, Scherwitz LW, Doody RS, Kesten D, McLanahan SM, Brown SE, DePuey G, Sonnemaker R, Haynes C, Lester J, McAllister GK, Hall RJ, Burdine JA, Gotto AM. Effects of stress management training and dietary changes in treating ischemic heart disease. JAMA. 1983; 249:54–59
Ornish DM, Brown SE, Scherwitz LW, et al. Can lifestyle changes reverse coronary atherosclerosis? The Lifestyle Heart Trial. The Lancet. 1990; 336:129–133.

p. 341
"What was most striking about the Lifestyle Heart Trial..."
Gould KL, Ornish D, Scherwitz L, et al. Changes in myocardial perfusion abnormalities by positron emission tomography after long-term, intense risk factor modification. JAMA. 1995; 274:894–901.

"the research was later extended to eight medical centers…"
Koertge J, Weidner G, Elliott-Eller M, Scherwitz L, Merritt-Worden TA, Marlin R, Lipsenthal L, Guarneri M, Finkel R, Saunders DE, Jr, McCormac P, Scheer JM, Collins RE, Ornish D. Improvement in medical risk factors and quality of life in women and men with coronary artery disease in the Multicenter Lifestyle Demonstration Project. Am J Cardiol. 2003 Jun 1; 91(11):1316–22.

"Both men and women were able to avoid bypass surgery…"
Ornish D. Avoiding revascularization with lifestyle changes: The Multicenter Lifestyle Demonstration Project. Am J Cardiol. 1998 Nov 26; 82(10B):72T–76T.

"Dean Ornish is compiling data on over 2000 patients…"
Dean Ornish, personal communication.

p. 342
"A controlled trial conducted at the Yoga Institute…"
Yogendra J, Yogendra HJ, Ambardekar S, Lele RD, Shetty S, Dave M, Husein N. Beneficial effects of yoga lifestyle on reversibility of ischaemic heart disease: caring heart project of International Board of Yoga. J Assoc Physicians India. 2004 Apr; 52:283–9.

"A randomized controlled trial of 93 patients…"
Mahajan AS, Reddy KS, Sachdeva U. Lipid profile of coronary risk subjects following yogic lifestyle intervention. Indian Heart J. 1999 Jan–Feb; 51(1):37–40.

"Two other Indian studies…"
Khare KC, Rai S. Study of lipid profile in post myocardial infarction subjects following yogic life style intervention. Indian Practitioner. 2002 Jun; 55(6):369–73.
Singh RB, Singh NK, Rastogi SS, Mani UV, Niaz MA. Effects of diet and lifestyle changes on atherosclerotic risk factors after 24 weeks on the Indian Diet Heart Study. Am J Cardiol. 1993 Jun 1; 71(15):1283–8.

Chapter 20

p. 363
"Two studies examining the effectiveness of yoga…"
Patel CH. Yoga and bio-feedback in the management of hypertension. Lancet. 1973; 2(837):1053–5.
Patel C. 12-month follow-up of yoga and bio-feedback in the management of hypertension. Lancet. 1975 Jan 11; 1(7898):62–4.

"Other studies have also documented…"
Sundar S, Agrawal S, Singh V, Bhattacharya S, Udupa K, Vaish S. Role of yoga in management of essential hypertension. Acta Cardiol. 1984; 39:203–8.
Datey KK, Deshmukh SN, Dalvi CP, Vinekar SL. "Shavasan": A yogic exercise in the management of hypertension. Angiology. 1969 Jun; 20(6):325–33.

p. 364
"A small randomized controlled study, published in the year 2000..."
Murugesan R, Govindarajulu N, Bera TK. Effect of selected yogic practices on the management of hypertension. Indian Journal of Physiology & Pharmacology. 2000; 44:207–10.

"Prospective data are being collected on approximately two thousand people..."
Dean Ornish, personal communication.

"Transcendental Meditation (TM)..."
Alexander CN, Schneider RH, et al. Trial of stress reduction for hypertension in older African Americans. II. Sex and risk subgroup analysis. Hypertension. 1996 Aug; 28(2):228–37.

"Another randomized controlled study of TM..."
Barnes VA, Treiber FA, Johnson MH. Impact of transcendental meditation on ambulatory blood pressure in African-American adolescents. Am J Hypertens. 2004 Apr; 17(4):366–9.

"Devices that slow down breathing, mimicking pranayama..."
Viskoper R, Shapira I, et al. Nonpharmacologic treatment of resistant hypertensives by Device-Guided slow breathing exercises. Am J Hypertens. 2003 Jun; 16(6):484–7.

p. 375
"One major study found that the old standby water pills..."
The ALLHAT Officers and Coordinators for the ALLHAT Collaborative Research Group. Major outcomes in high-risk hypertensive patients randomized to angiotensin-converting enzyme inhibitor or calcium channel blocker vs diuretic: The Antihypertensive and Lipid-Lowering Treatment to Prevent Heart Attack Trial (ALLHAT). JAMA. 2002; 288:2981–2997.

Chapter 21

p. 379
"patients treated by doctors with fewer than five HIV patients..."
Kitahata MM, Koepsell TD, Deyo RA, et al. Physicians' experience with the acquired immunodeficiency syndrome as a factor in patients' survival. N Engl J Med. 1996; 334:701–706.

p. 380
"all behaviors that can further compromise immunity and put them at risk of progressing to AIDS."
Golub ET, Astemborski JA, Hoover DR, Anthony JC, Vlahov D, Strathdee SA. Psychological distress and progression to AIDS in a cohort of injection drug users. J Acquir Immune Defic Syndr. 2003 Apr 1; 32(4):429–34.

"A study of subjects on HIV medications found that twenty-four..."
Robinson FP, Mathews HL, Witek-Janusek L. Psycho-endocrine-immune response to mindfulness-based stress reduction in individuals infected with the human immunodeficiency virus: a quasiexperimental study. J Altern Complement Med. 2003 Oct; 9(5):683–94.

p. 381

"a ten-week program of CBSM..."
Antoni MH, Carrico AW, Duran RE, Spitzer S, Penedo F, Ironson G, Fletcher MA, Klimas N, Schneiderman N. Randomized clinical trial of cognitive behavioral stress management on human immunodeficiency virus viral load in gay men treated with highly active antiretroviral therapy. Psychosom Med. 2006 Jan–Feb; 68(1):143–51.

"A randomized controlled study on using yoga..."
Frederick M. Hecht, MD, personal communication.

p. 387

"a recording called 'Naad' by Sangeet Kaur..."
Available from Ancient Healing Ways, at 800-359-2940.

p. 390

"Reiki, involving light touch..."
Miles P. Preliminary report on the use of Reiki HIV-related pain and anxiety. Altern Ther Health Med. 2003 Mar–Apr; 9(2):36.

"Writing in a journal about emotionally charged events..."
Petrie KJ, Fontanilla I, et al. Effect of written emotional expression on immune function in patients with human immunodeficiency virus infection: a randomized trial. Psychosom Med. 2004 Mar–Apr; 66(2):2.

Chapter 22

p. 397

"There is evidence of a higher rate of major birth defects..."
Hansen M, Kurinczuk JJ, Bower C, Webb S. The risk of major birth defects after intracytoplasmic sperm injection and in vitro fertilization. N Engl J Med. 2002 Mar 7; 346(10):725–30.

"A recent systematic review of twenty-five similar studies..."
Hansen M, Bower C, Milne E, de Klerk N, Kurinczuk JJ. Assisted reproductive technologies and the risk of birth defects—a systematic review. Hum Reprod. 2005 Feb; 20(2):328–38.

p. 399

"a randomized controlled study of 184 women..."
Domar AD, Clapp D, Slawsby EA, Dusek J, Kessel B, Freizinger M. Impact of group psychological interventions on pregnancy rates in infertile women. Fertil Steril. 2000 Apr; 73(4):805–11.

"high levels of depression..."
Domar AD, Zuttermeister PC, Friedman R. The psychological impact of infertility: a comparison with patients with other medical conditions. J Psychosom Obstet Gynaecol. 1993; 14 Suppl:45–52.

"Women who entered the ten-week training program with severe depression..."
Domar AD, Friedman R, Zuttermeister PC. Distress and conception in infertile women: a complementary approach. J Am Med Womens Assoc. 1999 Fall; 54(4):196–8.

Chapter 23

p. 410
"demonstrated how a common blood pressure reflex..."
Cole RJ. Postural baroreflex stimuli may affect EEG arousal and sleep in humans. J Appl Physiol. 1989 Dec; 67(6):2369–75.

p. 413
"high levels of stress hormones..."
Vgontzas AN, et al. Chronic insomnia is associated with nyctohemeral activation of the hypothalamic-pituitary-adrenal axis: clinical implications. J Clin Endocrinol Metab. 2001 Aug; 86(8):3787–94.

p. 414
"Various yogic practices also appear to increase nighttime melatonin levels . . ."
Tooley GA, Armstrong SM, Norman TR, Sali A. Acute increases in night-time plasma melatonin levels following a period of meditation. Biological Psychology. 2000; 53:69–78.
Harinath K, Malhotra AS, Pal K, Prasad R, Kumar R, Kain TC, Rai L, Sawhney RC. Effects of Hatha yoga and Omkar meditation on cardiorespiratory performance, psychologic profile, and melatonin secretion. J Altern Complement Med. 2004 Apr; 10(2):261–8.

p. 415
"Research led by Gregg Jacobs, PhD..."
Jacobs GD, Benson H, Friedman R. Perceived benefits in a behavioral-medicine insomnia program: a clinical report. Am J Med. 1996 Feb; 100(2):212–6.

"Also at Harvard Medical School, Dr. Sat Bir Khalsa..."
Khalsa SB. Treatment of chronic insomnia with yoga: a preliminary study with sleep-wake diaries. Appl Psychophysiol Biofeedback. 2004 Dec; 29(4):269–78.

"A study by Dr. Lorenzo Cohen..."
Cohen L, Warneke C, Fouladi RT, Rodriguez MA, Chaoul-Reich A. Psychological adjustment and sleep quality in a randomized trial of the effects of a Tibetan yoga intervention in patients with lymphoma. Cancer. 2004 May 15; 100(10):2253–60.

p. 416
"randomized controlled trial of sixty-nine elderly people..."
Manjunath NK, Telles S. Influence of Yoga and Ayurveda on self-rated sleep in a geriatric population. Indian J Med Res. 2005 May; 121(5):683–90.

p. 417

"more effective than sleeping pills, particularly in the long run..."

Sivertsen B, Omvik S, Pallesen S, Bjorvatn B, Havik OE, Kvale G, Nielsen GH, Nordhus IH. Cognitive behavioral therapy vs zopiclone for treatment of chronic primary insomnia in older adults: a randomized controlled trial. JAMA. 2006 Jun 28; 295(24):2851–8.

Morin CM, Colecchi C, Stone J, Sood R, Brink D. Behavioral and pharmacological therapies for late-life insomnia: a randomized controlled trial. JAMA. 1999 Mar 17; 281(11):991–9.

Jacobs GD, Pace-Schott EF, Stickgold R, Otto MW. Cognitive behavior therapy and pharmacotherapy for insomnia: a randomized controlled trial and direct comparison. Arch Intern Med. 2004 Sep 27; 164(17): 1888–96.

p. 425

"diffused essential lavender oil helped elderly patients sleep longer..."

Hardy M, Kirk-Smith MD, Stretch DD. Replacement of drug treatment for insomnia by ambient odour. Lancet. 1995 Sep 9; 346(8976):701.

Chapter 24

p. 429

"A study, published in the *American Journal of Gastroenterology*..."

Choi YK, Johlin FC Jr, Summers RW, Jackson M, Rao SS. Fructose intolerance: an under-recognized problem. Am J Gastroenterol. 2003 Jun; 98(6):1348–53.

p. 430

"small randomized controlled study conducted at the All India..."

Taneja I, Deepak KK, et al. Yogic versus conventional treatment in diarrhea-predominant irritable bowel syndrome: a randomized control study. Appl Psychophysiol Biofeedback. 2004 Mar; 29(1):19–33.

p. 431

"The relaxation response, a technique developed by..."

Keefer L, Blanchard EB. The effects of relaxation response meditation on the symptoms of irritable bowel syndrome: results of a controlled treatment study. Behav Res Ther. 2001 Jul; 39(7):801–11.

"When ten of the original thirteen patients were surveyed..."

Keefer L, Blanchard EB. A one year follow-up of relaxation response meditation as a treatment for irritable bowel syndrome. Behav Res Ther. 2002 May; 40(5):541–6.

"Another randomized controlled study of one hundred patients..."

Kumar, Virendra. A study on the therapeutic potential of some hatha yogic methods in the management of irritable bowel syndrome. The Journal of the International Association of Yoga Therapists. 1992; 3:25–38.

p. 441

"Enteric-coated capsules containing peppermint oil..."

Pittler MH, Ernst E. Peppermint oil for irritable bowel syndrome: a critical review and meta-analysis. Am J Gastroenterol. 1998; 93(7):1131–5.

"treatment with a combination of Chinese herbs..."
Bensoussan A, Talley NJ, Hing M, Menzies R, Guo A, Ngu M. Treatment of irritable bowel syndrome with Chinese herbal medicine: a randomized controlled trial. JAMA. 1998 Nov 11; 280(18):1585–9.

Chapter 25

p. 446
"A randomized controlled trial of thirty-three women with hot flashes..."
Irvin JH, Domar AD, Clark C, Zuttermeister PC, Friedman R. The effects of relaxation response training on menopausal symptoms. J Psychosom Obstet Gynaecol. 1996; 17:202–7.

"Another randomized controlled study of thirty-three women..."
Freedman RR, Woodward S. Behavioral treatment of menopausal hot flushes: evaluation by ambulatory monitoring. Am J Obstet Gynecol. 1992; 167:436–9.

"A pilot study led by Dr. Beth Cohen..."
Cohen, BE, Kanaya AM, Macer JL, Shen H, Chang AA, Grady D. Feasibility and acceptability of restorative yoga for treatment of hot flushes: a pilot trial. Maturitas. 2007 Feb 20; 56(2): 198–204.

p. 456
"though a recent large study..."
Newton KM, Reed SD, LaCroiz AZ, Grothaus LC, Ehrlich K, Guiltinan J. Treatment of vasomotor symptoms of menopause with black cohosh, multibotanicals, soy, hormone therapy, or placebo: a randomized trial. Ann Intern Med. 2006; 145:869–79.

Chapter 26

p. 460
"stress is an important factor in increasing the likelihood of developing the disease..."
Li J, Johansen C, et. al. The risk of multiple sclerosis in bereaved parents: a nationwide cohort study in Denmark. Neurology. 2004 Mar 9; 62:726–729.

"...and in flare-ups after the initial onset."
Mohr DC, Hart SL, Julian L, Cox D, Pelletier D. Association between stressful life events and exacerbation in multiple sclerosis: a meta-analysis. BMJ. 2004 Mar 27; 328(7442):731. Epub 2004 Mar 19.

p. 461
"volunteers showed greater benefits than those they counseled..."
Cited in "Multiple Sclerosis" by Nidus Information Services, 2001.

p. 462
"Led by Barry Oken, MD..."
Oken BS, Kishiyama S, Zajdel D, Bourdette D, Carlsen J, Haas M, Hugos C, Kraemer DF, Lawrence J, Mass M. Randomized controlled trial of yoga and exercise in multiple sclerosis. Neurology. 2004 Jun 8; 62(11):2058–64.

p. 473

"decrease levels of chemical messengers..."

Mohr DC, Goodkin DE, Islar J, Hauser SL, Genain CP. Treatment of depression is associated with suppression of nonspecific and antigen-specific T(H)1 responses in multiple sclerosis. Arch Neurol. 2001 Jul; 58(7):1081–6.

"Treating depression also appears to reduce fatigue."

Mohr DC, Hart SL, Goldberg A. Effects of treatment for depression on fatigue in multiple sclerosis. Psychosom Med. 2003 Jul–Aug; 65(4):542–7.

Chapter 27

p. 478

"A 1992 *New England Journal of Medicine* study..."

Lichtman SW, Pisarska K, et al. Discrepancy between self-reported and actual caloric intake and exercise in obese subjects. N Engl J Med. 1992 Dec 31; 327(27):1893–8.

p. 480

"A study led by Dr. Alan Kristal..."

Kristal AR, Littman AJ, Benitez D, White E. Yoga practice is associated with attenuated weight gain in healthy, middle-aged men and women. Altern Ther Health Med. 2005 Jul–Aug; 11(4):28–33.

"A study by Dr. Anand Shetty..."

American Heart Association's 46th Annual Conference on Cardiovascular Disease Epidemiology and Prevention, American Heart Association, news release, March 3, 2006.

"In the Lifestyle Heart Trial..."

Ornish D, Scherwitz LW, Billings JH, Brown SE, Gould KL, Merritt TA, Sparler S, Armstrong WT, Ports TA, Kirkeeide RL, Hogeboom C, Brand RJ. Intensive lifestyle changes for reversal of coronary heart disease. JAMA. 1998 Dec 16; 280(23):2001–7.

p. 481

"Dr. Suzanne Engelman and colleagues..."

Engelman SR, Clance PR, Imes S. Self and body-cathexis change in therapy and yoga groups. Journal of the American Society of Psychosomatic Dentistry and Medicine. 1982; 29(3):77–88.

A C K N O W L E D G M E N T S

THIS BOOK WOULD NOT HAVE BEEN POSSIBLE without the love, help, and support of many people. First of all, my thanks to the teachers whose work is featured in the book, and the students whose stories are told, most of whom spent many hours being interviewed and answering follow-up questions. These real-life interactions of seasoned yoga teachers and the individuals they guided through yoga are the heart of this book. Several other teachers including Ana Forrest, Julie Gudmestad, Rod Stryker, and Leslie Kaminoff, as well as Dr. David Frawley, Dr. Dean Ornish, and Dr. Jon Kabat-Zinn, contributed generously with their time and knowledge.

I am indebted to the many people who have taught me yoga over the years, including Mary Dunn, Eleanor Williams, Candace Carey, James Murphy, Karin Stephan, Peentz Dubble, Amy Ipolitti, Sianna Sherman, Donald Moyer, and most especially Patricia Walden, who first inspired me to pursue the practice. Later on, a number of teachers helped me follow my interest in therapy, including Patricia and Mary, Gary Kraftsow, John Friend, and Dr. Tom Alden. I am indebted to many people in India I learned from. Special thanks to Dr. A. G. and Indra Mohan, Dr. S. V. Karandikar, Hansa and Dr. Jayadeva Yogendra of The Yoga Institute, Dr. Bindu Kutty and Dr. A. Vedamurthachar of the National Institute of Mental Health and Neuro Sciences (NIMHANS), Dr. Mukund Bhole, the staff and volunteers at Samskrita Bharati, Tantra master Dr. Ananth Atre, and Vedic scholar Sudhakara Sharma. From the Krishnamacharya Yoga Mandarim, I owe thanks to T. K. V. Desikachar, Kaustub Desikachar, Dr. Chandrasekaran, and D. K. Shidar. I am especially indebted to Dr. Shirley Telles, N. V. Ragurham, Dr. R. Nagarathna, Dr. H. R. Nagendra, Dr. Raghavendra Rao, Dr. Manoj Dash, and Falguni Harkisondas of the Swami Vivekananda Research Foundation for all their help over the years, and to Ayurvedic master A.C. Chandukkuty Vaidhyar and his son, Bency.

Many thanks to John Abbott and Kathryn Arnold of *Yoga Journal,* who first approached me in 2002 to become the magazine's medical editor and write a regular column. Later that year John asked me write a book for them on yoga therapy, which I was happy to do, as I'd already begun work on *Yoga as Medicine* two years before. Kathryn also offered editing suggestions and helpful advice on the book's photo shoot. Special thanks to yoga teacher Jason Crandell for his help teaching the restorative sequence to the student in the headache chapter. Thanks, too, for various favors from my nephew Sean McCall, Sarah and Ty Powers, Reed Wulsin, Dr. Carrie Demers, Dr. David Coulter, Saraswati Clere, Carlos Pomeda, Dr. Douglas Brooks, Elizabeth Eliades, Sue Luby, William Broder, Grace Jebara, Hillari Dowdle, Chandra Easton, Scott Blossom, Koren Paalman, Jaki and Allan Nett, Chris Saudek, Eleanor Williams, Dr. Jarvis Chen, Jolyon Cowen, Joan Arnold, Dr. Tom Birch, Steve and Val Smith, Ted Surman, Roopesh Arrakkal, Suzanne Gordon, Steve Hubble, as well as Dr. Sapna Velayudan, K. P. Balakrishnan and all my friends at Surya Ayurvedics in Arimpur (Thrissur) Kerala.

Several people helped me learn about published and unpublished research on yoga, or provided me with copies of hard-to-locate studies: Trisha Lamb of the International Association of Yoga Therapists, Dr. Shirley Telles, Dr. W. Selvamurthy of India's Defence Institute of Physiological and Allied Sciences, Dr. Mukund Bhole, Gloria Goldberg, Marla Apt, Beth Sternlieb, Wyatt Townley, Bee Beckman, Dr. David Shannahoff-Khalsa, Dr. Kimberly Williams, Dr. Rolf Sovik, and especially Dr. Sat Bir Khalsa of Harvard Medical School, who shared with me dozens of studies that I'd been unable to track down. Thanks, too, to the many researchers who sent me reprints of their articles.

For the better part of a year while writing the book, during 2004 and 2005, I was honored to be a Scholar in Residence at the Kripalu Center for Yoga and Health in Lenox, Massachusetts. Special thanks to Stephen Cope, as well as Cathy Husid and Ila and Dinabandhu Sarley for making this invaluable experience possible. There is simply no way I could have been as productive and supported in writing the book anywhere else as I was there. The setting was gorgeous, and the many people I met there, the stories they told, and workshops I attended helped shape this book. My gratitude goes also to teachers who allowed me to attend workshops there, including Sarah Powers, Yoganand Michael Carroll, Russell Delman, Tias Little, Paul Cramer, Hilary Garavaltis, Dr. Robert Svoboda, Donna Eden, Dr. Marc Grossman, Cheri Huber, Suzie Hurley, Rama Berch, Sara Meeks, Alan Finger, and Bonnie Bainbridge Cohen.

A number of friends and colleagues read sections of the book and offered helpful commentary, including Andrea Kleinhuber, Richard Rosen, Joan Arnold, Vici Williams, Swami Shivananda Saraswati, Dr. Thomas Birch, Dr. Todd Patton (Srijan), Dr. Kimora, Shari Ser, Madeline Pearlmutter, Dr. Catalina Arboleda, Melitta Rorty, Josh Summers, James Vitale, Tricia Mickelberry, Dr. Tom Alden, and my brother Dr. Tony McCall. I'm deeply indebted to my brother Dr. Ray McCall, who read multiple versions of many chapters, and for years has brainstormed with me and been a fabulous sounding board, and to my friend Nina Zolotow, who read the entire book, helped rewrite the practice sequences in part 3, and offered many helpful editing suggestions.

Nina Zolotow was also the producer of the book's photo shoot, and functioned brilliantly in that role. She did everything from creating storyboards to buying the models' outfits to running a tight ship on the set. She helped pick a fantastic photographer, Michal Venera, and the models, Autumn Alvarez, Eric Small, Tracee Newell, Dr. Baxter Bell, Ashley Miller, and Donna Fone, all of whom were great. Thanks to stylist Chris McDonald who was excellent. Special thanks to Richard Rosen, the director of the Piedmont Yoga Studio in Oakland, California, who was the spotter during the shoot, and who lent us most of the blankets, bolsters, and other props we used.

I am particularly indebted to Beth Rashbaum of Bantam Dell, who is quite simply the best editor I've ever worked with, and I've worked with many. She is smart, passionate, incredibly knowledgeable, and always on the side of the book. From the beginning of our work together, she understood what I was trying to do, offered insightful commentary, and pushed me to make the book as good as it could be. Thanks, too, to Meghan Keenan and Glen Edelstein of Bantam Dell, and to copy editor Howard Mittelmark. I am also grateful to my agents Anne and Georges Borchardt for their consummate professionalism, good humor, and hard work.

My journey into yoga and the study of yoga therapy might not have happened without the support, generosity, and encouragement of my teacher, Patricia Walden. I can never repay all she has done for me. I also want to recognize Yogacharya B. K. S. Iyengar for his genius in yoga and yoga therapy and in bringing them to the world—and for training Patricia to be the extraordinary teacher she is. It was through his system that I came to yoga and fell in love with it, and through which I was introduced to yoga therapy. I'm also indebted to his children, Prashant and particularly Geeta for her generous teaching to me in both the US and India.

Finally, and most of all, my love and gratitude goes to my mother, Betty McCall, to whom this book is dedicated, who died during the final weeks of editing after a long and good life. She knew this book was for her, and I hope that some of the good karma she set in motion will live on through it.

INDEX

anxiety and panic attacks, 3, 5, 12; active relaxation for, 149; asana to avoid, 149; awareness of thought patterns, 136–37; breathing practices, 1:2 ratio and, 141; contraindications, special considerations, and modifications, 149–50; contributing factors, 137, 148; delayed healing and, 134; focus on the breath for, 135–36; gastrointestinal problems and, 428; gratitude and diminishing, 137; holistic approach, 137, 148; inverted pose caution, 149; Iyengar yoga and, 150; meditation caution, 98; monkey mind and, 137; overview, 134; real-life example, 133–34, 139–40, 150; Rolf Sovik's approach, 130–47; scientific evidence of yoga's benefits, 28, 137–39; seated meditation for, 146–47; twisting poses and restriction of breath, 142; vital exhaustion and, 149

apana, 331

Apanasana: for IBS, 439, *439*

Arms Overhead pose (Urdhva Hastasana), *22*, 22–23; for depression, 278; for IBS, 433

aromatherapy: for anxiety and panic attacks, 148

arthritis and rheumatic disorders, 3, 5, 6, 151–68; contraindications, special considerations, and modifications, *164*, 164–65; diet and, 76, 167; footwear and, 166; holistic approach, 166–67; how yoga can help, 152–54; Iyengar yoga for, 106, 151–68; joint-replacement surgery, 165, 167; Marian Garfinkel's approach, 156–64; misalignment and, 152, 153, 158; muscle relaxation for, 12; overview, 152; pain medication and yoga practice, 165; pain relief and, 43, 166; posture and, 32; real-life example, 151–52, 153, 156–64, 167–68; scientific evidence of yoga's benefits, 28, 151, 155–56; stress and, 49, 154; supplements for, 166; surgery and yoga practice, 165; visualization for, 164

Artist's Way, The (Cameron), 174

asana (poses), xiii, 8, 14; as aerobic, 39, 113, 339, 362, 446, 477; for anxiety and panic attacks, 141–46, 149; for arthritis and rheumatic disorders, 156–64; Ashtanga yoga primary series, 481, 488; for asthma, 180, 181, 182–83, 185; Ayurveda doshas and choice of, 83; for back pain, 192, 196–203, 204; for beginning yoga practice, 85; for bone strength, *38*, 38–39, 446; building endurance with, 31; for building tapas, *22*, 22–23, *23*; cancer patients,

seated postures for, 213–16; for CFS, 249–56; for constipation, 438, 440; contraindicated for back pain, 203, 204; contraindicated for CTS, 237–38; contraindicated for diarrhea, 440; contraindicated for headache, 331; contraindicated for heart disease, 354; contraindicated for HIV/AIDS, 391; contraindicated for hot flashes, 455; contraindicated for insomnia, 425; contraindicated for osteoporosis, 455; contraindicated for obesity, *488–89*, 488–89; counter for support during, 291–93; for CTS, 233–36; for depression, 268–78; for diabetes, 288–95; examples of each major category, *14–15*; for fibromyalgia, 304–11; flood of emotions during, 98; for headache, 326–29, 450; with head wrap, 325, *325*, *372*, 372; for heart disease, 342–54; heating and cooling principles, 330; for high blood pressure, 367–72; for HIV/AIDS, 383–89; for IBS, 429, 433–39; for infertility, 399–405; for insomnia, 413, 418–23; inverted poses, dizziness caution, 180; inverted poses, pressure in the head and, 149; inverted postures, high blood pressure caution, 373–74; for menopause, 457; menstruation, adaptations during, *99*, 99; for MS, 462–72; for MS, caution, 466, 470, 472; for muscle cramps, 414; muscle strengthening of, 31; playing the edge, 93, 288, 432; as preventative medicine, 58, 154; reducing fatigue with, 31; for stress reduction, 58–68; on a table or platform, 157; twisting and restriction of breath, 142; Viniyoga adaptations, 249; for weight loss, 481–87; working at the wall and, 271. *See also specific poses*

Ashtanga yoga, 106, 108, 318, 475, 476, 477; direction of gaze (drishti), 108; health problems not suited for, 108, 183; pranayama and, 108; primary series, 481, 488; root lock (mula bandha) and, 108; solar plexus lock (uddiyana bandha), 108; Ujjayi breath exercise and, 108; Website, 481; for weight loss, 481–87

asthma, 5, 114, 150, 169–86; asana for asthma attack, *182*, 182; Barbara Benagh's approach, 176–81; best time for yoga practice, 123; contraindications, special considerations, and modifications, 181–83; diet and, 185; dysfunctional breathing and yoga, 171–74; environmental allergies and, 184; food allergies and, 185; holistic approach, 184; indoor

blinking: left/right breathing and, 62

blood: cortisol and blood sugar levels, 49; left/right breathing and blood sugar levels, 62; stress and clotting of, 42, 48; twisting poses ("wring and soak"), 36; yoga and improved return of venous blood, 37; yoga and lowered blood sugar levels, 41; yoga and lowered hemoglobin A1c, 41, 285; yoga and raising pH, 36; yoga and thinning of, 42; yoga practice and oxygenation, 36, 446

Boat pose (Navasana): contraindicated for back pain, 203; contraindicated for hot flashes, 455

bodywork: for back pain, 205; for CTS, 232–33, *233*, 239; for headache, 333; for HIV/AIDS, 390; for MS, 473; neglected by Western medicine, 77; types of, 77–78, 120

bone density and strength, 3; calcium supplements for, 85; cortisol and lowering, 49; menopause and, 445; posture and spinal fractures, 33; prescription drugs for, 456; weight bearing asanas and, *38*, 38–39; yoga and improved, 38–39; yoga and reduction in hip fractures, 31; yoga's ability to lower stress hormones and, 39. *See also* posture

bowel function, 8, 42. *See also* irritable bowel syndrome (IBS)

Bow pose (Dhanurasana): for weight loss, 481

brain: cortisol and memory loss, 50; left/right breathing and hemisphere stimulation, 62; meditation and brain waves, 26; neuroplasticity of, 21; tumors, 318; yoga and activation of left prefrontal cortex, 42; yoga and changes in neurotransmitter levels, 42; yoga and improved function, 41–42; yogis' ability to alter brain waves, 26–27

Brand, Erin, 207–8, 223–24

breast cancer, 29, 207–8; HRT and, 444; lymphedema, yoga modifications and, 220–21, *221*; scientific evidence of yoga's benefits, 211, 212

Breath Awareness exercise: for headache, *330*, 330; for MS, *471*, 471

breathing: abdominal breathing, 135; anxiety or panic attacks and, 135–36, 137, 149; apana and headache relief, 331; asthma and dysfunctional, 171–74; "attentive" and angina pain, 340; back pain and, 192; breath holding, 171, 172; breathing assessment, 56; carpal tunnel syndrome and, 229; chanting and increased length of exhalation, 41; chest breathing, 135, 171, 402; complete breath

technique to help CHF, 36, 340; diaphragmatic, 55–56; fibromyalgia and, 303–4, 311; heart disease and, 340; left/right breathing, 62; mouth breathing, 171, 172, 173, 185–86; mouth vs. nostril, 36; nasal congestion restricting, what to do, 136; optimal, 136; overbreathing, 171, 172–73; poor posture and, 137; practices, 1:2 ratio of exhalation to inhalation, 141, 175; reverse, or paradoxical, 55–56, 171, 173; stress, effects of, 54; svadhyaya (self-study) and, 174; yoga and health benefits, 35–36, 176–81. *See also* asthma; pranayama (breathing techniques)

Breathing with Arm Movement: for IBS, *433*, 433

Bridge pose (Setu Bandha Sarvangasana): for diabetes, *294*, 294; for heart disease, 356

Buteyko, Konstantin, 169

calcium: cortisol and decrease of, 39; supplements of, 85, 456

Camel pose (Ustrasana): for weight loss, 481

Cameron, Julia, 174

cancer, 5, 6, 207–24; asana risks, 220; back pain and, 196; contraindications, special considerations, and modifications, 220–21; diet and, 222; holistic approach, 222–23; how yoga can help, 209–10; indoor pollution and, 80; Integral yoga and, 112; Jnani Chapman's approach, 212–20; overview, 208–9; overweight or obesity and, 476; pain and, 209, 222; quality of life therapies, 222; real-life example, 207–8, 223–24; sangha (community), support groups as, 209; scientific evidence of yoga's benefits, 28, 210–12; side effects of cancer therapy, control of, 20, 223; sleep study, 415–16; spiritual well-being and, 210; stress and, 49; svadhyaya (self-study) and, 210

cardiovascular system, 3, 4, 39, 339. *See also* heart disease

carpal tunnel syndrome (CTS), 89, 225–40, *227*; alternative medical treatments for, 239; contraindications, special considerations, and modifications, 237–38; diabetes and, 227; Eleanor Williams's exercises, 240; emotions and, 226, 230; Garfinkel study on, 18, 230; holistic approach, 239; how yoga can help, 227–30; hypothyroidism and, 227; Iyengar yoga for, 106, 151; medication for, 239; muscle relaxation for, 12; overview, 226–27; pain relief, 43; posture and, 32, *228*, 228; real-life example, 225–26,

Cow Face pose (Gomukhasana): for high blood pressure, 367

craniosacral therapy, 78, 103, 120

Cranz, Galen, 195

Crocodile Breathing: for anxiety and panic attacks, *140*, 140–41

Cross Bolsters. *See* Supported Bridge pose (Setu Bandha Sarvangasana)

Cross-Legged Twist (Parsvasuk hasana): for anxiety and panic attacks, *142*, 142–43

Cross-Legged Twist (Sukasana): for infertility, 404

Csikszentmihalyi, Mihaly, 52

Davidson, Richard, 32, 42, 266

death and dying: yoga and facing, 393–94

Deep Relaxation pose. *See* Savasana (Deep Relaxation pose)

deep tissue massage, 239

depression, 3, 12, 42, 261–80, 339, 380; acupuncture, 279; aerobic exercise, 279; antidepressants for, 222, 263–64, 266, 279, 314; anxiety and panic attacks and, 148; Ayurveda categories, 267–68; breathing and, 270; cancer patients and, 222; CFS and, 244; contraindications, special considerations, and modifications, 277–78; cortisol and, 49; diagnosing, 263; holistic approach, 279; increased serotonin levels and yoga, 42; infertility and, 399, 408; insomnia and, 412; Iyengar yoga for, 106; MBSR and, 266–67; meditation caution, 98; MS and, 473; overview, 262–64; overweight or obesity and, 476; Patricia Walden's approach, 268–78; posture and, 264–65; psychotherapy and, 279; real-life example, 261–62, 268–78, 280; recovery affected by, xii; scientific evidence of yoga's benefits, 28, 265–67; seasonal affective disorder (SAD), 102–3; stress and, 49, 264; supplements for, 279, 314

Desikachar, Kausthub, 108

Desikachar, T. K. V., 90, 103, 107–8, 121, 207, 213, 242, 281

Devi, Nischala Joy, 70, 112, 213, 295, *335*, 335–36; on anger, 338–39; approach to heart disease, 342–54; audio tapes by, 357; on heart disease, 336–37, 339; Ornish's Lifestyle Heart Trial and, 335–36, 340, 341, 342

devotional practices. *See* Bhakti yoga

dharana (concentration), 17

dharma (life purpose), 75; CFS and, 246

dhyana (meditation), 17. *See also* meditation

diabetes, xii, 3, 5, 6, 281–98; anxiety and panic attacks and, 148; Ayurveda and, xii, 285–86; balance, risk of falls, and, 298; belly fat and, 49; carpal tunnel syndrome and, 227; contraindications, special considerations, and modifications, 297–98; diet and, 296; health risks of, 283, 284–85, 297–98; holistic approach, 296; how yoga can help, 283–84; karma yoga for, 295; nervous system problems (peripheral neuropathy), 283–84; overview, 282–83; overweight and obesity and, 476, 477; real-life example, 281–82, 286–87, 295, 298; reducing complications of, 41; reducing stress hormones and, 12; Sandra Summerfield Kozak's approach, 286–95; scientific evidence of yoga's benefits, 284–85; stress and, 49, 283; types of, 282; vegetarian diet and lowered risk, 84, 284; yoga and lowered blood sugar levels, 41, 284–85; yoga and lowered hemoglobin A1c, 41, 285; yoga and lowering need for medication, 43, 91, 297

Diamond, Seymour, 323

diarrhea, 42, 431, 440, 441 (*see also* irritable bowel syndrome [IBS])

diet, 18, 84–86; anxiety and panic attacks and, 148; arthritis and rheumatic disorders and, 167; asthma and, 185; Ayurveda diet, for hot flashes, 455; Ayurveda doshas and choices of foods, 83; cancer and, 222, 224; for CFS, 259; for CTS, 239; dairy products and mucus, 76; for diabetes, 296, 298; eating as form of meditation, 85; environmental pollutants in, 79; feedback from your body and choices of foods, 76–77; fish, 79, 148; food allergies and, 185, 429; food as a divine gift, 481; foods that commonly trigger migraines, 322; fresh, locally grown foods in, 84–85, 148; for headache, 333; for heart disease, 356; for high blood pressure, 374–75; how to eat, 85, 491; for IBS, 440–41; for immune system, 390; importance of changes in, 85; karmic implications, 79; for menopause, 456; for MS, 473; nightshade vegetables and arthritis, 76, 167; organic foods, 79; overweight and obesity and, 477; prana in, 84; supplements in, 85; vegetarian, 79, 84, 175, 284, 337, 357; for weight loss, 480, 490; yoga and healthier choices, 44, 74–75. *See also* herbs and spices direction of gaze (drishti), 18, 108

Dolphin pose: for CTS, *238*, 238

Domar, Alice, 399, 405

Domar Center for Complementary Health Care, 405

Douillard, John, 81

Down Syndrome, 6

Downward-Facing Dog (Adho Mukha Svanasana): for building tapas, *23*, 23; contraindicated for high blood pressure, 374; for depression, 275, *275*; with head wrap, for high blood pressure, 369; for increased bone density, 38; for infertility, 404; for menopause, 454; modifications for lymphedema, 221, *221*; modified, for CTS, *238*, 238; substitution for high blood pressure, 369; substitutions for, 483; for weight loss, *483*, 483

drug withdrawal: scientific evidence of yoga's benefits, 28

duhkha (suffering): yoga and reduction in, 44, 47

Dunn, Mary, 42, 103, 117, 228

Dworkis, Sam, 114, 299, *299*; approach to fibromyalgia, 299, 303–11, 315–16; MS and, 299, 461

Eagle pose (Garudasana): for high blood pressure, 367

eating disorders: scientific evidence of yoga's benefits, 28

Eischen, Roger, 102, 114, 118

Eisenberg, Deedee, 102–4, 114, 118

Elbow pose (Pincha Mayurasana): for menopause, 454, *454*

Eliot, Robert, 135

energetic locks (bandha), 18

Engelman, Suzanne, 481

environmental pollutants and health, 78–80; air pollution, 79–80; asthma and, 184, 185; fish and, 79; in food chain, 79; indoor pollution, 80; male infertility and, 408

epilepsy: Bikram/hot yoga caution, 109; scientific evidence of yoga's benefits, 28

Equal Standing Pose (Samasthiti): for CFS, *249*, 249

Eric Small Adaptive Iyengar Yoga Program, 458

Eric Small Living Well with MS program, 458

Establishing Neutral Alignment exercise, *231*, 231

Extended Exhalation Breath: for cancer patients, 218

Extended Side Angle (Utthita Parsvakonasana): for diabetes, 293, *293*; for infertility, 404; supported, for MS, *466*, 466; for weight loss, *485*, 485

Utthita Hasta Padangusthasana: contraindicated for overweight and obesity, 488, *488*

ExTension (Dworkis), 299

eyebrow tug exercises, *11*, 11–12, *12*, 334

eyes: diabetes and retinal problems, 296, 297; headaches and, 324–25, 334; head wrap and, *325*, 325; high blood pressure and, 365, 366; HIV/AIDS and, 391; indoor pollution and, 80; left/right breathing and intraocular pressure, 62

Eyes on the Side of Your Head, *58*, 58

Faber, Michael, 428, 430, 441–42

faith, 18, 21, 23, 265, 461. *See also* Ishvara pranidhana (faith in a higher power)

Farmer, Angela, 169

fatigue, 3; causes, 243; indoor pollution and, 80; Iyengar yoga for, 256; posture and, 32; reducing, yoga and, 31. *See also* chronic fatigue syndrome (CFS); multiple sclerosis (MS)

Feathered Pipe Ranch, 119, 206

feet: yoga and improved function, 37

Feldenkrais Method, 78, 103, 116, 166, 205, 239

Feuerstein, Greg, 10

fibrinogen and fibrin (clotting factors), 42

Fibromyalgia Network, 301, 314–15

fibromyalgia syndrome, 244, 299–316; best time for yoga practice, 123, 313; Bikram/hot yoga caution, 109; breathing and, 303–4, 311; contraindications, special considerations, and modifications, 313; diagnosing, 300, 301; holistic approach, 314–15; how yoga can help, 301–3; insomnia and, xii, 300–301, 302, 314; Iyengar restorative poses and, *312*, 312; pain relief and, 314; real-life example, 299–300, 304–11, 315–16; Recovery yoga and, 114; Sam Dworkis's yoga therapy for, 304–11; scientific evidence of yoga's benefits, 28, 303; support groups for, 302–3; yoga and pain relief, 43, 302

Fish pose (Matsyasana): for heart disease, 349, *349*

flatulence, 431, 440. *See also* irritable bowel syndrome (IBS)

flexibility, 3, 4; joint health and, 36–37; risk of injury and, 94; yoga and health benefits, 30, 31 food allergies, 185, 429

Forrest, Ana, 237–38, 248, 486; on fibromyalgia, 311

Forrest yoga, 113

Forward Bend (Paschimottanasana): contraindicated for osteoporosis, 455; for fibromyalgia, *312*, 312

Framingham Heart Study, 70

Freeman, Richard, 475, *475*; approach to weight loss, 477, 478–79, 481–87, 490–92

Friedell, Aaron, 340

Friend, John, 105, 111, 331, *395*, 395; chanting taught by, 404; hands-on adjustments and assists, 404–5; "inner spiral" and, 403; yoga therapy for infertility, 395–96, 399–405, 407

Front Body Stretch (Purvottanasana): supported, on two chairs, for MS, *469*, 469–70

Full Circular Rotation of the Shoulders: for cancer patients, 216, *216*

Garfinkel, Marian, 18, 151, *151*; arthritis and yoga, 153, 155; arthritis therapy by, 156–64; carpal tunnel syndrome study, 18, 230; use of platform for asanas, 157

Garland pose (Malasana): contraindicated for arthritis, 164

geometric designs (yantra), 18, 68

Green, Elmer and Alyce, 26–27

Green, Felicity, 102–3

Gross, Ron, 336–37, 339, 341, 343–54, 357–58

Gudmestad, Julie, 320, 488

Guided Relaxation (smile meditation), 51–52; as Tantric practice, 113

Guru Ram Das Center, 377, 378

gym yoga, 113

Hackborn, Dick, 359–60, 366, 375–76

Half Locust pose (Salabasana): for heart disease, 347, *347*

Half Lotus pose (Ardha Padmasana): for HIV/AIDS, 383, *383*, 384

Half Moon pose (Ardha Chandrasana): for depression, *270*, 270–71; for IBS, *434*, 434

Half Plow pose (Ardha Halasana): for headache, *328*, 328; for menopause (hot flashes), *450*, 450–51; supported, for HIV/AIDS, 389

Half Spinal Twist (Ardha Matsyendrasana): for anxiety and panic attacks, *143*, 143; for heart disease, *350*, 350

Half Standing Forward Bend (Ardha Uttanasana): for arthritis and rheumatic disorders, 158, *158*; for high blood pressure, *369*, 369

Hands in Prayer (Namaste): for IBS, 435, *435*

hands-on adjustments and assists, 18; Anusara yoga and, 111

Handstand: contraindicated for CTS, 237; contraindicated for MS, 472

Harrigan, J. M., 138

Hartz, Arthur, 246

hatha yoga, 8, 106; anxiety reduction and, 139; Ashtanga yoga and, 108; classes vs. therapeutic yoga, 118–19; contraindicated for infertility, 407

Hatha Yoga Pradipika, 3, 16

Hay, Louise, 378

headaches, 317–34; acupressure, 333; acupuncture, 333; anger as predictor of, 323; asana for, 326–29, 450; Ayurveda constitutions and, 318, 330; caused by yoga, 320; caution on diagnosing of cause, 318, 319–20; cluster, 331; contraindications, special considerations, and modifications, 331; diary for triggers of, 321–22; diet for, 333; drug treatment, 332; holistic approach, 332–33; how yoga can help, 321–23; indoor pollution and, 80; Iyengar yoga and, 102–3; life-threatening illness and, 318; migraines, 5, 317–18, 319, 322, 331; muscle relaxation for, 12; overview, 318–20; posture and, 32, 333; pratyahara for, 321; preventative treatment, 332–33; real-life example, 317–18, 324–31, 333–34; Rodney Yee's approach, 324–31, 333–34; scientific evidence of yoga's benefits, 28, 323–24; sinus, Neti Kriya for, 80, 319; stress and, 49; stress reduction for, 321; svadhyaya (self-study) for, 322; tension, 3, 318–19; triggers, 321–22; use of pain relievers and "rebound" headaches, 319, 332

Head Movement, Horizontal: for cancer patients, 215, *215*

Head Movement, Vertical: for cancer patients, 214, *214*

Headstand (Sirsasana), *90*; avoiding falls, 96–97; cautions, 272; cautions with thoracic outlet syndrome (TOS), 90; contraindicated for CFS, 257; contraindicated for high blood pressure, 373; contraindicated for infertility, 407; contraindicated for osteoporosis, 455; for depression, 272, *272*; for headache, 330; for insomnia, 413, *418*, 418; as "king of the asana," 90; modified, for menopause, 455; supported, for HIV/AIDS, 389

Head Tilting: for cancer patients, 215, *215*

Head to Knee (Janu Sirsasana): for infertility, 404

Head-to-Knee pose (Janu Sirsasana): contraindicated for back pain, 203, *203*; for insomnia, *422*, 422

head wrap, *325*, 325, *372*, 372

Healing Back Pain: The Mind-Body Connection (Sarno), 190

Healing Path of Yoga, The (Devi), 335

healing relationships: Viniyoga and, 107; yoga and fostering, 43–44

healing touch, 222

heart disease, 6, 335–58; anger and, 44, 336, 338–39; arterial blockage and, 339–40; attacks and clots, 42; "attentive" breathing and angina pain, 340; Ayurvedic constitutional types and, 338; baroreceptor sensitivity and heart rate variability and, 41; belly fat and, 49; Bikram/hot yoga caution, 109; cholesterol-lowering drugs and, 337; contraindications, special considerations, and modifications, 354–55; depression following heart attack, 339; diet for, 356; flu shots and, 356; high blood pressure and, 41; holistic approach, 356–57; how yoga can help, 338–40; indoor pollution and, 80; inflammation and, 337–38; Integral yoga and, 112; karma yoga for, 339; lack of vacations and increased risk, 70; low-dose aspirin for, 356; lowering blood pressure with yoga and, 12; menopause and, 446; mouth and teeth, cleaning, 357; Nischala Joy Devi's yoga therapy for, 342–54; as number one killer, 208, 337, 446; Ornish program and angina pain, 341; overview, 337–38; overweight and obesity and, 476, 477; posture and, 32; real-life example, 336–37, 343–54, 357–58; risk factors, 49; scientific evidence of yoga's benefits, 28, 340–42; stress and, 49, 338; stress test before starting vigorous yoga forms, 96; supplements for, 357; symptoms in women vs. men, 338; type A personality and, 336, 337, 338, 342, 358; vegetarian diet and lowered risk, 84; web of causation, 4; yoga and improved levels of cholesterol and triglycerides, 42; yoga survey results, 5

Heart of Yoga, The (Desikachar), 103–4

heart rate: left/right breathing and, 62; m[...] and lowering, 69; variability, 40; variabili[...] ing and improved, 41

Hecht, Frederick, 381

hemorrhoids, 5

Hendricks, Gay, 169

herbs and spices, 18; ashwagandha, 258; Ayurveda, 258; bilberry, 296; black cohosh, 456–57; cancer therapy side effects and, 223; chamomile, 148; Chinese medicine (TCM), 223, 258, 441; cinnamon, 296; contraindicated for infertility, 409; dong quai, 457; evening primrose oil, 457; ginger, 167, 185, 223, 473; ginseng, 296; lavender oil, 425; marijuana, 223, 390, 473; passion flower, 148; peppermint, 441; red clover, 457; St. John's wort, 279; Siberian ginseng, 258; triphala, 473; turmeric, 167, 185, 473; valerian, 223, 425; willow bark tea, 204

high blood pressure, 3, 5, 12, 38, 41, 359–76, 446; Aadil Palkhivala's approach, 365–74; breathing techniques for, 364, 366, 367, 374; chanting for, 366; contraindications, special considerations, and modifications, 373–74; contributing factors, 49, 361–62, 476; diet, 374–75; health risks of, 41, 361; holistic approach, 374–75; how yoga can help, 362–63; karma yoga for, 375; medication and male infertility, 408; meditation and lowering, 69, 364; muscle tightness and, 366; notebook for, 363; overview, 360–62; prescription drugs for, 375; Purna yoga and, 114; real-life example, 359–60, 366, 375–76; salt sensitivity, 375; scientific evidence of yoga's benefits, 28, 363–64; stress and, 41, 362–63; svadhyaya (self-study) and, 363; vegetarian diet and, 84; weight loss and, 41; yoga and lowering need for medication, 43, 91

Himalayan Institute, 113, 139, 392

Hippocrates, 91

HIV/AIDS, xii, 3, 377–94; alternative therapies for, 390; breathing techniques, 392; chanting for, 382; choice of physician and, 379; contraindications, special considerations, and modifications, 391–92; depression and, 380; diet, 390; holistic approach, 390–91; how yoga can help, 379–80; improved immune function and, 379–80; "Massage for the Lymphatic System" kriya, 382–87; meditation for,

yoga's benefits, 28, 430–31; stress and, 42, 429; supplements for, 441; svadhyaya (self-study) for, 430

Ishvara pranidhana (faith in a higher power), 21, 23, 125; as calming, 137

Iyengar, B. K. S., ix, xviii, 46, 89, 95, 106, 107, 111, 151, 261, 264, 281, 359, 443, 458, 474, 475; on depression, 262, 264, 277; head wrap and, 325; inverted poses, 331; Legs-Up-the-Wall pose (Viparita Karani), variation, *64*, 64; recommendations for heart disease, 354; restorative yoga and, 63; on taking a step (intention), 127

Iyengar, Geeta, 46, 103

Iyengar, Prashant, 58, 92

Iyengar Institute, Pune, India, 46, 92, 102–3, 107

Iyengar yoga, xviii, 90, 106–7; for anxiety and panic attacks, 150; for arthritis, 151–68; B. K. S. Iyengar Yoga Studio, Philadelphia, 151; cancer survivors and, 211; for CFS, *256*, 256; classes vs. therapeutic yoga, 118–19; eight-limbed path of yoga and, 106; for headaches and upper body strain, 102–3; health problems best addressed by, 106; for heart disease, 356; for HIV/AIDS, 389; infertility and, 406; props used in, 106, 118; restorative yoga, 106; for SAD, 102–3; teachers of, 102–3; teacher training and certification, 106–7. *See also* Garfinkel, Marian; yoga teacher

Jacobs, Gregg, 415

Jain, S[uresh] C., 175, 284

Japanese medicine, 77

Jivamukti yoga, 108, 225, 476

joints: Establishing Neutral Alignment exercise, 231, *231*; instability and pregnancy, 100–101; misalignment and, 94, 152, 153, 158, 231, 487; MS and, 460; overweight and obesity and, 476; pain, HIV/AIDS and, 392; Pumping the Wrist, *232*, 232; safety of poses and, 92, 94; synovial fluid, 36–37; yoga and health benefits, 36–37

journal and journaling: as complement to psychotherapy, 174; food and exercise diary, 478; for headache triggers, 321–22; for high blood pressure, 363; for HIV/AIDS, 390; for IBS symptoms, 430; "morning pages," 174; Phoenix Rising Yoga Therapy (PRYT) and, 110; plan for yoga for life and, 127–28; sleep diary, 415; of symptoms and factors affecting, 76–77

Kabat-Zinn, Jon, 32, 43, 69, 138–39, 155–56, 303, 323, 432

Kabir Baug, Pune, India, 119

Kado, Deborah, 32

Kaivalyadhama ashram, Lonavla, India, 175

Kaliappan, K. V., 323

Kaminoff, Leslie, 92–93, 94, 183, 298

Kapalabhati breathing, 101, 109; after Neti Kriya, 80; for asthma, 181–82; contraindicated for cancer patients, 221; contraindicated for heart disease, 354; contraindicated for high blood pressure, 374; contraindicated for insomnia, 425; for diabetes, 286–87

Kaplan, Kenneth, 303

Karandikar, Dr., 119, 129

karma yoga, 18, 75, 86, 112; for cancer survivors, 209; for diabetes, 295; diet and, 79; for heart disease, 295, 339; for high blood pressure, 375; for MS, 461, 474

Kaur, Sangreet, 387

Keshavadas, Sant, 281

Khalsa, Sat Bir, 415

Khalsa, Shanti Shanti Kaur, xii, 69, 111–12, 115, 117, *377*, 377–78; approach to HIV/AIDS, 381–89, 391–94; use of "Naad" recording, 387

kinesiology, 116

Kneeling pose (Vajrasana): for CFS, 254, *254*

knee problems: arthritis and rheumatic disorders and, 153; Ashtanga/power yoga caution, 107; misalignment and, 153 (*see also* arthritis and rheumatic disorders); not crossing legs when sitting, 158; real-life example, 151–52, 153, 156–64, 167–68; scientific evidence of yoga's benefits, 155. *See also* joints

Knee to Chest pose: contraindicated for osteoporosis, 455; for heart disease, 346, *346*; for high blood pressure, 367

Kozak, Sandra Summerfield, xii, 281, *281*; approach to diabetes, 281–82, 283, 286–95; diabetes and Ayurvedic concepts, 285–86; on weight loss asanas, 487

Kraftsow, Gary, xii, 105, 107–8, 242, *242*; approach to CFS, 242–43, 245–46; Pancha Maya model and, 247–49

ful absorption) and, 52; scientific evidence of yoga's benefits, 212; spirituality optional in, 7; Transcendental Meditation (TM), 40, 44, 364, 415; transformation (of self) and, 69; for weight loss, 491; where to place your focus, 218. *See also* specific meditation exercises

Meditation on the Breath, 53–54

Meeks, Sara, 455

melanoma, 212

menopause, 3, 5, 443–57; acupuncture for, 457; asana for, 447–54, 457; asana for hot flashes, 448, 450–51; asana that can cause hot flashes, 455; in Ayurveda, hot flashes as pitta problem, 455; bioidentical hormones and, 445; breathing techniques for, 452–53, 454; contraindications, special considerations, and modifications, 455–56; diet for, 456; Elise Miller's approach, 447–54; heart disease and, 446; herbal remedies, 457; holistic approach, 456–57; how yoga can help, 445–46; HRT and, 444–45; loss of bone density, 445; loss of muscle mass, 445–46; meditation for, 454, *454*; overview, 444–45; prescription drugs for bone strength, 456; real-life example, 443–44, 445, 447; sangha (community) and, 457; scientific evidence of yoga's benefits, 28, 446–47; smoking and, 456; stress and, 445; supplements for, 456

menstruation: asana adaptations during, 99; asana adaptations during, *99*; asana to avoid, 99; problems alleviated, yoga survey results, 5; yoga during, cautions, 98–99

mental and psychological well-being, xvi, 44, 47; breathing practices, caution, 97–98; calm mind, 55; cancer survivors and yoga therapy, 211; equanimity, 3, 44, 358; left/right breathing and, 62; meditation caution, 98; mood enhancement, 44; sattvic, or clear, state of mind, 59, 84; self-esteem, 44; serenity and peace, xvii, 4, 302; yoga and fibromyalgia, 302; Yoga Nidra to relax the mind, 68. *See also* anxiety and panic attacks

mental retardation, 28

Michalsen, Andreas, 138

Miller, Elise Browning, *443*, 443; approach to menopause, 447–54, 457

Mohan, A. G. and Indra, 108, 119

monkey mind, 53, 54, 137

monoamine oxidase, 42

Monro, Robin, 4–5, 155, 285

mood enhancement, 3, 44, 446, 460. *See also* depression

Mountain pose (Tadasana): for CFS, 249, *249*; for CTS, *231*, 231; for depression, 278; used for Eyes on the Side of Your Head exercise, *58*, 58; widening stance for safety, 97, *97*

Moving Inward: The Journey to Meditation (Sovik), 139

Moving Toward Balance (Yee and Zolotow), 317

moxibustion, 120

Muktananda, Swami, 281

multiple sclerosis (MS), 3, 299, 458–74; alternative therapies for, 473; asanas for, 462–72; balance improvement for, 460; Bikram/hot yoga caution, 109; breathing techniques for, 460, 471; chanting, 463–64; contraindications, special considerations, and modifications, 472; depression and, 473; diagnosing, 460; diet for, 473; Eric Small's approach, 462–72; herbs and spices, 473; holistic approach, 472–73; how yoga can help, 460–61; karma yoga for, 461, 474; online support groups, 473; overview, 459–60; pain, treatment of, 472; real-life example, 459, 463, 471, 473–74; satya (honesty) and, 474; scientific evidence of yoga's benefits, 28, 462; strap used in exercises, 466; stress and, 49, 460; svadhyaya (self-study) for, 474; tapas (discipline) and yoga practice, 461

muscle cramps, 414

muscle strength, 3, 30, 31; asana for, 38–39, 321; dieting and loss of muscle mass, 477; imagery and improved, 43; menopause and loss of mass, 445–46

myofascial release, 78, 205, 239; for CTS, 232–33, *233*; for headache, 333

"Naad" (Sangreet Kaur), 387

nadis (channels for prana), 29; ida and pingala, 62

Nadi Shodhana. *See* Alternate Nostril Breathing (Nadi Shodhana)

Nagaratha, R., 119, 175

Nagendra, H. R., 175

Namaste. *See* Hands in Prayer (Namaste)

Naoi, Akira, 120

nausea. *See* cancer

Neck Movements: for heart disease, 343, *343*

Nelson, Sonia, 103–4

nervous system: ANS (autonomic nervous system), 39, 40, 190, 429; back pain and, 190; baroreceptor sensitivity and, 40; breath to achieve relaxation of, 55; calming, 4, 35, 39–40; diabetes and, 283–84; digestive function and, 429; eyebrow tug, two experiential exercises, 11, 11–12, 12; "fight or flight" response, 39, 48; heart rate variability and, 40; high blood pressure and, 365; insomnia and, 413; left/right breathing and, 62; Nadi Shodhana (alternate nostril breathing) and balancing, 62; noisy workplace and stimulation of stress response, 57; PNS (parasympathetic nervous system), 39, 40, 48, 54, 190, 413, 429; pranayama (breathing techniques) cautions, 97–98; SNS (sympathetic nervous system), 39, 40, 48, 54, 61, 111, 301, 413; stress and, 429; stress response and fibromyalgia, 301; stress response and high blood pressure, 41; "the relaxation response," 40, 64, 415, 431; yoga and improved function, 40; Yoga Nidra to relax, 68

Neti Kriya, 80–81, 81; before bedtime, 423–24; for sinus headaches, 80, 319

niyamas (spiritual observances), 13, 21, 78

obsessive-compulsive disorder (OCD), 28, 43

One-Legged Forward Bend (Janu Sirsasana): for headache, 329, 329

1:1 Breathing: for asthma, 180

1:2 Breathing: for asthma, 180

Ornish, Dean, 112; on arterial blockage, 339–40; high blood pressure study, 364; Lifestyle Heart Trial, 335, 339, 340–42, 480; lifestyle program, 285, 357; Program for Reversing Heart Disease, 207; studies on prostate cancer, 210–11; weight loss study, 480

Osher Center for Integrative Medicine, 207

osteoarthritis (OA). See arthritis and rheumatic disorders

osteopathic manipulation, 315

osteoporosis: asana cautions, 455; prescription drugs for, 456; risk of injury and, 455; scientific evidence of yoga's benefits, 28; stress and, 49; weight bearing asanas and increased bone density, 38–39

overweight and obesity, 475–92; apple-shaped body type, 477; asana to avoid and modifications, 488–89, 488–89; awareness and, 481; body image,

self-image, and, 480–81; in children, stress and, 49; contraindications, special considerations, and modifications, 487; cortisol and belly fat, 49, 338, 477; cortisol and binge eating, 49; diet and, 477; food and exercise diary, 478; health risks of, 476; how yoga can help, 477–80; infertility and, 408; injury risks, 487; meditation for, 478–79; overview, 476–77; real-life example, 475–76, 481–82, 489–92; Richard Freeman's approach, 481–87; samskaras and, 478; scientific evidence of yoga's benefits, 480–81; seeing clearly and, 478; stress and, 478; stress-related eating and, 49, 477; vegetarian diet and lowered risk, 84; yoga survey results, 5

pain (chronic): angina and yogic techniques, 340, 341; cancer and, 209, 222; fibromyalgia and, 302; headaches, medication for, 332; heat or cold applications, 166; HIV/AIDS, 392; importance of proceeding slowly, 156; meditation for relief of, 43, 460; MS and, 472; NSAIDs for, 166, 314; painkillers for, 205, 314; scientific evidence of yoga's benefits, 28; topical medications, 166, 314; yoga and reduction in suffering, 44, 47; yoga and relief of, 43, 152–53. See also arthritis and rheumatic disorders; back pain

Palkhivala, Aadil, 97–98, 114, 190, 359, 359, 360; approach to high blood pressure, 365–74; categories of hypertension conceptualized by, 365; on Downward-Facing Dog, 448; on Savasana, 371

Palming Exercise, 57, 57–58

Pancha Maya model: CFS and, 247–49; five layers of the Upanishads (koshas), 247

pancreatitis, 28, 42

Parkinson's disease, 106

Patanjali, 407; balancing effort and ease, 112, 463; cultivating the opposite thought, 136, 270; eight-limbed path of yoga, 13, 52, 106; five yamas and five niyamas of yoga, 13, 78, 91; Kriya yoga, 21, 125, 125–27; levels of samadhi, 52; on regular yoga practice, 21; seeing clearly, 126; "the hollow of the throat" meditation, 392

Patel, Chandra, 363

Pattabhi Jois, K., 1, 106, 107, 108, 475

Paul, Ken, 169, 176–81, 185–86

Pelvic Awareness exercise: for infertility, 400, 400–401

Pelvic Tipping exercise: for infertility, 403, 403

Phoenix Rising Yoga Therapy (Lee), 427

Phoenix Rising Yoga Therapy (PRYT), 110, 427; breathing techniques and, 432; IBS therapy, 428, 431–32

Piedmont Yoga Studio, 317

Pigeon (Eka Pada Rajakapotasana): for infertility, 404

piriformis syndrome, 225

placebo effect, 44–45

Plato, 71

pleural effusion, 28

Plow pose (Halasana), *90;* cautions with thoracic outlet syndrome (TOS), 90; for depression, *278,* 278; for HIV/AIDS, 385, *385;* support for, 450

postoperative recovery, 20, 28

post-polio syndrome, 28

posture, 8; arthritis and rheumatic disorders and, 153–54; back pain and, 32, 188, 190–92, *191;* bowel function problems and poor, 42; breathing and, 137, 171–72; carpal tunnel syndrome and, 228; C-shaped slump, *228,* 228; depression and, 264–65; exercise using yoga strap, *34,* 34; good, *33;* headaches and, 333; improved, xvi; incorrect seating and, 229; kyphosis (rounded back), 32–33, *33,* 250; MS and, 460; rope jacket to prevent slouching, *35,* 35, 240, *240;* yoga and health benefits, 30, 32–33

power yoga, xv, 108, 225, 299–300, 477; contraindicated for asthma, 183; risk of injury and, 108

Prabhakar, S., 324

prana (vital force), 29; apana (downward force of), 331; in food, 84

pranayama (breathing techniques), xiii, xvii, 8, 16; for anxiety and panic attacks, 139–41, *140;* for asthma, 176–81; awareness and safety of, 98; for balancing the nervous system, 62; before rising for the day, 124; for cancer patients, 218, 220; cautions, 97–98, 177; for CFS, 245–46, 250–51, 255–56; contraindicated for cancer patients, 221; contraindicated for heart disease, 354; contraindicated for high blood pressure, 374; contraindicated for HIV/AIDS, 391; as defined in Patanjali's *Yoga Sutras,* 16; for depression, 277–78; for diabetes, 286–87; diaphragmatic breathing, 55–56; during your daily routine, 124; guidance of an experienced teacher recommended, 98; for headache, 330; for heart disease, 352–53; heart disease caution, 352; for high blood pressure, 364, 374; for IBS, 433; for improved

cardiovascular functioning, 339; for infertility, 402–3; for insomnia, 414, 420–21; for menopause, 452–53, 454; for MS, 460, 471; Neti Kriya before, 81; Phoenix Rising Yoga Therapy (PRYT) and, 432; during pregnancy, 101; for stress reduction, 56. *See also* Bhramari (Bee Breath); Kapalbhati breathing; Ujjayi breath exercise

pratyahara (withdrawal of the senses), 16; for headache relief, 321; tuning out external phenomena with, 57; Ujjayi breath exercise, 16–17; use of head wrap and, 372

Prayer Pose (Namaste): for CTS, 233, *233;* for high blood pressure, 367

pregnancy: back pain and, 191–92; Bikram yoga and, 109; breathing techniques during, 101; forward bends, form for, *100,* 100; hot yoga, avoidance of, 100, 109; reintroducing practice following delivery, 101; Savasana adaptation for, *101,* 101; Savasana and, 60; scientific evidence of yoga's benefits, 28; yoga during and after, cautions, 100–101

preventative medicine, 3, 58–68, 154, 380

Priddy, Connie, 443–44, 445, 447, 457

proprioception: bodywork and improved, 78 (*see also* awareness); recognizing "the spark before the flame," 38; yoga and improved, 38, 193

props (blankets, mats, blocks, etc.), 18; Aadil Palkhivala's yoga therapy and, 367; blocks, 122; cylindrical bolster, 63, 122; eyebag, 122; getting started, needs, *122,* 122–23; Iyengar yoga and, 106, 118; metal chair, 122; posture exercise using yoga strap, *34,* 34; for restorative yoga, 63–68; strap for restorative yoga sequence, 65, 122; for therapeutic yoga, 20; yoga mat, 122

prostate cancer, 210–11

psoriasis, 32, 134, 152

psychotherapy: for anxiety and panic attacks, 148; anxiety and panic attacks and, 148; for arthritis and rheumatic disorders, 166; for cancer patients, 222; for CFS, 244; for depression, 222, 279; for fibromyalgia, 314; for HIV/AIDS, 391; for HIV/AIDS patients, 75; insomnia and, 415; journaling and, 174; Kripalu yoga and, 109, 110

Pumping the Wrist, 232, *232*

Purna yoga, 114

Pursed-Lip Exhaling: for asthma, 179, *179*

Push-Up pose (Chaturanga Dandasana): contraindicated for CTS, 237; modified, for CTS, 238, *238;* for weight loss, 484, *484*

Rabago, David, 80
Rama, Swami, 26–28, 38, 76, 139
Ramana Maharshi, 24
Ram Das, 377
Randolph, Patrick, 303
Ranganathan, Vinoth, 43
Rao, Raghavendra, 212
Reclining Cross-Legged pose (Supta Svastikasana): for depression, 268, *268*
Reclining or Reclined Cobbler's pose. *See* Supported Cobbler's pose (Supta Baddha Konasana)
Recovery yoga, 114
Recovery Yoga (Dworkis), 299
reflexology, 78
Reiki, 77, 222, 390
Relax and Renew: Restful Yoga for Stressful Times (Lasater), 187
relaxation exercises. *See* stress reduction
Relaxation pose. *See* Savasana (Deep Relaxation pose)
restless leg syndrome, 301, 402
restorative yoga, 106; for arthritis, 156–64; for CFS, *256,* 256; chest openers, 183, *183,* 211, 356; for digestive problems, 438; eyes covered during, 325, *325;* for fibromyalgia, *312,* 312; for headache, 324; for HIV/AIDS, 389; for insomnia, 416–17; instruction from a teacher used to working with props, 66; Legs-Up-the-Wall pose (Viparita Karani), 64, *64;* for MS, 462; series of poses with cumulative effects, 65, *65;* supported Savasana, *63,* 63. *See also* Iyengar yoga
Revolved Side Angle pose (Parivrtta Parsvakonasana): using chair, for MS, *468,* 468
Revolved Triangle pose (Parivrtta Trikonasana): for back pain, *201,* 201; for CFS, *253, 253;* use of block with, 201
rheumatoid arthritis (RA). *See* arthritis and rheumatic disorders
Rocking and Rolling: for IBS, *437,* 437; as self-nurturing, 437
Rocking Chair Pose: for anxiety and panic attacks, *144,* 144

Rolfing, 78, 239
root lock (mula bandha), 108; infertility and, 396, 400

Sada Sat Kaur, 388
safety, 89–101; alerting yoga teacher to your health condition or medications, 91–92; asana, cautions and, 90; avoiding falls, 96–97, 298; balancing effort (sthira) with ease (sukha), 92; balancing poses, who should avoid, 97, 298; breathing, as indication of overdoing practice, 92; contraindications, awareness of, 91; dehydration, avoiding, 96; first do no harm (ahimsa), 91–92; flexibility and risk of injury, 94; good pain vs. bad pain, 93–94; hands-on adjustments and, 95; hot and humid conditions, 96; injury risks, 91, 93, 298; joints and, 92; medication, doses change, caution about, 91; meditation caution, 98; osteoporosis concerns, 455; playing the edge, 93; power yoga, related styles, and risk of injury, 108; pranayama (breathing techniques) cautions, 97–98; signs of overdoing practice, 92; stress test before starting vigorous yoga forms, 96, 354; transitions in and out of poses, injury risk and, 95; trying too hard, 92–93; yoga class and, 94–95; yoga during and after pregnancy, 100–101; yoga during menstruation cautions, 98–99, *99*
Sagan, Carl, 29
samadhi (blissful absorption), 17, 52
samskaras, 20–21; anxiety and, 137; developing healthy, 125, 128–29, 137; eating too quickly as, 430; insomnia and, 414, 417; monkey mind and, 53; overweight and obesity and, 478; poor posture as, 153–54; reducing mental intrusion of, 50; repetition as key to, 24
Sandbag Breathing: for anxiety and panic attacks, 139–40, *140*
sangha (community), 18; cancer patients and, 209; CFS and, 246, 256; fibromyalgia and, 302–3; for menopause, 457; religious faith and, 75; yoga teachers, studios, and social support for healing, 44
Sankalpa (intention), 126–27
Sarno, John, 190
Satchidananda, Swami, 112, 207, 218, 220, 335, 340, 443
"Sat Nam Wahe Guru" (Singh Kaur), 388
sattvic, or clear, state of mind, 59, 84

Smith Farm Center, 207

snoring: mouth breathing and, 36

Sobel, Dava, 193

So Ham Meditation, 69; for anxiety and panic attacks, 147

solar plexus lock (uddiyana bandha), 108

Sovik, Mary Gail, 139

Sovik, Rolf, 113, *133*, 133, 137; approach to anxiety and panic attacks, 134, 137, 139–47; "breathing in a tight spot," 142

spinal column: ankylosing, 119; ankylosing spondylitis, 119; author's yoga practice for, 119–20; fractures and back pain, 196; posture and spinal fractures, 33; weight bearing asanas and increased bone density in, 38–39; yoga and nourishing intervertebral disks, 37. *See also* back pain; posture

spiritual well-being, 3, 4; cancer patients and, 210; yoga and reduction in suffering, 44, 47; yoga and spiritual growth, 44

Staff pose (Dandasana): contraindicated for back pain, 203; for CTS, *236*, 236; for high blood pressure, 367

Standing Backbend: for IBS, 435, *435*

Standing Balance: for anxiety and panic attacks, 145, *145*

Standing Forward Bend (Uttanasana): for CFS, *250*, 250, 253; for IBS, 436, *436*; for infertility, 404; jumping, into Downward-Facing Dog, 482, *482*; for menopause, *449*, 449; modified for postural hypotension, 257; with Namaste, for IBS, 435, *435*

Standing Half Forward Bend (Ardha Uttanasana): for lymphedema, 220, *221*

Standing Twist (Marichyasana): for diabetes, 293, *293*

stress: arthritis and rheumatic disorders and, 154; beneficial type, 48; blood clotting and, 42, 48, 338; bowel function problems and, 42; breath and, 54; breathing assessment, 56; cancer patients and, 209; CFS and, 245; chronic and susceptibility to disease, 50; depression and, 264; factor in illness, 7, 40, 49–50; fibromyalgia syndrome and, 301; heart disease and, 44, 338; high blood pressure and, 41, 362–63; infertility and, 398, 408; MS and, 460; muscle spasms and, 58; overwork and, 70; raised levels of cholesterol, triglycerides, and, 42; reverse, or

paradoxical, breathing as sign of, 55–56; sensory overload and, 56–57; in tongue, 60; unconscious muscular gripping and, 42–43

stress hormones: benefits of, 48; blood clotting and, 338; harmful effects of, 39–40, 41, 49–50, 245, 338; insomnia and, 413; meditation and lowering, 69; stress-related eating and, 49, 477; weight gain and, 339; yoga's ability to lower, 12, 39, 42, 338, 339

stress reduction, 3, 7, 42, 48–70; asana for, 8–9, 58–68; breathing and, 53–54, 55, 62; cognitive-behavioral stress management (CBSM), 381; exercises for, *57*, 57–58; eyebrow tug exercises, *11*, 11–12, *12*; headaches and, 321; for IBS, 429; for infertility, 397–98; for insomnia, 414; left/right breathing and, 62; making time to relax, 70; meditation for, 40, 51–52, 68–69; for menopause, 445; mindfulness based (MBSR), 138, 156, 193, 212, 266–67, 303, 323; reducing mental samskaras, 50; samadhi (blissful absorption) and, 52; "the relaxation response," 40, 64, 415, 431; vacations for, 70; yoga and release of unconscious muscular gripping, 42–43, 265; Yoga Nidra, 67–68; yoga's effectiveness, 245, 362

stroke, 12, 41, 42, 49, 359–60

Structural yoga therapy, 113

Stryker, Rod, 16, 50, 52, 68, 113

Sun Salutation: adaptation for CTS, 18, *19*; contraindicated for hot flashes, 455; contraindicated for insomnia, 425; for depression, 277; modified, for cancer patients, 220; modified, for diabetes, 288–89, *289*; modified, for fibromyalgia, 310–11; in power yoga and related styles, 108; for weight loss, 481, 482

Supine Cobbler's pose (Supta Baddha Konasana), *65*, 65

Supine Cross-Legged pose (Supta Svastikasana), *65*, 65

Supine Hand to Foot pose (Supta Padangusthasana): for arthritis and rheumatic disorders, *163*, 163; for high blood pressure, 367; to the side, for arthritis and rheumatic disorders, 162, *162*; for weight loss, *488*, 488

Supine Hip Rotator Stretch: for back pain, 199, *199*

Supine Twist (Jathara Parivrtta): for CFS, *254*, 254

Supine Twist with Bent Knees (Jathara Parivartanasana): for fibromyalgia, *312*, 312

supplements (nutritional): 5-HTP, 279; antioxidants, 85; for anxiety, 148; for arthritis and rheumatic disorders, 166–67; calcium, 85, 456; for CFS, 259; chromium, 296; Coenzyme Q10, 259, 296, 357, 390; containing several related forms of the same vitamin, 85; for CTS, 239; for depression, 279, 314; for diabetes, 296; digestive enzymes, 441; glucosamine and chondroitin, 166; for headache, 333; for heart disease, 356, 357; for HIV/AIDS, 390; for IBS, 441; magnesium, 148, 296, 456; for menopause, 456; for MS, 473; MSM, 166; multivitamin, 85, 390; niacin, 357; omega-3 fatty acids, 85, 148, 259, 279, 333, 356, 473; SAMe, 166, 279, 314; vitamin B complex, 148, 279, 357; vitamin B6, 239; vitamin D, 85, 167, 456; vitamin E, 457

Supported Bridge pose (Setu Bandha Sarvangasana), *65*, 65; for asthma, *182*, 183; for CFS, *256*, 256; for depression, *269*, 269; for HIV/AIDS, 389; for infertility, 406, *406*; for menopause, *451–52*, 451–52; during menstruation, *99*, 99

Supported Camel pose (Ustrasana): for depression, 273, *273*

Supported Cobbler's pose (Supta Baddha Konasana): for asthma, 183, *183*; for headache, *326*, 326; for heart disease, 356; for IBS, 438; for infertility, *406*, 406; for MS, 471; on a table, for arthritis and rheumatic disorders, 157, *157*

Supported Downward-Facing Dog (Adho Mukha Svanasana), *65*, 65; for depression, *269*, 269–70; for HIV/AIDS, 389; for insomnia, 418, *418*; for menopause, *447*, 447–48

Supported Forward Bends: for asthma attack, 182, *182*

Supported Half-Standing Forward Bend (Ardha Uttanasana), *65*, 65

Supported Headstand (Sirsasana): for HIV/AIDS, 389

Supported Inverted Staff pose (Viparita Dandasana): for depression, *273*, 273–74; over chair seat, for depression, *274*, 274

Supported Shoulderstand (Salamba Sarvangasana). *See* Chair Shoulderstand (Salamba Sarvangasana)

svadhyaya (self-study), 21, 23, 125, 126; cancer patients and, 210; for correct form of asana, 94; for depression, 265; food and exercise diary as, 478; for headache, 322; for high blood pressure, 363; for IBS, 430; journal keeping and, 76–77; for MS, 474; of your breathing, 174

Svaroopa yoga, 113

Svatmarama, 3

Swami Vivekananda Yoga Research Foundation, 155, 175, 212, 381, 416

Swinging Twist: for IBS, *434*, 434

Tadasana. *See* Mountain pose (Tadasana)

Talukdar, B., 175

tamasic state (dullness of mind), 59

Tantra, 86, 112–13; ancients and, 75; for anxiety and panic attacks, 133–49; Ayurvedic herbs and dietary advice, 113; cleansing exercises (kriyas) and, 113; Himalayan Institute, 113, 139. *See also* Sovik, Rolf; Stryker, Rod

tapas (discipline), 47, 125, 127, 461; awareness and, 137; building with asanas, *22*, 22–23, *23*; the mind and, 23; taking a step, 127

Taylor, Michael, 432

Telles, Shirley, 416

Thai yoga massage, 78

therapeutic touch, 77, 222

Thom, Camille, 360

thoracic outlet syndrome (TOS), 89–90; asana to avoid, 90, *90*; various recommendations, author's experience, 119–20

Thornton, Flora, 458

Thorson, Kristin, 301–2, 313

Three-Part Breathing (Dheerga Svasam): for heart disease, 352, *352*

Thunderbolt pose (Vajrasana): for HIV/AIDS, 383, *383*, 384

thyroid disease: anxiety and panic attacks and, 148

Tibetan yoga, 211, 415–16

Tigunait, Pandit Rajmani, 392

Trager work, 78, 333

transformation (of self), 20–21, 112–13; Kriya yoga and, *125*, 125–29

Tree pose (Vrksasana), *31*, 31; for anxiety and panic attacks, *146*, 146; avoiding falls, 96–97; contraindicated for arthritis, *164*, 164; for diabetes, *291*; modified for overweight and obesity, 488; using wall for safety, 97, *97*

Windmill pose: for fibromyalgia, *309*, 309

Wind-Releasing Pose to Leg Lift (Apanasana to Modified Supta Padangusthasana): for CFS, *255*, 255

Woolery, Alison, 266

yamas (ethical guidelines), 13; ahimsa (non-harming), 91–92; satya (honesty), 474

Yee, Rodney, 123, 317, *317*; approach to headaches, 318, 324–31, 333–34; use of head wrap, 325

yin yang, 62

Yoga Alliance, 115

Yoga and Multiple Sclerosis (Small), 458

yoga as medicine: ahimsa (nonharming) principle and, 13, 77–78, 91–92; asana, 14, *14–15* (see also asana [poses]); Ayurveda to complement, 83–84, 107; balance and, 8–9; choosing a style, 114; claims about, caveats, 29–30; common misconceptions, 6–7; as complementary medicine, 4, 46–47, 71; continuum effects, 8; dhyana (meditation), 17 (see also meditation); diet and, 18, 74–75; diseases and disorders improved by, 3, 5, 6, 8, 28 (see also *specific diseases*); eight-limbed path of yoga, 13, 52, 106; encourages involvement in your own healing, 45, 74–75; environmental health and, 78–80; future of, 493–96; health care, yogic approach, 75–84; health care decisions and, 76–77; herbs and, 18; as holistic medicine, 4, 71–75; how it works to improve health, forty ways, 30–45; how to find a teacher or therapist, 114–20; imagery, 18, 43; lack of fitness and ability to do, 6; life transformation and, 20–21, 112–13, 125–29; love and healing, 44, 86; multipronged approach preferred, 85; for optimizing health, 4; personalization for maximum effectiveness, 46; as preventative medicine, 3, 58–68, 154; private lessons, 115; relaxation effect, 8; ritual, 18; roots of, as medicine, 10–11; seeing clearly and, 126, 478; as "slow medicine," 8; social aspect of, 246; spiritual dimension, 7, 18, 21, 23; styles of, 102–14; symptom relief, 8; therapeutic yoga, 18–20, 43–44; therapeutic yoga vs. conventional medicine, 72–73; for very ill patients, 20, 63, 68; what it is, 7–10; what to expect in your first session, 118; yamas (ethical guidelines), 13; yoga philosophy

(jnana yoga), 18, 478; yogic tools (list), 18; on your own, 115

Yoga Biomedical Trust, 4–5, 155, 285, 446, 480

yoga centers, 119

yoga class: in gyms or health clubs, 113; hands-on adjustments, 95; hot and humid conditions, 96; staying safe in, 94–95; styles of yoga that work best in class setting, 118–19; therapeutic yoga vs., 18–20, 43–44

Yoga for Scoliosis (Miller), 443

Yoga for Transformation (Kraftsow), 242

Yoga for Wellness (Kraftsow), 242

Yoga Institute, Mumbai, India, 119

Yoga: Mastering the Basics (Sovik and Anderson), 139

Yogananda, Paramahansa, 340

Yoga Nidra, 67–68; for anxiety and panic attacks, 149; for cancer patients, 209, 218–20; for depression, 280

yoga philosophy (jnana yoga), 18, 478

Yoga: The Poetry of the Body (Yee and Zolotow), 317

yoga practice, 121–29; accrued benefits, 45; apparel for, 123; bare feet for, 123, 298; daily practice of asanas, xvi; empty stomach and, 123; establishing a personal practice, 121–22; following surgery, 165; frequency of, 24, 87; hands-on adjustments and assists, 18; keeping a journal (notebook), 127–28; Kriya yoga (yoga of action) applied, *125*, 125–27; as lifelong vs. to treat symptoms, 129; pain medication and, 165; props to start with, *122*, 122–23; quick poses for yoga moments, *124*, 124; resistance to, and seeing clearly, 126; safety of, 89–101 (see also safety); scheduling tip, 124; temperature concerns, 123, 125; when to practice, 123–24; where to practice at home, 125

Yoga Sutras (Patanjali), 13, 21, 92, 106, 136, 270, 392, 463

yoga teachers, 43–44; alerting to your health condition or medications, 91–92; Anusara yoga, 105, 111, 395; Ashtanga yoga, 108, 475; Bikram yoga, 109; diagnosis of illness and, caution, 116; experience needed in, 116; flexibility of approach, 117; found in gym classes, 113, 115; how to find a teacher or therapist, 114–20; Integral yoga, 112, 207, 443; Iyengar yoga, 42, 46, 58, 92, 102–3, 106–7, 114, 117, 225, 228, 240, 261, 281, 312, 410, 443, 458; Kripalu yoga, 109–10, 174, 220, 229; Kundalini